THE PARAMEDIC EXAM REVIEW

•

BOB ELLING, MPA, REMT-P

KIRSTEN M. ELLING, BS, REMT-P

THOMSON

DELMAR LEARNING

Australia Canada Mexico Singapore Spain United Kingdom United States

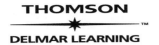

The Paramedic Exam Review, 2nd Edition
Bob Elling & Kirsten Elling

Vice President, Technology and Trades ABU:
David Garza

Director of Learning Solutions:
Sandy Clark

Managing Editor:
Larry Main

Acquisitions Editor:
Alison Pase

Product Manager:
Jennifer A. Starr

Marketing Director:
Deborah S. Yarnell

Marketing Manager:
Erin Coffin

Marketing Coordinator:
Patti Garrison

Director of Production:
Patty Stephan

Production Manager:
Stacy Massuci

Content Project Manager:
Jennifer Hanley

Technology Project Manager:
Kevin Smith

Editorial Assistant:
Maria Conto

Library of Congress Cataloging-in-Publication Data

Elling, Bob.
  The paramedic review / Bob Elling, Kirsten M. Elling ; technical reviewer, Terry Devito. — 2nd ed.
     p. ; cm.
  Includes bibliographical references and index.
  ISBN-13: 978-1-4180-3818-2 (alk. paper)
  ISBN-10: 1-4180-3818-0 (alk. paper)
  1. Emergency medical technicians—Examinations, questions, etc.
I. Elling, Kirsten M. II. Title.
  [DNLM: 1. Emergency Medical Services—Examination Questions.
2. Emergency Medical Technicians—Examination Questions. 3. Emergency Treatment—Examination Questions. WX 18.2 E46p 2007]
  RC86.9.E43 2007
  616.02'5076—dc22
                              2006037511

Dedication

This work is dedicated to Kirsten and my daughters Laura and Caitlin.
May you always maintain humility as your accomplishments meet the stars.

—BOB ELLING

In memory of my mother Inge Nicholson, 1940–2000, whose love and support I miss very much;
To my husband Bob, whose support and inspiration continue to drive me to
continuously improve patient care in the field.

—KIRSTEN M. ELLING

Special Thanks

Our deepest thanks to our close friend and colleague Mikel A. Rothenberg, MD
for all his hard work, insight, and guidance during the development of
the companion text, Why-Driven EMS Review.

Contents

About the Authors

Bob Elling, MPA, REMT-P

Bob has been involved in EMS since 1975. He is an active paramedic with Colonie EMS and the Times Union Center, both in upstate NY. He has served as National Faculty for the American Heart Association (AHA), and Regional Faculty for the NYS Bureau of EMS. Bob is also a Professor of Management for Andrew Jackson University, faculty for Hudson Valley Community College (HVCC) paramedic program, as well as the BLS Guidelines 2005 editor/writer for AHA. He has also served as a paramedic and lieutenant for NYC EMS, Program Director for the Institute of Prehospital Emergency Medicine of HVCC, Associate Director of the NYS EMS Program, and the Education Coordinator for PULSE: Emergency Medical Update. Bob is an author/coauthor of many Delmar Learning titles in addition to *The Paramedic Exam Review*, 2e, including: *Principles of Assessment in EMS*, *Why-Driven EMS Review*, 2e, and *The EMT-Intermediate Exam Review.*

Kirsten M. Elling, BS, REMT-P

Kirsten (Kirt) Elling is a career paramedic who works in the Town of Colonie in upstate New York. She began work in EMS in 1988 as an EMT/firefighter and has been a National Registered paramedic since 1991. She has been an EMS educator since 1990 and teaches basic and advanced EMS programs at the Institute of Prehospital Emergency Medicine in Troy, New York. Kirsten serves as Regional Faculty NYS DOH, Bureau of EMS and Regional Faculty American Heart Association, Northeast region. In addition to *The Paramedic Exam Review*, 2e, Kirsten is the author/coauthor of the following: Numerous scripts for the EMS training video series PULSE: Emergency Medical Update; *EMT-Basic Exam Review*; *Why-Driven EMS Review*, 2e; *Principles of Assessment for the EMS Provider*; contributing author of the Paramedic Lab Manual for the IPEM, and an adjunct writer for the 1998 revision of the National Highway Traffic Safety Administration, EMT-Paramedic and EMT-Intermediate: National Standard Curricula.

Preface

Intent of This Book

The Paramedic Exam Review, second edition, is the perfect resource for preparing for the National Registry written exam. This book is a valuable tool to help review your knowledge, and practice the content requirements in order to build confidence for the actual exam. Intended as a review for both state and national examinations, the book is designed to follow the organizational chapter format of the 1999 Edition of the DOT Paramedic curriculum and is updated to the 2005 American Heart Association Guidelines.

Why We Wrote This Book

Paramedic training has evolved quite a bit since I first completed the program at the Institute of Albert Einstein Medical School in "da-Bronx" back in 1978. I remember the first day of class when Dr. J. and the instructor coordinator wheeled in a hand truck piled high with papers that we used as our textbook. Most of the materials consisted of the yet-unpublished draft of the Paramedic book that Nancy Caroline, M.D. had just completed for the U.S. DOT and lots of interesting articles from the medical journals. These days, it is hard to find a 15-module trained medic still working in the field. Both Kirsten, my co-author and partner, and I have seen the curriculum become more enriched and sophisticated in 1985 with the six division program and then again in 1998 with the latest revision. Working as paramedics and EMS educators for the past 16 years and 30 years respectively, both Kirsten and I have seen medic training evolve firsthand. Today there are many choices of books, magazines, video, workbooks, and Web sites for instructors to use to prepare their students for the streets.

We sincerely hope you will enjoy *The Paramedic Exam Review*, second edition, and benefit from the test-taking review to expand your knowledge base. After all, when the real test occurs, in the field, our patients rely on us to be prepared. See you in the streets!

—*Bob & Kirsten Elling*

Features of This Book

- *Accessible for both Certification and Refresher Exams*   These questions allow you to study for the exam whether you are a candidate for paramedic certification, or a current paramedic working to renew certification.

- *Organized to the DOT Curriculum*   The chapter order follows that of the curriculum for ease of reference and use. Early in this project we also made a decision that the questions would only be the multiple choice style with the standard format of three distractors and one correct answer to each question. Since this book will be used to prepare for both state and national paramedic examinations, it makes the most sense to use the format and style of questions used on these types of exams, in order to provide the best possible practice and build confidence for the actual exam.

- *Over 3100 questions*   We suggest you tackle a chapter at a time and after taking each exam, check the answer key and mark the ones you need to review. The more time you spend using the practice questions, the better your chances for success on the exam.

- *Rationale*   The rationale for correct answers provides you with the necessary feedback for understanding the context of the question, and, if applicable, a point of reference for review.

New to This Edition

- *Section on Test-Taking Strategies*   Appendix B provides you with valuable advice on developing best practices for completing and achieving success on your paramedic exam.

- *New Scenario-Based Questions*   Practice crucial critical-thinking skills that will be required on the job as a paramedic.

- *10% New Questions*   A fresh approach to the content ensures that the questions remain up to date with the latest information required on the state and national paramedic exams.

- *Updated to the 2005 AHA Guidelines*   The questions provide technical information that remains updated to the latest procedures outlined by the 2005 Edition of the American Heart Association guidelines.
- *Interactive CD-ROM*   The CD-ROM included in the back of the book is now interactive and provides two practice exams that simulate the actual paramedic exam. Each question is identified by a topic for context, and provides immediate feedback, including rationale for both correct and incorrect answers, to help you practice for the exam and highlight areas requiring further study.

Acknowledgements

The authors and publisher would like to extend appreciation to the following experts for their thorough review of the content. Their comments proved invaluable to the revision of this book:

Linda Anderson
Director, Paramedic Education
Santa Rosa Junior College
Windsor, CA

David McDonald
Program Faculty
Greenville Technical College
Greenville, SC

Mike McLaughlin
Director of Health Occupations
Kirkwood Community College
Cedar Rapids, IA

Gordon Kokx
Associate Professor
College of Southern Idaho
Twin Falls, ID

1

The Well-Being of the EMS Provider

1. _____ is defined as a state of complete physical, mental, and social well being.

   a. Health
   b. Wellness
   c. Fitness
   d. Nutrition

2. The components of wellness include physical well-being, proper nutrition, and:

   a. vaccinations.
   b. past medical history.
   c. mental and emotional health.
   d. compliance with prescribed medications.

3. Proper nutrition involves an understanding of nutrients the body needs, as well as the principles of:

   a. mental health.
   b. emotional well-being.
   c. exercise.
   d. weight control.

4. According to the Surgeon General's Report on Nutrition and Health, diet-related diseases account for over _____ of all deaths in the United States.

   a. one-quarter
   b. one-third
   c. one-half
   d. two-thirds

5. Poor diet and nutrition can be attributed to the development of degenerative diseases such as:

   a. gout.
   b. anxiety.
   c. diabetes.
   d. chronic lung disease.

6. The diets of EMS providers are often complicated by meals that are rushed, interrupted, and:

   a. provide limited access to choices of food types.
   b. provide increased susceptibility to lactose intolerance.
   c. low in cholesterol.
   d. high in vitamins and complex carbohydrates.

7. For the EMS provider who is making a conscious effort to eat better at work, which of the following activities should be avoided?

   a. Preparing meals at home in advance.
   b. Expanding the range of foods from your normal choices.
   c. Stopping for fast food when you are hungry and did not bring a meal.
   d. Bringing along a small cooler with fresh fruits or vegetable snacks.

8. Which of the following modifications to a diet is considered to be a reasonable and healthy change?

   a. Watching the fat content, not the calories.
   b. Making small changes with a slow transition.
   c. Drinking less fluid before and during meals.
   d. Watching only the calories, not the fat content.

9. Which of the following tips about snacking is most accurate?

   a. Low-fiber snacks are better for dental health.
   b. Snacking will make you fat and should be avoided.
   c. Waiting until you are starving before you eat a snack will better satisfy your hunger.
   d. Snacks can fill the voids between meals and should be a part of your food plan.

10. Being physically fit involves a combination of elements, including aerobic conditioning, strength, endurance, and:

    a. attitude.
    b. monitoring your heart rate.
    c. having a personal trainer.
    d. being able to run several miles a week.

11. Before starting a fitness program, it is a good idea to get a physical examination by a physician because:

    a. a physician will identify any specific limitations to consider.
    b. most gyms require medical clearance before joining.
    c. athletic trainers require medical clearance before working with new clients.
    d. your physician will prescribe steroids to help you increase muscle mass.

12. Which of the following immunizations may be recommended rather than required for some paramedics?

    a. rubella
    b. hepatitis B
    c. Lyme disease
    d. tetanus and diphtheria

13. Being physically fit has many benefits, including:

    a. decreased metabolism.
    b. decreased resistance to injury and illness.
    c. improved personal appearance and self-image.
    d. increased blood pressure and resting heart rate.

14. Routine aerobic exercise lasting at least twenty minutes, three times a week, improves the cardiac stroke volume of the heart while increasing:

    a. the resting heart rate.
    b. wear and tear on the heart.
    c. nutritional fortitude.
    d. physical endurance.

15. _____ are regular changes in mental and physical characteristics that occur in the course of a day.

    a. Anxieties
    b. Circadian rhythms
    c. Addictions
    d. Stimulants

16. Major industrial accidents, such as the Exxon Valdez oil spill, have been attributed partly to errors made by:

    a. fatigued night-shift workers.
    b. smokers who suffered a stroke.
    c. stressed, obese shift workers.
    d. overdose on No Doz®.

17. When considering the risk assessment for cardiovascular disease, the paramedic should take into account:

    a. blood pressure.
    b. personal hygiene.
    c. exposure to the sun.
    d. proper lifting techniques.

18. To avoid contact with a potentially infectious body fluid found on a piece of your equipment, you remove the substance. You use a product that is designed to kill all forms of microbial life, except high numbers of bacterial spores. This level of cleaning is called:

    a. low-level disinfection.
    b. intermediate-level disinfection.
    c. high-level disinfection.
    d. sterilization.

19. Which of the following is considered an unsafe practice rather than a proper lifting technique?

    a. Bending at the hips.
    b. Avoiding any twisting when lifting.
    c. Using caution and knowing your limits.
    d. Keeping the load close to your body.

20. A low-priority call at a two-story apartment building for an elderly woman who fell has suddenly turned into a hostile scene. The patient is conscious and confused, with an obvious fracture to the left ankle. She is refusing transport, throwing objects, and spitting. Which of the following actions is most appropriate for this scenario?

    a. Stand your ground while waiting for the police.
    b. Retreat to your ambulance until the police arrive.
    c. Leave yourself an exit and be prepared to retreat.
    d. Force a mask onto the patients face, then physically restrain her.

21. A frequent and typical profile of an ambulance collision is one that occurs in the:

    a. daytime, on clear, dry roads.
    b. night, involving intoxicated drivers.
    c. winter, while driving on snow and ice.
    d. fall, when the roads are covered with wet leaves.

22. Knowledge of the proper use of lights and sirens, as well as the public's typical reactions, includes the understanding that:

    a. these devices guarantee you the right of way.
    b. there are limitations with the use of lights and sirens.
    c. the public has to yield the right of way.
    d. driving an emergency vehicle requires a special course.

23. Which of the following actions can reduce the risks associated with driving an emergency vehicle?

    a. Using lights and sirens on training drills.
    b. Using a police escort whenever possible.
    c. Avoiding the use of flashing lights at night and in fog.
    d. Driving with due regard for the safety of other drivers.

24. When developing strategies to help reduce or eliminate ambulance collisions, you should consider which of the following?

    a. Provide instruction on the use of global positioning systems (GPS).
    b. Ensure that vehicle operators know the proper way to change a tire.
    c. Test all drivers on their knowledge of standard operating procedures (SOPs).
    d. Ensure that only the most senior operators drive with the siren and lights on.

25. For which emergency vehicle operation topic should each emergency service have an SOP?

    a. What to do when a collision occurs.
    b. How to load and unload a stretcher.
    c. How to deal with uncooperative drivers.
    d. How to avoid inclement weather conditions.

26. Safety equipment that EMS personnel use at the scene of a collision may include:

    a. head protection, such as a helmet.
    b. eye protection, such as safety goggles or shields.
    c. a turnout coat to protect from sharp objects.
    d. all of the above.

27. Twenty minutes after the cessation of smoking a cigarette, which of the following physical changes occurs?

    a. The pulse rate increases.
    b. The blood pressure increases.
    c. The blood pressure decreases.
    d. The body temperature of the hands and feet decreases.

28. At one year after the cessation of cigarette smoking, the excess risk of coronary heart diseases is decreased to _____ of a smoker.

    a. one-fourth
    b. one-third
    c. one-half
    d. two-thirds

29. Which of the following is inaccurate about the cessation of cigarette smoking?

    a. Even heavy smokers can benefit significantly by stopping.
    b. For longtime smokers, stopping is not of any benefit.
    c. At five to ten years after quitting, the stroke risk is reduced to that of nonsmokers.
    d. Nicotine is a drug that causes addiction.

30. All the following are accurate about the effects of nicotine, *except*:

    a. nicotine has no effect on nerve cells.
    b. withdrawal is difficult with nicotine.
    c. nicotine can act as a stimulant.
    d. nicotine can act as a sedative.

31. A/an _____ is a compulsive need for, and use of, a habit-forming substance.

    a. anxiety
    b. addiction
    c. agonist
    d. stimulant

32. Which of the following statements is most correct in reference to stress?

    a. Stress is associated with positive events.
    b. Stress is only associated with negative events.
    c. Stress is an unnatural and unnecessary emotion.
    d. Stress is a harmful emotion that should be avoided.

33. The three distinct phases of a stress response include:

    a. anxiety, panic, and relief.
    b. alarm, denial, and acceptance.
    c. alarm, resistance, and exhaustion.
    d. physical, emotional, and behavioral.

34. A person can become desensitized or adapted to extreme stressors. This is a result of an increase in the:

    a. level of resistance in the resistance phase of the stress reaction.
    b. production of epinephrine in the alarm reaction phase.
    c. norepinephrine released during the denial phase.
    d. glucose production from a pituitary response.

35. As stress continues, and coping mechanisms are exhausted, the body will have an increased:

    a. release of adrenocorticotrophic hormones.
    b. pulse rate and blood pressure.
    c. resistance to stressors.
    d. susceptibility to physical and psychological ailments.

36. Which of the following is a cognitive sign or symptom of stress?

   a. anger
   b. disorientation
   c. chest tightness
   d. aching muscles and joints

37. An emotional sign or symptom of stress may include:

   a. depression.
   b. panic reaction.
   c. poor concentration.
   d. increased smoking.

38. Which of the following is a physical sign or symptom of stress?

   a. nausea and vomiting
   b. feeling overwhelmed
   c. fighting with coworkers
   d. increased alcohol consumption

39. You are evaluating a patient with multiple general complaints. During your interview and physical assessment, you have learned that this patient is experiencing withdrawal, is smoking more than usual, and displays hyperactivity. These are all _____ signs and symptoms of stress.

   a. cognitive
   b. physical
   c. emotional
   d. behavioral

40. _____ is an example of an environmental stress trigger.

   a. Siren noise
   b. Inclement weather
   c. Confined workspace
   d. All of the above

41. An example of a psychosocial stress trigger is:

   a. a conflict with a supervisor or coworker.
   b. a rapid scene response.
   c. life and death decision-making.
   d. hyperventilation syndrome.

42. Personality and emotional stress in EMS providers is often caused by a trigger such as:

   a. feelings of guilt.
   b. changes in eating habits.
   c. changes in sleep patterns.
   d. cardiac rhythm disturbances.

43. _____ is an active process of confronting the stress or the cause of the stress.

   a. Putting up defenses
   b. Coping
   c. Exposure
   d. Gaining experience

44. _____ is a technique used to manage stress.

   a. Circadian rhythms
   b. Controlled breathing
   c. Guided hyperactivity
   d. Sleep deprivation

45. _____ is an organized process that enables emergency personnel to vent feelings and facilitates understanding of stressful situations.

   a. Coping for EMS providers (CEMSP)
   b. EMS problem solving (EMSPS)
   c. Emergency EMS distress (EEMSD)
   d. Critical incident stress management (CISM)

46. One of the indications that a coworker may be experiencing a crisis-induced stress reaction would be:

   a. getting plenty of rest.
   b. focusing on the positives.
   c. signs of gastrointestinal distress.
   d. maintaining a good sense of humor.

47. A characteristic example of an incident that might provoke a crisis-induced stress reaction in an EMS provider would be:

   a. a prolonged incident.
   b. defusing a large-scale incident.
   c. line-of-duty death or serious injury.
   d. successful reversal of a cardiac arrest.

48. A practice to avoid when trying to reduce crisis-induced stress would be:

   a. getting plenty of rest.
   b. replacing fluids and food.
   c. increased cigarette smoking.
   d. limiting exposure to the provoking incident.

49. During the grieving process, it is not unusual for families to vent their anger on the paramedic. As long as there is no perceived physical harm to you, it is best to:

   a. allow them to express their feelings as best as you can.
   b. walk away, as it could get personal.
   c. give them your opinion based on your experience.
   d. let them argue with the police instead.

50. In which developmental age group do children begin to understand the finality of death?

   a. 3 to 6 years old
   b. 6 to 9 years old
   c. 9 to 12 years old
   d. adolescence

51. Which of the following statements about helping children deal with grief is most accurate?

   a. It is less distressing for the child to see that "everything is normal."
   b. Tell the truth and be straightforward when talking about the death of a loved one.
   c. Shielding a child from grief may protect her in the long run.
   d. A child seeing his father cry over the mother's death is an unnecessary burden on the child.

52. The stages of the grieving process will vary for any given individual; however, most will experience all of the stages, beginning with:

   a. anger.
   b. shock.
   c. denial.
   d. bargaining.

53. Prevention of disease transmission by the EMS provider includes all the following, *except*:

   a. protection against airborne pathogens.
   b. protection against blood-borne pathogens.
   c. following recommended guidelines for proper cleaning and disinfection.
   d. sterilizing all ambulance equipment on a regular basis.

54. A/an _____ is contact with a potentially infectious body fluid substance that may be carrying a pathogen.

   a. exposure
   b. removal
   c. reaction
   d. preventive measure

55. The procedure used to manage an exposure includes:

   a. conducting the incident investigation.
   b. conducting a period risk assessment.
   c. completing the required medical follow-up.
   d. safeguarding against potential disciplinary action.

56. When documenting an exposure, the paramedic should include:

   a. periodic risk assessment.
   b. ongoing exposure control training.
   c. actions taken to reduce chances of infection.
   d. obtaining proper immunization boosters.

57. _____ is cleaning the surface of objects with a specific agent designed to kill pathogens that may have come in contact with the object.

   a. Cleaning
   b. Disinfection
   c. Sterilization
   d. Isolation precaution

58. BSI is an acronym for body substance isolation procedures, which are a series of practices designed to:

   a. prevent lapses in immunizations.
   b. improve screening for exposures.
   c. improve personal hygiene habits.
   d. prevent contact with body substances such as blood and urine.

59. There are a number of ways to positively deal with excessive stress, such as:

   a. alcohol.
   b. biofeedback.
   c. decreasing exercise.
   d. overeating.

60. All the following are used to treat stress, *except*:

   a. vaccination.
   b. patient education.
   c. medication.
   d. psychotherapy.

Exam #1 Answer Form

	A	B	C	D			A	B	C	D
1.	❏	❏	❏	❏		26.	❏	❏	❏	❏
2.	❏	❏	❏	❏		27.	❏	❏	❏	❏
3.	❏	❏	❏	❏		28.	❏	❏	❏	❏
4.	❏	❏	❏	❏		29.	❏	❏	❏	❏
5.	❏	❏	❏	❏		30.	❏	❏	❏	❏
6.	❏	❏	❏	❏		31.	❏	❏	❏	❏
7.	❏	❏	❏	❏		32.	❏	❏	❏	❏
8.	❏	❏	❏	❏		33.	❏	❏	❏	❏
9.	❏	❏	❏	❏		34.	❏	❏	❏	❏
10.	❏	❏	❏	❏		35.	❏	❏	❏	❏
11.	❏	❏	❏	❏		36.	❏	❏	❏	❏
12.	❏	❏	❏	❏		37.	❏	❏	❏	❏
13.	❏	❏	❏	❏		38.	❏	❏	❏	❏
14.	❏	❏	❏	❏		39.	❏	❏	❏	❏
15.	❏	❏	❏	❏		40.	❏	❏	❏	❏
16.	❏	❏	❏	❏		41.	❏	❏	❏	❏
17.	❏	❏	❏	❏		42.	❏	❏	❏	❏
18.	❏	❏	❏	❏		43.	❏	❏	❏	❏
19.	❏	❏	❏	❏		44.	❏	❏	❏	❏
20.	❏	❏	❏	❏		45.	❏	❏	❏	❏
21.	❏	❏	❏	❏		46.	❏	❏	❏	❏
22.	❏	❏	❏	❏		47.	❏	❏	❏	❏
23.	❏	❏	❏	❏		48.	❏	❏	❏	❏
24.	❏	❏	❏	❏		49.	❏	❏	❏	❏
25.	❏	❏	❏	❏		50.	❏	❏	❏	❏

	A	B	C	D		A	B	C	D
51.	❏	❏	❏	❏	56.	❏	❏	❏	❏
52.	❏	❏	❏	❏	57.	❏	❏	❏	❏
53.	❏	❏	❏	❏	58.	❏	❏	❏	❏
54.	❏	❏	❏	❏	59.	❏	❏	❏	❏
55.	❏	❏	❏	❏	60.	❏	❏	❏	❏

2

Roles and Responsibilities of the EMS Provider

1. The first civilian ambulance service was started in _____ in 1865.

   a. New York City
   b. Cincinnati
   c. Philadelphia
   d. Chicago

2. In _____ the first known air medical transport occurred during the retreat of the Serbian army from Albania.

   a. 1915
   b. 1930
   c. 1955
   d. 1962

3. In 1958 Peter Safar, MD demonstrated the effectiveness of:

   a. public access defibrillation.
   b. mouth-to-mouth ventilation.
   c. seat belts to save lives in motor vehicle collisions.
   d. electricity to convert ventricular fibrillation to an organized rhythm.

4. In 1960 _____ was first shown to be an effective treatment method for cardiac arrest.

   a. intubation
   b. epinephrine administration
   c. sodium bicarbonate
   d. cardiopulmonary resuscitation (CPR)

5. In 1966 landmark legislation called the _____ created the U.S. Department of Transportation (DOT) as a cabinet-level department.

   a. White Paper
   b. Highway Safety Act
   c. Committee on Traffic Safety report
   d. EMT–Ambulance curriculum

6. In 1970 the _____ was established with DOT to provide leadership to the EMS community and states, as well as federal agencies involved in EMS.

   a. television show *EMERGENCY!*
   b. Board of Directors of the National Registry of EMTs
   c. Emergency Medical Services Systems Act
   d. National Highway Traffic Safety Administration

7. In 1974 DOT published the "KKK-A-1822" Federal:

   a. educational standards.
   b. Emergency Medical Dispatch system.
   c. Ambulance Specifications.
   d. Standards for CPR.

8. In 1983 the American College of Surgeons identified the:

   a. standard equipment to be carried on BLS ambulances.
   b. standard equipment to be carried on ALS ambulances.
   c. first trauma training program.
   d. first trauma care system.

9. The _____ EMT–Basic curriculum included the use of the automated external defibrillator as a skill taught to the EMT–B, rather than reserved for only the advanced levels of EMTs.

   a. 1985
   b. 1990
   c. 1995
   d. 1998

10. A/an _____ is a coordinated effort to bring together a minimum of ten key components to reduce out-of-hospital morbidity and mortality.

   a. EMS curriculum
   b. NHTSA Act
   c. EMS system
   d. emergency medical dispatch flowchart

11. Permission that is granted by a government authority to practice in a profession, business, or activity is called:

    a. certification.
    b. licensure.
    c. public access.
    d. registration.

12. A _____ is a document testifying to the fulfillment of the requirements for practice in the field.

    a. certification
    b. licensure
    c. public access
    d. registration

13. Which of the following is not one of the four national levels of out-of-hospital training that is recognized by the National Registry of Emergency Medical Technicians?

    a. First Responder
    b. EMT–Basic
    c. Critical Care Technician
    d. EMT–Paramedic

14. The level of provider that is not intended to be utilized as the minimum staffing for an ambulance is the:

    a. First Responder.
    b. Critical Care Technician.
    c. EMT–A.
    d. EMT–B.

15. The roles and responsibilities of the _____ include: providing safety, initial assessment and treatment, including immediate resuscitative measures, and portraying a professional and positive appearance.

    a. First Responder
    b. EMT–Intermediate
    c. EMT–Paramedic
    d. All the above

16. One of the roles of the National Registry of Emergency Medical Technicians (NREMT) is:

    a. eradicating the process of state-to-state reciprocity.
    b. contributing to the development of professional standards.
    c. issuing licensure to the EMS provider once competency has been verified.
    d. providing constructive feedback in association with verifying competency.

17. Select the statement that is most accurate regarding paramedic recertification.

    a. All states require recertification through the same process.
    b. The current EMT–Paramedic curriculum contains recertification curricula.
    c. The current EMT–Paramedic curriculum does not contain recertification curricula.
    d. The medical director of an EMS agency can determine how recertification is to be accomplished.

18. _____ is the legal recognition of training obtained in another state.

    a. Recertification
    b. Challenging
    c. Reciprocity
    d. National Registration

19. One of the benefits of participating in continuing education is that it:

    a. provides positive feedback.
    b. guarantees reciprocity to other states.
    c. improves your image in the public's eyes.
    d. refreshes knowledge and skills, and introduces new material.

20. What is the single most important attribute of an EMS provider?

    a. integrity
    b. indifference
    c. good personal hygiene
    d. good time management

21. Select the most accurate statement about healthcare professionals.

    a. Smoking in public is viewed as a positive attribute by society.
    b. Society's expectations of healthcare professionals are high, both on and off duty.
    c. Working as part of a team is not an essential attribute for the healthcare profession.
    d. When the public sees you without your seat belt on while driving the ambulance, your public image is unaffected.

22. _____ are moral principles of one's practice in his or her profession.

    a. Standards of care
    b. Ethics
    c. Peer review
    d. Professional conduct

23. Constructive feedback by other EMS providers in a genuine effort to improve future performance is called:

    a. quality control.
    b. quality improvement.
    c. peer review.
    d. the standard of care.

24. After turning a patient over to the emergency department (ED) staff and giving a verbal report, you complete your documentation for the call. As usual, you are conscientious about providing accurate documentation and completing all necessary paperwork. This attribute is an example of:

    a. integrity.
    b. empathy.
    c. good time management.
    d. working well with others.

25. You are on the scene with an elderly female patient who had a syncopal event, but is now awake and alert. She denies dyspnea and chest pain, and admits to having recent fainting spells. She lives alone and is worried about leaving her home and not being able to return. Your assessment findings are that she is hypotensive and has a third-degree heart block. As you begin treatment, you also address the patient's concern and provide an understanding of her feelings. This is an example of behavior demonstrating:

    a. ethics.
    b. empathy.
    c. sympathy.
    d. self-motivation.

26. _____ acknowledges the patient's circumstances and how serious they must be without the provider becoming emotionally involved.

    a. Empathy
    b. Sympathy
    c. Pity
    d. Kindness

27. Examples of demonstrating self-confidence include:

    a. consulting with Medical Direction after the patient's condition deteriorates.
    b. having a good understanding of your limitations.
    c. calling for backup after realizing the patient you are lifting is too heavy.
    d. being able to call for help once you are overwhelmed.

28. A neat and professional appearance, and being well groomed and clean, are important and:

    a. very subjective qualities of an EMT–B.
    b. an indication of your competency and skills.
    c. show diplomacy to the patient and his family.
    d. help to instill confidence in the patient and his family.

29. An example of the paramedic who demonstrates good time management skills is one who:

    a. is accepting of all learning opportunities.
    b. attends a required continuing education class.
    c. shows enthusiasm for learning and continuous improvement.
    d. is dressed appropriately and prepared to work when the shift begins.

30. The best opportunity for a patient to have a positive outcome begins with the paramedic who:

    a. is prepared to work alone.
    b. shows up on time for work.
    c. works well as a team member.
    d. is accepting of constructive feedback.

31. _____ is defined as tact and skill in dealing with people.

    a. Respect
    b. Diplomacy
    c. Teamwork
    d. Communication

32. Which of the following examples of behavior demonstrates unprofessionalism rather than a teamwork effort?

    a. Disagreeing with a coworker in private.
    b. Disagreeing with a coworker in public.
    c. Remaining flexible and open to changes.
    d. Communicating in an effort to solve problems.

33. Patients are at a disadvantage when thrust into the health-care system because of a sudden illness or injury; this is why part of the responsibility of the paramedic is to:

    a. let their neighbors know which hospital you took them to.
    b. let them use your cell phone to call a friend.
    c. take their wallet or purse for safekeeping.
    d. be an advocate for your patient.

34. For the paramedic who is making an effort to be conscientious about patient advocacy activities, which of the following should be avoided?

    a. Placing the patient's needs ahead of your own.
    b. Telling a patient who smokes that he is really stupid for doing so.
    c. Placing your safety and the safety of the crew ahead of your patient's.
    d. Explaining to an unrestrained patient injured in a motor vehicle collision that being belted during a collision is a safer practice.

35. Examples of behavior demonstrating patient advocacy include:

    a. placing the patient's safety above your own.
    b. protecting the patient's confidentiality.
    c. rushing a patient report to get out of work on time.
    d. allowing personal bias to influence patient care.

36. An important attribute for the paramedic is being careful in the delivery of services to the patient. An example of this would be:

    a. consistently adhering to a nutritional diet.
    b. getting to know all the residents in your district.
    c. protecting the patient's furniture while moving your stretcher through the living room.
    d. helping to implement legislation that provides protection from liability for EMS providers when dealing with unusual situations.

37. The primary role of the Medical Director of an EMS agency is to:

    a. ensure quality patient care.
    b. oversee all continuing education.
    c. delineate the quality control process.
    d. evaluate and revise patient access to definitive care.

38. _____ are guidelines for the management of specific patient-presenting problems.

    a. Diagnosis
    b. Algorithms
    c. Protocols
    d. Definitive care standards

39. The role of the Medical Director has expanded over the past decade and now typically includes:

    a. participating in the development of continuing education.
    b. developing policies and procedures for billing patient services.
    c. providing interface between EMS systems and the families of patients.
    d. ensuring the proper utilization of safety equipment by EMS personnel.

40. Potential benefits of online (direct) medical control include:

    a. the ability to obtain real-time direction and orders.
    b. interfacing with a physician for more effective treatment.
    c. treatment orders that are more efficient.
    d. quicker access to definitive care.

41. Off-line (indirect) medical control primarily relies on:

    a. judgment.
    b. protocols.
    c. ACLS algorithms.
    d. advanced directives.

42. If a physician stops at the scene of your call and offers assistance, which of the following should you do before consenting to allow his assistance?

    a. Confirm that the person is actually a medical doctor and not a Ph.D.
    b. Confirm that the physician is willing to come to the hospital with you and the patient.
    c. Let the physician speak to your medical control so they can work together.
    d. All of the above.

43. EMS providers are responsible for being prepared to work in the field as a paramedic in which of the following ways?

    a. By getting a college education.
    b. By having a lawyer on retainer for potential lawsuits.
    c. By personally knowing many residents in the area where you work.
    d. By conforming to the standards of a healthcare professional providing quality patient care.

44. When making the determination about the appropriate disposition for your patient, which of the following factors regarding the hospitals in your area should be considered?

    a. clinical capabilities
    b. discharge capacity
    c. rehabilitation resources
    d. availability of critical care beds

45. When returning the ambulance to service after a call, one of the primary responsibilities of the paramedic and crew is:

    a. filling any oxygen tanks used on the call.
    b. disinfecting all items used on the call.
    c. performing a complete equipment checklist.
    d. replacing disposable items available from the hospital.

46. Which of the following is the most practical benefit of having paramedics teach in the community?

    a. It enhances the visibility and positive image of paramedics and their agencies.
    b. It ensures the safety of all the children in the community.
    c. It ensures proper utilization of safety helmets.
    d. It helps to get the elderly compliant with medication use.

47. Examples of citizen involvement in EMS systems include all the following, *except*:

    a. learning how to access EMS.
    b. training and being willing to do bystander CPR.
    c. training to be a career paramedic/firefighter.
    d. fund-raising and lobbying for EMS improvements.

48. As the "scope of practice" evolves, the paramedic may be utilized in nontraditional activities such as:

    a. patient well care visits.
    b. assisting with daily living activities.
    c. assisting with physical therapy.
    d. minor surgical procedures.

49. The expanded scope pilots have been utilized to bring medically trained healthcare professionals to the patients when they are underserved or:

    a. in a hospice program.
    b. the transportation alternatives are very costly.
    c. dental or chiropractic services are not affordable.
    d. they cannot prepare their own meals.

50. In the document *EMS Agenda for the Future*, integration of health services specifically refers to the:

    a. allocation of funding for HMOs.
    b. development of paramedic jobs in private home care.
    c. integration of EMS with other healthcare providers to deliver quality care.
    d. implementation of laws that provide protection from liability for EMS providers.

51. In the document *EMS Agenda for the Future*, EMS research is developing strategies to:

    a. address the portion of the population with special needs.
    b. develop a system of reciprocity for EMS provider credentials.
    c. develop information systems that provide linkage between various healthcare services.
    d. expand the EMS role in public health and involve EMS in community health monitoring activities.

52. Legislation and regulation recommendations for the future of EMS are focused on:

    a. authorizing and funding a leading federal EMS agency.
    b. ensuring the adequacy of EMS education programs.
    c. developing laws for the accreditation of EMS education programs.
    d. developing laws that provide liability insurance for all career and volunteer EMS providers.

53. System Finance in EMS is striving for which of the following?

    a. To commission the development of government-funded healthcare.
    b. Collaboration with other healthcare providers and insurers to enhance patient care efficiency.
    c. To compensate EMS on the basis of volume.
    d. To provide immediate access to the Medicare approval process.

54. In the document *EMS Agenda for the Future*, strategies for human resources include:

    a. conducting EMS occupation health research.
    b. formalizing paramedicine as a subspecialty of home healthcare.
    c. requiring appropriate credentials for all physicians who provide online medical direction.
    d. enhancing the ability of EMS systems to triage calls and providing resource allocation that is tailored to patients' needs.

55. A key proposal for Medical Direction in the future is to:

    a. require appropriate credentials for all those who provide online medical direction.
    b. develop a system for reciprocity of EMS physician credentials.
    c. ensure that Medical Directors are allocated federal funding for participating in an EMS system.
    d. appoint national EMS Medical Directors.

56. In the document *EMS Agenda for the Future*, strategies for educational systems include:

    a. accrediting only college-based EMS education.
    b. promulgating and updating standards for EMS dispatch.
    c. acknowledging that public education is a critical EMS activity.
    d. developing, bridging, and transitioning EMS programs with all health professions' education.

57. Goals for EMS public education for the future include:

    a. relying on HMOs to get the message out.
    b. collaborating efforts with federally funded programs.
    c. exploring and evaluating public education alternatives.
    d. supporting legislation that results in injury prevention.

58. A major goal for the future in EMS communications systems is to:

    a. acknowledge that public education is a critical EMS activity.
    b. assess the effectiveness of resource attributes for EMS dispatching.
    c. provide the 9-1-1 emergency telephone service to all global positioning system (GPS) monitors.
    d. develop models for EMS evaluations that incorporate consumer input.

59. One of the major goals for the future in the clinical care aspect of EMS is to:

   a. evaluate EMS effects on various medical conditions.
   b. evaluate EMS standards for higher earning potentials.
   c. obtain legal advice on how to obtain informed consent.
   d. commit to a common definition of what constitutes baseline community EMS care.

60. One of the goals that EMS information systems is striving for in the future is to:

   a. incorporate task analyses to configure staffing of patient transfers.
   b. employ new care techniques and technology after they are shown to be effective.
   c. develop a mechanism to generate and transmit data that are valid, reliable, and accurate.
   d. facilitate the exploration of potential uses of advancing communication technology.

61. In the document *EMS Agenda for the Future*, one of the elements of the evaluation components is to:

   a. value peer review and publishing research.
   b. establish proactive relationships between EMS and other healthcare providers.
   c. determine EMS effects for multiple outcome categories and cost-effectiveness.
   d. update geographically integrated and functionally based EMS communications networks.

62. Continuous quality improvement (CQI) is a process that is designed to:

   a. focus on specific problem individuals within an organization.
   b. uncover problems and provide solutions.
   c. correct life-threatening patient conditions.
   d. monitor the work performance of field paramedics.

63. Research in EMS is important for all the following reasons, *except*:

   a. research helps to enhance recognition and respect for EMS professionals.
   b. outcome studies are needed to assure the continued funding for EMS system grants.
   c. changes in professional standards, training, and equipment need to be based on empirical data.
   d. research can be influenced by biases.

64. The role of EMS providers in data collection is to enthusiastically participate and honestly comply with the study requirements without:

   a. changing the sample size.
   b. obtaining informed consent.
   c. changing the initial hypothesis.
   d. negatively affecting patient care.

65. One of the basic principles of research is understanding:

   a. what a randomized and controlled group is.
   b. how to change patient care standards.
   c. those populations that are to be researched.
   d. that there are no limitations within a study.

66. Which of the following is not one of the typical steps in the procedure for conducting research in EMS?

   a. Collect the funding needs for the hypothesis development.
   b. Prepare the question to be studied.
   c. Describe who the populations to be studied will be.
   d. Obtain legal advice on how to obtain informed consent.

67. The general areas of prehospital research include: answering clinically important questions, arriving at conclusions based on scientifically sound procedures, and:

   a. obtaining informed consent.
   b. making decisions based on traditions or opinions.
   c. providing results that lead to system improvements.
   d. arriving at conclusions based on questionable ethical procedures.

68. When assessing the validity of research findings, all of the following questions should be critically considered, *except*:

   a. was the research peer-reviewed?
   b. who developed the hypothesis?
   c. what types of data were collected?
   d. were the data properly analyzed?

69. _____ is unrecognized in the DOT curriculum as an EMS provider level.

   a. EMT–Basic
   b. Cardiac rescue technician (CRT)
   c. EMT–Intermediate
   d. EMT–Paramedic

70. A _____ is a "calling" requiring specialized preparation and specific academic preparation.

   a. validation
   b. credential
   c. profession
   d. business

71. Which of the following is inaccurate about the public image of healthcare workers?

    a. Your image and behavior in the public's eye are insignificant.
    b. EMS providers are very visible role models whose behaviors are closely observed.
    c. Your actions in public represent the image of your peers as well as your own.
    d. If people see you not wearing your seat belt, they may think that seat belts are really unnecessary.

72. Empathy is an attribute the paramedic would typically demonstrate to:

    a. him- or herself.
    b. the general public.
    c. the EMS profession.
    d. patients and their families.

73. Which of the following is an example of behavior that demonstrates self-motivation by the paramedic?

    a. Not accepting constructive feedback, because there is no such thing.
    b. Taking advantage of all learning opportunities.
    c. Taking on selective tasks as recommended by supervision.
    d. Making corrections to improve work performance when advised.

74. At times the paramedic must be the diplomat, which means saying and doing things that are considered by some to be:

    a. status quo.
    b. newsworthy.
    c. political suicide.
    d. politically correct.

75. Why is it necessary for paramedics to be good communicators?

    a. It is a prerequisite for an EMS provider.
    b. Because many patients cannot communicate verbally.
    c. Most of what paramedics do involves communication skills.
    d. Good communication skills keep the paramedic from being overbearing.

Exam #2 Answer Form

	A	B	C	D		A	B	C	D
1.	❏	❏	❏	❏	26.	❏	❏	❏	❏
2.	❏	❏	❏	❏	27.	❏	❏	❏	❏
3.	❏	❏	❏	❏	28.	❏	❏	❏	❏
4.	❏	❏	❏	❏	29.	❏	❏	❏	❏
5.	❏	❏	❏	❏	30.	❏	❏	❏	❏
6.	❏	❏	❏	❏	31.	❏	❏	❏	❏
7.	❏	❏	❏	❏	32.	❏	❏	❏	❏
8.	❏	❏	❏	❏	33.	❏	❏	❏	❏
9.	❏	❏	❏	❏	34.	❏	❏	❏	❏
10.	❏	❏	❏	❏	35.	❏	❏	❏	❏
11.	❏	❏	❏	❏	36.	❏	❏	❏	❏
12.	❏	❏	❏	❏	37.	❏	❏	❏	❏
13.	❏	❏	❏	❏	38.	❏	❏	❏	❏
14.	❏	❏	❏	❏	39.	❏	❏	❏	❏
15.	❏	❏	❏	❏	40.	❏	❏	❏	❏
16.	❏	❏	❏	❏	41.	❏	❏	❏	❏
17.	❏	❏	❏	❏	42.	❏	❏	❏	❏
18.	❏	❏	❏	❏	43.	❏	❏	❏	❏
19.	❏	❏	❏	❏	44.	❏	❏	❏	❏
20.	❏	❏	❏	❏	45.	❏	❏	❏	❏
21.	❏	❏	❏	❏	46.	❏	❏	❏	❏
22.	❏	❏	❏	❏	47.	❏	❏	❏	❏
23.	❏	❏	❏	❏	48.	❏	❏	❏	❏
24.	❏	❏	❏	❏	49.	❏	❏	❏	❏
25.	❏	❏	❏	❏	50.	❏	❏	❏	❏

	A	B	C	D			A	B	C	D
51.	❏	❏	❏	❏		64.	❏	❏	❏	❏
52.	❏	❏	❏	❏		65.	❏	❏	❏	❏
53.	❏	❏	❏	❏		66.	❏	❏	❏	❏
54.	❏	❏	❏	❏		67.	❏	❏	❏	❏
55.	❏	❏	❏	❏		68.	❏	❏	❏	❏
56.	❏	❏	❏	❏		69.	❏	❏	❏	❏
57.	❏	❏	❏	❏		70.	❏	❏	❏	❏
58.	❏	❏	❏	❏		71.	❏	❏	❏	❏
59.	❏	❏	❏	❏		72.	❏	❏	❏	❏
60.	❏	❏	❏	❏		73.	❏	❏	❏	❏
61.	❏	❏	❏	❏		74.	❏	❏	❏	❏
62.	❏	❏	❏	❏		75.	❏	❏	❏	❏
63.	❏	❏	❏	❏						

3

Illness and Injury Prevention

1. _____ is the study of occurrence of disease.

   a. Morbidity
   b. Mortality
   c. Incidence
   d. Epidemiology

2. The extent of an injury or illness is called:

   a. morbidity.
   b. mortality.
   c. incidence.
   d. epidemiology.

3. What is the leading cause of overall deaths in the United States?

   a. heart disease
   b. malignant tumors
   c. cerebrovascular diseases
   d. COPD

4. Which of the following is most accurate about causes of death when broken down by gender, age, and race?

   a. Accidents are the leading cause of death for ages one to forty-four.
   b. Those who marry have a higher mortality rate than those who do not.
   c. Life expectancy for males has recently surpassed that of females.
   d. Cerebrovascular disease is the leading cause of death for those over sixty years of age.

5. Which of the following is an effect that has occurred as a result of early release/discharge of patients from the hospital?

   a. Home healthcare will reduce the overall lifetime cost of injuries.
   b. There are more expectations for EMS services to provide care for patients being managed in the home setting.

   c. This cost-cutting trend is going to decrease the reliance on EMS.
   d. More hospitals will rely on EMS to care for and transport patients that have had outpatient procedures.

6. The leading cause of death for white males age fifteen to twenty-four is:

   a. accidents.
   b. homicide.
   c. HIV infection.
   d. suicide.

7. _____ is defined as a real or potential hazardous situation that puts individuals at risk for sustaining an injury.

   a. Harm's way
   b. Injury surveillance
   c. Injury prevention
   d. Injury risk

8. An important part of any injury surveillance program is the timely dissemination of the data to those who need to use it for:

   a. prevention and control efforts.
   b. obtaining funding through grants.
   c. treatment of patients.
   d. reversal of management plans.

9. _____ injury prevention are activities involved in the care of an injury that has already occurred to prevent it from getting worse.

   a. Primary
   b. Secondary
   c. Tertiary
   d. Productive

10. Activities that are involved in the rehabilitation of an injured person, such as preventing infections, are known as:

    a. a teachable moment.
    b. tertiary injury prevention.
    c. sensible ongoing care.
    d. productive quality care.

11. You have decided that it is sensible to be involved in injury and illness prevention efforts in the community where you live and work. One of the ways to act on this decision is to:

    a. visit each school in the community.
    b. pick a cause that best suits your interests.
    c. visit each nursing home in the community.
    d. always wear your seat belt, on and off duty.

12. Which of the following statements about bicycle-related head injuries is most accurate?

    a. The solution to preventing these injuries is to make better helmets.
    b. The lack of parental supervision is the primary contributing factor to these injuries.
    c. Over 95% of victims of bicycle-related head injuries were not wearing helmets when injured.
    d. Reducing speed limits in residential communities is the solution to preventing these types of injuries.

13. In addition to public education in the prevention of drowning, which of the following is a recommended solution for prevention?

    a. Assuring adequate supervision of adults who drink while boating.
    b. Legislation banning any alcohol consumption while in or near water.
    c. Requiring that personal flotation devices (PFDs) be worn whenever children or adults who cannot swim are on or near water.
    d. Legislation requiring that all school-age students receive swimming lessons for two years.

14. The key strategy for reducing deaths from motor vehicles is:

    a. reducing speed limits in school zones.
    b. mandating lower speed limits on the highways.
    c. advocating for more vehicles to include airbags.
    d. getting everyone in the vehicle to wear seat belts.

15. In 1970 the Poison Prevention Act required the U.S. Consumer Product Safety Commission to require the:

    a. use of residential smoke detectors.
    b. use of carbon monoxide detectors in commercial properties.
    c. installation of locks for the storage of toxic substances in schools.
    d. use of child-resistant packaging of toxic substances for in-home use.

16. According to the U.S. Poison Control Centers, more than 90% of poison exposures occur in:

    a. schools.
    b. hospitals.
    c. homes.
    d. work facilities.

17. A strategy for fire prevention safety that you can use at home is to:

    a. practice family fire escape plans every six months.
    b. get everyone in your family to stop smoking as soon as possible.
    c. change the batteries on carbon monoxide and smoke alarms every five years.
    d. increase the amount of coverage on your homeowner's or renter's insurance.

18. A key strategy to reduce injury and death that occur from motorcycle collisions is to:

    a. educate riders to always wear a helmet and protective gear.
    b. educate motor vehicle drivers to give way to riders.
    c. increase insurance rates for riders who drink and drive.
    d. offer insurance discounts for riders who drive slower.

19. Two key strategies for playground safety are adult supervision and:

    a. making hourly inspections for equipment in need of repair.
    b. making sure that any surface that children may fall onto is soft and padded.
    c. ensuring that all playground surfaces have shredded rubber to cushion a fall.
    d. ensuring that all playground surfaces use fine sand or pea gravel to cushion a fall.

20. Select the most accurate statement about common injuries related to falls.

   a. Toddlers should not be allowed to sit in shopping carts.
   b. Every adult age sixty-five or older will fall at least once each year.
   c. Injuries from falls affect the very young and the elderly more severely.
   d. The use of handrails when walking on stairs will eliminate any chance of falling.

21. Which of the following practices should be avoided as a strategy for prevention of falls among the elderly?

   a. Installing metal grates on windows in high-rise buildings.
   b. Installing tiles in kitchens and baths.
   c. Eliminating throw rugs and other trip hazards.
   d. Using shopping carts with straps for holding toddlers.

22. Which of the following is often a frequent cause of strangulation among infants and children?

   a. locks on bathroom doors
   b. unattended child in a vehicle
   c. drawstrings on curtains or blinds
   d. shopping carts with straps for holding infants

23. Key strategies for the prevention of firearm injuries and fatalities include all the following, *except*:

   a. disassembling the National Rifle Association.
   b. gun control and proper storage.
   c. training and licensing of handgun owners.
   d. mandates for trigger locks and loading indicators.

24. Of the approximately 82,000 auto–pedestrian injuries that occur annually, over _____ of those include children who often receive serious brain injury.

   a. 10,000
   b. 20,000
   c. 35,000
   d. 50,000

25. A key strategy for injury prevention and pedestrian safety is to:

   a. avoid drinking and walking.
   b. have a good sense of timing.
   c. avoid crossing the road with small children.
   d. wear reflective clothing both day and night.

26. One of the most effective ways EMS providers can provide leadership in the area of illness and injury prevention is to:

   a. say they are in support of prevention programs.
   b. set examples in all activities of the organization.
   c. give an in-service training program on injury prevention.
   d. advocate for state laws requiring helmet use.

27. An EMS leader has the responsibility to protect individual EMS providers from injury while on duty. One of the things that a leader is expected to do is:

   a. seek out financial resources to sponsor injury prevention programs.
   b. develop sensible policies and procedures promoting safety in all work activities.
   c. mandate each employee to teach injury prevention in one of the local schools or nursing homes.
   d. direct participation in a wellness program for EMS providers, but not for management and office staff.

28. An example of an exposure to a potential injury for the paramedic at the scene of a call is:

   a. day care centers.
   b. unconscious patients.
   c. extreme ambient temperatures.
   d. a broken or faulty blood pressure cuff.

29. An example of a resource that the paramedic should be aware of as part of an injury prevention program is:

   a. retirement options.
   b. child protective services.
   c. utility reimbursement resources.
   d. recreation options for the elderly.

30. One concept of effective communication that the paramedic can use as part of the on-scene education strategy for injury prevention is:

   a. to avoid being objective.
   b. recognizing the teachable moments.
   c. being judgmental about safety issues.
   d. to avoid consideration of ethnic, religious, or social diversity.

31. When a paramedic documents a safety hazard, which of the following should be included?

   a. primary care provided
   b. primary injury data
   c. information required by the EMS agency
   d. all of the above

32. _____ is/are an example of primary injury data.

    a. Scene conditions
    b. Time of response
    c. Past medical history
    d. Medications and allergies

33. Which of the following is associated with an overall lower risk of death?

    a. higher education attainment
    b. residing in warm climates
    c. residing in cold climates
    d. occupation in healthcare

34. Paramedics are in an ideal position to be frontline advocates for injury and disease prevention because:

    a. of the support provided by private sector groups.
    b. of their perspective offered in out-of-hospital care.
    c. of their knowledge of communicable diseases.
    d. all EMS leaders are progressive with injury prevention.

35. _____ is an effort to keep an injury from ever occurring.

    a. Incidence prevention
    b. Injury surveillance
    c. Primary injury prevention
    d. Accident Watch®

Exam #3 Answer Form

	A	B	C	D			A	B	C	D
1.	❏	❏	❏	❏		19.	❏	❏	❏	❏
2.	❏	❏	❏	❏		20.	❏	❏	❏	❏
3.	❏	❏	❏	❏		21.	❏	❏	❏	❏
4.	❏	❏	❏	❏		22.	❏	❏	❏	❏
5.	❏	❏	❏	❏		23.	❏	❏	❏	❏
6.	❏	❏	❏	❏		24.	❏	❏	❏	❏
7.	❏	❏	❏	❏		25.	❏	❏	❏	❏
8.	❏	❏	❏	❏		26.	❏	❏	❏	❏
9.	❏	❏	❏	❏		27.	❏	❏	❏	❏
10.	❏	❏	❏	❏		28.	❏	❏	❏	❏
11.	❏	❏	❏	❏		29.	❏	❏	❏	❏
12.	❏	❏	❏	❏		30.	❏	❏	❏	❏
13.	❏	❏	❏	❏		31.	❏	❏	❏	❏
14.	❏	❏	❏	❏		32.	❏	❏	❏	❏
15.	❏	❏	❏	❏		33.	❏	❏	❏	❏
16.	❏	❏	❏	❏		34.	❏	❏	❏	❏
17.	❏	❏	❏	❏		35.	❏	❏	❏	❏
18.	❏	❏	❏	❏						

Medical/Legal Issues

1. A state's EMS Act, which defines the governmental agency taking the lead in supervising the EMS and issuing certifications, is an example of _____ law.

   a. civil
   b. common
   c. legislative
   d. administrative

2. The statutes that are voted on and passed by the city council, county board, state legislature, or U.S. Congress are called _____ law.

   a. legislative
   b. civil
   c. tort
   d. common

3. A jury panel composed of a selection of people from the community is often referred to as a/an:

   a. appellate jury.
   b. legislative body.
   c. "jury of your peers."
   d. party of legal action.

4. The rules and regulations that outline the specifics of the enacting EMS law in each state are called the:

   a. standard operating procedure (SOP).
   b. EMS code.
   c. state protocols.
   d. Practice Act.

5. Precedents are often decided in a court of law based upon _____ law.

   a. criminal
   b. tort
   c. case
   d. administrative

6. A paramedic found to be purposely hurting patients by withholding essential medications would be charged in a/an _____ court.

   a. small claims
   b. criminal
   c. civil
   d. administrative

7. When a plaintiff sues a paramedic for a breach of confidentiality in which she felt harm was caused to her reputation in the community, this action would take place in _____ court.

   a. criminal
   b. administrative
   c. civil
   d. case law

8. The person or institution (corporation) being sued is called the:

   a. plaintiff.
   b. responder.
   c. claimant.
   d. defendant.

9. A less formal legal process, which involves a judge and attorneys but no jury, is called a/an:

   a. civil trial.
   b. hearing.
   c. common law action.
   d. appellate court.

10. In a trial court, the _____ is responsible for deciding the facts of the case as presented by the competing attorneys.

    a. judge
    b. jury
    c. hearing officer
    d. respondent's attorney

11. If a party to a legal action is not satisfied with the results of the case in a trial court, the decision:

    a. is conclusive and final.
    b. may be appealed to a higher court.
    c. cannot be overruled by another court.
    d. is automatically remanded to a higher court.

12. A/an _____ is convened to help decide if the district attorney or prosecutor has enough evidence to indict an individual to stand trial for a crime.

    a. appellate court
    b. civil court
    c. grand jury
    d. higher court

13. Deviation from the accepted standard of care is called:

    a. abandonment.
    b. negligence.
    c. confidentiality.
    d. a civil tort.

14. When a plaintiff's objective is to receive a financial award for damages that were allegedly caused by the paramedic, this is conducted in a/an:

    a. grand jury.
    b. criminal court.
    c. civil court.
    d. administrative hearing.

15. If the paramedic has an established duty to act and does not comply with that duty, this is referred to as a/an:

    a. error of commission.
    b. breach of duty.
    c. error of omission.
    d. infraction of decorum.

16. The failure to do a required act or duty, such as CPR on a patient who has been down for five minutes prior to your arrival, is called:

    a. nonfeasance.
    b. breach.
    c. malfeasance.
    d. non-reliance.

17. In a malpractice case against a paramedic, the plaintiff's lawyer must prove:

    a. proximate cause.
    b. the presence of an advanced directive.
    c. the absence of an advanced directive.
    d. lack of moral judgment related to societal standards.

18. When an expert witness is called to testify in a malpractice case, it is usually to establish:

    a. proximate cause.
    b. that a duty was present.
    c. that there was a breach of duty.
    d. that commission incurred.

19. If a paramedic was found to have administered an excessive dose of Lasix to a drug addict in order to get "pleasure" out of watching the patient urinate all over himself, this is an example of:

    a. proximate cause.
    b. gross negligence.
    c. abandonment.
    d. commission of duty.

20. The termination of a paramedic/patient care relationship before assuring that a healthcare provider of equal or higher training will continue care is called:

    a. false imprisonment.
    b. confidentiality.
    c. malpractice.
    d. abandonment.

21. Detaining a patient without her consent or legal authority is considered:

    a. abandonment.
    b. false imprisonment.
    c. slander.
    d. kidnapping.

22. A crime in which a patient, her character, or her reputation is injured by false statements of another person is called:

    a. false imprisonment.
    b. libel.
    c. slander.
    d. abandonment.

23. A crime in which a person, her character, or her reputation is injured by the false written statements of another person is called:

    a. libel.
    b. slander.
    c. graffiti.
    d. confidentiality.

24. The granting of medical privileges by a physician either online or off-line is called:

    a. libel.
    b. delegation.
    c. confiscation.
    d. scope of practice.

25. The range of duties and skills a paramedic is expected to perform when necessary is called the:

    a. scope of practice.
    b. delegated authority.
    c. protocol.
    d. negligence per se.

26. The Latin term _____ means "the thing speaks for itself."

    a. vini veni vechi
    b. semper fi
    c. res ipsa loquitor
    d. negligence per se

27. Negligence shown because the law was violated and an injury occurred is called:

    a. res ipsa locquitor.
    b. causation implied.
    c. negligence per se.
    d. contributory negligence.

28. In a rear-end collision, the driver sustained a neck injury. Despite wearing a seat belt, the headrest was improperly positioned, which most likely contributed to the injury. At sentencing, the judge reduces the award to the injured party; this may be because of:

    a. negligence per se.
    b. government immunity.
    c. abandonment.
    d. contributory negligence.

29. One of the first steps taken in the most basic process of civil litigation is:

    a. the trial.
    b. an investigation.
    c. the discovery phase.
    d. serving of the defendant.

30. The period during the pretrial phase when opposing sides get the opportunity to obtain the facts and information from the other side in preparation for the trial is called:

    a. interrogations.
    b. discovery.
    c. settlement.
    d. deposition.

31. The damages and award that are to be given to the plaintiff are called the:

    a. settlement.
    b. interrogatory.
    c. sentencing.
    d. deposition.

32. Written answers to a list of questions about charges are called:

    a. interrogatories.
    b. settlement.
    c. deposition.
    d. discovery.

33. The responsibility for one's own actions is also called:

    a. immunity.
    b. per se negligence.
    c. liability.
    d. malpractice.

34. The time limit within which a lawsuit may be filed is called the:

    a. penalty clause.
    b. statute of limitations.
    c. maximum penalty.
    d. government immunity option.

35. Generally, _____ years is a good period to save records for interactions with adult patients.

    a. three
    b. five
    c. seven
    d. nine

36. When an adult patient agrees to your care, this is called _____ consent.

    a. expressed
    b. informed
    c. implied
    d. detailed

37. After full disclosure or explanation, the patient is said to have given _____ consent.

    a. expressed
    b. implied
    c. involuntary
    d. informed

38. Another name for implied consent is the:

    a. writ of Hypheas.
    b. emergency doctrine.
    c. mental health law.
    d. nolo de solvo.

39. Can an unemancipated minor refuse care?

    a. No.
    b. Yes.
    c. Sometimes.
    d. Yes, but only when a parent cannot be contacted.

40. When a minor can refuse care or give consent, this is officially called:

   a. naturalization.
   b. emancipation.
   c. regionalization.
   d. authorization.

41. A refusal of medical care is considered legal when:

   a. the patient signs a release.
   b. the Medical Director was contacted.
   c. a parent or family member was contacted.
   d. full disclosure was provided to an alert patient.

42. When a patient refuses any part of medical care or transport for evaluation that you deem necessary, despite all of your efforts to convince the patient otherwise, it may be helpful to:

   a. ask the police to threaten the patient with arrest.
   b. get the patient to sign a release.
   c. consult medical control.
   d. avoid a conflict and return to service.

43. Can intoxicated patients refuse care?

   a. Yes; if they do not want transport, just leave them.
   b. Yes, unless they are minors.
   c. No; persons with altered mental status are not considered able to make a competent decision.
   d. No; they can only make decisions of implied consent.

44. Can the paramedic determine how intoxicated a patient may be?

   a. Yes.
   b. Not without additional training.
   c. Only if the Medical Director is involved.
   d. Yes, after ruling out medical causes of the altered behaviors.

45. If a patient who is refusing care becomes unconscious, can the paramedic treat him?

   a. Yes, under the informed consent provision.
   b. Yes, under the emergency doctrine.
   c. Not without the police present.
   d. Not without permission of medical control.

46. Who can take a patient away against his will for evaluation in a hospital?

   a. a spouse
   b. a mental health officer
   c. the paramedic
   d. the medical control physician

47. When a police officer agrees that a patient who is refusing your care may be harmful to himself, he/she can order the patient to the hospital under:

   a. executive powers.
   b. protective custody.
   c. mental health laws.
   d. offensive consent.

48. You are called to the scene of a private residence. The patient is an elderly man whose two daughters meet you at the door and proceed to tell you how he is acting crazy and is so much trouble to care for. They would like you to take him to the hospital. If the patient refuses to go and is alert with no life threats, what should you do?

   a. Just take him in restraints.
   b. Involve the police for some assistance.
   c. Call medical control to get an order to take him in.
   d. Call a mental health officer.

49. The federal rules on sexual harassment are found in the:

   a. state harassment code.
   b. Civil Rights Act.
   c. OSHA regulations.
   d. NFPA guidelines.

50. A living will is a document that states the type of life-saving medical treatment a patient wants or does not want to be employed in case of:

   a. terminal illness.
   b. coma.
   c. persistent vegetative state.
   d. all of the above.

51. A _____ allows a person to designate an agent in cases where the person is unable to make decisions for himself.

   a. living will
   b. healthcare proxy
   c. patient self-determination act
   d. release

52. In which of the following cases it is legal for the paramedic or an EMS agency to release confidential information about a patient to others?

   a. When a third party requires the information for billing.
   b. When the receiving hospital requests the patient's name over the radio.
   c. When the patient's lawyer goes to the EMS office and verbally requests it.
   d. When a spouse calls on the phone asking for a fax of the billing information.

53. _____ is/are the use of sheets, tape, or leather padded restraints to reduce the potential harm to a patient who is unruly or violent.

   a. Humane restraints
   b. Hog tying
   c. Prove binding
   d. Mummy wrapping

54. The paramedic has a/an _____ responsibility to resuscitate all potential organ donors so that others may benefit from the organs.

   a. legal
   b. ethical
   c. moral
   d. religious

55. It is important for the paramedic to write the patient care report (PCR) "in the course of business" for all of the following reasons, *except*:

   a. completing the paperwork at a later time looks suspicious.
   b. the information is fresh in the paramedic's mind.
   c. the information has to be quickly available for billing.
   d. a copy needs to go to the ED to be placed in the patient's record.

56. Punitive damages are designed to punish the defendant for:

   a. her harmful actions.
   b. the extended response time.
   c. the delay in responding to the patient's needs.
   d. discourteous language used.

57. Which of the following is a typical example of compensable damages that the paramedic may be required to pay as a result of a malpractice suit?

   a. college tuition
   b. public assistance
   c. medical expenses
   d. retirement contributions

58. Who has the burden of proof in a lawsuit?

   a. defendant
   b. plaintiff
   c. responder
   d. hearing officer

59. _____ is the range of skills and knowledge the paramedic is trained in.

   a. Scope of practice
   b. Standard of care
   c. Protocol
   d. Code of ethics

60. The _____ makes certain types of information collected by public agencies available to the media, legal council, or the public upon demand.

   a. "standards of care"
   b. Burden of Proof Act
   c. Freedom of Information Act
   d. innocent until proven guilty pretext

61. The paramedic is responsible for the actions of the intern under the _____ concept.

   a. "cloak of secrecy"
   b. medical extender
   c. Good Samaritan
   d. "borrowed servant"

62. Except for the unconscious patient, all EMS providers must get the patient's consent for treatment or they could be charged with:

   a. battery and assault.
   b. sexual harassment.
   c. false imprisonment.
   d. no charges can be filed in this case.

63. In determining whether or not an ambulance operator was exercising due regard in the use of signaling equipment, the courts will consider which of the following?

   a. Was the given signal audible and/or visible to motorist and pedestrians?
   b. Does the insurance company require the use of lights and sirens for all calls?
   c. Does the insurance company require the use of lights and sirens for emergency calls?
   d. Does the insurance company require the use of lights and sirens for all nonemergency calls?

64. According to the American Heart Association (AHA), successful completion of an AHA course:

    a. warrants acceptable quality of care delivered to patients by the provider.
    b. authorizes the provider to perform the procedures learned in the course.
    c. ensures that the performance of procedures learned in the course is of the highest standard.
    d. does not warrant performance or quality, or authorize a person to perform any procedures on a patient.

65. A _____ is a document testifying that one has fulfilled certain requirements, such as a course of instruction.

    a. certificate
    b. license
    c. permit
    d. regents insignia

66. Select the most accurate statement regarding the use of lights and sirens during an emergency response.

    a. The use of lights and sirens during an emergency response gives the operator complete immunity.
    b. The operator of the emergency vehicle assumes the extra burden of driving with due regard for others.
    c. The emergency vehicle operator will be held to a lower standard than the average driver in the eyes of the law.
    d. The use of lights and sirens during an emergency response gives the operator and EMS agency complete immunity.

67. The Americans with Disabilities Act (ADA) is a federal law designed to protect qualified persons with disabilities, such as one who _____, from discrimination in employment.

    a. is pregnant
    b. uses illegal drugs
    c. has hearing impairment
    d. fractured an ankle on the job

68. If an ambulance is involved in a collision en route to the hospital with a patient, is it necessary to stop?

    a. No.
    b. Yes.
    c. Only if someone is injured as a result of the collision.
    d. Only when the collision is more than five minutes from the hospital.

69. The _____ is the federal law that has an impact on issues such as on-call pay, comp time, and long shift and overtime pay.

    a. Family and Medical Leave Act (FMLA)
    b. Fair Labor Standards Act (FLSA)
    c. Federal Insurance Contributions Act (FICA)
    d. Occupational Safety and Health Administration (OSHA)

70. One of the major roles of the Occupational Safety and Health Administration (OSHA) is to:

    a. enforce regulations within employment by federal agencies.
    b. encourage the improvement of existing safety and health programs.
    c. assure that self-employed workers are covered by OSHA regulations.
    d. enforce safety regulations and fine noncompliant farmers where only family members are employed.

71. It is good practice to wear an ID tag and introduce yourself to your patient by name and level of training because:

    a. it is the polite thing to do.
    b. she will know who to sue if she feels treatment was inappropriate.
    c. she will know to send a tip and thank-you letter.
    d. patients have a right to know who you are and your level of training.

72. The Medical Director's liability for prehospital care falls into the two categories of:

    a. training and continuing education.
    b. online and off-line supervision.
    c. quality improvement and quality assurance.
    d. omission and commission.

73. The best way for a paramedic to avoid a lawsuit is to:

    a. always be respectful and pleasant to patients, their families, and their property.
    b. practice good medicine and be a competent caregiver.
    c. accurately document the assessment and management of the patient clearly on the PCR.
    d. all of the above.

74. The first responsibility the paramedic has at a crime scene is to:

    a. protect potential evidence.
    b. provide care for the patient.
    c. protect herself and the crew.
    d. notify law enforcement if not already done.

75. In an effort to maintain the paramedic–patient relationship, which of the following pieces of information must be kept confidential?

    a. gunshot and stab wounds
    b. signs of suspected abuse
    c. signs of a communicable disease
    d. observations made of the patient's residence

Exam #4 Answer Form

	A	B	C	D			A	B	C	D
1.	❏	❏	❏	❏		27.	❏	❏	❏	❏
2.	❏	❏	❏	❏		28.	❏	❏	❏	❏
3.	❏	❏	❏	❏		29.	❏	❏	❏	❏
4.	❏	❏	❏	❏		30.	❏	❏	❏	❏
5.	❏	❏	❏	❏		31.	❏	❏	❏	❏
6.	❏	❏	❏	❏		32.	❏	❏	❏	❏
7.	❏	❏	❏	❏		33.	❏	❏	❏	❏
8.	❏	❏	❏	❏		34.	❏	❏	❏	❏
9.	❏	❏	❏	❏		35.	❏	❏	❏	❏
10.	❏	❏	❏	❏		36.	❏	❏	❏	❏
11.	❏	❏	❏	❏		37.	❏	❏	❏	❏
12.	❏	❏	❏	❏		38.	❏	❏	❏	❏
13.	❏	❏	❏	❏		39.	❏	❏	❏	❏
14.	❏	❏	❏	❏		40.	❏	❏	❏	❏
15.	❏	❏	❏	❏		41.	❏	❏	❏	❏
16.	❏	❏	❏	❏		42.	❏	❏	❏	❏
17.	❏	❏	❏	❏		43.	❏	❏	❏	❏
18.	❏	❏	❏	❏		44.	❏	❏	❏	❏
19.	❏	❏	❏	❏		45.	❏	❏	❏	❏
20.	❏	❏	❏	❏		46.	❏	❏	❏	❏
21.	❏	❏	❏	❏		47.	❏	❏	❏	❏
22.	❏	❏	❏	❏		48.	❏	❏	❏	❏
23.	❏	❏	❏	❏		49.	❏	❏	❏	❏
24.	❏	❏	❏	❏		50.	❏	❏	❏	❏
25.	❏	❏	❏	❏		51.	❏	❏	❏	❏
26.	❏	❏	❏	❏		52.	❏	❏	❏	❏

	A	B	C	D		A	B	C	D
53.	❑	❑	❑	❑	65.	❑	❑	❑	❑
54.	❑	❑	❑	❑	66.	❑	❑	❑	❑
55.	❑	❑	❑	❑	67.	❑	❑	❑	❑
56.	❑	❑	❑	❑	68.	❑	❑	❑	❑
57.	❑	❑	❑	❑	69.	❑	❑	❑	❑
58.	❑	❑	❑	❑	70.	❑	❑	❑	❑
59.	❑	❑	❑	❑	71.	❑	❑	❑	❑
60.	❑	❑	❑	❑	72.	❑	❑	❑	❑
61.	❑	❑	❑	❑	73.	❑	❑	❑	❑
62.	❑	❑	❑	❑	74.	❑	❑	❑	❑
63.	❑	❑	❑	❑	75.	❑	❑	❑	❑
64.	❑	❑	❑	❑					

5

Ethical Issues for the EMS Provider

1. In the EMS community, global ethical conflicts are typically resolved by utilizing standards of care and:

   a. treatment protocols.
   b. maintaining a high degree of suspicion.
   c. involving a family member whenever possible.
   d. avoiding having family involved whenever possible.

2. Ethics are defined as:

   a. a system of principles governing moral conduct.
   b. not acting in a rude or crude manner.
   c. never cheating on your taxes.
   d. a true measure of honesty.

3. Morals relate to _____ standards and ethics relate to _____ standards.

   a. high; objective
   b. subjective; high
   c. personal; societal
   d. societal; personal

4. Which of the following questions should the paramedic consider when confronted with an ethical dilemma?

   a. "What is in the EMS agency's best interest?"
   b. "How will I keep from getting sued?"
   c. "How can my interest best be preserved?"
   d. "What is in the patient's best interest?"

5. How can a refusal of medical assistance involve ethical decisions?

   a. Once the standard of care has been applied, there are no ethical issues.
   b. Ethics are not really a factor when the patient has given informed consent.
   c. Ethics can affect the extent to which you should persuade a patient to receive treatment.
   d. Ethics can affect how much your agency will bill a patient for services after the patient refuses transport.

6. Some states have laws to provide immunity from _____ for the paramedic who begins CPR on a patient with a DNAR order.

   a. liability
   b. willful disregard
   c. wanton disregard
   d. malicious disregard

7. For the patient to be able to be well informed in his decisions regarding care, the paramedic, as a rule, should be honest and:

   a. have a family member involved when possible.
   b. use language/terms the patient can understand.
   c. ask the patient to sign for consent for treatment.
   d. avoid having family involved whenever possible.

8. When the paramedic is faced with a global ethical conflict, which of the following should he avoid using to help resolve the conflict?

   a. standards of care
   b. treatment protocols
   c. retrospective reviews of medical decisions
   d. preplanned wills

9. The American Medical Association's (AMA) Code of Medical Ethics states that patients have the right to:

   a. refuse payment when they are dissatisfied with care rendered.
   b. name the physician who will not do their surgery.
   c. waive their ethical options.
   d. make decisions on healthcare.

10. In which of the following areas might a paramedic have to make an ethical decision?

   a. implied consent
   b. billing
   c. privacy disclosure
   d. reporting suspected child abuse

11. In EMS systems with multiple hospitals and ill-defined transport protocols, the paramedic should use which of the following to influence the patient's decision on where to be transported?

   a. capabilities of the hospital
   b. the closest hospital to the patient's residence
   c. the fastest trip to the hospital
   d. the hospital that accepts the patient's insurance

12. Which of the following is an example of a prehospital ethical decision the paramedic may be confronted with?

   a. deciding to stay home from work when injured
   b. dealing with a patient who is experiencing a behavioral emergency
   c. deciding whether or not to stop to render assistance when not on duty
   d. receiving and confirming a physician order that seems medically acceptable

13. Select the most accurate statement about ethics in the EMS profession.

   a. There is really no difference between ethics and morals.
   b. Ethics involve larger issues than a paramedic's practice.
   c. Every treatment decision the paramedic makes is based on ethics.
   d. Making a medication error and reporting it is an example of unethical behavior.

14. Criteria that are used for allocating scarce EMS resources include: need based upon established criteria, earned based upon an established criteria awarding points or value, and:

   a. true parity.
   b. hardship.
   c. distribution.
   d. prerequisite.

15. _____ is an attempt to make a comparison of all variables in an effort to arrive at a similarity.

   a. True parity
   b. Objective standard
   c. Subjective parity
   d. True standard

16. The paramedic is ethically accountable to all of the following, *except*:

   a. the patient.
   b. the patient's advanced directives.
   c. the Medical Director.
   d. fulfilling the standard of care.

17. When answering an ethical question regarding a patient, which of the following should be considered?

   a. passion
   b. good faith
   c. sentiment
   d. sympathy

18. When the paramedic is making a determination of "what is in the patient's best interest," which of the following should be considered first?

   a. the patient's statements
   b. input from the patient's lawyer
   c. unsigned advanced directives
   d. input from the patient's physician

19. A husband called 9-1-1 when he found his wife unresponsive. You arrived and began resuscitation efforts, but shortly thereafter the patient's son arrives and tells you that the patient did not want any type of resuscitation. There is no Do Not Attempt Resuscitation order (DNAR) for the patient. What should you do next?

   a. Stop CPR and call the coroner.
   b. Call the patient's physician for his advice.
   c. Ask the police to keep the son away.
   d. When in doubt, resuscitate.

20. _____, as we know it today, stands for soundness of moral principle and character, uprightness, and honesty.

   a. Ethics
   b. Integrity
   c. Candor
   d. Sincerity

21. An example of unethical behavior would be:

   a. treating and transporting a patient with no health insurance.
   b. witnessing a coworker do something unethical and saying nothing.
   c. transporting a trauma arrest patient to the nearest hospital instead of a trauma center.
   d. transporting a patient to a hospital that is not the closest because it has more appropriate resources for the patient.

22. Society attempts to resolve global ethical conflicts by using preplans such as wills and advanced directives to make a patient's wishes known, and by:

   a. preprogramming the phone to dial 9-1-1.
   b. using enhanced 9-1-1 and emergency medical dispatch.
   c. creating laws protecting patient's rights.
   d. researching prospective medical decisions.

23. Which of the following is an example of an ethical dilemma the paramedic may experience as a physician extender?

   a. An indirect (off-line) protocol is not in the patient's best interest.
   b. An indirect (off-line) protocol is contraindicated but morally right.
   c. Receiving a direct (online) order that is not part of standing orders.
   d. Receiving a direct (online) order that is medically acceptable but morally wrong.

24. When a patient wants to refuse treatment or transport, but the paramedic believes the patient needs immediate care, the paramedic can avoid an ethical dilemma by:

   a. using value judgment.
   b. acting in the patient's best interest.
   c. letting the patient sign a waiver of care.
   d. preemptively calling a personal lawyer after the call.

25. When we discuss and study ethical principles, this practice serves to:

   a. maintain a high degree of integrity.
   b. strengthen and validate our own inner value system.
   c. define a futile situation and who makes the decision.
   d. prevent incorrect documentation or record tampering.

Exam #5 Answer Form

	A	B	C	D		A	B	C	D
1.	❏	❏	❏	❏	14.	❏	❏	❏	❏
2.	❏	❏	❏	❏	15.	❏	❏	❏	❏
3.	❏	❏	❏	❏	16.	❏	❏	❏	❏
4.	❏	❏	❏	❏	17.	❏	❏	❏	❏
5.	❏	❏	❏	❏	18.	❏	❏	❏	❏
6.	❏	❏	❏	❏	19.	❏	❏	❏	❏
7.	❏	❏	❏	❏	20.	❏	❏	❏	❏
8.	❏	❏	❏	❏	21.	❏	❏	❏	❏
9.	❏	❏	❏	❏	22.	❏	❏	❏	❏
10.	❏	❏	❏	❏	23.	❏	❏	❏	❏
11.	❏	❏	❏	❏	24.	❏	❏	❏	❏
12.	❏	❏	❏	❏	25.	❏	❏	❏	❏
13.	❏	❏	❏	❏					

6

General Principles of Pathophysiology

1. Pathophysiology is defined as:

   a. the study of disease.
   b. an abnormality of function or a structural problem.
   c. a description of how a disease develops from its onset.
   d. the study of how normal physiological processes are altered by disease.

2. The cause of a disease is referred to as the:

   a. pathogenesis.
   b. etiology.
   c. pathology.
   d. prognosis.

3. When the symptoms of a disease rapidly worsen, this is referred to as:

   a. remission.
   b. iatrogenic.
   c. exacerbation.
   d. prognosis.

4. Iatrogenic causes of injury or illness indicate that the cause, or significant contribution to the cause, is:

   a. heredity.
   b. impaired immunity.
   c. nutritional imbalance.
   d. the actions of a healthcare provider.

5. A group of symptoms or conditions that may be caused by a disease or various related medical problems is called a/an:

   a. toxidrome.
   b. infection.
   c. syndrome.
   d. malignancy.

6. A decreased size in the cell leading to a decrease in the size of the tissue and organ is called:

   a. atrophy.
   b. hypertrophy.
   c. acceleration.
   d. cellular adaptation.

7. Atrophy, hyperphasia, and neoplasia are forms of:

   a. muscular dysfunction.
   b. dysplasia.
   c. cellular adaptation.
   d. dysfunction syndrome.

8. An increase in the actual number of cells by hormonal stimulation is called:

   a. hypertrophy.
   b. dysplasia.
   c. metaplasia.
   d. hyperplasia.

9. An alteration in the size and shape of cells, as in a developing tumor, is called:

   a. dysplasia.
   b. hyperplasia.
   c. metaplasia.
   d. hypertrophy.

10. The development of a new type of cell with an uncontrolled growth pattern is called:

    a. neoplasia.
    b. hyperplasia.
    c. metaplasia.
    d. hypertrophy.

11. The ability of microorganisms to cause disease is called:

    a. toxicity.
    b. infectability.
    c. carcinogenesis.
    d. virulence.

12. Many bacteria have a capsule that is designed to:

    a. hide the microorganism from its host.
    b. make it easier to infect the organism.
    c. protect it from ingestion and destruction by phagocytes.
    d. prevent destruction by a virus.

13. When large amounts of endotoxins are present in the body, the patient may develop:

   a. renal failure.
   b. septic shock.
   c. hypovolemic shock.
   d. liver dysfunction.

14. When white blood cells release endogenous pyrogens, it causes:

   a. the production of additional white blood cells.
   b. septic shock.
   c. the body to lower its temperature.
   d. fever to develop.

15. One major difference between viruses and bacteria is that:

   a. viruses are not encapsulated, and bacteria are.
   b. viruses do not produce exotoxins or endotoxins.
   c. there is a symbiotic relation between viruses and bacteria.
   d. bacteria cause a decreased synthesis of macro-molecules, and viruses do not.

16. The body's most common reaction to the presence of bacteria is:

   a. inflammation.
   b. hemorrhage.
   c. hyperplasia.
   d. increased capillary pressure.

17. An example of an injurious genetic factor affecting the cell is:

   a. sepsis.
   b. hepatitis C.
   c. Down syndrome.
   d. mineral deficiency.

18. Why is good nutrition required by the cells?

   a. It helps the nerve cells to rejuvenate.
   b. It helps the cells in fighting off diseases.
   c. It helps the muscle cells multiply.
   d. It decreases the production of energy in the cells.

19. The cellular environment is associated with the:

   a. ability of the bladder to store urine.
   b. changes in cell distribution with aging.
   c. movement of potassium into the cells.
   d. movement of potassium out of the cells.

20. How much of the body's weight is fluid?

   a. 10–12%
   b. 30–40%
   c. 50–70%
   d. 70–90%

21. Where, in the body, can most of the fluid be found?

   a. in the fluid between the cells
   b. intracellular fluids
   c. extracellular fluids
   d. in the bladder

22. How much fluid does the average adult take in each day?

   a. 1,500 ml
   b. 2,500 ml
   c. 3,500 ml
   d. 4,500 ml

23. When a person loses large quantities of water, he also loses the major extracellular cation:

   a. sodium.
   b. calcium.
   c. potassium.
   d. chloride.

24. Lymph fluid is a part of _____ fluid.

   a. interstitial
   b. intracellular
   c. extracellular
   d. transcellular

25. The movement of a substance from an area of higher concentration to an area of lower concentration is called:

   a. osmosis.
   b. filtration.
   c. active transport.
   d. diffusion.

26. When a cell membrane ingests a substance, this is called:

   a. exocytosis.
   b. pinocytosis.
   c. endocytosis.
   d. phagocytosis.

27. The engulfing of solid particles by a cell membrane is called:

   a. exocytosis.
   b. pinocytosis.
   c. endocytosis.
   d. phagocytosis.

28. The pressure that develops when two solutions of different concentrations are separated by a semipermeable membrane is called _____ pressure.

   a. intracranial
   b. osmotic
   c. colloid
   d. oncotic

29. Of the following age groups, which males have the greatest total body water percentage?

   a. ten to eighteen
   b. eighteen to forty
   c. forty to sixty
   d. over sixty

30. A solution with a lower solute concentration than the blood is referred to as a/an _____ solution.

   a. hypertonic
   b. hypotonic
   c. isotonic
   d. neotonic

31. When a helper molecule, found within the membrane, helps the movement of a substance from areas of higher concentration to areas of lower concentration, this is called:

   a. facilitated diffusion.
   b. active transport.
   c. osmosis.
   d. filtration.

32. Which of the following plasma proteins is responsible for maintaining osmotic pressure?

   a. albumin
   b. globulin
   c. fibrinogen
   d. prothrombin

33. The pressure generated by dissolved proteins in the plasma that are too large to penetrate the capillary membrane is called:

   a. tissue colloidal osmotic pressure.
   b. capillary hydrostatic pressure.
   c. tissue hydrostatic pressure.
   d. capillary colloidal osmotic pressure.

34. The pressure that pushes water out of the capillary into the interstitial space is referred to as the:

   a. tissue colloidal osmotic pressure.
   b. capillary colloidal osmotic pressure.
   c. capillary hydrostatic pressure.
   d. tissue hydrostatic pressure.

35. An accumulation of excess fluids in the interstitial space is called:

   a. edema.
   b. lymph.
   c. cellular swelling.
   d. engorgement.

36. Fluid that accumulates in the peritoneal cavity is referred to as:

   a. ascites.
   b. sacral edema.
   c. intestinal swelling.
   d. pitting edema.

37. Edema can be caused by:

   a. increased capillary pressure.
   b. decreased colloidal osmotic pressure.
   c. lymphatic vessel obstruction.
   d. all of the above.

38. When a patient has an extensive burn injury, swelling is caused by:

   a. increased capillary pressure.
   b. decreased colloidal osmotic pressure.
   c. dehydration.
   d. lymphatic vessel obstruction.

39. When edematous tissue, such as in the ankles, is compressed with a finger, the fluid is pushed aside causing a temporary impression. This is referred to as:

   a. lymphatic edema.
   b. pitting edema.
   c. ascites.
   d. acute pulmonary edema (APE)

40. What is the main function of the sodium/potassium pump?

   a. To pump sodium into the cells.
   b. To move potassium out of the cells.
   c. To exchange three sodium ions for every two potassium ions.
   d. To exchange two sodium ions for every three potassium ions.

41. The tension exerted on cell size caused by water movement across the cell membrane is referred to as:

   a. tonicity.
   b. oncotic pressure.
   c. osmotic pressure.
   d. colloid pressure.

42. Cells with an osmolarity of 280 mOsm/L will neither shrink nor swell. This is because they:

   a. are considered hypotonic solutions.
   b. are high in both sodium and potassium.
   c. have the same osmolarity as intracellular fluid.
   d. are considered hypertonic solutions.

43. When a cell is placed in a _____ solution, it will shrink as the water is _____ the cell.

   a. hypotonic; pushed into
   b. hypotonic; pulled out of
   c. hypertonic; pushed into
   d. hypertonic; pulled out of

44. When a cell is placed in a hypotonic solution that has a _____ osmolarity than ICF, it will _____.

   a. lower; shrink
   b. lower; swell
   c. higher; shrink
   d. higher; swell

45. The most common cation in the body is:

   a. calcium.
   b. potassium.
   c. sodium.
   d. chloride.

46. Although the average adult ingests between 6 and 15 grams of sodium per day, the required amount is:

   a. 100 mg.
   b. 500 mg.
   c. 1000 mg.
   d. 4 mg.

47. Angiotensin II is responsible for:

   a. dilating the renal blood vessels.
   b. increasing kidney blood flow.
   c. stimulating sodium reabsorption.
   d. increasing the glomerular filtration rate.

48. The protein enzyme that is released by the kidney into the blood stream in response to changes in blood pressure is called:

   a. renin.
   b. epinephrine.
   c. tensin.
   d. aldosterone.

49. Angiotensin II is responsible for stimulating the secretion of the hormone _____, which acts on the kidney to increase the reabsorption of sodium into the blood.

   a. adenosine
   b. aldosterone
   c. epinephrine
   d. norepinephrine

50. When a patient has excess body water loss without a proportionate sodium loss, she is said to be:

   a. hyponatremic.
   b. hypernatremic.
   c. dehydrated.
   d. edematous.

51. One of the most severe manifestations of hypernatremia is:

   a. oliguria.
   b. seizures and coma.
   c. decreased salivation.
   d. dry and flushed skin.

52. Which of the following is a classic cause of hyponatremia?

   a. sepsis
   b. esophageal varices
   c. vomiting and diarrhea
   d. intra-abdominal hemorrhage

53. An athlete who has had excessive sweating for a three-hour period, and has only been drinking water to rehydrate, may suffer the symptoms of:

   a. hypovolemia.
   b. hypertension.
   c. hyponatremia.
   d. hypernatremia.

54. The major intracellular cation, which is critical to many of the functions of the cell, is:

   a. sodium.
   b. potassium.
   c. chloride.
   d. calcium.

55. A patient may become hypokalemic from:

   a. excessive vomiting or diarrhea.
   b. a diet deficient in sodium.
   c. excessive eating.
   d. decreased sweating.

56. ECG changes associated with a deficiency in potassium may include:

   a. depressed P wave.
   b. widening QRS complex.
   c. low T wave and sagging ST segment.
   d. peaked T waves and depressed ST segment.

57. When a patient has an elevated serum potassium level, this can be caused by:

    a. decreased potassium intake.
    b. excess use of diuretics.
    c. renal failure.
    d. treatment with angiotensin.

58. The clinical manifestations of hyperkalemia include:

    a. paresthesia and intestinal colic.
    b. a feeling of euphoria.
    c. excessive urination.
    d. muscle overactivity.

59. A hyperkalemic patient may exhibit ECG changes such as:

    a. peaked ST segments.
    b. depressed T waves.
    c. widened QRS.
    d. peaked P waves.

60. Where is the vast majority of the body's calcium found?

    a. kidneys
    b. teeth
    c. liver
    d. bones

61. The purpose of calcium is to provide:

    a. strength and stability to bones.
    b. increased conduction through muscles.
    c. enhanced renal effectiveness.
    d. maintenance of the blood pressure.

62. How does calcium enter the body?

    a. through the lungs
    b. by way of the bones
    c. through the GI tract
    d. through the skin

63. Hypocalcemia can be caused by:

    a. renal failure.
    b. decreased pH.
    c. decreased fatty acids.
    d. vomiting and diarrhea.

64. Other causes of hypocalcemia include:

    a. hypermagnesemia.
    b. rapid transfusion of citrated blood.
    c. decreased pH.
    d. excess vitamin D.

65. A patient with hypocalcemia often presents with:

    a. skeletal muscle cramps.
    b. absence of tetany.
    c. hypertension.
    d. hypoactive reflexes.

66. A patient who has frequent skeletal muscle cramps, abdominal spasms, and cramps, as well as frequent fractures, may benefit by supplementing his diet intake of:

    a. sodium.
    b. calcium.
    c. zinc.
    d. potassium.

67. Osteomalacia and carpopedal spasms have been found to be manifestations of:

    a. hyponatremia.
    b. hyperkalemia.
    c. hypophosphatemia.
    d. hypocalcemia.

68. Hypercalcemia can be caused by:

    a. increased pH.
    b. excess calcium in the diet.
    c. insufficient calcium in the diet.
    d. decreased levels of parathyroid hormone.

69. Kidney stones, constipation, and polyuria are sometimes a manifestation of:

    a. hypocalcemia.
    b. hyponatremia.
    c. hypercalcemia.
    d. hypokalemia.

70. A shortening QT interval and A-V block on the ECG sometimes is found with which condition?

    a. hypercalcemia
    b. hyponatremia
    c. hypokalemia
    d. hyperkalemia

71. Hypophophatemia is an abnormally low level of phosphate in the body and can be caused by:

    a. seizures.
    b. heat stroke.
    c. potassium deficiency.
    d. diabetic ketoacidosis.

72. The clinical manifestation of hypophosphatemia includes:

    a. impaired red blood cell function.
    b. hyperflexia.
    c. hemolytic anemia.
    d. excessive hunger.

73. Often patients who experience trauma and have kidney failure are at risk to develop:

    a. hypokalemia.
    b. hyperphosphatemia.
    c. hypocalcemia.
    d. hyponatremia.

74. Malnutrition or starvation can be caused by which of the following conditions?

    a. hypocalcemia
    b. hypomagnesemia
    c. hypercalcemia
    d. hyponatremia

75. Positive Babinski's sign, positive Chvostek's sign, and positive Trousseau's sign may be found in the patient who has:

    a. hypomagnesemia.
    b. hypercalcemia.
    c. hypernatremia.
    d. hyponatremia.

76. A muscular spasm resulting from pressure applied to nerves and vessels of the upper arm is called _____ sign.

    a. Babinski's
    b. Chvostek's
    c. Trousseau's
    d. Cushing's

77. What is the normal pH range of the body?

    a. 7.15–7.25
    b. 7.25–7.35
    c. 7.35–7.45
    d. 7.45–7.55

78. A blood pH _____ than 7.45 is called _____.

    a. greater; acidosis
    b. greater; alkalosis
    c. greater; neutral
    d. less; alkalosis

79. Sepsis, diabetic ketoacidosis, and salicylate poisoning may cause:

    a. respiratory acidosis.
    b. metabolic acidosis.
    c. metabolic alkalosis.
    d. respiratory alkalosis.

80. When CO_2 retention leads to increased levels of pCO_2, the patient develops:

    a. respiratory acidosis.
    b. respiratory alkalosis.
    c. metabolic acidosis.
    d. metabolic alkalosis.

81. Patients who experience a medical condition causing hypoventilation may develop:

    a. metabolic acidosis.
    b. metabolic alkalosis.
    c. respiratory acidosis.
    d. respiratory alkalosis.

82. When a patient has been hyperventilating from an anxiety attack, the patient may ultimately develop:

    a. metabolic acidosis.
    b. metabolic alkalosis.
    c. respiratory acidosis.
    d. respiratory alkalosis.

83. Analyzing disease risk involves reviewing all of the following, *except*:

    a. genetic histories of populations.
    b. rates of incidence.
    c. prevalence.
    d. mortality.

84. An example of a disease that is more prevalent in males is:

    a. osteoporosis.
    b. Parkinson's disease.
    c. breast cancer.
    d. rheumatoid arthritis.

85. Acquired hypersensitivity is called a/an:

    a. rheumatic fever.
    b. cancer.
    c. asthma.
    d. allergy.

86. You are treating a patient who tells you he had a recent strep throat, and he has a history of myocarditis and arthritis. Which of the following conditions could he most likely have?

    a. Parkinson's disease
    b. rheumatic fever
    c. lung cancer
    d. diabetes

87. Which of the following signs or symptoms is an atypical finding associated with cancer?

    a. recent weight gain
    b. difficulty swallowing
    c. nagging cough or hoarseness
    d. change in bowel or bladder habits

88. A hypersensitivity reaction causing constriction of the bronchi, wheezing, and dyspnea is a chronic illness called:

    a. diabetes.
    b. anemia.
    c. asthma.
    d. cardiomyopathy.

89. The leading cause of chronic illness in children is:

    a. diabetes.
    b. chicken pox.
    c. cancer.
    d. asthma.

90. The leading cause of cancer deaths in both males and females combined is from _____ cancer.

    a. rectal
    b. brain
    c. lung
    d. breast

91. The difference between Type I and Type II diabetes is:

    a. Type I develops as a disease in adults.
    b. Type II does not become hypoglycemic.
    c. Type I requires exogenous insulin.
    d. Type II requires injected insulin.

92. Why do diabetic patients need to *inject* insulin?

    a. So they can take an entire day's dose at once.
    b. Their digestive juices would destroy oral forms.
    c. Pills do not counteract low blood pressure.
    d. It is cheapest in this form.

93. What organ is responsible for the production of insulin?

    a. kidney
    b. liver
    c. spleen
    d. pancreas

94. Exposure to benzene and bacterial toxins can cause the patient to develop:

    a. hemophilia.
    b. hematochromatosis.
    c. drug-induced anemia.
    d. septal hypertrophy.

95. Select the statement that is most correct about mitral valve prolapse condition.

    a. The cause is unknown.
    b. The condition is more prevalent in men.
    c. Management of this condition is focused on surgical repair.
    d. The mitral valve leaflets balloon into the right atrium during systole.

96. Long QT syndrome is a cardiac conduction system abnormality that:

    a. is inherited.
    b. there is no treatment for.
    c. is not associated with other diseases.
    d. occurs as a result of abnormal iron retention by the liver.

97. A sex-linked hereditary disorder most commonly passed on from an asymptomatic mother to a male child is:

    a. anemia.
    b. hemophilia.
    c. ALS.
    d. hematochromatosis.

98. Incurable diseases of the heart, which ultimately lead to congestive heart failure or acute coronary syndrome (ACS), include:

    a. stroke.
    b. cardiomyopathies.
    c. mitral valve prolapse.
    d. hematochromatosis.

99. The disease mortality rate for _____ is significantly higher than that of other diseases.

   a. cancer
   b. accidents
   c. HIV/AIDS
   d. cardiovascular disease

100. What is the leading cause of stroke in the prehospital setting?

   a. brain aneurysm
   b. diabetes
   c. cigarette smoking
   d. hypertension

101. A disorder of protein metabolism that primarily affects males, leading to inflammation of the joints, is called:

   a. arthritis.
   b. lactose intolerance.
   c. gout.
   d. ulcerative colitis.

102. Chronic hypertension is a devastating disease that affects the cardiovascular system by:

   a. increasing the blood supply.
   b. changing the size and shape of the heart.
   c. causing the right ventricle to work harder than the left.
   d. increasing the blood volume pumped through the body.

103. Why is smoking a risk factor for stroke?

   a. The carbon dioxide levels run higher.
   b. It damages the lung cells.
   c. Nicotine causes vasoconstriction.
   d. It paralyzes the brain tissues.

104. The medical term for kidney stones is:

   a. uric acid crystals.
   b. renal calculi.
   c. hematuria.
   d. renal calcium.

105. Kidney stones are most common in _____ between the ages of _____.

   a. males: fifty and seventy
   b. females: thirty and seventy
   c. males: thirty and fifty
   d. females: fifty and seventy

106. A disorder affecting the rectum and colon, causing inflammation, lesions, and ulcerations of the mucosal layer, is called:

   a. lactose intolerance.
   b. irritable bowel syndrome.
   c. ulcerative colitis.
   d. Crohn's disease.

107. Patients who are unable to break down the complex carbohydrates found in ice cream have:

   a. renal calculi.
   b. lactose intolerance.
   c. ulcerative colitis.
   d. irritable bowel syndrome.

108. A group of disorders that occurs in areas of the upper GI tract that are normally exposed to acid pepsin secretions is referred to as:

   a. peptic ulcers.
   b. muscular dystrophy.
   c. Crohn's disease.
   d. Huntington's disease.

109. Cholelithiasis is the medical term for:

   a. kidney stones.
   b. peptic ulcers.
   c. gallstones.
   d. Crohn's disease.

110. When the flow of bile is obstructed, the patient may be suffering from:

   a. renal calculi.
   b. lactose intolerance.
   c. gallstones.
   d. Huntington's disease.

111. Each of the following is considered a health risk associated with obesity, *except*:

   a. hyperlipidemia.
   b. hypotension.
   c. gallbladder disease.
   d. insulin resistance.

112. Morbidly obese patients often have sleep apnea and:

   a. lactose intolerance.
   b. hypolipidemia.
   c. multiple sclerosis.
   d. respiratory function impairment.

113. A rare hereditary disorder involving chronic progressive chorea, psychologic changes, and dementia is called:

    a. Crohn's disease.
    b. Huntington's disease.
    c. multiple sclerosis.
    d. muscular dystrophy.

114. You are treating a patient who has a disease that manifests itself with acute episodes of paresthesia, optic neuritis, diplopia, or gaze paralysis. You suspect he may have a history of:

    a. multiple sclerosis.
    b. Huntington's disease.
    c. muscular dystrophy.
    d. Alzheimer's.

115. A patient who has stage 2 Alzheimer's disease may exhibit:

    a. indifference to food and inability to communicate.
    b. memory loss and lack of spontaneity.
    c. impaired cognition and abstract thinking.
    d. inability to taste spicy food and disorientation to time and date.

116. The most common cause of cardiogenic shock is:

    a. anaphylaxis.
    b. a ventricle septal defect.
    c. an extensive acute myocardial infarction.
    d. multiple organ dysfunction syndrome following a severe traumatic injury.

117. _____ is an example of a condition that can cause obstructive shock.

    a. Anaphylaxis
    b. Heart failure
    c. Pericardial tamponade
    d. Ventricular septal defect

118. Causes of hypovolemic shock include:

    a. heart failure.
    b. ventricular septal defect.
    c. electrolyte loss from dehydration.
    d. pericardial tamponade.

119. What is MODS?

    a. a disease of the brain
    b. advice for managing shock
    c. multiple organ dysfunction syndrome
    d. mutation of disease syndrome

120. When a patient who receives a blood transfusion from another person has a reaction to the red blood cells, this is called an _____ reaction.

    a. allergic
    b. isoimmune
    c. autoimmune
    d. inflammation

121. _____ is one of the local effects of an inflammation response.

    a. Fever
    b. Vasodilation
    c. Leukocytosis
    d. Decreased capillary permeability

122. A system response to acute inflammation is:

    a. fever.
    b. vasodilation.
    c. the development of exudates.
    d. increased capillary permeability.

123. The type of immunity that you acquire by getting a disease and developing immunity afterward is _____ immunity.

    a. natural
    b. acquired
    c. nonspecific
    d. cell-mediated

124. The system that plays a vital role in attracting white blood cells to the site of the infection is called:

    a. bradykinin.
    b. imunocascade.
    c. complement.
    d. macrophage.

125. The role of _____ during inflammation is to engulf foreign matter and bacteria.

    a. phagocytes
    b. monocytes
    c. macrophages
    d. eosinophils

Exam #6 Answer Form

	A	B	C	D			A	B	C	D
1.	❏	❏	❏	❏		27.	❏	❏	❏	❏
2.	❏	❏	❏	❏		28.	❏	❏	❏	❏
3.	❏	❏	❏	❏		29.	❏	❏	❏	❏
4.	❏	❏	❏	❏		30.	❏	❏	❏	❏
5.	❏	❏	❏	❏		31.	❏	❏	❏	❏
6.	❏	❏	❏	❏		32.	❏	❏	❏	❏
7.	❏	❏	❏	❏		33.	❏	❏	❏	❏
8.	❏	❏	❏	❏		34.	❏	❏	❏	❏
9.	❏	❏	❏	❏		35.	❏	❏	❏	❏
10.	❏	❏	❏	❏		36.	❏	❏	❏	❏
11.	❏	❏	❏	❏		37.	❏	❏	❏	❏
12.	❏	❏	❏	❏		38.	❏	❏	❏	❏
13.	❏	❏	❏	❏		39.	❏	❏	❏	❏
14.	❏	❏	❏	❏		40.	❏	❏	❏	❏
15.	❏	❏	❏	❏		41.	❏	❏	❏	❏
16.	❏	❏	❏	❏		42.	❏	❏	❏	❏
17.	❏	❏	❏	❏		43.	❏	❏	❏	❏
18.	❏	❏	❏	❏		44.	❏	❏	❏	❏
19.	❏	❏	❏	❏		45.	❏	❏	❏	❏
20.	❏	❏	❏	❏		46.	❏	❏	❏	❏
21.	❏	❏	❏	❏		47.	❏	❏	❏	❏
22.	❏	❏	❏	❏		48.	❏	❏	❏	❏
23.	❏	❏	❏	❏		49.	❏	❏	❏	❏
24.	❏	❏	❏	❏		50.	❏	❏	❏	❏
25.	❏	❏	❏	❏		51.	❏	❏	❏	❏
26.	❏	❏	❏	❏		52.	❏	❏	❏	❏

	A	B	C	D			A	B	C	D
53.	❑	❑	❑	❑		82.	❑	❑	❑	❑
54.	❑	❑	❑	❑		83.	❑	❑	❑	❑
55.	❑	❑	❑	❑		84.	❑	❑	❑	❑
56.	❑	❑	❑	❑		85.	❑	❑	❑	❑
57.	❑	❑	❑	❑		86.	❑	❑	❑	❑
58.	❑	❑	❑	❑		87.	❑	❑	❑	❑
59.	❑	❑	❑	❑		88.	❑	❑	❑	❑
60.	❑	❑	❑	❑		89.	❑	❑	❑	❑
61.	❑	❑	❑	❑		90.	❑	❑	❑	❑
62.	❑	❑	❑	❑		91.	❑	❑	❑	❑
63.	❑	❑	❑	❑		92.	❑	❑	❑	❑
64.	❑	❑	❑	❑		93.	❑	❑	❑	❑
65.	❑	❑	❑	❑		94.	❑	❑	❑	❑
66.	❑	❑	❑	❑		95.	❑	❑	❑	❑
67.	❑	❑	❑	❑		96.	❑	❑	❑	❑
68.	❑	❑	❑	❑		97.	❑	❑	❑	❑
69.	❑	❑	❑	❑		98.	❑	❑	❑	❑
70.	❑	❑	❑	❑		99.	❑	❑	❑	❑
71.	❑	❑	❑	❑		100.	❑	❑	❑	❑
72.	❑	❑	❑	❑		101.	❑	❑	❑	❑
73.	❑	❑	❑	❑		102.	❑	❑	❑	❑
74.	❑	❑	❑	❑		103.	❑	❑	❑	❑
75.	❑	❑	❑	❑		104.	❑	❑	❑	❑
76.	❑	❑	❑	❑		105.	❑	❑	❑	❑
77.	❑	❑	❑	❑		106.	❑	❑	❑	❑
78.	❑	❑	❑	❑		107.	❑	❑	❑	❑
79.	❑	❑	❑	❑		108.	❑	❑	❑	❑
80.	❑	❑	❑	❑		109.	❑	❑	❑	❑
81.	❑	❑	❑	❑		110.	❑	❑	❑	❑

	A	B	C	D		A	B	C	D
111.	❏	❏	❏	❏	119.	❏	❏	❏	❏
112.	❏	❏	❏	❏	120.	❏	❏	❏	❏
113.	❏	❏	❏	❏	121.	❏	❏	❏	❏
114.	❏	❏	❏	❏	122.	❏	❏	❏	❏
115.	❏	❏	❏	❏	123.	❏	❏	❏	❏
116.	❏	❏	❏	❏	124.	❏	❏	❏	❏
117.	❏	❏	❏	❏	125.	❏	❏	❏	❏
118.	❏	❏	❏	❏					

7

Pharmacology

1. Any chemical substance that, when taken into a living organism, produces a biologic response affecting one or more of that organism's processes or functions is a:

   a. solution.
   b. drug.
   c. antigen.
   d. antibody.

2. The term for the study of how a drug is altered as it travels through the body is:

   a. pharmacokinetics.
   b. pharmacodynamics.
   c. pharmaceutics.
   d. antagonism.

3. The study of how and why a drug works, specifically its biochemical and physiologic effects, is called:

   a. pharmacodynamics.
   b. pharmaceutics.
   c. pharmacokinetics.
   d. pharmacopoeia.

4. The chemical breakdown of a drug while in the body is called:

   a. absorption.
   b. distribution.
   c. elimination.
   d. biotransformation.

5. The general properties of a drug include all the following, *except*:

   a. therapeutic.
   b. prophylactic.
   c. diagnostic.
   d. research.

6. Drug-induced physiologic changes in a body function or process are known as a/an:

   a. drug action.
   b. side effect.
   c. half-life.
   d. idiosyncrasy.

7. A drug that stimulates a receptor is called a/an:

   a. agonist.
   b. antagonist.
   c. sympatholytic.
   d. sympathomimetic.

8. The major mechanism by which a drug affects the body is by joining with receptors located on the:

   a. red blood cells.
   b. target organs or tissues.
   c. white blood cells.
   d. mast cells.

9. A drug that mimics the functions of the sympathetic nervous system is called a/an:

   a. agonist.
   b. antagonist.
   c. sympatholytic.
   d. sympathomimetic.

10. An example of an emergency-use drug that is also a sympathetic nervous system neurotransmitter is:

    a. dopamine.
    b. amiodarone.
    c. dobutamine.
    d. procainamide.

11. ACLS drugs, such as epinephrine, dopamine, and dobutamine, belong to a group of drugs called:

    a. fibrins.
    b. ionospheres.
    c. sympatholytics.
    d. sympathomimetics.

12. Antiadrenergic drugs that block the function of the sympathetic nervous system are called:

    a. fibrins.
    b. ionospheres.
    c. sympatholytics.
    d. sympathomimetics.

13. Cholinergic receptors respond to the neurotransmitter:

    a. acetylcholine.
    b. epinephrine.
    c. norepinephrine.
    d. nortriptyline.

14. Drugs that block cholinergic receptors and parasympathetic response are called parasympatholytics. In the prehospital setting, the most commonly used parasympatholytic is:

    a. metaprolol.
    b. atenolol.
    c. dobutamine.
    d. atropine.

15. For a drug to get inside a cell or body part, the two primary means of transportation are active and passive transport. The difference between the two is that active transport requires:

    a. energy produced through a chemical reaction.
    b. a change in homeostasis.
    c. the formation of genetic repressors.
    d. energy to produce and displace phosphatide.

16. When repeated doses of a drug lead to toxicity in a patient, this condition is known as a:

    a. side effect.
    b. habituation.
    c. hypersensitivity.
    d. cumulative effect.

17. When a patient takes a medication and has an unexpected response that most patients would *not* have, this is called a/an:

    a. idiosyncrasy.
    b. side effect.
    c. toxicity.
    d. cumulative effect.

18. A physiologic blockade that protects the brain from exposure to various drugs is called:

    a. cerebral spinal fluid.
    b. blood-brain barrier.
    c. meninges.
    d. collateral barrier.

19. The name of a drug that is assigned by the U.S. Adopted Name Council is the _____ name.

    a. official
    b. generic
    c. trade
    d. brand

20. Angiotensin-converting enzyme (ACE) inhibitors work primarily by inhibiting:

    a. renin from releasing sodium.
    b. angiotensin I from converting angiotensin II.
    c. sodium and water retention.
    d. acetylcholine.

21. Chemical assay is a test that determines a drug's:

    a. ingredients.
    b. reliability.
    c. half-life.
    d. mechanism of injury.

22. The Pure Food and Drug Act of 1906 required drug manufacturers to:

    a. test a drug for effectiveness.
    b. test a drug for safety.
    c. label all ingredients.
    d. label all dangerous ingredients in drug products.

23. The Federal Drug Administration (FDA) is responsible for all of the following, *except*:

    a. testing of drugs.
    b. marketing of drugs.
    c. availability of drugs.
    d. drug enforcement.

24. Most pediatric medication doses are administered according to body weight because:

    a. children metabolize drugs faster than adults.
    b. the total body weight affects the distribution of the drug.
    c. children require more medication than adults because of immature liver function.
    d. children require more medication than adults because of immature kidney function.

25. A drug's ability to join with a receptor is known as:

    a. affinity.
    b. ability.
    c. selective response.
    d. agonist.

26. A drug that joins partially with a receptor and prevents a reaction is called a/an:

    a. partial antagonist.
    b. partial agonist.
    c. agonist.
    d. antagonist.

27. The two types of sympathetic receptors in the body are:

    a. dopaminergic and adrenergic.
    b. adrenergic and cholinergic.
    c. iatrogenic and dopaminergic.
    d. cholinergic and inhibitoric.

28. Diffusion, filtration, and osmosis are all means of:

    a. drug actions.
    b. precipitation.
    c. active transport.
    d. passive transport.

29. The pressure that develops when two solutions of different concentrations are separated by a semipermeable membrane is called _____ pressure.

    a. osmotic
    b. hydrostatic
    c. hypertonic
    d. hypotonic

30. The term for the combined effect of drugs taken at the same time altering the expected therapeutic effect of each is known as:

    a. systemic action.
    b. therapeutic antagonism.
    c. drug interaction.
    d. mechanism of action.

31. When two drugs are used together to produce a desired effect that is much better than only one drug alone could produce, this is referred to as what type of synergism?

    a. additive effect
    b. potentiation
    c. competitive effect
    d. physiologic effect

32. You are interviewing a patient and find that the patient has been taking barbiturates regularly. Today he has also been drinking alcohol. What type of synergistic effect would you expect to find in this patient?

    a. additive
    b. potentiation
    c. competitive
    d. therapeutic

33. A patient who has ingested poison was given activated charcoal. The charcoal will bind and absorb to toxins present in the GI tract to inactivate and then excrete them. This chemical process is known as:

    a. loading dose.
    b. tolerance.
    c. hypersensitivity.
    d. antagonism.

34. A paramedic is about to administer adenosine to a patient experiencing SVT. The paramedic chooses a large venous access and will administer this medication in a *rapid* IV push, followed by a rapid flush, to achieve the correct therapeutic effect. Which of the following terms best refers to the specific reason for this therapeutic effect?

    a. idiosyncrasy
    b. adverse reaction
    c. half-life
    d. side effect

35. The Harrison Narcotic Act of 1914 was the first act passed by a nation that:

    a. controlled the sale of narcotics and drugs that cause dependence.
    b. required drug manufacturers to label certain dangerous ingredients on the packages.
    c. empowered the government to enforce safety standards on the production of narcotics.
    d. required proof of both safety and efficacy before a new narcotic could be approved for use.

36. Controlled substances are divided into five schedules depending on their potential for abuse. Which of the following schedules would a cough preparation containing an opioid be listed in?

    a. I
    b. II
    c. IV
    d. V

37. Before a new drug is approved by the FDA for use, the drug has to complete _____ phases to ensure its safety and efficacy.

    a. three
    b. four
    c. six
    d. eight

38. Defects in drug products can result in lawsuits. For drug product liability to exist, which of the following criteria must be met?

    a. The defect occurred after it left the manufacturer.
    b. The defect occurred before it left the manufacturer.
    c. The product was not used for its intended purpose.
    d. The defect was reported by a healthcare professional.

39. Drugs are classified by their chemical class, mechanism of action, or:

   a. potency.
   b. therapeutic effect.
   c. solid or liquid form.
   d. potential for abuse.

40. Drugs that are administered in higher doses often have:

   a. the tendency to delay hepatic metabolism.
   b. a slower absorption rate than lower doses.
   c. a quicker absorption rate than lower doses.
   d. the same absorption rate as lower doses.

41. What is the difference between a loading dose and a maintenance dose of a drug?

   a. A loading dose is typically a single dose of a drug.
   b. A loading dose is typically administered by IV drip.
   c. A maintenance dose will never lose its half-life.
   d. A maintenance dose is only administered by IV drip.

42. You are assessing a patient with an altered mental status (AMS), and you find that the patient takes Lasix, potassium, and Colace. The potassium bottle is old and empty. Based only on the medications of the patient, what might be the cause of the patient's AMS?

   a. dehydration
   b. hypertension
   c. diabetes
   d. thyroid

43. A sixty-six-year-old female patient is experiencing severe side effects (slow heart rate and low blood pressure) from a new medication. Her past medical history (PMH) includes stroke, COPD, kidney failure, and diverticulitis. Based on her PMH, which of the following is the probable cause of the side effects?

   a. decreased pulmonary function
   b. decreased renal function
   c. neurologic dysfunction
   d. decreased GI motility

44. A drug reference, and the only official book of drug standards in the United States that only lists drugs that have met high standards of quality, purity, and strength, is the:

   a. Physician's Desk Reference (PDR).
   b. US Pharmacopoeia.
   c. Hospital Formulary (HF).
   d. FDA's Drug Reference.

45. Because the stomach has a pH of approximately 1.4 and the small intestine a pH of 5.3, a drug's chemical acidity will determine where it is absorbed. Which drugs will be better absorbed in the stomach than in the intestine?

   a. All drugs are absorbed in the intestine.
   b. Drugs that are neutral.
   c. Drugs with a weak base.
   d. Drugs with weak acidity.

46. IM drug administration should be avoided in the patient suspected of having an ACS because:

   a. the pain of injection may worsen the MI.
   b. it may elevate diagnostic enzyme levels.
   c. the drug will not be absorbed fast enough to be of benefit.
   d. total drug volumes are too large for cardiac patients.

47. You are administering an aerosolized medication to a patient for an asthma attack. How can you avoid inhaling the medication yourself?

   a. Have the patient take deep breaths and hold them.
   b. Wear a face mask.
   c. Ask the patient to exhale in a direction away from you.
   d. Plug the end of the nebulizer oxygen tubing.

48. Drugs are metabolized in the body by various organs and tissues. Which of the following is not involved in this process?

   a. liver
   b. lungs
   c. heart muscle
   d. intestinal mucosa

49. The adverse mental or physical condition affecting a patient through the outcome of treatment by a practitioner is called:

   a. iatrogenic.
   b. assay.
   c. disregard.
   d. identity crises.

50. The method for making sure a drug dosage and reliability are accurate is called:

   a. standardization.
   b. classification.
   c. cataloging.
   d. bioassay.

Exam #7 Answer Form

	A	B	C	D		A	B	C	D
1.	❏	❏	❏	❏	26.	❏	❏	❏	❏
2.	❏	❏	❏	❏	27.	❏	❏	❏	❏
3.	❏	❏	❏	❏	28.	❏	❏	❏	❏
4.	❏	❏	❏	❏	29.	❏	❏	❏	❏
5.	❏	❏	❏	❏	30.	❏	❏	❏	❏
6.	❏	❏	❏	❏	31.	❏	❏	❏	❏
7.	❏	❏	❏	❏	32.	❏	❏	❏	❏
8.	❏	❏	❏	❏	33.	❏	❏	❏	❏
9.	❏	❏	❏	❏	34.	❏	❏	❏	❏
10.	❏	❏	❏	❏	35.	❏	❏	❏	❏
11.	❏	❏	❏	❏	36.	❏	❏	❏	❏
12.	❏	❏	❏	❏	37.	❏	❏	❏	❏
13.	❏	❏	❏	❏	38.	❏	❏	❏	❏
14.	❏	❏	❏	❏	39.	❏	❏	❏	❏
15.	❏	❏	❏	❏	40.	❏	❏	❏	❏
16.	❏	❏	❏	❏	41.	❏	❏	❏	❏
17.	❏	❏	❏	❏	42.	❏	❏	❏	❏
18.	❏	❏	❏	❏	43.	❏	❏	❏	❏
19.	❏	❏	❏	❏	44.	❏	❏	❏	❏
20.	❏	❏	❏	❏	45.	❏	❏	❏	❏
21.	❏	❏	❏	❏	46.	❏	❏	❏	❏
22.	❏	❏	❏	❏	47.	❏	❏	❏	❏
23.	❏	❏	❏	❏	48.	❏	❏	❏	❏
24.	❏	❏	❏	❏	49.	❏	❏	❏	❏
25.	❏	❏	❏	❏	50.	❏	❏	❏	❏

Medication Administration

1. You are working the v-fib algorithm on a patient in cardiac arrest; you have intubated, started an IV, given shocks, and administered 1 mg epinephrine, and now you call medical control for further direction. Up to this point, all the skills you have performed have been done as:

   a. direct orders of medical control.
   b. indirect orders of medical control.
   c. quality management.
   d. quality improvement.

2. The "six rights of medication administration" are used by healthcare providers in an effort to:

   a. avoid making medication administration errors.
   b. gain patient consent for emergency treatment.
   c. assure that the patient is informed of his rights.
   d. remember when to document a PCR.

3. A chemical product designed for topical application to kill bacteria is a/an:

   a. antimicrobiotic.
   b. antibiotic.
   c. antiseptic.
   d. disinfectant.

4. A chemical or physical agent approved by the Environmental Protection Agency (EPA) to prevent infection by killing bacteria is a/an:

   a. antimicrobiotic.
   b. antibiotic.
   c. antiseptic.
   d. disinfectant.

5. Which of the following is an example of a sharp?

   a. an open vial
   b. an open ampule
   c. a used angio-catheter
   d. a three-way stop cock

6. Which of the following is the most common complication associated with drawing blood samples?

   a. local infection
   b. systemic infection
   c. nerve or muscle damage
   d. miscannulation of an artery instead of a vein

7. You are looking at a patient's prescription medication bottle and the dose reads 40 mg b.i.d. How often should the medication be taken?

   a. once a day
   b. four times a day
   c. twice a day
   d. twice a night

8. Which of the following routes of drug administration injects the medication under the dermis into connective tissue or fat?

   a. enteral
   b. epidural
   c. subcutaneous
   d. intramuscular

9. The three systems of measure used for drug administration include the metric system, the apothecary system, and the _____ method.

   a. household
   b. English
   c. Mayan
   d. Egyptian

10. In the metric system of measure, the basic unit of mass (weight) is the:

    a. kilo.
    b. ounce.
    c. gram.
    d. pound.

11. You are adjusting your drip rate to run approximately one drop every two seconds. This is the standard rate used when an IV is kept in place for purposes other than replacing fluids, and is often referred to as:

    a. KVO.
    b. TKO.
    c. either KVO or TKO.
    d. neither KVO or TKO.

12. One of the primary advantages of giving drugs by parenteral route in emergencies is that:

    a. it is most convenient.
    b. it is the most economical.
    c. IV access is always available.
    d. absorption effects are more predictable.

13. When a drug is administered to be dissolved between the cheek and gum, what type of route is this?

   a. buccal
   b. ingestion
   c. sublingual
   d. intra-atricular

14. When diazepam is administered per rectum, by what route of administration has this drug been given?

   a. enteral
   b. parenteral
   c. transdermal
   d. subcutaneous

15. The injection of a drug into the spinal canal on or outside the dura mater that surrounds the spinal column is called a/an:

   a. subdural.
   b. epidural.
   c. intrapleural.
   d. intravenous.

16. Convert 3,500 mg to grams:

   a. 0.35 grams
   b. 3.5 grams
   c. 35 grams
   d. 350 grams

17. Convert 1,200 mcg to grams:

   a. 0.0012 grams
   b. 0.012 grams
   c. 0.12 grams
   d. 1.2 grams

18. Convert 2.5 liters to milliliters:

   a. 2.5 ml
   b. 25 ml
   c. 250 ml
   d. 2,500 ml

19. Convert a patient's weight of 198 pounds to kilograms:

   a. 86 kg
   b. 92 kg
   c. 90 kg
   d. 99 kg

20. Convert 66 kilograms to pounds:

   a. 140 lb
   b. 142 lb
   c. 145 lb
   d. 146 lb

21. You need to administer 1.5 mg/kg of lidocaine to your patient who weighs 176 pounds. The drug comes packaged as 100 mg in 10 ml. How much lidocaine do you need to administer?

   a. 265 mg
   b. 120 mg
   c. 100 mg
   d. 80 mg

22. In reference to question 21, how many milliliters of the lidocaine will you need to administer to deliver 1.5 mg/kg?

   a. 20.65
   b. 12
   c. 10
   d. 4

23. Medical control gives you an order to administer a 300 ml bolus over thirty minutes using a 10 gtt drip set. How many drops per minute will it take to infuse the bolus?

   a. 10 gtt/min
   b. 100 gtt/min
   c. 30 gtt/min
   d. 300 gtt/min

24. You are to administer D-50 to an unresponsive diabetic patient. The D-50 comes in a 50 ml (preload) syringe, and you will administer all of it. How many grams of dextrose will you administer?

   a. 5
   b. 25
   c. 50
   d. 500

25. Medical control advises you to administer D-25 to a diabetic pediatric patient. The only dextrose you have on hand is D-50. What do you need to do to administer the proper concentration?

   a. Hang a drip of D-50.
   b. Infuse half the dose of D-50 without diluting.
   c. Dilute the D-50 by one-half, then administer.
   d. Tell medical control you cannot help the patient.

26. Following a bolus of lidocaine, you now need to set up an IV drip of 3 mg per minute. You have 200 mg of lidocaine, a 50 ml bag of normal saline, and a 60 gtt drip set. How many drops (gtts) per minute will you need to run to administer a 3 mg/min drip?

   a. 15 gtts
   b. 30 gtts
   c. 45 gtts
   d. 60 gtts

27. You are given an order to administer 5 mg of morphine sulfate to a patient. You have on hand two vials, each containing 4 mg in 2 ml. How many ml of the drug will you have remaining after administering the correct dose?

   a. 0.5 ml
   b. 1 ml
   c. 1.5 ml
   d. 2 ml

28. Convert a temperature of 98.6° Fahrenheit to Celsius and select the correct answer.

   a. 37°
   b. 39.5°
   c. 40.2°
   d. 41.6°

29. A drug package that is a small glass container with a rubber stopper by which the drug is withdrawn by a needle and syringe is a/an:

   a. ampule.
   b. vial.
   c. preloaded cartridge.
   d. small volume nebulizer.

30. Which of the following medications is administered enterally in the prehospital setting?

   a. epinephrine
   b. nitro paste
   c. nitro spray
   d. aspirin

31. Which of the following is least accurate about medication administration by (PO) oral route?

   a. The absorption rate is fast.
   b. The absorption rate is slow.
   c. NPO in the field is common due to nausea and vomiting.
   d. PO medications are easy to take.

32. Which of the following is true about medication administration by (PR) rectal route?

   a. PR is the preferred route for pediatric medications.
   b. PR is the preferred route for seizure patients.
   c. PR allows for rapid absorption.
   d. The absorption rate is unpredictable.

33. When reviewing your paperwork, you realize you made an error while charting a medication administration dose. The proper way to correct this error is to:

   a. erase the error and rewrite the correct dose.
   b. use a single line to mark out the error, make the change, and initial it.
   c. write over the error to fix it.
   d. never change or correct medications errors.

34. When using a blood pressure cuff as a tourniquet to start an IV, the cuff is inflated to occlude venous blood flow, but not arterial flow. What is the appropriate range of inflation for this procedure?

   a. 140–160 mmHg
   b. 120–130 mmHg
   c. 90–110 mmHg
   d. 70–80 mmHg

35. You have administered 25 mg of Benadryl® IVP to a patient experiencing an allergic reaction to a bee sting. Suddenly the patient becomes hypotensive. The hypotension is probably a result of:

   a. an incorrect dose of Benadryl®.
   b. a reaction from the bee sting.
   c. the incorrect route of medication administration.
   d. a potentiation effect of the medication.

36. Which of the following metric units is the largest prefix?

   a. kilo
   b. micro
   c. centi
   d. milli

37. Medical control has given you an order to administer an amiodarone drip. The order is for 150 mg of amiodarone into a 50 ml bag, to be run in over ten minutes with a macro 10 gtt drip set. How many drops per minute will you need to run?

   a. 15 gtt/min
   b. 45 gtt/min
   c. 50 gtt/min
   d. 150 gtt/min

38. You have a patient in severe bronchospasm, and medical control has given you an order for a magnesium sulfate drip. The order is 2 grams into 50 ml over twenty minutes with a macro 10 gtt drip set. How many drops per minute will you need?

   a. 4 gtt/min
   b. 25 gtt/min
   c. 40 gtt/min
   d. 250 gtt/min

39. You have a 500 ml bag of IV D5W. How many grams of dextrose (sugar) are in this bag?

    a. 5
    b. 20
    c. 25
    d. 50

40. Medical control gives you an order to run a dopamine drip at 5 mcg/kg/min. The patient weighs 100 kg and you have a concentration of 1600 mcg/ml mixed in a 250 ml bag with a micro drip set. How many drips per minute do you run?

    a. 19
    b. 30
    c. 45
    d. 63

41. Medical control gives you the order to administer 0.02 mg/kg of atropine to a child who weighs 12 pounds. The minimum loading dose of atropine is 0.1 mg. What is the correct dose for this child?

    a. 0.1 mg
    b. 0.15 mg
    c. 1.0 mg
    d. 1.5 mg

42. You are running a micro drip at one drop every two seconds. How many minutes will it take for a 50 ml bag of normal saline to run out completely?

    a. 25
    b. 30
    c. 50
    d. 100

43. You are running a 1-liter bag of normal saline through a 10-gtts administration set at 60 gtts/min. During a twenty-minute transport time to the hospital, how much fluid will be infused?

    a. 10 ml
    b. 20 ml
    c. 60 ml
    d. 120 ml

44. You are going to administer 0.25 mg/kg of diltiazem over two minutes to a patient with an uncontrolled atrial fibrillation. The patient weighs 200 pounds, and the package of medication has 25 mg in 5 ml. How many milligrams will you administer?

    a. 4 mg
    b. 8 mg
    c. 16 mg
    d. 23 mg

45. In reference to question 44, what is the smallest size of syringe you can use to administer the entire dose in one injection?

    a. 1 cc
    b. 5 cc
    c. 20 cc
    d. 30 cc

46. You are going to administer 150 mg of lidocaine over ten minutes. How many mg per minute will you infuse?

    a. 10
    b. 15
    c. 1.0
    d. 1.5

47. A male patient is bleeding from a traumatic injury and has lost 3.5 pints of blood. If his total blood volume is 6 quarts, what percent of his blood volume has he lost?

    a. 10
    b. 20
    c. 25
    d. 30

48. You have started an IV with a macro drip set at 10 gtt/ml. Medical control tells you to give one liter bag at a rate of 250 ml/hr. How many drops per minute will you need to infuse?

    a. 4 gtts/min
    b. 10 gtts/min
    c. 33 gtts/min
    d. 42 gtts/min

49. You are administering oxygen via a non-rebreather mask to a patient at 12 lpm. The tank contained 350 liters of oxygen when you began. How many minutes can you continue at the current rate before running completely out of oxygen?

    a. 25
    b. 29
    c. 33
    d. 39

50. You are going to give a subcutaneous injection to a patient. Which of the following needles would be the most appropriate for this administration?

    a. 19-ga and 1.5-inch needle
    b. 23-ga and 0.5-inch needle
    c. 18-ga angio
    d. 20-ga biopsy needle

Exam #8 Answer Form

	A	B	C	D			A	B	C	D
1.	❏	❏	❏	❏		26.	❏	❏	❏	❏
2.	❏	❏	❏	❏		27.	❏	❏	❏	❏
3.	❏	❏	❏	❏		28.	❏	❏	❏	❏
4.	❏	❏	❏	❏		29.	❏	❏	❏	❏
5.	❏	❏	❏	❏		30.	❏	❏	❏	❏
6.	❏	❏	❏	❏		31.	❏	❏	❏	❏
7.	❏	❏	❏	❏		32.	❏	❏	❏	❏
8.	❏	❏	❏	❏		33.	❏	❏	❏	❏
9.	❏	❏	❏	❏		34.	❏	❏	❏	❏
10.	❏	❏	❏	❏		35.	❏	❏	❏	❏
11.	❏	❏	❏	❏		36.	❏	❏	❏	❏
12.	❏	❏	❏	❏		37.	❏	❏	❏	❏
13.	❏	❏	❏	❏		38.	❏	❏	❏	❏
14.	❏	❏	❏	❏		39.	❏	❏	❏	❏
15.	❏	❏	❏	❏		40.	❏	❏	❏	❏
16.	❏	❏	❏	❏		41.	❏	❏	❏	❏
17.	❏	❏	❏	❏		42.	❏	❏	❏	❏
18.	❏	❏	❏	❏		43.	❏	❏	❏	❏
19.	❏	❏	❏	❏		44.	❏	❏	❏	❏
20.	❏	❏	❏	❏		45.	❏	❏	❏	❏
21.	❏	❏	❏	❏		46.	❏	❏	❏	❏
22.	❏	❏	❏	❏		47.	❏	❏	❏	❏
23.	❏	❏	❏	❏		48.	❏	❏	❏	❏
24.	❏	❏	❏	❏		49.	❏	❏	❏	❏
25.	❏	❏	❏	❏		50.	❏	❏	❏	❏

Life Span Development

1. The average weight of a newborn at birth is:

    a. 2.5–3.0 kg.
    b. 3.0–3.5 kg.
    c. 4.0–4.5 kg.
    d. 4.5–5.0 kg.

2. During the first week of life, a baby will lose _____ % of its body weight due to excretion of extracellular fluid present at birth.

    a. 2–5
    b. 5–10
    c. 10–15
    d. 15–20

3. The average weight of an infant is double its birth weight by what age?

    a. one year
    b. three months
    c. four to six months
    d. nine to twelve months

4. When a newborn's cardiovascular system has made the shift from fetal circulation to normal infant circulation, which of the following has occurred?

    a. The foramen ovale has opened.
    b. The ductus venosus has opened.
    c. The ductus arteriosus has opened.
    d. The ductus arteriosus has closed.

5. Infants are primarily obligate nose breathers until what age?

    a. four weeks
    b. three months
    c. six weeks
    d. six months

6. Of the following statements about the infant's pulmonary system, which is true?

    a. Diaphragmatic breathing causes the airways to be more easily obstructed.
    b. Accessory muscles of respiration are prone to barotraumas.
    c. The alveoli are numerous with increased collateral ventilation.
    d. The ribs are positioned horizontally, causing diaphragmatic breathing.

7. At what age do the posterior fontanelles close on an infant?

    a. three months
    b. six months
    c. twelve months
    d. eighteen months

8. At what age do the anterior fontanelles usually close on an infant?

    a. three to six months
    b. six to nine months
    c. nine to eighteen months
    d. two years

9. Which of the following factors can lead to abnormally fast bone growth in an infant?

    a. poor general health
    b. abnormal sleep cycle
    c. abnormal thyroid hormone levels
    d. formula supplemented with calcium and iron

10. What is the average annual weight gain, in kilograms, for a toddler?

    a. one
    b. two
    c. three
    d. four

11. A four-year-old boy puts on his father's golf shoes and attempts to take a few practice swings with one of his father's golf clubs. In psychologic terms, what type of behavior is the child displaying?

    a. magical thinking
    b. modeling
    c. separation anxiety
    d. sibling rivalry

12. In which age group do children primarily develop self-esteem?

    a. toddler
    b. preschool
    c. school age
    d. adolescence

13. When a young teenage male experiences a change in voice quality, this is an example of a typical stage of:

   a. primary sexual development.
   b. secondary sexual development.
   c. a growth spurt.
   d. menarche.

14. Which of the following statements is true about endocrine system changes that take place during adolescence?

   a. Gonadotropins released by the pituitary gland promote the production of testosterone.
   b. Interstitial cell-stimulating hormone causes acne.
   c. Muscle mass increases from the release of lutenizing hormone.
   d. Body fat decreases from the release of follicle-stimulating hormone.

15. Changes that occur during late adulthood within the respiratory system that lead to decreased respiratory function include a/an:

   a. decrease in elasticity of the diaphragm.
   b. increase in chest wall resolution.
   c. decrease in alveolar pressures.
   d. increase in pulmonic vascular strength.

16. The elderly often have an ineffective cough reflex caused by:

   a. exposure to cigarette smoke.
   b. weakening of the chest wall.
   c. lower production of cortisol.
   d. atrophy of the pituitary gland.

17. A major change in the endocrine system function during late adulthood is a/an:

   a. increase in insulin production.
   b. decrease in insulin production.
   c. increase in thyroid hormone production.
   d. decrease in red blood cell (RBC) production.

18. Older adults are often prescribed medications in lower doses than younger adults because of changes in metabolism caused by:

   a. increased acid reflux.
   b. increased GI obstruction.
   c. vitamin deficiencies.
   d. changes in renal function.

19. You are transferring an elderly nursing home resident to the hospital for an injury from a fall. The patient is lying in bed, conscious, and complaining of pain in her right wrist. The wrist is swollen and bruised. As you transfer the patient to the stretcher, you see that she wearing an adult diaper. One of the primary reasons elderly adults develop stool incontinence is that:

   a. they are prone to fluid retention.
   b. they are prone to urinary tract infections.
   c. their muscular sphincters become less effective with age.
   d. they are unable to digest food as effectively as younger patients.

20. Which of the following statements about adolescent growth spurts is most accurate?

   a. More boys than girls experience growth spurts.
   b. Growth spurts begin with enlargement of the chest and trunk.
   c. Growth spurts begin with enlargement of the feet and hands.
   d. Most boys are finished growing before most girls.

21. In which age group are the kidneys unable to concentrate urine?

   a. infancy
   b. toddler
   c. adolescence
   d. late adulthood

22. The "startle" reflex is a normal reflex in the first year of life. It consists of a rapid abduction and extension of the arms, followed by adduction of the arms. This reflex is also known as the _____ reflex.

   a. moro
   b. palmar grasp
   c. suckling
   d. rooting

23. At birth, the infant immune system is relatively undeveloped. Antibodies transferred from the mother maintain passive immunity through what age?

   a. six months
   b. one year
   c. eighteen months
   d. two years

24. A heart rate of less than _____ bpm in a newborn is abnormal.

   a. 140
   b. 120
   c. 110
   d. 100

25. You have just assisted in the delivery of a newborn, and the respiratory rate after one minute is 20. This is considered a/an _____ finding.

    a. normal
    b. abnormal
    c. critical
    d. insignificant

26. You are assessing an infant that is eleven months old. You do not know the child's exact weight, but you can estimate that the child's weight is _____ its birth weight.

    a. double
    b. triple
    c. quadruple
    d. five times

27. Baby teeth begin to erupt at _____ months.

    a. one to three
    b. five to seven
    c. twelve to eighteen
    d. eighteen to twenty-four

28. The amount of time remaining in a person's life before he is expected to die is referred to as the life:

    a. span.
    b. profile.
    c. expansion.
    d. expectancy.

29. What is the leading cause of death among early adults?

    a. cancer
    b. accidents
    c. ACS
    d. suicide

30. In what age group does cardiovascular disease become a major concern?

    a. adolescent
    b. early adulthood
    c. middle adulthood
    d. late adulthood

31. The _____ syndrome occurs when all of a parent's children become old enough to leave home.

    a. biological clock
    b. desolation
    c. life span
    d. empty nest

32. _____ is the total duration of one life, from birth to death.

    a. Life expectancy
    b. Life profile
    c. Development
    d. Life span

33. With the effects of aging, the baroreceptors within blood vessels lose their sensitivity. As a result, late adults are more sensitive to _____ changes.

    a. climate
    b. orthostatic
    c. elevation
    d. nutritional

34. It is not uncommon for a blood pressure reading to be falsely high in late adults because of the effects of:

    a. arteriosclerosis.
    b. postural hypotension.
    c. orthostatic changes.
    d. gravity.

35. As the heart ages, the myocardium is less able to respond to exercise because the muscle is:

    a. dehydrated.
    b. hypertrophied.
    c. less elastic.
    d. more elastic.

36. Degeneration of the cardiac conduction system may lead to a combination of brady- and tachydysrhythmias, often called "tachy–brady" syndrome or _____ syndrome.

    a. Wolff–Parkinson–White
    b. Sick–sinus
    c. Wilson–Mikity
    d. Witzelsucht

37. With aging, there is a decreased functional blood volume and a decrease in the levels of RBCs caused by:

    a. polypharmacy.
    b. poor nutrition and malabsorption.
    c. dehydration.
    d. hypothyroidism.

38. _____ decreases the oxygen-carrying capacity of the blood, thus worsening an already tenuous cardiac function in the late adult.

    a. Atrial valve disease
    b. Diabetes
    c. Anemia
    d. Cardiomegaly

39. Which of the following statements is true about the changes in the respiratory system in late adulthood?

    a. There is an increase in generalized lung capacity.
    b. There is a decrease in upper respiratory infections.
    c. There is an increase of normal mucous membrane linings.
    d. There is a loss of normal mucous membrane linings.

40. Because of a decrease in _____ in the late adult, the development of serious diseases with very few clinical signs or symptoms may occur.

    a. pain perception
    b. kinesthetic sense
    c. visual acuity
    d. proprioception

41. Normal changes in the nervous system during late adulthood result in disturbances of the:

    a. sleep–wake cycle.
    b. myelin sheath.
    c. psychosomatic process.
    d. leukapheresis cycle.

42. You are transporting an elderly female to the hospital for a local infection that is in need of immediate care. The patient is alert and, during the ride, your conversation turns to a discussion about the patient's height. She tells you that she is several inches shorter than she was as a young adult. What is one of the primary reasons for the change in height that comes with aging?

    a. perpetual hypocalcemia
    b. trauma injury to the spine
    c. osteoporosis of the spine
    d. loss of neurons and neurotransmitters

43. In which age group does the body reach peak physical conditioning?

    a. school-age
    b. adolescence
    c. early adulthood
    d. middle adulthood

44. Normal behavioral "milestones," such as the development of self-concept, self-esteem, and morals typically occur in which age group?

    a. preschool
    b. school-age
    c. adolescence
    d. early adulthood

45. At what age does the hearing sense reach peak (maturity) levels?

    a. one to two years
    b. three to four years
    c. five to six years
    d. seven to eight years

46. Which one of the four parenting styles described by psychologists is characterized by the parent(s) showing tolerance toward the child's impulses and using a minimal amount of punishment, while making few demands on the child to act maturely?

    a. authoritarian
    b. authoritative
    c. permissive-indulgent
    d. permissive-indifferent

47. Normal behavioral "milestones" for the toddler and preschool child include all the following, *except*:

    a. development of basics of language.
    b. understanding of cause and effect.
    c. understanding of body image.
    d. television may affect behavior.

48. _____ is a term for normal hearing loss caused by aging.

    a. Tympanitis
    b. Otomylitis
    c. Kinesthesia
    d. Presbycusis

49. The late adult is less equipped to handle bodily stresses such as severe infection because of:

    a. an increase in thyroid hormone production.
    b. an increase in insulin production.
    c. a decrease in cortisol production.
    d. a decrease in financial status.

50. Changes in the myocardium in the late adult include:

    a. loss of normal cardiac pacemaker cells.
    b. enhanced automaticity.
    c. increased syncytium.
    d. decreased syncytium.

Exam #9 Answer Form

	A	B	C	D			A	B	C	D
1.	❏	❏	❏	❏		26.	❏	❏	❏	❏
2.	❏	❏	❏	❏		27.	❏	❏	❏	❏
3.	❏	❏	❏	❏		28.	❏	❏	❏	❏
4.	❏	❏	❏	❏		29.	❏	❏	❏	❏
5.	❏	❏	❏	❏		30.	❏	❏	❏	❏
6.	❏	❏	❏	❏		31.	❏	❏	❏	❏
7.	❏	❏	❏	❏		32.	❏	❏	❏	❏
8.	❏	❏	❏	❏		33.	❏	❏	❏	❏
9.	❏	❏	❏	❏		34.	❏	❏	❏	❏
10.	❏	❏	❏	❏		35.	❏	❏	❏	❏
11.	❏	❏	❏	❏		36.	❏	❏	❏	❏
12.	❏	❏	❏	❏		37.	❏	❏	❏	❏
13.	❏	❏	❏	❏		38.	❏	❏	❏	❏
14.	❏	❏	❏	❏		39.	❏	❏	❏	❏
15.	❏	❏	❏	❏		40.	❏	❏	❏	❏
16.	❏	❏	❏	❏		41.	❏	❏	❏	❏
17.	❏	❏	❏	❏		42.	❏	❏	❏	❏
18.	❏	❏	❏	❏		43.	❏	❏	❏	❏
19.	❏	❏	❏	❏		44.	❏	❏	❏	❏
20.	❏	❏	❏	❏		45.	❏	❏	❏	❏
21.	❏	❏	❏	❏		46.	❏	❏	❏	❏
22.	❏	❏	❏	❏		47.	❏	❏	❏	❏
23.	❏	❏	❏	❏		48.	❏	❏	❏	❏
24.	❏	❏	❏	❏		49.	❏	❏	❏	❏
25.	❏	❏	❏	❏		50.	❏	❏	❏	❏

10

Airway Management and Ventilation

1. Which of the following structures is/are considered to be part of the lower airways?

   a. alveoli
   b. vocal cords
   c. cricoid ring
   d. thyroid cartilage

2. In the pediatric patient, the smallest diameter of the airway is located at the:

   a. epiglottis.
   b. pyriform fossae.
   c. ring in the trachea.
   d. cricothyroid membrane.

3. Which of the following is most correct about the differences between adult and pediatric airways?

   a. Infants and children have a more flexible trachea than adults.
   b. The epiglottis of infants and children is more rigid than an adult's.
   c. The mouth and nose of an adult are more easily obstructed than an infant's or child's.
   d. The epiglottis of an adult is proportionately larger and floppier than a pediatric epiglottis.

4. Which of the following is most correct about the tongues of infants and children?

   a. The tongue is difficult to manipulate during intubation.
   b. The tongue is easy to manipulate during intubation.
   c. They are proportionately smaller and take up less space in the mouth.
   d. They are proportionately larger and take up more space in the mouth.

5. Which of the following structures is considered part of the upper airway?

   a. carina
   b. trachea
   c. cricoid ring
   d. ethmoid bone

6. The function of the upper airway is to:

   a. warm, filter, and humidify the air we breathe.
   b. facilitate oxygenation at the cellular level.
   c. service pulmonary circulation through ventilation.
   d. exchange oxygen and carbon dioxide in the nares.

7. The function of the lower airway is to:

   a. warm, filter, and humidify the air we breathe.
   b. facilitate conversion of oxygen to energy.
   c. exchange oxygen and carbon dioxide at the cellular level.
   d. equalize pulmonary pressures.

8. _____ is the movement of carbon dioxide out of the lungs, and _____ is the movement of oxygen into the lungs.

   a. Ventilation; oxygenation
   b. Ventilation; perfusion
   c. Perfusion; ventilation
   d. Oxygenation; ventilation

9. The combined pressure of all atmospheric gases is the total pressure. At sea level the pressure, measured in torr, should add up to _____ torr, and the percentage should equal _____ %.

   a. 100; 90
   b. 100; 75
   c. 760; 100
   d. 760; 96

10. The partial pressure of oxygen in the atmosphere at sea level is _____ torr.

   a. 597.0
   b. 159.0
   c. 3.7
   d. 0.3

11. Which of the following is correct about the difference between the concentrations of alveolar and atmospheric gas?

    a. There is less nitrogen and oxygen in the alveolar gas.
    b. There is more nitrogen and oxygen in the alveolar gas.
    c. There is less water and carbon dioxide in the alveolar gas.
    d. There is no difference in concentrations.

12. The major controlling factors over the respiratory rate are the central nervous system (CNS) and the:

    a. patient's mental status.
    b. patient's metabolic status.
    c. age of the patient.
    d. patient's heart rate.

13. What area in the CNS is the primary involuntary respiratory center?

    a. medulla
    b. vagus nerve
    c. chemoreceptor
    d. baroreceptor

14. The pons has the secondary control center of respirations called the _____ center.

    a. secondary
    b. backup
    c. chemoreceptor
    d. apneustic

15. Chemoreceptors control respiration by measuring the pH of the blood and:

    a. surfactant.
    b. pulmonary pressure.
    c. CSF.
    d. blood pressure.

16. Chemoreceptors are most plentiful in the carotid sinus and:

    a. aortic arch.
    b. medulla.
    c. pons.
    d. pneumotaxic center.

17. Normally the primary stimulus to breathe is a _____ in the blood.

    a. low concentration of carbon dioxide
    b. high concentration of carbon dioxide
    c. low concentration of oxygen
    d. high concentration of oxygen

18. In chronic COPD patients, the normal stimulus to breathe may fail because of:

    a. the use of steroids.
    b. excessive mucus production.
    c. trapped or retained CO_2.
    d. excessive surfactant production.

19. You are assessing a fifty-six-year-old female with a complaint of sudden onset of difficulty breathing. She has a history of COPD and is on oxygen 24/7 by cannula at 2 lpm. She is alert and denies chest pain but gets dizzy when standing. The physical exam shows skin that is cyanotic, warm, and dry; lung sounds are clear; and the distal pulse is tachy/regular. She has retractions of the sternocleidomastoid muscles but no peripheral edema or jugular vein distention. Select the statement that is most accurate about this patient.

    a. There is a great possibility that this patient will need to be intubated.
    b. Long-term use of high-flow oxygen will not be harmful to this patient.
    c. The risk of under-oxygenating this patient is greater than the risk of suppressing the stimulus to breathe.
    d. This patient is a CO_2 retainer and is likely to deteriorate to respiratory arrest if given a light level of oxygen.

20. Your patient is a fifty-nine-year-old male with shortness of breath. He states that he has been sick for several days, and each day he feels worse. It is obvious that he is a smoker, but he denies having a COPD history. After your physical exam, you begin treatment and transport to rule out pneumonia. How can cigarette smoking be a direct contributing factor to developing pneumonia for this patient?

    a. Smoking causes bronchospasm and bronchoconstriction.
    b. Smoking inhibits the normal movement of mucus out of the lung.
    c. Smoking causes inflammation of the lung tissue, blocking the small airways.
    d. Smoking causes overgrowth of mucus glands and excess secretion of mucus that blocks the airway.

21. The condition that is characterized by a lack of oxygen in the tissues of the body is called:

    a. anaerobic metabolism.
    b. anoxia.
    c. hypoxemia.
    d. hypoxia.

22. _____ is a lack of oxygen in the blood.

   a. Anaerobic metabolism
   b. Anoxia
   c. Hypoxemia
   d. Hypoxia

23. The paramedic should consider any patient with a neurologic emergency to be _____ until proven otherwise.

   a. hyperventilating and alkalotic
   b. hypoventilating and hypoxemic
   c. obstructed
   d. acidotic

24. _____ is an atypical cause of laryngeal spasm.

   a. Post-extubation
   b. Cold water submersion
   c. Cerebrovascular accident
   d. An overly aggressive intubation attempt

25. In response to a call for difficulty breathing, you are assessing a patient whom you suspect has pneumonia. What should be your first consideration when dealing with this patient?

   a. The patient is contagious.
   b. The patient may deteriorate to respiratory arrest.
   c. Pneumonia can precipitate congestive heart failure.
   d. The patient requires high-flow oxygen immediately.

26. Which of the following is an atypical complication associated with aspiration?

   a. severe allergic reaction
   b. destruction of lung tissue
   c. exposure of pathogens into the lungs
   d. foreign body airway obstruction (FBAO)

27. The bulb syringe, V-Vac®, or foot pump unit are all examples of _____ devices.

   a. battery-powered airway
   b. oxygen-powered suction
   c. manual suction
   d. AC- or DC-powered suction

28. Oxygen-powered suction units work well, but the biggest disadvantage is that they:

   a. are difficult to clean.
   b. are expensive.
   c. are heavy and difficult to carry.
   d. deplete your oxygen source rapidly.

29. Sterile suction technique is necessary when:

   a. performing any type of patient suctioning.
   b. suctioning the nose only.
   c. suctioning the tracheobronchial region.
   d. the patient has an OPA in place.

30. Suctioning can cause vagal stimulation by:

   a. changing the intrathoracic pressure.
   b. tickling the back of the throat.
   c. creating a hypoxic state.
   d. irritating the carotid sinuses.

31. Oral airways are hard plastic tubes designed to:

   a. prevent the tongue from obstructing the glottis.
   b. facilitate oral suctioning.
   c. facilitate oral tracheal intubation.
   d. guarantee that the airway will remain open.

32. One major disadvantage of using the nasopharyngeal airway (NPA) is that:

   a. you cannot suction through them.
   b. they do not provide a secured airway.
   c. they cannot be used on a conscious patient.
   d. they can only be used on an unconscious patient.

33. Which of the following is correct about the bevel on the end of a nasal airway?

   a. The bevel helps to facilitate suctioning.
   b. The bevel is designed to face the nasal septum.
   c. The bevel is a measuring device.
   d. The bevel follows the natural curvature of the nasopharynx.

34. Only water-soluble jelly is used when lubricating airway tubes, because other products are not biodegradable and can:

   a. cause laryngeal edema.
   b. cause excessive slipping of the airway adjuncts.
   c. collect in the lung tissue, causing a chemical aspiration pneumonia.
   d. interfere with surfactant production.

35. Pulsus paradoxus is present when the _____ BP drops more than 10 mmHg with _____

   a. systolic; inspiration.
   b. systolic; expiration.
   c. diastolic; inspiration.
   d. diastolic; expiration.

36. Pulsus paradoxus is seen in COPD patients and patients with pericardial tamponade, and may occur:

    a. in an allergic reaction.
    b. during an asthma attack.
    c. with pneumonia.
    d. with a URI.

37. A cough, sneeze, and hiccup are all examples of:

    a. abnormal breathing patterns.
    b. temporary impairment of the respiratory muscles.
    c. protective reflexes used by patients to modify their respirations.
    d. inadequate ventilation associated with impairment of the nervous system.

38. _____ is an involuntary deep breath that increases opening of alveoli, preventing atelectasis. This occurs, on average, once every hour.

    a. Coughing
    b. Sighing
    c. Hiccuping
    d. A gag reflex

39. Your unit has been called for an ALS transport of a patient with kidney failure. As you listen to the verbal report from the nurse, you observe that the patient is unconscious and has deep, gasping respirations. What respiratory pattern is most likely occurring with this patient?

    a. Biot's
    b. agonal
    c. Kussmaul's
    d. Cheyne-Stokes

40. It is 4:00 P.M. when you respond to a call for a patient in severe respiratory distress. The patient is a sixty-six-year-old female who is sitting on the edge of her chair in a sniffing position, working hard to breathe. She has a nasal cannula on and is cyanotic with sternal retractions. You hear audible wet gurgling and wheezing. She is in this position because it:

    a. helps to make it easier to breathe.
    b. increases the opening of the alveoli.
    c. gradually increases the tidal volume.
    d. aids in the clearing of the bronchi and bronchioles.

41. Gastric distention results when a rescuer is giving too much ventilatory volume or when the:

    a. patient has an inspiratory effort.
    b. airway is not properly opened.
    c. patient aspirates.
    d. patient is not intubated.

42. Gastric distention increases the risk of regurgitation and potential for aspiration, as well as:

    a. creating resistance to bag mask ventilation.
    b. making an intubation more difficult.
    c. increasing the potential for laryngospasm.
    d. increasing the potential for bronchospasm.

43. The noninvasive method for managing gastric distention includes being prepared for the patient to vomit and:

    a. slowly applying pressure to the epigastric region.
    b. rapidly suctioning the hypopharynx until the patient is relieved.
    c. stimulating the gag reflex with the rigid suction tip.
    d. performing cricoid pressure and pressing on the stomach.

44. Which of the following statements regarding the use of a gastric tube is most accurate?

    a. It interferes with intubation.
    b. It is tolerated by conscious patients.
    c. It is only used on unconscious patients.
    d. It causes severe esophageal irritation and bleeding.

45. Naso- or orogastric intubation causes vagus nerve stimulation and may lead to:

    a. atrial flutter.
    b. heart block.
    c. atrial fibrillation.
    d. supraventricular tachycardia.

46. While inserting a nasogastric tube in a patient with severe gastric distention, you observe that the patient's heart rate is decreased significantly. Which of the following would be appropriate to correct the problem?

    a. Terminate the procedure.
    b. Continue the procedure and then hyperventilate the patient.
    c. Ask the patient to stop talking.
    d. Administer Phenergan for nausea.

47. If your efforts to correct the bradycardia in the patient described in question 46 have not worked and the heart rate remains low, your next step would involve:

    a. administering atropine.
    b. terminating the procedure.
    c. administering Phenergan for nausea.
    d. asking the patient to cough.

48. Managing the airway of a patient can be hazardous because of the:

   a. potential for a spinal injury.
   b. potential for breaking teeth.
   c. potential lawsuit by the patient when harm is done.
   d. exposure to body fluids.

49. Oxygen tanks are pressurized vessels that can be very dangerous if dropped. The weakest point is the _____, which could break and send the pressurized vessel flying like a missile.

   a. bottom of the tank
   b. valve stem
   c. hydrostate plate
   d. spine of the tank

50. Oxygen cylinders need to be hydrostatically tested every five years. However, if the tank has a star after the test date, it is good for a/an _____-year period.

   a. eight
   b. ten
   c. twelve
   d. fifteen

51. When handling oxygen cylinders, the use of adhesive tape to mark or label tanks is not recommended because the materials in these products may:

   a. react with the oxygen, causing a fire.
   b. react with the oxygen and cause an explosion.
   c. cause the pressurized vessel to fly like a missile.
   d. make the tank sticky and difficult to handle.

52. Select the statement that is most accurate about oxygen tanks, pressure, and regulators.

   a. High-pressure regulators are used to transfer oxygen directly to patients.
   b. The pressure of the tank is usually around 3,500 psi when the tank is full.
   c. A therapy regulator is designed to be attached to the cylinder stem or wall of the ambulance.
   d. A therapy regulator is generally set at 100 PSI, and the actual delivery to the patient is adjustable to liters per minute.

53. The maximum pressure recommended for positive pressure ventilation should not exceed _____ cm of water pressure.

   a. 15
   b. 30
   c. 50
   d. 100

54. On which of the following patients would a demand-valve device be most appropriate?

   a. trauma arrest patient
   b. respiratory arrest patient
   c. medical cardiac arrest patient
   d. exacerbated congestive heart failure patient

55. On a call for a patient with respiratory distress, you are caring for a patient with a laryngectomy. Select the most accurate statement about the airway management for this patient.

   a. When ventilating a partial laryngectomy patient, you need to cover the mouth.
   b. When ventilating a *complete* laryngectomy patient, you do not need to cover the mouth.
   c. When performing rescue breathing on a laryngectomy patient, you give ventilations into the mouth.
   d. The end of the stoma should never be removed, nor should any airway adjuncts be attached.

56. What is the potential hazard of using a bag mask with a pop-off valve?

   a. Pop-off valves are difficult to close and open.
   b. Pop-off valves are difficult to size to patients.
   c. Ventilations can exit the pop-off valve without getting air into the patient.
   d. It is more difficult to get a mask seal.

57. After a cervical collar is applied to a patient, it can be removed for intubation or to correct a problem in the airway only when:

   a. two hands provide manual in-line immobilization.
   b. a second paramedic is available to assist.
   c. the head is taped to a long backboard.
   d. the front of a collar is removed.

58. Which of the following is an indication for the use of intermittent positive pressure breathing (IPPB)?

   a. when a patient is noncompliant or combative
   b. when a patient has poor tidal volume
   c. when a patient needs a high volume of high-concentration oxygen
   d. when the patient is a small child

59. One of the advantages of using IPPB is:

   a. that it allows for an easy mask seal.
   b. it reduces the risk of overinflation.
   c. there is no chance for barotrauma.
   d. there is no chance for gastric distention.

60. You are treating a seventy-two-year-old resident in a nursing home for difficulty breathing. The staff tells you that she was fine in the morning and suddenly had deterioration in mental status and respiratory effort. The patient is alert to voice, and is pale, warm, and dry. Lung sounds are diminished in the bases, and wheezing is present in the apices. Distal pulse is tachy/irregular, and her blood pressure is 180/100. You put her on a non-rebreather while your partner sets up a nebulizer treatment. You start an IV, and, after a few minutes of treatment, her SpO$_2$ has increased from the low 80s to the low 90s. The patient denies chest pain and tells you with difficulty that she doesn't feel much better. What noninvasive airway management/ventilation device or technique would be most comfortable and most likely effective for this patient?

    a. biphasic positive airway pressure
    b. nasal cannula with a partial-rebreather mask
    c. assisted ventilations with a bag mask device
    d. small volume nebulizer attached to a bag mask device

61. All of the following are advantages of an automatic transport ventilator (ATV), *except* that they:

    a. are lightweight and portable.
    b. can minimize airway pressures.
    c. can reduce the risk of distension.
    d. can eliminate the risk of aspiration.

62. Which of the following is an indication for the use of an ATV?

    a. conscious patients who are combative
    b. patient with an obstructed airway
    c. patient with a pneumothorax
    d. unconscious patients who are sedated

63. _____ refers to positive pressure ventilation in a patient using either a tight-fitting nasal or face mask, but without endotracheal intubation.

    a. Continuous inflation flow
    b. Esophageal obturator
    c. Noninvasive ventilation
    d. Noninvasive transthoracic perfusion

64. The major advantage to the use of CPAP and BiPAP devices is that:

    a. intubation may be avoided where it may have previously been required.
    b. there is no wasting of oxygen.
    c. it is available to all prehospital providers.
    d. it does not require continuing education.

65. Collapse of the smaller airways and alveoli caused by hypoventilation or obstruction is called:

    a. pneumotaxis.
    b. atelectasis.
    c. hemotaxis.
    d. pneumothorax.

66. Which of the following patient conditions is a common cause of the condition described in question 65?

    a. epistaxis
    b. fractured ribs
    c. allergic reaction
    d. a pediatric on a ventilator

67. When inserted too far, why is the ET tube more likely to slide into the right mainstem bronchus than the left?

    a. The left mainstem is harder to see.
    b. The left mainstem is often occuled with mucus.
    c. The right mainstem bronchus is straighter.
    d. The right mainstem is more rigid than the left.

68. The _____ is used to help visualize the vocal cords during intubation with a laryngoscope.

    a. Berman maneuver
    b. Rothberg maneuver
    c. tripod position
    d. sniffing position

69. The patient you have intubated, because of a near respiratory arrest, appears to be improving and attempting to remove the ET tube. Which of the following is appropriate for the paramedic to manage the patient?

    a. Be prepared to suction the patient.
    b. Anticipate the need to reintubate the patient.
    c. Consider physical and chemical restraint in consult with medical control.
    d. All of the above.

70. During a lengthy extrication process of an unconscious patient who was trapped in a vehicle, you intubated and started an IV. En route to the nearest trauma center ten minutes away, the patient begins to awaken and attempts to pull out the endotracheal tube. What is the most significant risk for the patient who attempts to extubate herself?

    a. hemothorax
    b. pneumothorax
    c. aspiration of vomitus
    d. tension pneumothorax

71. What is the complication associated with performing the Sellick maneuver?

   a. When pressure is applied improperly, airway obstruction results.

   b. When performed improperly, atelectasis may develop.

   c. The early release of pressure can result in obstruction.

   d. The late release of pressure can result in aspiration.

72. When performing the Sellick maneuver, pressure is applied on the _____ of the cartilages, and maintained until after the ET tube is inserted and _____

   a. lateral edge; the tube is measured.

   b. top edge; the cuff is inflated.

   c. bottom edge; the tube is measured.

   d. lateral edge; the cuff is inflated.

73. The use of the laryngeal mask airway (LMA) should be avoided when the patient:

   a. is elderly.

   b. has chest trauma.

   c. has been sedated.

   d. is an infant or small child.

74. Which of the following airway devices is considered a direct, rather than an indirect, method of advanced airway device?

   a. EOA

   b. PTL

   c. LMA

   d. ETT

75. Digital or tactile intubation is a technique that may be helpful when:

   a. there is a suspected cervical spine injury.

   b. the tongue is extra large.

   c. secretions are copious.

   d. bleeding into the airway is uncontrolled.

76. Retrograde intubation is a technique that should only be performed by properly trained providers and:

   a. involves an invasive procedure beyond intubation.

   b. requires the use of an uncuffed endotracheal tube.

   c. can only be performed with the use of rapid sequence induction.

   d. should only be considered for patients with suspected cervical spine injury.

77. Pulse oximetry is a noninvasive technique that uses a/an _____ light beam to measure the oxygen saturation of the blood.

   a. effervescent

   b. luminescent

   c. infrared

   d. ultraviolet

78. Pulse oximetry is known to provide false readings under certain conditions. Which of the following is the correct explanation for the false readings?

   a. Any condition that impairs venous blood flow will cause false readings.

   b. When the skin is too thick to absorb the luminescent light, a false reading will occur.

   c. Any condition that causes an altered hemoglobin molecule can cause a false reading.

   d. The principle of pulse oximetry assumes blood temperature is normothermic, so abnormally high temperatures cause false readings.

79. You are treating a patient who called EMS because she has been vomiting blood (bright red blood clots). She is pale and diaphoretic and tells you that she has been sick for a week. Her vital signs are respiratory rate of 24/nonlabored, pulse rate of 130/irregular, BP of 88/50, and SpO_2 of 99%. Why is the pulse oximetry reading likely to be unreliable?

   a. The hemoglobin concentration is low due to shock.

   b. Pale and diaphoretic skin can impede the light beam reading.

   c. Low blood pressure enhances the light beam through the fingertip.

   d. Low blood pressure diminishes the light beam through the fingertip.

80. Which of the following devices is used for detection of exhaled CO_2 via the paper filter method?

   a. pulse oximetry

   b. colormetric

   c. capnography

   d. capnometer

81. Before obtaining an accurate end-tidal CO_2 reading, it is recommended that the patient be ventilated five to six times to:

   a. wash out any residual $EtCO_2$ that may be present in the esophagus.

   b. rule out the presence of a pulmonary embolism.

   c. give the meter a chance to warm up.

   d. make sure the patient is hyperoxygenated.

82. The most common conditions for false capnography readings include all the following, *except*:

    a. non-perfusing patients.
    b. premature neonates.
    c. presence of a pulmonary embolism.
    d. ingestion of fruits prior to obtaining a reading.

83. A/An _____ is a syringe-like device that may be helpful in verifying tracheal, versus esophageal, intubation.

    a. esophageal-gastric tube airway
    b. esophageal intubation detector
    c. Beck airway flow monitor
    d. esophageal obturator airway

84. During transport to the hospital with a cardiac arrest patient, you observe that the patient has become difficult to ventilate. Which of the following should you check first?

    a. Verify lung sounds.
    b. Check the pulse oximeter reading.
    c. Check the capnograph reading.
    d. Check the pulse.

85. The fire department is working on a vehicle extrication with an unconscious young male driver who is trapped. Your initial assessment reveals that the patient has a large contusion on the forehead, his teeth are clenched, he is breathing abnormally, and he has a weak and rapid distal pulse. You begin ventilations with a bag mask device as your partner prepares your equipment to nasally intubate the patient. The major advantage of using nasotracheal intubation for this patient is that:

    a. the technique does not require the use of a laryngoscope.
    b. correct tube placement is more effectively verified than an orally placed tube.
    c. the patient cannot pull the tube or accidentally dislodge it once it is secured.
    d. the tube is more easily placed in a patient with a suspected spinal injury than an orally placed tube.

86. The major disadvantage of nasotracheal intubation is that it:

    a. is a blind technique.
    b. is more difficult to verify tube placement.
    c. does not work with spinal cord injured patients.
    d. often has false-positive capnography readings.

87. Devices such as the Beck Airway Airflow Monitor (BAAM) and the Endotrol® tube are effective in facilitation of:

    a. orotracheal intubation.
    b. nasotracheal intubation.
    c. sterile suctioning.
    d. CO_2 monitoring.

88. _____ is a last resort airway technique when a patient has a complete airway obstruction or in whom endotracheal intubation is otherwise impossible.

    a. laryngeal mask airway (LMA)
    b. Needle decompression
    c. Needle cricothyrotomy
    d. Rapid sequence intubation

89. Translaryngeal cannula ventilation (TLCV) is a means of providing ventilation through a large-bore needle that is directly inserted:

    a. through the cricothyroid membrane.
    b. in the second intercostal space on the midclavicular chest.
    c. in the fifth intercostal space on the midaxillary chest.
    d. in the laryngectomy patient's stoma.

90. The neuromuscular blocking agent succinylcholine (SUX) is contraindicated in patients with massive tissue injury because of the:

    a. side effects associated with hypovolemia.
    b. effects of prolonged muscular tremors.
    c. risk of hypokalemia.
    d. risk of hyperkalemia.

91. Your patient is a two-year-old infant in respiratory arrest. Your partner is ventilating with a bag mask while you prepare to intubate the child. You choose an uncuffed tube for this intubation because:

    a. cuffed tubes make visualization of the vocal cords more difficult.
    b. uncuffed tubes are easier to place than cuffed tubes.
    c. the cricoid cartilage narrows in the trachea and serves as a functional cuff.
    d. it is easier to verify tube placement with an uncuffed tube.

92. The patient you are evaluating for a syncopal event has started to seize, and his teeth are clenched. Which of the following airway devices is appropriate for this patient?

    a. LMA
    b. nasotracheal intubation
    c. nasal airway
    d. nasogastric tube

93. Which of the following situations would most likely invite a paramedic to the courtroom?

    a. use of the wrong size LMA that resulted in laryngitis
    b. use of a pediatric pop-off device that prevented adequate oxygenation of a patient
    c. recognition of a misplaced endotracheal tube, which was subsequently extubated in the field by the paramedic in charge
    d. documentation of a normal pulse oximetry reading by the paramedic on a patient who was really sick

94. Upon arrival at the scene of an MVC, you find that the driver is slumped over the steering wheel. You manually stabilize his cervical spine and see that he struck his neck on the rim of the steering wheel. Which of the following airway problems can you expect with this patient?

    a. laryngeal edema
    b. fractured larynx
    c. laryngeal spasm
    d. all of the above

95. Further evaluation of the patient described in question 94 reveals that he is unresponsive to painful stimuli and has slow, shallow, and stridorous respiration at a rate of 10 bpm. His distal pulse is rapid and weak, and his skin is ashen and cool. What action should you take next?

    a. Suction the airway and insert a nasal airway.
    b. Place a cervical collar and perform a rapid extrication.
    c. Insert an oral airway and start an IV prior to extrication.
    d. Have your partner contact medical control to obtain an order for a possible emergency needle cricothyrotomy.

96. Your EMS service is conducting an update on advanced airway devices. One of the devices that is being discussed is the LMA. A significant benefit of the use of the LMA as an advanced airway device is that:

    a. it has no face mask seal to maintain.
    b. it can be used on conscious patients.
    c. it increases anatomical dead air space.
    d. once properly inserted, it completely protects against aspiration.

97. Your patient is a twenty-four-year-old female asthmatic in severe respiratory distress. She called EMS when she could not get relief from her metered dose inhalers (Combivent and albuterol). The patient appears exhausted and cyanotic, and auscultation of her lungs reveals no air movement on inspiration or expiration. What should you do next?

    a. Obtain a pulse oximetry reading.
    b. Administer a nebulizer treatment through a nonrebreather mask.
    c. Insert an oral airway and provide rapid ventilations with a bag mask device.
    d. Assist ventilations with a bag mask device slowly and gently over two seconds.

98. Rapid sequence induction (RSI) can be a safe way of providing airway access and is an ideal airway management procedure for which type of patient?

    a. traumatic cardiac arrest patient
    b. conscious, uncooperative patient in respiratory failure
    c. unconscious, hypothermic patient with slow and shallow respirations
    d. unresponsive patient in respiratory arrest preceded by an asthma attack

99. The RSI can produce muscular tremors called fasciculations, which are produced by:

    a. narcotic sedatives.
    b. temporary hypoxia.
    c. benzodiazepine sedatives.
    d. neuromuscular blocking agents.

100. Which of the following airway devices is not an appropriate device for a patient with high airway pressures?

    a. LMA
    b. Combitube
    c. orotracheal tube
    d. nasotracheal tube

Exam #10 Answer Form

	A	B	C	D		A	B	C	D
1.	❏	❏	❏	❏	26.	❏	❏	❏	❏
2.	❏	❏	❏	❏	27.	❏	❏	❏	❏
3.	❏	❏	❏	❏	28.	❏	❏	❏	❏
4.	❏	❏	❏	❏	29.	❏	❏	❏	❏
5.	❏	❏	❏	❏	30.	❏	❏	❏	❏
6.	❏	❏	❏	❏	31.	❏	❏	❏	❏
7.	❏	❏	❏	❏	32.	❏	❏	❏	❏
8.	❏	❏	❏	❏	33.	❏	❏	❏	❏
9.	❏	❏	❏	❏	34.	❏	❏	❏	❏
10.	❏	❏	❏	❏	35.	❏	❏	❏	❏
11.	❏	❏	❏	❏	36.	❏	❏	❏	❏
12.	❏	❏	❏	❏	37.	❏	❏	❏	❏
13.	❏	❏	❏	❏	38.	❏	❏	❏	❏
14.	❏	❏	❏	❏	39.	❏	❏	❏	❏
15.	❏	❏	❏	❏	40.	❏	❏	❏	❏
16.	❏	❏	❏	❏	41.	❏	❏	❏	❏
17.	❏	❏	❏	❏	42.	❏	❏	❏	❏
18.	❏	❏	❏	❏	43.	❏	❏	❏	❏
19.	❏	❏	❏	❏	44.	❏	❏	❏	❏
20.	❏	❏	❏	❏	45.	❏	❏	❏	❏
21.	❏	❏	❏	❏	46.	❏	❏	❏	❏
22.	❏	❏	❏	❏	47.	❏	❏	❏	❏
23.	❏	❏	❏	❏	48.	❏	❏	❏	❏
24.	❏	❏	❏	❏	49.	❏	❏	❏	❏
25.	❏	❏	❏	❏	50.	❏	❏	❏	❏

	A	B	C	D		A	B	C	D
51.	❏	❏	❏	❏	76.	❏	❏	❏	❏
52.	❏	❏	❏	❏	77.	❏	❏	❏	❏
53.	❏	❏	❏	❏	78.	❏	❏	❏	❏
54.	❏	❏	❏	❏	79.	❏	❏	❏	❏
55.	❏	❏	❏	❏	80.	❏	❏	❏	❏
56.	❏	❏	❏	❏	81.	❏	❏	❏	❏
57.	❏	❏	❏	❏	82.	❏	❏	❏	❏
58.	❏	❏	❏	❏	83.	❏	❏	❏	❏
59.	❏	❏	❏	❏	84.	❏	❏	❏	❏
60.	❏	❏	❏	❏	85.	❏	❏	❏	❏
61.	❏	❏	❏	❏	86.	❏	❏	❏	❏
62.	❏	❏	❏	❏	87.	❏	❏	❏	❏
63.	❏	❏	❏	❏	88.	❏	❏	❏	❏
64.	❏	❏	❏	❏	89.	❏	❏	❏	❏
65.	❏	❏	❏	❏	90.	❏	❏	❏	❏
66.	❏	❏	❏	❏	91.	❏	❏	❏	❏
67.	❏	❏	❏	❏	92.	❏	❏	❏	❏
68.	❏	❏	❏	❏	93.	❏	❏	❏	❏
69.	❏	❏	❏	❏	94.	❏	❏	❏	❏
70.	❏	❏	❏	❏	95.	❏	❏	❏	❏
71.	❏	❏	❏	❏	96.	❏	❏	❏	❏
72.	❏	❏	❏	❏	97.	❏	❏	❏	❏
73.	❏	❏	❏	❏	98.	❏	❏	❏	❏
74.	❏	❏	❏	❏	99.	❏	❏	❏	❏
75.	❏	❏	❏	❏	100.	❏	❏	❏	❏

Therapeutic Communications and History Taking

1. Like many professions, _____ is an integral component of the EMS profession.

   a. encoding
   b. communication
   c. sign language
   d. diet

2. The best way to assess the mental status of your patient, to see if he is conversing normally, is to:

   a. speak with him.
   b. obtain a glucose reading.
   c. obtain a pulse oximetry reading.
   d. ask a family member if the patient is acting normal.

3. In the communication process, the message moves through various forms, including: verbal, nonverbal, encoding, and:

   a. receiver.
   b. translator.
   c. interpreter.
   d. forecaster.

4. A _____ history is all the medical events and conditions that have ever occurred to the patient.

   a. complete health
   b. focused
   c. past medical
   d. SAMPLE

5. A focused history is the chronologic history of the patient's:

   a. surgeries.
   b. present illness.
   c. medication use.
   d. family history.

6. During the patient interview, the paramedic should attempt to obtain the following information about a patient's current event.

   a. What is the patient's marital status?
   b. What is the patient's general outlook?
   c. Is this event similar to any previous events?
   d. Will a similar event occur in the near future?

7. The acronym OPQRST is used to remember the set of questions used to obtain information about the patient's:

   a. past medical history.
   b. complete health history.
   c. use of OTC medications.
   d. present illness or injury.

8. Use the acronym SAMPLE to remember the set of questions used to obtain information about the patient's:

   a. past medical history.
   b. focused history.
   c. childhood history.
   d. present illness or injury.

9. Which of the following pieces of patient information is irrelevant to the paramedic in the field?

   a. recent surgery
   b. recent illness
   c. change in daily living activities
   d. tonsillectomy in childhood

10. Why should the paramedic avoid asking a patient leading questions?

    a. Leading questions are a form of negative communication.
    b. Some patients may tell you what you want to hear rather than the truth.
    c. Leading questions can provide a sense of false reassurance for the patient.
    d. Asking open-ended questions will always get a better response than leading questions.

11. Why is it important for the paramedic to be empathetic when obtaining a health history?

    a. Showing empathy helps to obtain more cooperation from the patient.
    b. Empathy helps the family to trust you with the patient.
    c. It is a way of showing respect to the patient.
    d. It helps the patient to communicate with the next healthcare provider.

12. Which of the following is a disrespectful use of terms for the patient?

    a. using the patient's proper name
    b. calling the patient "honey"
    c. using the patient's nickname with permission
    d. using the patient's first name with permission

13. Although paramedics are taught to ask direct questions of the patient, which of the following is an example of a good open-ended question to ask a patient?

    a. What do you for relaxation?
    b. Why did you call us here today?
    c. How does that make you feel?
    d. Why do you feel that your doctor is unable to help you?

14. When you are not getting the answer to questions that appear obvious, consider that the patient may be:

    a. pregnant.
    b. falsely reassured.
    c. not ill or injured.
    d. embarrassed.

15. During an interview with a patient having chest pain, you ask the patient, "How is the pain different today?" This is an example of a/an _____ question.

    a. direct
    b. closed
    c. leading
    d. open-ended

16. When is it better to ask direct questions of the patient?

    a. when a behavioral problem is suspected
    b. when specific information is required
    c. when the patient's family is present
    d. when the patient has no specific complaint

17. Which of the following cultures may consider direct eye contact during an interview to be impolite or aggressive?

    a. Italian
    b. German
    c. Native American
    d. New Yorker

18. Why should the paramedic avoid providing false reassurance when the situation is serious?

    a. The patient will sue if she finds out the truth.
    b. The patient will suffer harm.
    c. The paramedic could lose her certification.
    d. The paramedic could lose the patient's trust.

19. Which of the following is an example of a leading question?

    a. Do you have sharp chest pain?
    b. Are you pregnant?
    c. Do you have a history of diabetes?
    d. When did you last take your medication?

20. Which of the following is an example of a condescending question to be avoided during an interview?

    a. How much did you have to drink tonight?
    b. You don't smoke, do you?
    c. Do you take your medications every day?
    d. When was your last menstrual period?

21. In an effort to keep a patient from becoming more anxious during a patient interview, the paramedic should:

    a. shun nonverbal communication.
    b. avoid facilitation whenever possible.
    c. stay away from silence as an interview technique.
    d. avoid the use of complicated medical terminology.

22. An example of a negative communication technique that the paramedic should avoid with patients and their families is:

    a. reflection.
    b. inattentiveness.
    c. asking for clarification when a patient's response is ambiguous.
    d. being conscious of the amount of physical space between you and the patient.

23. _____ is the way you speak, and how your posture and your actions are used to encourage the patient to say more.

    a. Empathy
    b. Confrontation
    c. Facilitation
    d. Reflection

24. To repeat or echo the patient's own words as a way of encouraging the flow of conversation without interrupting the patient's concentration is referred to as:

    a. interpretation.
    b. clarification.
    c. facilitation.
    d. reflection.

25. _____ is reasoning based not on what you observed from the patient, but on what you have concluded from the information you have compiled.

    a. Interpretation
    b. Clarification
    c. Empathy
    d. Silence

26. Which of the following conditions is least likely to be an obstacle during a patient interview?

    a. a patient who is blind
    b. a patient who is overtalkative
    c. a patient who is symptomatic
    d. a patient who is developmentally disabled

27. A rolled piece of paper in a plastic container, which contains medical information about a patient, is a/an:

    a. MedicAlert tag®.
    b. Prescription bottle.
    c. Vial of Life®.
    d. Emergency Lifeline®.

28. When treating a patient who only speaks a foreign language that you do not, and no interpreter is immediately available, which of the following can you do to best facilitate care?

    a. Use positive body language while you begin care.
    b. Wait for a translator before initiating care.
    c. Ask police for assistance.
    d. Call the paramedic supervisor.

29. While caring for a blind patient, it is appropriate to announce yourself, to explain as much as possible, and to:

    a. secure the seeing eye dog for your protection.
    b. speak while facing the patient.
    c. interact with the patient the same as with a seeing patient.
    d. ask permission to touch the patient before actually touching him.

30. You are caring for a patient who is very angry and is taking his anger out on you. Which of the following should you avoid doing?

    a. getting angry in return
    b. doing a quick pat down for weapons
    c. keeping the situation calm
    d. requesting police

31. Sleep disorders, appetite disturbances, the inability to concentrate, and lack of energy are all signs of:

    a. fear.
    b. confusion.
    c. depression.
    d. abuse.

32. When interviewing a patient who is extremely talkative, but is not providing you with the information you need, which of the following techniques might be useful in obtaining what you need?

    a. Ignore the patient.
    b. Ask the patient to stop talking and listen.
    c. Try using diversion tactics.
    d. Try using direct "yes" or "no" questions.

33. _____ and history taking are a significant portion of the patient interview.

    a. Dispatch information
    b. A rapid response time
    c. Establishing a rapport with the patient
    d. Professional appearance

34. During an interview with a patient in severe respiratory distress, you ask the patient to "nod yes or shake no" to answer your questions. This is an example of asking questions that are:

    a. direct.
    b. leading.
    c. patronizing.
    d. open-ended.

35. Which of the following is not considered part of a health history?

    a. religious beliefs
    b. career status
    c. daily living activities
    d. current vital signs

36. Information obtained from the patient or bystanders about the current event, including what led up to it, is called:

    a. chief complaint.
    b. focused history.
    c. signs and symptoms.
    d. positive feedback.

37. _____ is part of the communication process rather than a communication technique.

   a. Silence
   b. Encoding
   c. Listening
   d. Explanation

38. _____ may be found on necklaces, bracelets, and anklets, and provide vital medical information such as a medical condition or reaction.

   a. Dog tags®
   b. Lucky charms®
   c. MedicAlert tags®
   d. Coils

39. Once you have arrived at the ED with a hearing-impaired patient, the _____ requires that the hospital provide a sign interpreter within thirty minutes of the patient's arrival.

   a. American's with Disabilities Act (ADA)
   b. Veteran's Administration (VA)
   c. Centers for Disease Control (CDC)
   d. American Sign Language (ASL) bill

40. When caring for a hearing-impaired patient, be sure to face the patient when you are speaking and to:

   a. speak very slowly.
   b. use a family member to communicate.
   c. exaggerate your speech.
   d. look to see if his hearing aid is on.

Exam #11 Answer Form

	A	B	C	D			A	B	C	D
1.	❑	❑	❑	❑		21.	❑	❑	❑	❑
2.	❑	❑	❑	❑		22.	❑	❑	❑	❑
3.	❑	❑	❑	❑		23.	❑	❑	❑	❑
4.	❑	❑	❑	❑		24.	❑	❑	❑	❑
5.	❑	❑	❑	❑		25.	❑	❑	❑	❑
6.	❑	❑	❑	❑		26.	❑	❑	❑	❑
7.	❑	❑	❑	❑		27.	❑	❑	❑	❑
8.	❑	❑	❑	❑		28.	❑	❑	❑	❑
9.	❑	❑	❑	❑		29.	❑	❑	❑	❑
10.	❑	❑	❑	❑		30.	❑	❑	❑	❑
11.	❑	❑	❑	❑		31.	❑	❑	❑	❑
12.	❑	❑	❑	❑		32.	❑	❑	❑	❑
13.	❑	❑	❑	❑		33.	❑	❑	❑	❑
14.	❑	❑	❑	❑		34.	❑	❑	❑	❑
15.	❑	❑	❑	❑		35.	❑	❑	❑	❑
16.	❑	❑	❑	❑		36.	❑	❑	❑	❑
17.	❑	❑	❑	❑		37.	❑	❑	❑	❑
18.	❑	❑	❑	❑		38.	❑	❑	❑	❑
19.	❑	❑	❑	❑		39.	❑	❑	❑	❑
20.	❑	❑	❑	❑		40.	❑	❑	❑	❑

12

Techniques of Physical Examination

1. Which of the following paramedic skills is considered more of a manual dexterity skill than a cognitive skill?

    a. assessing vital signs
    b. assessing mental status
    c. obtaining a focused history
    d. making a priority treatment decision

2. Putting on gloves and wearing a face mask and a gown are examples of:

    a. taking standard precautions.
    b. performing an assessment.
    c. components of a physical examination.
    d. developing a rapport with the patient.

3. Which technique of physical examination is typically the first method used when assessing a patient's chest wall for symmetry?

    a. auscultation
    b. visual inspection
    c. percussion
    d. palpation

4. An example of a patient's specific characteristic that is apparent on visual inspection is:

    a. wheezing.
    b. personal hygiene.
    c. bruits.
    d. crepitus.

5. _____ is a form of assessment that utilizes listening skills combined with tapping on various body areas to determine the size, position, and consistency of underlying structures.

    a. Doppler
    b. Palpation
    c. Percussion
    d. Ultrasound

6. One step that the paramedic can take to reduce a patient's anxiety, fear, and muscle tensing prior to palpation is to:

    a. warm hands before touching the patient.
    b. establish medical control.
    c. begin transport and turn the lights down low.
    d. apply oxygen by non-rebreather.

7. Evaluating the patient for levels of distress, age, gender and skin color, temperature, and condition are examples of things the paramedic looks for to determine:

    a. the patient's chief complaint.
    b. the general appearance of the patient.
    c. when to question a patient's family about history.
    d. how to recognize a sensory dysfunction.

8. When auscultating for apical heart sounds, the paramedic should place the bell of the stethoscope at the:

    a. fifth intercostal space at the midclavicular line on the left chest.
    b. midaxillary line at the fourth intercostal space on the left chest.
    c. just above the left nipple line.
    d. two inches to the left of the suprasternal notch.

9. While a new EMT–B is assessing a blood pressure on a patient who is morbidly obese, you notice that the blood pressure cuff is too small for the patient's arm. What reading would you expect to get under this circumstance?

    a. an accurate reading
    b. an inaccurately high reading
    c. an inaccurately low reading
    d. no reading

10. While taking a blood pressure, the sounds heard with a stethoscope that indicate the systolic and diastolic readings are called:

    a. pulse pressures.
    b. pulsus paradoxus.
    c. apical pulse.
    d. Korotkoff's sounds.

11. When taking a blood pressure by palpation, the paramedic will palpate a distal pulse while first inflating and then deflating the cuff in order to obtain a _____ pressure.

   a. pulse
   b. systolic
   c. diastolic
   d. mean arterial

12. The method of obtaining a blood pressure by palpation is often used because:

   a. ambient noise is too loud to hear pulse sounds.
   b. the paramedic is too lazy to use a stethoscope.
   c. taking a blood pressure by auscultation takes too long.
   d. a trained provider is not available to take it.

13. A paramedic is about to take a blood pressure on a patient's right arm when she tells him that she has had a mastectomy on the right side. The paramedic now takes the blood pressure on the left arm because taking a blood pressure on the right arm may be painful for the patient, as well as:

   a. cause the patient to experience a TIA.
   b. precipitate a blood clot.
   c. cause an inaccurate reading.
   d. give the patient a reason to sue the paramedic.

14. While assessing a patient's legs for the presence of edema, the paramedic notes that edema is severe and pitting +4. The paramedic recognizes that this condition is significant and indicates a problem with patient's heart, lungs, or:

   a. spleen.
   b. kidneys.
   c. gallbladder.
   d. liver.

15. Assessing the elasticity of the skin (turgor) can indicate the patient's state of hydration. Another possible reason for having an increased skin turgor is that the patient has:

   a. obesity.
   b. ingested methanol.
   c. Cushing's syndrome.
   d. connective tissue disease.

16. The presence of jugular vein distension (JVD) in a patient sitting at a 90° position is an abnormal finding and may indicate serious pathology such as severe right heart failure, pericardial tamponade, or:

   a. tension pneumothorax.
   b. thyroid storm.
   c. hypertensive crises.
   d. hypovolemia.

17. The presence of unilateral JVD is abnormal and may indicate which of the following conditions?

   a. liver disease
   b. excessive alcohol use
   c. local vein blockage or restriction
   d. congestive heart failure

18. To assess the hepatojugular reflex on a patient, the paramedic begins by placing the patient in which position?

   a. Trendelenburg position
   b. semi-Fowler's with the head at a 30° angle
   c. high-Fowler's with the head at a 10° angle
   d. semi-recumbent

19. While assessing a patient's hepatojugular reflex, the paramedic notes an increase of 1.5 cm in JVD. This finding may indicate right heart failure or:

   a. an ACS.
   b. unstable angina.
   c. stable angina.
   d. fluid overload.

20. A device consisting of a light source projected through a cone-shaped device that is placed into an orifice to visualize the inner structures is called a/an:

   a. otoscope.
   b. ophthalmoscope.
   c. penlight.
   d. Doppler.

21. A device consisting of a light source and several lenses that is used to look at the eye is called a/an:

   a. otoscope.
   b. ophthalmoscope.
   c. penlight.
   d. Doppler.

22. Pulse oximetry is used to assess the oxygen saturation of a patient's:

    a. hematocrit.
    b. central venous pressure.
    c. capillary venous pressure.
    d. hemoglobin.

23. A patient who is in shock may have pulse oximetry readings that are:

    a. indicative of an ACS.
    b. consistent with altered mental status.
    c. falsely low.
    d. falsely high.

24. When percussing the chest of a patient with a disease, such as the accumulation of fluid in the lungs, the paramedic may expect to hear what type of sound?

    a. dull or flattened tone
    b. hyperresonance
    c. intonation
    d. sonority

25. A paramedic is assessing a patient for carotid bruits and hears them on the patient's left side. The paramedic knows that the left carotid artery is occluded at least:

    a. one-quarter to one-half.
    b. one-half to two-thirds.
    c. one-third.
    d. 20%.

26. The most helpful finding the paramedic can provide to the ED about a patient's bowel sounds is which of the following?

    a. hyperactive sounds
    b. hypoactive sounds
    c. absence of sounds
    d. normal sounds

27. After performing deep palpation on a patient's abdomen, the paramedic reported to the ED that the patient was positive for Murphy's sign. Which of the following conditions did the paramedic find during her examination?

    a. tenderness of the gallbladder
    b. enlarged liver
    c. enlarged spleen
    d. tenderness of the appendix

28. In which of the following cases would the pulse oximetry reading be most useful to the paramedic?

    a. SpO$_2$ 96% in a sixty-five-year-old female complaining of exertional dyspnea and who has a history of COPD.
    b. SpO$_2$ 88% in a three-year-old having an asthma attack.
    c. SpO$_2$ 98% in a thirty-year-old female complaining of weakness and who has a history of anemia.
    d. SpO$_2$ 100% in a nineteen-year-old male who just attempted suicide by CO exposure.

29. Whenever possible, avoid taking a blood pressure on an extremity that is:

    a. painful or injured.
    b. cool to the touch.
    c. wet or diaphoretic.
    d. presenting with pitting edema.

30. A _____ is a turbulent noise that sounds like swishing, which can be heard over arteries in the body that have become occluded.

    a. crackle
    b. bruit
    c. tic
    d. murmur

31. You are assessing a seventy-four-year-old patient complaining of shortness of breath, with a history of COPD and CHF. She is at home in bed and states that she has been unable to get up to take her medications for two days. During your physical examination, you look for the presence of edema. What area would be prominent with edema?

    a. ankles
    b. feet
    c. hands
    d. sacral area

32. Which of the following is a sign of a distressed patient?

    a. a baby with grunting respirations
    b. a teenager with loud bilateral bowel sounds
    c. a toddler crying after falling out of a shopping cart
    d. a sleepy baby after having a febrile seizure

33. _____ is an irregular body texture characterized by air trapped under the skin.

    a. Edema
    b. Crepitus
    c. Tenting
    d. Subcutaneous emphysema

34. In which of the following patients would a head-to-toe exam be the preferred method of physical examination?

    a. two-year-old infant with respiratory distress
    b. eighteen-year-old male in a motorcycle accident
    c. forty-eight-year-old female with abdominal pain
    d. seventy-two-year-old female with fears of being sent to a nursing home by her son

35. You are transporting a patient from a nursing home to the hospital for evaluation. On the chart, you read that the patient has had rhinorrhea for two days. What clinical finding would this indicate?

    a. watery discharge from the nose
    b. bloody nose
    c. CSF seeping from the ear canal
    d. excessive drooling without control

36. Ascultating for bruits in the carotid arteries in the out-of-hospital setting has been discouraged in recent years due to the possibility of:

    a. disrupting plaque and possibly causing a stroke.
    b. causing vasospasms and possibly causing a stroke.
    c. disrupting plaque and possibly causing a heart attack.
    d. causing a vasovagal response and a profound tachycardia.

37. To accurately assess a patient for the presence of JVD, the patient should be placed in which position?

    a. supine, with legs dangling
    b. sitting upright at 90°
    c. sitting up at 45°
    d. Trendelenburg position

38. To listen for vesicular breath sounds, place the diaphragm over the:

    a. second intercostal space at the midclavicular line.
    b. second intercostal space at the midaxillary line.
    c. anterior axillary line and midaxillary line at the fifth rib level.
    d. fifth posterior axillary line and midclavicular line.

39. Muffled or distant heart sounds may indicate the presence of:

    a. trapped air.
    b. fluid.
    c. bruits.
    d. a broken stethoscope.

40. Which of the following findings associated with the examination of the abdomen is an abnormal finding?

    a. non-tender on palpation
    b. absence of bowel sounds
    c. presence of bowel sounds
    d. muscle tensing on palpation

41. A term for local or generalized abnormal accumulation of fluids in body tissues is:

    a. bloat.
    b. tenting.
    c. subcutaneous emphysema.
    d. edema.

42. When assessing a patient with bruising, the most significant clinical feature of the bruise is:

    a. the color or age.
    b. the shape.
    c. how the patient got it.
    d. how long it will last.

43. HEENT is an acronym used to recall all the areas to be examined about the:

    a. extremities.
    b. trunk.
    c. airway.
    d. head.

44. The most significant clinical finding about a person's hearing is:

    a. the absence of hearing.
    b. the presence of tinnitus.
    c. acute changes in hearing.
    d. the use of a hearing aid.

45. Deep palpation of the abdomen is an assessment technique that is:

    a. used to appreciate the size of the liver.
    b. never used in the out-of-hospital setting.
    c. used to determine the presence of an abdominal aortic aneurism.
    d. performed by depressing the palm of one hand, one to two inches deep, into the abdomen.

46. Assessment of the patient's range of motion is associated with the:

    a. eyes.
    b. spine.
    c. airway.
    d. extremities.

47. An $EtCO_2$ device measures the amount of _____ during each breath at the end of:_____.

    a. carbon dioxide; inspiration.
    b. carbon monoxide; inspiration.
    c. carbon dioxide; exhalation.
    d. carbon monoxide; exhalation.

48. _____ is a term used when assessing a patient's skin for state of hydration.

    a. Hydrolysis
    b. Edema
    c. Turgor
    d. Rigidity

49. The bell of the stethoscope is best used for listening to _____ sounds.

    a. heart
    b. fetal
    c. bowel
    d. breath

50. The presence of ascites upon physical examination is an abnormal finding on which area of the body?

    a. head
    b. neck
    c. abdomen
    d. extremities

Exam #12 Answer Form

	A	B	C	D		A	B	C	D
1.	❏	❏	❏	❏	26.	❏	❏	❏	❏
2.	❏	❏	❏	❏	27.	❏	❏	❏	❏
3.	❏	❏	❏	❏	28.	❏	❏	❏	❏
4.	❏	❏	❏	❏	29.	❏	❏	❏	❏
5.	❏	❏	❏	❏	30.	❏	❏	❏	❏
6.	❏	❏	❏	❏	31.	❏	❏	❏	❏
7.	❏	❏	❏	❏	32.	❏	❏	❏	❏
8.	❏	❏	❏	❏	33.	❏	❏	❏	❏
9.	❏	❏	❏	❏	34.	❏	❏	❏	❏
10.	❏	❏	❏	❏	35.	❏	❏	❏	❏
11.	❏	❏	❏	❏	36.	❏	❏	❏	❏
12.	❏	❏	❏	❏	37.	❏	❏	❏	❏
13.	❏	❏	❏	❏	38.	❏	❏	❏	❏
14.	❏	❏	❏	❏	39.	❏	❏	❏	❏
15.	❏	❏	❏	❏	40.	❏	❏	❏	❏
16.	❏	❏	❏	❏	41.	❏	❏	❏	❏
17.	❏	❏	❏	❏	42.	❏	❏	❏	❏
18.	❏	❏	❏	❏	43.	❏	❏	❏	❏
19.	❏	❏	❏	❏	44.	❏	❏	❏	❏
20.	❏	❏	❏	❏	45.	❏	❏	❏	❏
21.	❏	❏	❏	❏	46.	❏	❏	❏	❏
22.	❏	❏	❏	❏	47.	❏	❏	❏	❏
23.	❏	❏	❏	❏	48.	❏	❏	❏	❏
24.	❏	❏	❏	❏	49.	❏	❏	❏	❏
25.	❏	❏	❏	❏	50.	❏	❏	❏	❏

13

Overview: Patient Assessment

1. The components of the paramedic's patient assessment begin with the:

   a. initial assessment.
   b. focused history.
   c. scene size-up.
   d. general impression.

2. Components of the initial assessment include mental status (MS), ABCs, and:

   a. vital signs.
   b. scene safety.
   c. scene size-up.
   d. general impression.

3. When the paramedic obtains a baseline set of vital signs, she obtains the respiratory rate and effort, heart rate and quality, and:

   a. mental status.
   b. circulatory status.
   c. blood glucose level.
   d. core body temperature.

4. The patient's mental status, emotional state, physical condition, and _____ may change the usual progression of the assessment.

   a. location of the call
   b. DNAR status
   c. the presence of a healthcare proxy
   d. gender

5. Because of the dynamics of prehospital assessment, clinical judgment and experience will direct when specific steps should be:

   a. redefined.
   b. overhauled.
   c. omitted, deferred, or repeated.
   d. developed.

6. Which of the following is a component of scene size-up?

   a. assessing the need for appropriate PPE
   b. performing initial extrication
   c. assessing the patient's level of distress
   d. estimating the patient's age

7. While forming a general impression of the patient, the paramedic should include:

   a. a determination of the MOI.
   b. the call for extrication assistance.
   c. an observation of the patient's environment.
   d. the patient's past medical history.

8. The components of forming a general impression of the patient include all the following, *except* determining the patient's:

   a. gender.
   b. approximate age.
   c. health history.
   d. level of distress.

9. The initial assessment guides the decision making for the remaining steps in evaluation, treatment, and:

   a. ongoing assessment.
   b. focused history and physical examination.
   c. detailed physical examination.
   d. transportation.

10. For most adult patients, the paramedic will perform a physical assessment that is:

    a. inclusive of all of the body systems.
    b. performed the same way on all patients.
    c. focused on the patient's chief complaint.
    d. always completed in a head-to-toe fashion.

11. The detailed physical examination is another name for the:

    a. ABCDE.
    b. head-to-toe exam.
    c. toe-to-head exam.
    d. vectored physical exam.

12. On which of the following patients would you perform the detailed physical examination?

   a. pediatric asthma patient
   b. geriatric isolated extremity injury
   c. trauma patient with significant MOI
   d. responsive medical patient

13. For which of the following patients should spinal precautions be taken?

   a. asymptomatic patient after a trip and fall
   b. wrist pain after falling from a standing position
   c. asymptomatic after a fall of approximately three times the patient's height
   d. isolated knee pain after a fall while skiing

14. All the following are criteria for significant MOI, for which spinal precautions should be taken, *except*:

   a. an explosion within a confined space.
   b. motor vehicle rollover.
   c. asymptomatic after ejection from a car.
   d. minor damage to the front end of a car where the airbag deployed.

15. _____ is the process of obtaining a baseline assessment, repeating the assessment, and then using the information to reevaluate the patient's condition or modify treatment.

   a. Trending
   b. Diagnosis
   c. Rapid assessment
   d. Triage

16. The components of the _____ are directed at a quick and gross head-to-toe assessment of the body, similar to the detailed physical examination, yet not as thorough.

   a. initial assessment
   b. rapid trauma assessment
   c. focused physical examination
   d. ongoing exam

17. ECG, SpO$_2$, and blood glucose levels are examples of _____ information that becomes even more essential to the assessment process when caring for an unresponsive patient.

   a. physical
   b. conclusive
   c. diagnostic
   d. subjective

18. Each patient will require a different level of ongoing assessment based on:

   a. the patient's advanced directives.
   b. the need for spinal precautions.
   c. the age of the patient.
   d. the severity of the specific complaint.

19. Obtaining a patient's consent to treatment and respecting the patient's autonomy in the decision-making process are _____ components of the patient assessment.

   a. clinical
   b. diagnostic
   c. nonessential
   d. legal and ethical

20. In the unresponsive patient, _____ becomes a higher priority due to airway maintenance.

   a. positioning
   b. the blood glucose level
   c. the blood alcohol level
   d. bystander information

21. You are assessing a patient with an isolated ankle injury. Which of the following exams would be most appropriate for this patient?

   a. focused trauma examination
   b. rapid trauma examination
   c. detailed physical examination
   d. head-to-toe exam

22. The purpose of the initial assessment is to _____, and to find and manage any life-threatening conditions.

   a. assess for potential hazards
   b. determine the patient's mental status
   c. obtain baseline vital signs
   d. obtain patient consent

23. You are evaluating a patient who has a chief complaint of respiratory distress. On which of the following body systems, besides the respiratory system, should you focus your exam?

   a. neurologic and cardiac
   b. cardiac and musculoskeletal
   c. gastric and behavioral
   d. endocrine and musculoskeletal

24. To evaluate the mental status of an unconscious patient, check for deep pain response and:

    a. pulse.
    b. ECG.
    c. reflexes.
    d. glucose.

25. Good documentation of the patient on the prehospital care report (PCR) is part of the _____ component of patient assessment.

    a. legal
    b. moral
    c. ethical
    d. protocol

Exam #13 Answer Form

	A	B	C	D
1.	❑	❑	❑	❑
2.	❑	❑	❑	❑
3.	❑	❑	❑	❑
4.	❑	❑	❑	❑
5.	❑	❑	❑	❑
6.	❑	❑	❑	❑
7.	❑	❑	❑	❑
8.	❑	❑	❑	❑
9.	❑	❑	❑	❑
10.	❑	❑	❑	❑
11.	❑	❑	❑	❑
12.	❑	❑	❑	❑
13.	❑	❑	❑	❑

	A	B	C	D
14.	❑	❑	❑	❑
15.	❑	❑	❑	❑
16.	❑	❑	❑	❑
17.	❑	❑	❑	❑
18.	❑	❑	❑	❑
19.	❑	❑	❑	❑
20.	❑	❑	❑	❑
21.	❑	❑	❑	❑
22.	❑	❑	❑	❑
23.	❑	❑	❑	❑
24.	❑	❑	❑	❑
25.	❑	❑	❑	❑

14

Scene Size-Up and the Initial Assessment

1. The second component of an assessment in the field is:

   a. scene size-up.
   b. initial assessment.
   c. open the airway.
   d. provide high-flow oxygen.

2. One step the paramedic can take at the scene of a residential call in order to make it safe is to:

   a. make use of doorstops.
   b. quickly suction the patient's airway.
   c. notify dispatch of estimated scene time.
   d. take and maintain c-spine stabilization.

3. Which of the following MOIs is nonsignificant for most adult and pediatric patients?

   a. near drowning
   b. gunshot wound (GSW)
   c. fall from a height of 30 feet
   d. trip and fall from a standing position

4. The injury pattern commonly seen in children who have been hit by a motor vehicle, which includes injury to the legs, chest, and head, is known as:

   a. Waddell's triad.
   b. Cushing's blow.
   c. Warren's impact.
   d. Ryan's compression.

5. Getting a general impression of a patient is sometimes referred to as:

   a. the look test.
   b. the patient interview.
   c. prioritizing.
   d. the nature of illness.

6. The acronym AVPU is used in the initial assessment to:

   a. determine the patient's mental status.
   b. determine the patient's chief complaint.
   c. assess the need for an additional ambulance.
   d. determine the MOI.

7. The first and foremost priority for the paramedic on calls is:

   a. dispatching information.
   b. the patient's chief complaint.
   c. recognizing hazards.
   d. the MOI.

8. Which of the following clues indicate there may be hazardous materials involved in the incident?

   a. The family's pet dog is barking at the front door.
   b. Three out of four family members are complaining of headache.
   c. Power lines are down on the scene of a motor vehicle collision.
   d. There is advance notice of infestation at the scene of a call.

9. What does the term "secure" scene mean?

   a. The area is closed off to the public.
   b. The media is barred from entering the scene.
   c. The area is a crime scene.
   d. A potentially violent scene is safe for EMS.

10. Which of the following examples is a potential threat to the paramedic in a typical residential area?

    a. a nighttime response to a house that has no lights on
    b. a response to a house with no one to let you in, but a woman is calling out "I can't get up"
    c. a standby at a fire scene of a fully involved structure fire
    d. a response to a suicide attempt with police on-scene

11. You and your crew are working with the fire department to extricate the driver of a midsized vehicle who is trapped under the steering wheel after striking a tree with great force. The patient is in respiratory distress with a rapidly decreasing mental status. The decision has been made to rapidly extricate the patient; during the move, a handgun falls from the patient's clothing. What immediate action should be taken to keep the scene safe?

    a. Back away from the patient and let the police officer remove the gun.
    b. Continue to remove the patient and do not let anyone touch the gun.
    c. Assign a firefighter to remove the gun from the vehicle and continue to move the patient.
    d. Immediately remove the patient's clothing to assure no other weapons are present prior to moving him any further.

12. Before a scene is secure, where should EMS respond?

    a. staging area
    b. standby in quarters
    c. to get restock at the nearest station to the call
    d. to the nearest police department

13. Which of the following is an example of a potentially infectious process at the scene that may involve a hazard to the paramedic?

    a. a crying baby
    b. a patient with a bad cough
    c. the odor of vomitus at the scene
    d. the presence of insulin syringes at the scene

14. Which of the following is an example of an unstable scene that the paramedic can easily stabilize, if recognized?

    a. Put out a small engine fire with a fire extinguisher.
    b. Engage the emergency brake on a car that has been left in neutral.
    c. Disarm a perpetrator at a crime scene.
    d. Stand between a wife and her abusive husband.

15. What is one of the most common and greatest hazards to the paramedic?

    a. needle stick injuries
    b. exposure to TB
    c. exposure to hazardous materials
    d. working in traffic at the scene of a collision

16. A common MOI associated with sports such as basketball, skiing, soccer, and racquetball is:

    a. ejection.
    b. penetration.
    c. twisting of the knee.
    d. a rapid acceleration force.

17. Which of the following examples depicts a mechanism of injury (MOI) rather than a common nature of illness (NOI) that a paramedic would recognize during the scene size-up and initial assessment?

    a. seizure
    b. poisoning
    c. attempted hanging
    d. altered mental status

18. When the paramedic understands the _____, he can make some predictions or be more attuned to specific injury patterns.

    a. past medical history
    b. chief complaint
    c. mechanism of injury
    d. nature of illness

19. The _____ is your first impression of the patient as you approach her, and has been referred to as the "assessment from the doorway."

    a. scene size-up
    b. general impression
    c. initial assessment
    d. MOI

20. While working in an incident command situation, which of the following actions is inappropriate for the paramedic to take?

    a. Report to the incident commander upon arrival.
    b. Obtain a quick report and assignment for your crew.
    c. Complete the assignment and search for the next patient.
    d. Complete the assignment and report back to command.

21. You are assessing the level of consciousness of a patient who is wearing a helmet and appears to have been involved in a serious motorcycle collision. The patient's eyes are closed, and he has abnormal breathing. When you speak to him, he does not answer, but when you touch him, he moans and tries to move his arms. The patient's initial level of consciousness should be recorded as:

    a. alert.
    b. verbal.
    c. painful.
    d. unresponsive.

22. While assessing a patient for a painful response, which of the following is an appropriate response?

    a. withdrawing from pain
    b. no response
    c. flexing the arm
    d. extending the arm

23. The level of consciousness or mental status of an infant is best assessed by:

    a. calling medical control to consult for advice.
    b. using the Broselow tape for pediatrics.
    c. how loud the infant cries.
    d. asking the parent or caregiver to determine if the response is normal.

24. _____ is the degree of alertness, wakefulness, or arousibility of the patient.

    a. Mental response
    b. Level of consciousness
    c. Emotion
    d. Reaction

25. Decerebrate neurologic posturing is illustrative of _____ brain functioning.

    a. absence of
    b. low-level
    c. mid-level
    d. high-level

26. Neurologic posturing is most commonly caused by herniation and compression of the brainstem, or:

    a. the effects of advanced Alzheimer's.
    b. metabolic causes.
    c. hyperventilation by the patient.
    d. injury to the lumbar spine.

27. Even if a patient is responsive and alert, he may still have serious airway compromise, such as a/an:

    a. broken jaw.
    b. abscessed tooth.
    c. cervical spine injury.
    d. postnasal drip.

28. Anytime a patient has received a high-energy impact from the clavicles or superior to the clavicles, the paramedic must consider the possibility of:

    a. low blood sugar.
    b. hypoxia.
    c. neck injury.
    d. hypovolemia.

29. _____ is the appropriateness of the patient's thinking.

    a. Mental status
    b. Level of response
    c. Emotion
    d. Reaction

30. _____ volume is the amount of gas inspired or expired in a minute.

    a. Adequate
    b. Inadequate
    c. Tidal
    d. Minute

31. The neck of an infant should not be hyperextended when opening the airway, as this can:

    a. cause the infant to swallow the tongue.
    b. close the airway.
    c. interfere with nose breathing.
    d. cause cervical spinal injury.

32. During the initial assessment of an unconscious child, the pulse is taken at the _____ for the "quick check" to determine if the patient has a pulse.

    a. radial artery
    b. brachial artery
    c. carotid artery
    d. carotid vein

33. Assessing the _____ pulse is more useful in the initial assessment of a patient because it gives information about the effectiveness of the _____ circulation.

    a. radial; distal
    b. brachial; central
    c. carotid; central
    d. femoral; core

34. What is assessed about the patient's skin during the initial assessment?

    a. color and pigmentation
    b. color, temperature, and condition
    c. pulse oximetry
    d. the presence of urticaria

35. Which of the following skin colors is an abnormal finding associated with hepatic or renal failure?

    a. red
    b. pale
    c. jaundice
    d. cyanosis

36. When assessing the skin of patients with varying degrees of skin pigmentation, the paramedic should look at the _____, as the normal skin color is similar in most persons.

    a. ears
    b. axilla
    c. tongue
    d. palms or soles

37. In which of the following is capillary refill a reliable sign?

    a. fifty-five-year-old male with COPD
    b. twenty-five-year-old female with anemia
    c. fourteen-year-old male with hypothermia
    d. three-year-old asthmatic

38. The primary reason for prioritizing a patient for treatment and transportation considerations at the completion of the initial assessment is:

   a. to identify and manage immediate life-threatening conditions.
   b. that this task has the highest priority in the first few minutes of a call.
   c. to determine the need for rapid transport and definitive care at the hospital.
   d. to determine when a critical patient should be stabilized on scene or transported rapidly.

39. Where is severe trauma stabilized?

   a. on scene
   b. in the ambulance
   c. in the ED
   d. in the OR

40. Which of the following steps may be skipped or expedited during the care of a critical trauma patient?

   a. use of a short board immobilization device
   b. use of a long board immobilization device
   c. bleeding control for life-threatening external bleeding
   d. airway control

41. The _____ assessment is a name for what is done in the ambulance en route to the hospital and includes reassessment of vital signs and interventions.

   a. detailed
   b. focused
   c. ongoing
   d. vectored

42. A/An _____ exam is an examination that attempts to look at a specific patient problem and not examine every body part, which could take a long time and not be in the patient's best interest.

   a. detailed
   b. focused
   c. ongoing
   d. initial

43. The initial assessment is repeated in the ongoing assessment in cases where the patient's:

   a. condition may be changing rapidly.
   b. condition shows an improved mental status from the baseline.
   c. condition includes a nonsignificant MOI.
   d. blood glucose returns to normal.

44. _____ is establishing a pattern of assessment findings, which will help the paramedic determine if the patient's condition is getting worse or better.

   a. Diagnosing
   b. Trending
   c. Documenting
   d. Prioritizing

45. Medical patients are classified into two groups within the medical category of assessment-based management. These two groups are:

   a. significant and nonsignificant.
   b. responsive and unresponsive.
   c. critical and noncritical.
   d. adult and child.

46. Trauma patients are classified into two groups within the trauma category of assessment-based management. These two groups are _____ MOI.

   a. significant and nonsignificant
   b. conscious and unconscious
   c. adult and child
   d. alpha and delta

47. When a patient has both a medical and a trauma problem, which is treated first?

   a. medical
   b. trauma
   c. any immediate threat to life
   d. medical control decides

48. What is the best treatment the paramedic can provide for the patient with internal bleeding?

   a. Start two large bore IVs.
   b. Apply MAST/PASG pants and inflate.
   c. Administer analgesia for pain.
   d. Provide rapid transport to an OR.

49. Which of the following injuries or conditions is an example of a critical patient?

   a. low-grade fever
   b. sickle cell crisis
   c. productive cough
   d. possible cervical neck injury

50. Which of the following injuries or conditions is an example of a stable patient?

   a. patella dislocation
   b. respiratory distress
   c. compensated shock
   d. rising intracranial pressure

Exam #14 Answer Form

	A	B	C	D			A	B	C	D
1.	❏	❏	❏	❏		26.	❏	❏	❏	❏
2.	❏	❏	❏	❏		27.	❏	❏	❏	❏
3.	❏	❏	❏	❏		28.	❏	❏	❏	❏
4.	❏	❏	❏	❏		29.	❏	❏	❏	❏
5.	❏	❏	❏	❏		30.	❏	❏	❏	❏
6.	❏	❏	❏	❏		31.	❏	❏	❏	❏
7.	❏	❏	❏	❏		32.	❏	❏	❏	❏
8.	❏	❏	❏	❏		33.	❏	❏	❏	❏
9.	❏	❏	❏	❏		34.	❏	❏	❏	❏
10.	❏	❏	❏	❏		35.	❏	❏	❏	❏
11.	❏	❏	❏	❏		36.	❏	❏	❏	❏
12.	❏	❏	❏	❏		37.	❏	❏	❏	❏
13.	❏	❏	❏	❏		38.	❏	❏	❏	❏
14.	❏	❏	❏	❏		39.	❏	❏	❏	❏
15.	❏	❏	❏	❏		40.	❏	❏	❏	❏
16.	❏	❏	❏	❏		41.	❏	❏	❏	❏
17.	❏	❏	❏	❏		42.	❏	❏	❏	❏
18.	❏	❏	❏	❏		43.	❏	❏	❏	❏
19.	❏	❏	❏	❏		44.	❏	❏	❏	❏
20.	❏	❏	❏	❏		45.	❏	❏	❏	❏
21.	❏	❏	❏	❏		46.	❏	❏	❏	❏
22.	❏	❏	❏	❏		47.	❏	❏	❏	❏
23.	❏	❏	❏	❏		48.	❏	❏	❏	❏
24.	❏	❏	❏	❏		49.	❏	❏	❏	❏
25.	❏	❏	❏	❏		50.	❏	❏	❏	❏

15

Focused History and Physical Examination: Medical Patient

1. The focused history and physical examination of the medical patient are performed:

   a. immediately after the scene size-up has been performed.
   b. after the initial assessment has been completed.
   c. before the ABCs are managed.
   d. before the chief complaint has been attained.

2. The objective of the focused physical examination is to direct the assessment to:

   a. the patient's ABCs.
   b. gather a SAMPLE history.
   c. the patient's chief complaint.
   d. establish consent to treat the patient.

3. Your patient fell and possibly experienced a loss of consciousness while in the bathroom. She is alert and oriented when you perform your initial assessment, but she tells you that when she was on the floor she could not move or cry out for help. You suspect that the patient may have experienced a/an:

   a. TIA.
   b. ACS.
   c. hypertensive event.
   d. hypoglycemic event.

4. You have responded to a call for an unconscious female in the shopping mall. Security leads you to a department store restroom, where an alert forty-five-year-old female is lying on the floor complaining of abdominal pain and nausea. How should you proceed?

   a. Begin a rapid physical exam.
   b. Obtain a SAMPLE and focused history.
   c. Begin a focused physical exam of the abdomen.
   d. Determine if there is trauma associated with this event.

5. Obtaining the SAMPLE history of a medical patient will provide the paramedic with information about:

   a. a presumptive diagnosis.
   b. the need for a rapid physical exam.
   c. the events that preceded this episode.
   d. pertinent positive and negative findings.

6. While obtaining the focused history from a patient, the paramedic should gather a SAMPLE history, a history of the present illness (HPI), and:

   a. a list of the patient's possessions that she will be taking to the hospital.
   b. positive findings and pertinent negatives.
   c. a history of childhood vaccinations.
   d. the date of the patient's last tetanus shot.

7. A paramedic interviewing a patient has asked about chest pain associated with breathing, orthopnea, prolonged bed rest, and activity at onset. Based on these questions, what is most likely the patient's chief complaint?

   a. dizziness
   b. nausea and vomiting
   c. chest tightness
   d. difficulty breathing

8. An insulin-dependent diabetic patient is presenting with an altered mental status and a low blood sugar reading. Which of the following pieces of information from the SAMPLE history obtained from a family member is most important to the paramedic immediately?

   a. A—allergies
   b. M—medications
   c. P—past medical history
   d. L—last meal

9. The acronym "AEIOU-TIPS" is helpful to the paramedic when considering the causes of:

   a. chest pain.
   b. altered mental status.
   c. abdominal pain.
   d. shortness of breath.

10. While obtaining a focused history and physical examination on an elderly patient, it is common to discover:

    a. traumatic injury.
    b. measles.
    c. concurrent medical problems.
    d. poisoning.

11. When a medical patient is discovered to be unconscious, the paramedic performs an initial assessment
followed by the:

   a. rapid physical examination.
   b. focused history.
   c. ongoing assessment.
   d. SAMPLE history.

12. A fifty-four-year-old male has shortness of breath and
chest pain with deep inspiration. His skin color, temperature, and condition are pale, warm, and moist. Auscultation of the lungs reveals clear and dry sounds in all
fields. Vitals are: pulse of 100 bpm and slightly irregular, blood pressure of 130/68, and respiratory rate of 30
and labored. The paramedic begins treatment for this
patient by providing high-flow oxygen and a/an:

   a. diuretic.
   b. nitrate.
   c. bronchodilator.
   d. analgesic.

13. A patient with respiratory distress has denied having
chest pain, loss of consciousness, or a productive cough.
These are all examples of:

   a. past medical history.
   b. pertinent positive findings.
   c. pertinent negative findings.
   d. events leading up to this episode.

14. The frequency of performing ongoing assessments is
usually based on:

   a. medical versus trauma patient.
   b. good clinical judgment and experience.
   c. age of patient.
   d. past medical history.

15. During the patient interview, a patient admitted to having
a fever and productive cough for two days in addition to
a chief complaint of chest pain. This information, aside
from the chief complaint, is referred to as:

   a. the SAMPLE history.
   b. provocation.
   c. associated signs and symptoms.
   d. stimulus.

16. A twenty-four-year-old male has a chief complaint of
dizziness, but only when he moves his head. He also
has nausea, and his vital signs are stable. The only
other significant history is that of a recent head cold
that lasted several days. On which of the following
areas should the paramedic focus the exam?

   a. cardiac
   b. respiratory
   c. neurologic
   d. behavioral

17. During the typical time a paramedic has patient contact, she must attempt to quickly establish a positive
rapport with the patient in order to:

   a. make a patient transport decision.
   b. demonstrate professionalism to the patient.
   c. gain trust and cooperation from the patient.
   d. identify immediate life-threatening conditions.

18. Both the DOT EMT–Basic and Paramedic curriculum
differentiate medical patients by:

   a. responsiveness.
   b. stable versus critical.
   c. young versus old.
   d. chief complaint.

19. A seventy-eight-year-old female is complaining of
weakness, dizziness, and nausea. She denies having
chest pain or shortness of breath and is not diabetic.
Which of the following body systems should the paramedic focus on first?

   a. gastrointestinal
   b. genitourinary
   c. cardiac
   d. neurologic

20. The components of the focused physical examination
are guided by:

   a. scene size-up and baseline vital signs.
   b. priority dispatch, scene size-up, and the presence
      of a DNAR.
   c. initial assessment and absence of a DNAR.
   d. chief complaint, initial assessment, and the
      focused PE findings.

21. In many cases, making a precise diagnosis in the field
is difficult; therefore, the paramedic should strive to
recognize emergent signs and symptoms and then:

   a. begin transport and initiate treatment en route.
   b. stabilize and transport.
   c. transport to the nearest facility.
   d. contact medical control and transport.

22. During the initial assessment of an adult patient complaining of chest tightness, weakness, and lightheadedness, you find that he is pale and hypotensive.
When you apply oxygen and lay him down, you feel
that his skin is warm and dry. As your partner obtains
vital signs, you begin to focus your physical exam in
which direction?

   a. neurologic
   b. pulmonary
   c. abdominal
   d. cardiothoracic

23. In reference to question 22, as part of the focused physical exam the paramedic would:

    a. assess speech and facial symmetry.
    b. assess lung sounds and color of sputum.
    c. auscultate and palpate the abdomen.
    d. obtain an ECG and pulse quality.

24. When obtaining information about a presenting condition that is causing pain or discomfort for a patient, which of the following acronyms is commonly use by EMS providers?

    a. OPQRST
    b. SAMPLE
    c. DCAP-BTLS
    d. AEIOU-TIPS

25. A paramedic is assessing a patient who has had a loss of bowel control, decreased sensation in the legs bilaterally, and impaired coordination. Based on these problems, what type of medical problem might this patient be further evaluated for?

    a. cardiac
    b. neurologic
    c. behavioral disorder
    d. respiratory

26. A paramedic is assessing a patient who has a chief complaint of headache, nausea, and dizziness. The focused history revealed that the patient has had these symptoms for several days, and that the spouse and children have had similar complaints (but less severe). From the information obtained in the focused history, the paramedic should consider these to be associated symptoms of:

    a. food poisoning.
    b. possible CO poisoning.
    c. infestation in the home.
    d. family history of mental disorders.

27. When assessing a patient, the mnemonic DCAP-BTLS is used to help the paramedic remember to look for specific information about the patient's:

    a. skin.
    b. mental status.
    c. respiratory effort.
    d. trauma status.

28. In which of the following cases would the paramedic most likely perform a rapid physical examination?

    a. an unresponsive forty-year-old male
    b. a fifty-five-year-old female with crushing chest pain
    c. an eighteen-month-old who is post-ictal after a seizure and crying
    d. a sixteen-year-old experiencing an acute asthma attack

29. The components of the focused physical examination are guided by the chief complaint of the patient and:

    a. the dispatch information.
    b. findings from the initial assessment.
    c. the status of a patient's DNAR.
    d. all of the above.

30. When the paramedic assesses a patient for weakness or the ability of the patient to move a body part, which focused assessment is the EMS provider examining?

    a. behavioral
    b. neurologic
    c. head to toe
    d. rapid physical exam

31. Your patient has a chief compliant of severe nausea and vomiting. As you proceed to ask the patient more questions regarding his chief complaint, which of the following statements should you consider?

    a. Vomiting is always preceded by nausea.
    b. The vomiting reflex is located in the cerebral cortex.
    c. Intracranial pressure can stimulate the vomiting reflex.
    d. Nausea and vomiting are associated with very few disorders.

32. The difference between true vertigo and dizziness is that:

    a. vertigo is a vestibular disorder.
    b. there is no difference.
    c. only adults experience vertigo.
    d. vertigo is not associated with nausea.

33. The patient is complaining of lower back pain and dysuria. Which of the following body systems should the paramedic focus on first?

    a. gastrointestinal
    b. genitourinary
    c. cardiac
    d. neurologic

34. Some conscious patients are medicated to suppress vomiting in order to:

    a. promote vagus stimulation.
    b. prevent gastrointestinal blockage.
    c. prevent supraventricular tachycardia.
    d. prevent complications from dehydration.

35. Which statement best describes the difference between vomiting and regurgitation?

    a. There is no difference.
    b. Vomiting is an active process in conscious patients, and regurgitation is not.
    c. Vomiting is a passive process in unconscious patients, and regurgitation is not.
    d. Regurgitation is an active process in unconscious patients, and vomiting is not.

36. Sensory receptors that stimulate the vomiting reflex can be found in the:

    a. aortic arch.
    b. rectum.
    c. heart.
    d. stomach.

37. You respond to a residence for a twenty-nine-year-old male who fell in the bathroom. He has a laceration on the back of his head with active bleeding. His wife tells you that he was shaving when she heard him fall, and that he was unconscious for about ninety seconds. The first treatment step is to:

    a. take c-spine precautions.
    b. stop the bleeding.
    c. administer oxygen.
    d. start an IV.

38. In reference to question 37, the patient denies having chest pain or shortness of breath, but states that he felt dizzy just before passing out. The most likely cause of the fall may be from what type of syncope?

    a. pharmacologic
    b. neurologic
    c. vasovagal
    d. respiratory

39. _____ is a cause of noncardiac syncope.

    a. Angina
    b. Aortic stenosis
    c. Vasovagal stimulation
    d. Stokes-Adams syndrome

40. One of the most common drug classifications that causes syncope is:

    a. beta-blockers.
    b. cold medications.
    c. antacids.
    d. antibiotics.

41. An alert patient is complaining of a severe headache after experiencing a seizure for the first time. There is no apparent trauma visible from the seizure, pulse is 80 and regular, and respirations are 20 and nonlabored. The patient stated that he checked his sugar thirty minutes ago, and the blood sugar was 110 mg/dl. In continuing with the focused history and physical examination, what should the paramedic consider obtaining next?

    a. repeat blood glucose
    b. ECG
    c. breath sounds
    d. blood pressure

42. Vomiting, in itself, is not a medical diagnosis; however, prolonged or frequent vomiting can lead to serious complications such as:

    a. GI bleeding.
    b. limbic system disorders.
    c. cardiac stress.
    d. endogenous infections.

43. Cardiac patients are often medicated to prevent vomiting for the following reason:

    a. to prevent discomfort
    b. vagus stimulation
    c. dehydration
    d. hypoxia

44. One of the most common rooms in the home in which a patient becomes ill or injured is the:

    a. bathroom.
    b. garage.
    c. basement.
    d. attic.

45. During a detailed physical examination of a patient complaining of "almost passing out," the paramedic identifies a life-threatening condition. Which of the following did the paramedic most likely identify?

    a. nystagmus
    b. blood sugar of 80 mg/dl
    c. heart block
    d. orthostatic changes

46. When obtaining a history of the patient who has experienced a syncopal event, the paramedic should specifically ask about:

    a. pre-syncope information, such as what the patient ate today.
    b. post-syncope information, such as duration of LOC.
    c. recent electrolyte imbalances.
    d. the use of performance-enhancing drugs.

47. The most common causes of syncope are vasovagal faint, positional orthostatic hypotension, and:

    a. cardiac dysrhythmias.
    b. micturition.
    c. neurologic induced.
    d. dehydration.

48. Orthostatic hypotension is a common symptom in which of the following circumstances:

    a. prolonged bed rest
    b. blood loss of >100 cc
    c. the use of antihistamines
    d. male smoker, age twenty-five to fifty

49. Orthostatic vitals signs are not always significant or reliable, because most people will normally have subtle vital sign changes when going from a supine or sitting position to a standing position. A more significant finding is:

    a. an abnormal pulse oximetry reading.
    b. positional symptoms.
    c. the age of the patient.
    d. the presence of edema.

50. After interviewing a patient with a chief complaint of chest pain that increases ESL with movement and palpation of the chest, the paramedic obtained a history that included smoking, lack of exercise, and a family history of hypertension. Based on this information the paramedic should plan to treat the patient for:

    a. ACS.
    b. pleurisy.
    c. pneumonia.
    d. pericarditis.

Exam #15 Answer Form

	A	B	C	D		A	B	C	D
1.	❏	❏	❏	❏	26.	❏	❏	❏	❏
2.	❏	❏	❏	❏	27.	❏	❏	❏	❏
3.	❏	❏	❏	❏	28.	❏	❏	❏	❏
4.	❏	❏	❏	❏	29.	❏	❏	❏	❏
5.	❏	❏	❏	❏	30.	❏	❏	❏	❏
6.	❏	❏	❏	❏	31.	❏	❏	❏	❏
7.	❏	❏	❏	❏	32.	❏	❏	❏	❏
8.	❏	❏	❏	❏	33.	❏	❏	❏	❏
9.	❏	❏	❏	❏	34.	❏	❏	❏	❏
10.	❏	❏	❏	❏	35.	❏	❏	❏	❏
11.	❏	❏	❏	❏	36.	❏	❏	❏	❏
12.	❏	❏	❏	❏	37.	❏	❏	❏	❏
13.	❏	❏	❏	❏	38.	❏	❏	❏	❏
14.	❏	❏	❏	❏	39.	❏	❏	❏	❏
15.	❏	❏	❏	❏	40.	❏	❏	❏	❏
16.	❏	❏	❏	❏	41.	❏	❏	❏	❏
17.	❏	❏	❏	❏	42.	❏	❏	❏	❏
18.	❏	❏	❏	❏	43.	❏	❏	❏	❏
19.	❏	❏	❏	❏	44.	❏	❏	❏	❏
20.	❏	❏	❏	❏	45.	❏	❏	❏	❏
21.	❏	❏	❏	❏	46.	❏	❏	❏	❏
22.	❏	❏	❏	❏	47.	❏	❏	❏	❏
23.	❏	❏	❏	❏	48.	❏	❏	❏	❏
24.	❏	❏	❏	❏	49.	❏	❏	❏	❏
25.	❏	❏	❏	❏	50.	❏	❏	❏	❏

Focused History and Physical Examination: Trauma Patient

1. What are life-threatening conditions that require immediate intervention?

    a. any head injury
    b. any burn injury
    c. any injury that interferes with the ABCs
    d. all motorcycle collision injuries

2. Critical trauma patients have the best chance for survival if they can be stabilized in a surgical suite within _____ of the onset of injury.

    a. one hour
    b. 90 minutes
    c. two hours
    d. six hours

3. The maximum time the paramedic should spend on-scene with a critical trauma patient, barring any lengthy extrication, is _____ minutes.

    a. ten
    b. fifteen
    c. twenty
    d. thirty

4. For the noncritical trauma patient the concerns are similar to the critical trauma patient; however, _____ may not be required.

    a. determination of MOI
    b. the initial assessment
    c. assessment of the ABCs
    d. rapid transport

5. Proper evaluation of the _____ by the paramedic can help predict injuries that may or may not be readily apparent.

    a. ABCs
    b. MOI
    c. skin color, temperature, and condition
    d. vital signs

6. _____ is the abbreviation used to remember what is assessed about the patient's soft tissues.

    a. BTLS
    b. DCAP-BTLS
    c. GCS
    d. MOI

7. _____ physical examination is a complete head-to-toe exam for non-life- or limb-threatening injuries or significant MOI en route to the hospital.

    a. Detailed
    b. Focused
    c. Ongoing
    d. Rapid trauma

8. When should transport of the critical trauma patient be delayed while waiting for ALS to arrive?

    a. when the patient is unconscious
    b. only when the patient is fully immobilized
    c. only after MAST/PASG have been inflated
    d. transportation should not be delayed while waiting for ALS to arrive

9. The transportation decision is usually made after the scene assessment for MOI and the _____ have been completed.

    a. cervical collar application
    b. initial assessment
    c. radio report
    d. immobilization

10. You are assessing a trauma patient for a possible cervical injury; which of the following criteria would you give the most consideration when deciding to apply a cervical immobilization collar?

    a. the MOI
    b. the age of the patient
    c. the patient denies neck pain
    d. the patient had a loss of consciousness

11. How often should the ongoing assessment of the non-critical trauma patient be repeated?

    a. every five minutes
    b. every fifteen minutes
    c. only when a change in mental status is noted
    d. only when the patient becomes critical

12. A Level _____ trauma center may be a clinic rather than a hospital where the goal is to provide initial stabilization of the patient and then transfer to a higher level trauma center.

    a. I
    b. II
    c. III
    d. IV

13. A level _____ trauma center is a regional center that serves as a leader in trauma care for a specific geographic area.

    a. I
    b. II
    c. III
    d. IV

14. Which one of the following patients should be transported to the nearest hospital even if it is not a Level I trauma center?

    a. severe burns
    b. pediatric trauma
    c. pregnant trauma patient
    d. traumatic cardiac arrest

15. You are at the scene with a trauma patient who was involved in an MVC with extrication. The patient is a conscious but confused twenty-year-old male who was unconscious when you first arrived. The airway is open and he is breathing adequately, and he has a distal pulse that is 90/regular. His skin is pale, warm, and dry, and his BP is 150/100. Both lower legs are fractured, and the left is an open fracture. Transport to the trauma center takes forty-five minutes. Which of the following criteria would you use to request aeromedical transport for this patient?

    a. the fractures
    b. the transport time
    c. the age of the patient
    d. the loss of consciousness

16. The _____ is a numeric grading system that combines the GCS and measurements of cardiopulmonary function as a gauge of the severity of injury and a predictor of survival after blunt injury to the head.

    a. Cincinnati score
    b. Trauma Score
    c. CUPS
    d. Traumatic Brain Injury Scale

17. If a patient fell from a height of twenty feet and landed feet first, which of the following injuries could you predict the patient might have?

    a. fractures of the heels, ankles, and hips
    b. fractures of the heels, ankles, and clavicles
    c. lower extremity fractures and head injury
    d. lower and upper extremity fractures

18. Which of the following steps cannot be skipped or omitted during the care of a critical trauma patient?

    a. full spinal immobilization
    b. short board spinal immobilization
    c. bleeding control for venous bleeding
    d. hand fracture immobilization

19. Trauma is the number one killer of _____ in the United States.

    a. men
    b. women
    c. children
    d. geriatrics

20. Special consideration for assessment of the elderly trauma patient includes an understanding that decreased:

    a. brain mass lessens the risk for brain injury.
    b. body fat minimizes the body's protection (padding) against traumatic injury.
    c. stroke volume in the elderly helps to slow bleeding associated with traumatic injury.
    d. calcification of cartilage can increase pain tolerance, and it may take longer for the patient to develop pain when injury is present.

21. _____ is the most common cause of death in children.

    a. Spinal cord injury
    b. Head injury
    c. Abdominal trauma
    d. Chest trauma

22. The most common MOI in children is:

    a. falls.
    b. bicycle accidents.
    c. MVC.
    d. auto–pedestrian collisions.

23. Special consideration for assessment of the pediatric trauma patient includes an understanding that:

    a. the presence of rib fractures is a critical finding.
    b. the airway is less prone to obstruction than adults.
    c. growth plate injuries are rare and, when present, increase the risk of mortality.
    d. the abdomen is large and well padded, decreasing the risk of internal injuries.

24. Slowed peristalsis creates a full stomach in the pregnant trauma patient, and this increases the risk of:

    a. abdominal trauma.
    b. vomiting.
    c. hypotension.
    d. abruptio placenta.

25. In the third trimester pregnant trauma patient, a blood loss of _____ can occur before any signs of shock begin to develop.

    a. 10%
    b. 20%
    c. 30%
    d. 40%

26. The MOI is a rapid, head-first impact; injuries to consider include cranial, cervical spine, and:

    a. thoracic aortic disruption.
    b. crushed trachea.
    c. fractured ribs.
    d. fractured sternum.

27. You are assessing an unrestrained driver of a vehicle whose front end struck a tree. There is a foot of intrusion into the engine compartment, and the patient was found down and under the steering column. What predictable injury pattern is associated with this type of collision?

    a. chest and abdomen
    b. face, neck, and chest
    c. spine, knee, and lower legs
    d. head, humerus, ribs, and pelvis

28. As you assess a patient involved in an MVC, which of the following items that you observed as part of the scene size-up leads you to suspect underlying injuries to the patient?

    a. flat tires
    b. no air bag deployment
    c. broken steering wheel
    d. intrusion into the engine compartment

29. Striking one side of the head often causes blunt trauma to the brain in the area that was struck, as well as the opposite area of the brain. What type of injury is this called?

    a. contra coup
    b. coup contra coup
    c. traumatic brain ischemia
    d. contra coup constriction

30. _____ is an injury pattern in children, when struck by a vehicle, involving the legs, chest, and head.

    a. Waddell's triad
    b. SCIWORA
    c. Crushing
    d. Whipple's triad

31. The momentary acceleration of tissue laterally away from the projectile tract of a bullet in the body, which explains why exit wounds are usually larger than entrance wounds, is called:

    a. tumble.
    b. fragmentation.
    c. profile.
    d. cavitation.

32. It is estimated that the chance of a spinal injury increases up to _____ times by being ejected from a vehicle while not wearing a seat belt.

    a. 30
    b. 300
    c. 1,300
    d. 3,000

33. Striking the "temples" of the cranium with a blunt object can cause the middle meningeal artery to bleed and a/an _____ to develop.

    a. neoplasm
    b. leak of CSF in the ears
    c. subdural hematoma
    d. epidural hematoma

34. Secondary injuries from an MVC, where the driver went up and over the steering column/dash, include:

    a. face and head.
    b. head and neck.
    c. chest and abdomen.
    d. cervical spine.

35. You are caring for a critical trauma patient. Which of the following can be used to move the patient safely and quickly, and to minimize scene time?

    a. long backboard
    b. Kendrick Extrication Device (KED)
    c. short backboard
    d. blanket

36. Paradoxical motion, crepitation, and asymmetry are all abnormal findings the paramedic may find on the:

    a. head.
    b. chest.
    c. abdomen.
    d. pelvis.

37. Criteria for the designated transportation destination of trauma patients for a specific EMS agency can usually be found in:

    a. regional protocols.
    b. EMT-B and paramedic texts.
    c. hospital rules.
    d. state law.

38. Which of the following unique physiologic responses do children have to shock trauma?

    a. Children in shock decompensate slower than adults.
    b. Children in shock appear worse than they actually are.
    c. Children compensate for shock better than adults in late shock.
    d. Children compensate for shock better than adults in early shock.

39. Your patient is a five-year-old female who was struck by a car backing out of a driveway while she was riding her bike. The child is wearing a helmet, which is cracked. She is unconscious and breathing abnormally. Which of the following should you consider about pediatric trauma as you begin to assess this patient?

    a. Rib fractures are rare in pediatric trauma.
    b. Rib fractures frequently occur in pediatric trauma.
    c. Anterior airway structures make the airway less prone to obstruction.
    d. Children can sustain spinal cord injures without the same devastating results as adults.

40. Which of the following statements about trauma in the elderly is false?

    a. Aging immune systems put the elderly at risk for system infections.
    b. The use of MAOIs can interfere with the body's normal response to pain.
    c. Decreases in brain mass leave the brain at risk for injury from rapid deceleration forces.
    d. The use of beta-blockers can mask the signs of shock.

41. You are assessing a belted passenger involved in a moderate-speed MVC. Initially the patient had no complaint of injury or pain. Twenty minutes after the collision, the patient states that he feels dizzy, and he looks pale and diaphoretic. What condition do you suspect the patient has?

    a. potential spinal injury
    b. head injury
    c. intra-abdominal hemorrhage
    d. neurogenic shock

42. While responding to a call for a self-inflicted GSW, dispatch advises that the injury was to the head and face as reported by police. What do you anticipate will be the priority of care for this patient?

    a. complicated airway
    b. blood loss
    c. rapid transport
    d. spinal immobilization

43. A patient who was burned in a house fire sustained multiple injuries. Which of the following is the primary concern for the paramedic?

    a. third-degree burns on both hands
    b. first- and second-degree burns on the face and neck
    c. clothing charred into the chest and back
    d. wheezing present with a hoarse voice

44. After responding to the scene of a diving accident, you are treating a male patient who is unable to move any part of his body below the neck. You have him fully immobilized and are ready for transport. Where should you take him?

    a. the nearest hospital
    b. level I trauma center
    c. level II trauma center
    d. level III trauma center

45. While en route to the hospital with the patient from question 44, you determine that he has sensation to the shoulders but none below. Where do you suspect the spinal injury is?

    a. C1 and C2
    b. C3 and C4
    c. C6 and C7
    d. T1 and T2

Exam #16 Answer Form

	A	B	C	D		A	B	C	D
1.	❏	❏	❏	❏	24.	❏	❏	❏	❏
2.	❏	❏	❏	❏	25.	❏	❏	❏	❏
3.	❏	❏	❏	❏	26.	❏	❏	❏	❏
4.	❏	❏	❏	❏	27.	❏	❏	❏	❏
5.	❏	❏	❏	❏	28.	❏	❏	❏	❏
6.	❏	❏	❏	❏	29.	❏	❏	❏	❏
7.	❏	❏	❏	❏	30.	❏	❏	❏	❏
8.	❏	❏	❏	❏	31.	❏	❏	❏	❏
9.	❏	❏	❏	❏	32.	❏	❏	❏	❏
10.	❏	❏	❏	❏	33.	❏	❏	❏	❏
11.	❏	❏	❏	❏	34.	❏	❏	❏	❏
12.	❏	❏	❏	❏	35.	❏	❏	❏	❏
13.	❏	❏	❏	❏	36.	❏	❏	❏	❏
14.	❏	❏	❏	❏	37.	❏	❏	❏	❏
15.	❏	❏	❏	❏	38.	❏	❏	❏	❏
16.	❏	❏	❏	❏	39.	❏	❏	❏	❏
17.	❏	❏	❏	❏	40.	❏	❏	❏	❏
18.	❏	❏	❏	❏	41.	❏	❏	❏	❏
19.	❏	❏	❏	❏	42.	❏	❏	❏	❏
20.	❏	❏	❏	❏	43.	❏	❏	❏	❏
21.	❏	❏	❏	❏	44.	❏	❏	❏	❏
22.	❏	❏	❏	❏	45.	❏	❏	❏	❏
23.	❏	❏	❏	❏					

17

Assessment-Based Management

1. _____ is the cornerstone of patient care.

   a. Past medical history
   b. Assessment
   c. Field impression
   d. Scene size-up

2. It is estimated that 80% of a medical diagnosis is based on the:

   a. physical examination.
   b. medications.
   c. history.
   d. chief complaint.

3. You and your crew have been dispatched to a supermarket for a patient with an unknown problem. Upon your arrival, the store manager tells you that the patient has been wandering around the store acting confused and slurring his words. He brings you to an aisle where a male in his late fifties is sitting on a wheeled cart. He is conscious but confused, and he does have slurred speech. He cannot answer your questions. His skin is warm and dry with good color, and he has a strong distal pulse. Which of the following factors could impede a proper field assessment of this patient?

   a. gender
   b. environment
   c. advanced directives
   d. past medical history

4. Continuing with the patient in question 3, you assist him onto your stretcher and your crew obtains vital signs: respiratory rate is 20/nonlabored; pulse rate is 66, strong/regular; and BP is 144/100. There is no obvious injury, but the patient smells of body odor and dried urine. Where should you focus your assessment next?

   a. possible head injury
   b. rule out hypothermia
   c. rule out hypoglycemia
   d. behavioral emergency

5. Which of the following is an example of "labeling" a patient?

   a. frequent flyer
   b. unstable head injury
   c. gut instinct
   d. diabetic neuropathy

6. When obtaining a history from a patient, the paramedic should focus on the:

   a. organ systems associated with the complaint.
   b. family preference for treatment and hospital destination.
   c. length of time the patient has waited for treatment.
   d. medical conditions the patient's family members may have.

7. Which of the following statements about injury pattern recognition for the trauma patient is most correct?

   a. The paramedic's knowledge base of injury patterns needs to be similar to that of a trauma surgeon's.
   b. Recognition of various injury patterns can help the paramedic be better prepared to provide the proper emergency care.
   c. To become proficient in pattern recognition, a paramedic's knowledge base needs to be similar to an emergency physician's.
   d. It is the responsibility of the EMS agency's Medical Director to provide expanded and continuous training in injury pattern recognition.

8. What is the essential equipment that should initially be brought to the side of every patient?

   a. clipboard, pen, and stethoscope
   b. PPE, stethoscope, blood pressure cuff, and penlight
   c. Equipment to conduct the initial assessment of the patient's ABCs
   d. Cardiac monitor/AED, stretcher, blood pressure cull, and oxygen administration equipment.

9. It is important for the paramedic to understand that protocols are intended as:

a. the gold standard and should never be deviated from.
b. guidelines for care.
c. the basis of an action plan for all patients.
d. a cookbook list of what the paramedic must do.

10. Which of the following is a factor that could impede decision making or proper field assessment by the paramedic?

a. having a bias against people who do not have a similar background to her
b. having insufficient access to the patient's medical insurance records
c. taking the time to listen to the patient's associated complaints
d. treating distracting injuries after correcting life threats

11. When the paramedic has _____, he may miss vital pieces of information, which may short-circuit the information-gathering process.

a. insufficient manpower
b. a partner with less training or experience
c. a biased or prejudicial "attitude"
d. concerned family at the scene

12. The team leader is usually the paramedic who will:

a. talk to the family and bystanders.
b. act as the triage group leader in an MCI.
c. drive the crew to the hospital.
d. accompany the patient through definitive care.

13. Roles of the patient care provider member of the team usually include any of the following, *except*:

a. obtaining vital signs.
b. performing skills as designated by the team leader.
c. acting as the initial EMS command in an MCI.
d. gathering patient information.

14. Essential equipment that should be brought to the side of every patient includes:

a. equipment needed to conduct the initial assessment of the patient's priorities.
b. only the equipment needed to run an ACLS "code."
c. only what you can carry.
d. it is best to decide on each call what equipment to bring.

15. If a paramedic gives a poor oral presentation when giving a report on a patient, the paramedic suggests to the receiving healthcare provider that:

a. a poor assessment and care were made.
b. there is really nothing wrong with the patient.
c. the paramedic has other tasks of more importance.
d. the paramedic failed to establish trust and credibility with the patient.

16. The paramedic's ability to effectively communicate and transfer patient information is done with every patient encounter by all the following means, *except*:

a. writing on the PCR.
b. over the radio.
c. face to face.
d. dispatch information.

17. The paramedic's professional demeanor can be rated by the patient when he considers your:

a. level of training.
b. people skills and customer service.
c. medical performance.
d. amount of equipment you can carry.

18. In your general approach to any patient, you should display a calm, orderly demeanor. To avoid the appearance of confusion when working with multiple crew members, you should:

a. have and practice a preplan.
b. ignore non-life-threatening, distracting injuries.
c. carry the least amount of equipment to the patient.
d. consider the family's concern for the patient's welfare.

19. _____ is/are the staging of the events and actions of a call so that they happen smoothly.

a. Choreography
b. Algorithms
c. Protocols
d. Advanced directives

20. An example of how tunnel vision can obstruct the assessment process is:

a. responding to an anaphylactic call where the patient forgot to administer his Epi-pen®.
b. seeing a local drug abuser and immediately blaming his disorientation on the drugs rather than looking for a medical problem.
c. assessing a patient's MS-ABCs before attending to an open femur fracture with gross angulation.
d. assuming EMS command at the scene of an MCI where the fire department is on-scene first.

21. The paramedic must gather information as well as evaluate and synthesize that information. This is done in order to:

    a. diagnose a patient's illness.
    b. provide definitive care for the patient.
    c. educate the patient's family on future 9-1-1 calls for assistance.
    d. make the appropriate management decisions.

22. Why is it essential to proceed through the patient assessment in an organized fashion?

    a. It is necessary in order to explain each step to the patient.
    b. This approach will help you to follow protocols and standing orders.
    c. This approach will help you to limit the amount of time spent on-scene.
    d. An unorganized approach can lead to important information being overlooked.

23. Following a sequence when performing an assessment of the patient is most efficient because:

    a. the crew will know what they should do next.
    b. the patient will cooperate more easily.
    c. it allows for a complete and smooth assessment.
    d. it is easier to write up on the PCR.

24. Making treatment decisions based on the assessment involves consideration of the information gathered in the focused history, the physical exam, and:

    a. emergency medical dispatch procedures.
    b. existing treatment protocols.
    c. third-party caller information.
    d. the paramedic's ability to make a definitive field diagnosis.

25. Which of the following affects the quality of the history taken from the patient by the paramedic?

    a. the patient's knowledge about the healthcare system
    b. the paramedic's knowledge of a disease and its assessment findings
    c. local protocols and patient algorithms of a specific illness
    d. the Medical Director's level of involvement in QI/QA

26. What is the value of a complete physical examination?

    a. Performing a complete physical exam will build trust with the patient.
    b. Important information can be missed by performing a cursory physical exam.
    c. The attending physician at the destination hospital will be impressed by a complete physical exam.
    d. Performing a complete physical exam will keep you from being sued.

27. There is nothing wrong with the "Cookbook Practice" or using local protocol, as long as:

    a. you have a partner to ask for advice.
    b. your supervisor trusts your judgment.
    c. there is a "thinking cook."
    d. you know all the protocols by memory.

28. When two paramedics are working as a team, there can be simultaneous information gathering and treatment, which is:

    a. more efficient.
    b. less efficient.
    c. confusing to the patient.
    d. a problem for establishing patient rapport.

29. The paramedic can improve scene choreography by:

    a. utilizing distance learning.
    b. taking a course in MCI leadership.
    c. watching training videos.
    d. preplanning and practicing with her crew.

30. The patient care provider is responsible for providing scene "cover" by:

    a. shutting of the ambulance and taking the keys out of the ignition.
    b. setting up a cover for the crew working in the rain.
    c. watching everyone's back to make sure no one gets hurt.
    d. establishing a rehab sector for fire standbys.

Exam #17 Answer Form

	A	B	C	D			A	B	C	D
1.	❏	❏	❏	❏		16.	❏	❏	❏	❏
2.	❏	❏	❏	❏		17.	❏	❏	❏	❏
3.	❏	❏	❏	❏		18.	❏	❏	❏	❏
4.	❏	❏	❏	❏		19.	❏	❏	❏	❏
5.	❏	❏	❏	❏		20.	❏	❏	❏	❏
6.	❏	❏	❏	❏		21.	❏	❏	❏	❏
7.	❏	❏	❏	❏		22.	❏	❏	❏	❏
8.	❏	❏	❏	❏		23.	❏	❏	❏	❏
9.	❏	❏	❏	❏		24.	❏	❏	❏	❏
10.	❏	❏	❏	❏		25.	❏	❏	❏	❏
11.	❏	❏	❏	❏		26.	❏	❏	❏	❏
12.	❏	❏	❏	❏		27.	❏	❏	❏	❏
13.	❏	❏	❏	❏		28.	❏	❏	❏	❏
14.	❏	❏	❏	❏		29.	❏	❏	❏	❏
15.	❏	❏	❏	❏		30.	❏	❏	❏	❏

18

Ongoing Assessment and Clinical Decision Making

1. Which of the following is not a key aspect of the on-going assessment?

   a. trending
   b. time constraints
   c. scene size-up
   d. manpower

2. The hormonal "fight or flight" response to stress can affect the paramedic in which of the following ways?

   a. increased concentration
   b. improved muscular strength
   c. decreased visual senses
   d. improved critical thinking

3. Lights and sirens, pagers, phones, and traffic are all examples of:

   a. stimulants that improve critical thinking.
   b. stimulants of the "fight or flight" response for paramedics.
   c. distractions used in the standard approach to patient care.
   d. distractions for patients that provide structure for the paramedic.

4. Which of the following factors is most likely to alter the ongoing assessment in the unstable patient?

   a. short transport time
   b. the patient's gender
   c. an obvious injury pattern
   d. the patient's chief complaint

5. Which of the following statements about repeating the ongoing assessment is most correct?

   a. Ongoing assessment should only be repeated by a paramedic for critical trauma patients.
   b. The ongoing assessment should be repeated every ten minutes for the critical trauma patient.
   c. The ongoing assessment should be repeated every ten minutes for the noncritical trauma patient.
   d. The time interval for repeating the ongoing assessment for the critical trauma patient is the same for the critical medical patient.

6. _____ is the process of obtaining a baseline assessment and then repeating the assessment for comparison.

   a. Trending
   b. Palpation
   c. Pairing off
   d. Serial processing

7. During the management of the patient en route to the hospital, the earliest indicators of deterioration of a patient are often:

   a. subtle changes in the patient's blood pressure.
   b. subtle changes in the patient's mental status.
   c. changes in skin color.
   d. changes in the lung sounds.

8. Which of the following statements about measurements or observations obtained during management of the patient is most accurate?

   a. Isolated measurements are generally less helpful than changes over time.
   b. Isolated observations are significantly more helpful than acute changes over time.
   c. Treatment protocols are specifically designed for patients with acute assessment changes.
   d. Treatment protocols help the paramedic to anticipate observations that identify deterioration of a patient's mental status.

9. The cornerstone of being an effective paramedic is having the ability to:

   a. perform the ongoing examination on a bumpy street.
   b. avoid conflict with family members.
   c. drive all types of emergency vehicles.
   d. think and work under pressure.

10. One of the essential concepts of clinical decision making is:

   a. being a mentor to an EMT-Basic student.
   b. evaluating and processing information.
   c. scrutinizing the actions of the First Responders.
   d. gathering the patient's belongings for the transport.

11. Based on the ongoing assessment and evaluation, the paramedic may:

    a. formulate a new management plan.
    b. provide additional interventions.
    c. call medical control for consultation.
    d. all of the above.

12. Which of the following is a major difference between patient care in the out-of-hospital setting and in-hospital setting?

    a. Patients open up more to the ED staff than they do to paramedics.
    b. The hospital is a relatively controlled environment.
    c. Paramedics can perform skills that nurses cannot.
    d. The ongoing assessment is different in the hospital.

13. Which of the following is an example of a non-life-threatening condition the paramedic would address during an ongoing assessment?

    a. CVA
    b. fractured femur
    c. isolated extremity injury without neurologic compromise
    d. concurrent disease presentations

14. You are treating a fifty-two-year-old male patient with a complaint of chest pain 8/10 that radiates down the left arm. Vital signs are: respiratory rate of 22/nonlabored, pulse rate of 68/irregular, BP of 124/70, SpO_2 of 100%, and skin CTC is pale and moist. You have provided oxygen, administered aspirin and nitroglycerin, established an IV, and obtained a 12-lead ECG. You are now ready to transport. Which of the following aspects is most valuable to you in the ongoing assessment?

    a. repeating the ECG
    b. the patient's blood pressure
    c. the patient's level of discomfort
    d. the patient's oxygen saturation

15. One of the fundamental elements of critical thinking for the paramedic working in the out-of-hospital setting is:

    a. improving reflexes and muscular strength.
    b. avoiding distractions that impair critical thinking.
    c. following written protocols and never utilizing online medical control.
    d. achieving and maintaining an adequate body of medical knowledge.

16. Which of the following is not an aspect of critical thinking for the paramedic?

    a. criticizing the actions of the first responders
    b. differentiating between relevant and non-relevant information
    c. identifying and managing medical ambiguity
    d. documenting decision-making reasoning

17. During a call for an allergic reaction you realize that you have forgotten the new standing order dose for Benadryl®. Which of the following is the most appropriate action?

    a. Use the old standing order dose.
    b. Guess the dose, because it is too embarrassing to ask medical control.
    c. Look up the correct dose in your protocol book.
    d. Just give the epinephrine and say that you are out of Benadryl®.

18. _____ is one of the fundamental elements of critical thinking for the paramedic.

    a. Learning a second language
    b. Focusing on one task at a time
    c. Improving visual and auditory acuity
    d. Identifying and managing medical ambiguity

19. One of the benefits of protocols, standing orders, and patient care algorithms is that they:

    a. clearly define performance parameters.
    b. cover all aspects of the critically ill patient.
    c. cover all aspects of the critically injured patient.
    d. provide a solid legal, defensible back for the paramedic.

20. Which of the following is an advantage of protocols, standing orders, and patient care algorithms?

    a. They do not usually cover multisystem failures or nonspecific complaints.
    b. They do not usually cover concurrent disease processes.
    c. They can speed the application of critical interventions.
    d. They usually cover the "textbook" patient injury or illness.

21. In reference to clinical decision making, which of the following is not one of the "six Rs" of putting it all together?

    a. Read the patient.
    b. Read the scene.
    c. React.
    d. Rephrase.

22. You are assessing a male in his twenties who is lying on a couch and appears to be having a focal seizure. His eyes are open and he is staring to one side. He does not respond to you as you place an oxygen mask on his face. Which sequence of critical-thinking components should you follow with this patient?

    a. Collect information and formulate concepts, interpret and process information, apply treatment, reevaluate, and reflect.
    b. Apply treatment, reevaluate, reflect, collect information and formulate concepts, interpret and process information.
    c. Interpret and process information, reflect, apply treatment, reevaluate, collect information and formulate concepts.
    d. Reflect, reevaluate, apply treatment, collect information and formulate concepts, interpret and process information.

23. In reference to the "six Rs" of putting it all together, when the paramedic is "reading the scene" of an incident, which of the following is considered?

    a. location of the patient
    b. response to initial treatment
    c. getting insurance information
    d. interventions for life-threatening conditions

24. In reference to the "six Rs" of putting it all together, when the paramedic is "reading the patient" of an incident, which of the following is a primary consideration?

    a. identifying the chief complaint
    b. performing a detailed physical exam
    c. analyzing and comparing similar situations
    d. reassessing vitals signs after interventions

25. When multiple stimuli on the scene of a call start to cloud critical thinking, the paramedic can use which of the following mental tricks to avoid panicking?

    a. Stop and think before acting.
    b. Obtain insurance information.
    c. Reflect on what has occurred so far.
    d. Be optimistic and hope for the best outcome.

26. Behaviors that can aid the paramedic to make good decisions while working under pressure include using a systematic assessment process and:

    a. planning for the worst scenario.
    b. planning for the best possible outcome.
    c. reviewing the performance after the call.
    d. asking the patient to provide his past medical history.

27. An acute myocardial infarction in a thirty-nine-year-old male is an example of a patient situation that is:

    a. non-life-threatening.
    b. potentially life-threatening.
    c. critically life-threatening.
    d. fatal.

28. A patient involved in a motor vehicle collision with minor multisystem injuries is an example of a patient situation that is:

    a. non-life-threatening.
    b. potentially life-threatening.
    c. critically life-threatening.
    d. fatal.

29. In the clinical decision-making process, the paramedic should encourage the patient to actively participate in the process by doing any of the following, *except*:

    a. asking the patient to provide information.
    b. encouraging the patient to ask questions.
    c. asking the patient for a signature on a billing form.
    d. taking advantage of teaching moments.

30. Which of the following is an example of a potential teaching moment for the paramedic?

    a. an unrestrained victim of an MVC sustaining facial lacerations on the windshield
    b. a three-year-old child experiencing an anaphylactic reaction to a bee sting
    c. a fifty-five-year-old having an acute myocardial infarction
    d. an asthmatic having a severe asthma attack after three months without an attack

31. Which of the following acronyms is used to help paramedics determine treatment and transportation priority decisions?

    a. CUPS
    b. ALS
    c. PHTLS
    d. PALS

32. As the paramedic gains more experience over time, it is expected that she will be better able to:

    a. manage similar experiences.
    b. transport the patient to the nearest facility.
    c. work with less manpower on difficult calls.
    d. limit the amount of turnaround time at the hospital.

33. Key aspects of ongoing assessment include:

    a. observing the MOI.
    b. trending mental status and vital signs.
    c. starting an IV.
    d. obtaining a baseline ECG.

34. In the clinical decision-making process, one of the "six Rs" is "react," and this means that the paramedic should:

   a. call police backup.
   b. take a deep breath when experiencing sensory overload.
   c. discuss and analyze the call immediately after the call.
   d. treat as he goes, correcting life threats first.

35. When a paramedic becomes overwhelmed and critical thinking becomes clouded, which of the following is advised?

   a. Take a deep breath, revert back to assessing the ABCs.
   b. Call for a backup crew to transport the patient.
   c. Utilize the paramedic supervisor as a mentor.
   d. Call the paramedic supervisor and request to go home for the day.

Exam #18 Answer Form

	A	B	C	D		A	B	C	D
1.	❑	❑	❑	❑	19.	❑	❑	❑	❑
2.	❑	❑	❑	❑	20.	❑	❑	❑	❑
3.	❑	❑	❑	❑	21.	❑	❑	❑	❑
4.	❑	❑	❑	❑	22.	❑	❑	❑	❑
5.	❑	❑	❑	❑	23.	❑	❑	❑	❑
6.	❑	❑	❑	❑	24.	❑	❑	❑	❑
7.	❑	❑	❑	❑	25.	❑	❑	❑	❑
8.	❑	❑	❑	❑	26.	❑	❑	❑	❑
9.	❑	❑	❑	❑	27.	❑	❑	❑	❑
10.	❑	❑	❑	❑	28.	❑	❑	❑	❑
11.	❑	❑	❑	❑	29.	❑	❑	❑	❑
12.	❑	❑	❑	❑	30.	❑	❑	❑	❑
13.	❑	❑	❑	❑	31.	❑	❑	❑	❑
14.	❑	❑	❑	❑	32.	❑	❑	❑	❑
15.	❑	❑	❑	❑	33.	❑	❑	❑	❑
16.	❑	❑	❑	❑	34.	❑	❑	❑	❑
17.	❑	❑	❑	❑	35.	❑	❑	❑	❑
18.	❑	❑	❑	❑					

19

Communications

1. An example of electronic communication that is used by paramedics on many ALS calls is:

   a. triage.
   b. 10 codes.
   c. telephone interrogation.
   d. the code summary on a monitor-defibrillator unit.

2. When a citizen driving by a collision notices the patient and calls 9-1-1, this is called:

   a. notification.
   b. response.
   c. detection.
   d. occurrence.

3. When the paramedic confers with medical control over the field treatment of the patient, this is referred to as the _____ phase of communication.

   a. notification
   b. treatment
   c. preparation for the next call
   d. response

4. The basic model of communication includes which of the following steps?

   a. Receiver has a message.
   b. Receiver gives feedback.
   c. Sender decodes the message.
   d. Receiver sends the message.

5. On an EMS call the paramedic is required to interact with each of the following, *except*:

   a. emergency service personnel at the scene.
   b. the crew members and bystanders.
   c. the patient's family physician.
   d. the ED staff who will be taking over management of the patient.

6. Special radio codes:

   a. lead to a clearer understanding of the message.
   b. are necessary to avoid listeners.
   c. add an unnecessary level of complexity.
   d. should be used in public.

7. Newer cell phones are required to have a/an _____, which can help identify the location of a caller in an emergency.

   a. caller identification
   b. amplitude modulator
   c. global positioning device
   d. enhanced caller identification

8. The study of the meaning in language is called:

   a. diction.
   b. semantics.
   c. linguistics.
   d. context.

9. When talking with a child on an EMS call, it is important to:

   a. avoid technical terms.
   b. stretch the truth so it sounds better.
   c. use buzzwords.
   d. use only short words.

10. When speaking on a portable radio, you should depress the microphone for a moment prior to beginning to speak because:

    a. it will get everyone's attention.
    b. it helps to avoid cutting off the first few words.
    c. the radio will transmit louder.
    d. the receivers will be ready to hear you.

11. When an emergency occurs, why should the public avoid dialing "0" on their phones?

    a. The 9-1-1 system is more accurate.
    b. The operator may be unfamiliar with your community.
    c. The seven-digit line is easier to remember.
    d. The operator line is usually busy.

12. You are inside an office building taking care of a patient with severe respiratory distress. When you attempt to use your portable radio to call out, you get a buzzing noise and suspect that it is 60-cycle interference. Which of the following factors is most likely causing the radio interference?

    a. close proximity to computers
    b. thickness of the walls of the building
    c. metal skeletal structure of the building
    d. the cell phone the patient is using to call his family

13. When the EMD gives instructions on CPR compressions to the family member who called, this is known as:

    a. interrogation.
    b. pre-arrival instructions.
    c. radio dispatch.
    d. logistics coordination.

14. Part of the training of the emergency medical dispatcher (EMD) includes learning and using the "four cardinal rules of priority dispatching." One of four key questions the EMD must obtain an answer to is:

    a. is the patient conscious?
    b. what is the patient's date of birth?
    c. what prescription medications, if any, is the patient taking?
    d. has the patient ever called for an ambulance in the past?

15. The time between the receipt of the call and the time the call is given to the emergency unit to respond is called _____ time.

    a. response
    b. alerting
    c. dispatch
    d. queue

16. When analyzing the time segments of a call, it is important to remember that:

    a. scene time begins upon arrival at the patient's side.
    b. the scene time may be inaccurately lengthened.
    c. scene time ends once you load the patient on the stretcher.
    d. most times are usually inaccurate.

17. An example of a factor that may lengthen the actual scene time is:

    a. heavy traffic conditions.
    b. a lengthy extrication.
    c. the dispatch priority.
    d. a change in transport destination.

18. One example of a difference between 9-1-1 and an enhanced 9-1-1 system is:

    a. in enhanced 9-1-1, a computer displays the caller's phone number.
    b. the 9-1-1 system is no longer used.
    c. the enhanced system costs more money to make the call.
    d. in the enhanced system, there are fewer dispatch centers.

19. When called by someone who is in direct contact with the patient, this is referred to as:

    a. first-party caller.
    b. second-party caller.
    c. third-party caller.
    d. fourth-party caller.

20. The new roles of the Federal Communication Commission include:

    a. creating a model agency for the digital age.
    b. managing the electromagnetic spectrum.
    c. promoting competition in all communication markets.
    d. all of the above.

21. Who was the physician credited with the creation of meaningful change in the way dispatchers were trained in the past twenty years?

    a. Adam Cowley, MD
    b. David Boyd, MD
    c. Eugene Nagel, MD
    d. Jeff Clawson, MD

22. What medical breakthrough is referred to as zero-minute response time?

    a. Public Access Defibrillation
    b. pre-arrival instructions
    c. system status management
    d. rapid response vehicles

23. A system where the computer is used to assist the EMD in determining which units to deploy is called a/an:

    a. SSM.
    b. CAD.
    c. ALS.
    d. CSM.

24. The main purpose of a verbal report over the radio to the hospital is to:

    a. document on tape the patient's problem.
    b. document the run on tape for QI purposes.
    c. give them time to prepare for the patient.
    d. assess the need for diversion.

25. Which of the following pieces of information should the paramedic avoid giving over the radio as part of the report to the hospital?

    a. patient's name
    b. chief complaint
    c. baseline vital signs
    d. response to emergency interventions

26. In addition to the standard radio report, the paramedic report to medical control should also include:

    a. drugs administered on standing orders.
    b. a second set of vital signs.
    c. the patient's ETA.
    d. the patient's age.

27. The official listing of ten codes is prepared by:

    a. NFPA.
    b. OSHA.
    c. FEMA.
    d. APCO.

28. When speaking on a portable radio you should:

    a. only use the last names of patients.
    b. be courteous and say please and thank you.
    c. say each digit for clarity when transmitting a number.
    d. speak quickly with your lips about an inch from the microphone.

29. One major advantage of digital technology in communication for emergency responders is that:

    a. digital transmitters are not affected by typical sources of interference.
    b. digital transmitters do not require voice transmission time over the radio.
    c. technology makes it impossible for people with scanners to listen in on transmissions.
    d. technology reduces scene time by eliminating the need to talk to dispatch on the radio.

30. The number of repetitive cycles per second completed by a radio wave is called the:

    a. telemetry.
    b. frequency.
    c. amplitude modulation.
    d. call simplex.

31. When a radio transmits and receives on the same frequency, this is called:

    a. call simplex.
    b. duplex communications.
    c. telemetry.
    d. ultra-high frequency.

32. When the radio power of a portable is not strong enough to reach a base station, this system can be improved by the use of a/an:

    a. amplitude modulator.
    b. frequency modulator.
    c. duplex system.
    d. repeater.

33. Radio frequencies between 300 and 3,000 mHz are in the _____ band.

    a. AM
    b. VHF
    c. cellular
    d. UHF

34. The _____ band is less susceptible to interference than _____, so it is more frequently used in EMS communications.

    a. cellular; AM
    b. FM; AM
    c. AM; FM
    d. UHF; FM

35. Voice transmission is also referred to as:

    a. simplex.
    b. analog transmission.
    c. digital transmission.
    d. duplex.

Exam #19 Answer Form

	A	B	C	D		A	B	C	D
1.	❏	❏	❏	❏	19.	❏	❏	❏	❏
2.	❏	❏	❏	❏	20.	❏	❏	❏	❏
3.	❏	❏	❏	❏	21.	❏	❏	❏	❏
4.	❏	❏	❏	❏	22.	❏	❏	❏	❏
5.	❏	❏	❏	❏	23.	❏	❏	❏	❏
6.	❏	❏	❏	❏	24.	❏	❏	❏	❏
7.	❏	❏	❏	❏	25.	❏	❏	❏	❏
8.	❏	❏	❏	❏	26.	❏	❏	❏	❏
9.	❏	❏	❏	❏	27.	❏	❏	❏	❏
10.	❏	❏	❏	❏	28.	❏	❏	❏	❏
11.	❏	❏	❏	❏	29.	❏	❏	❏	❏
12.	❏	❏	❏	❏	30.	❏	❏	❏	❏
13.	❏	❏	❏	❏	31.	❏	❏	❏	❏
14.	❏	❏	❏	❏	32.	❏	❏	❏	❏
15.	❏	❏	❏	❏	33.	❏	❏	❏	❏
16.	❏	❏	❏	❏	34.	❏	❏	❏	❏
17.	❏	❏	❏	❏	35.	❏	❏	❏	❏
18.	❏	❏	❏	❏					

20

Documentation

1. In a medicolegal case review, poor documentation is:

   a. only a problem with new EMS personnel.
   b. an indication of poor assessment.
   c. usually caused by lack of training or supervision.
   d. a sign of laziness.

2. Which of the following statements about the documentation of patient care is most correct?

   a. Documentation serves as a legal record of the incident.
   b. A well-written prehospital care report (PCR) needs only the baseline set of vital signs.
   c. There is no standardization of data between different agencies and systems.
   d. Administrative data is listed on only the original copy of the PCR.

3. _____ has defined a minimum data set to be included in all prehospital care reports.

   a. NHTSA
   b. DOT
   c. State EMS
   d. DOH

4. Which of the items listed is an example of patient data?

   a. run times
   b. name of the service
   c. disposition of the call
   d. name of the crew members

5. Which of the items listed is an example of run data?

   a. nature of illness
   b. mechanism of injury
   c. location of the patient
   d. level of training of the crew members

6. All of the following are names for the out-of-hospital patient care documentation prepared by EMS personnel, *except* the:

   a. PCR.
   b. run sheet.
   c. ambulance call report.
   d. DNAR.

7. Which of the items listed is an example of patient demographic data?

   a. past medical history
   b. the patient's address
   c. time en route to the patient
   d. treatment self-administered prior to EMS arrival

8. Before a PCR can be used for quality improvement or educational purposes, what action must be taken?

   a. Obtain verbal consent from patient.
   b. Obtain written consent from patient.
   c. Remove patient's name from documentation.
   d. Remove paramedic's name from documentation.

9. Which of the following is most accurate about documentation of vital signs?

   a. Vital signs should be documented before and after a medication administration.
   b. Three sets of vital signs should be documented for every patient.
   c. Vital signs should be documented at least every ten minutes for critical patients.
   d. It is not difficult to make treatment decisions based on one set of vital signs.

10. Standard guidelines for documentation of out-of-hospital assessment and management include:

    a. always using print on the PCR.
    b. being objective, specific, and concrete.
    c. minimizing the use of abbreviations.
    d. avoiding the use of quotations.

11. The prefix ambi- means:

    a. around.
    b. both sides.
    c. dim, dull, or lazy.
    d. against, opposed to.

12. The suffix -plasia means:

    a. paralysis.
    b. surgical repair.
    c. painful condition.
    d. development, formation.

13. Because the paramedic will not be present to explain his findings to all who ultimately read the PCR, the form should be so complete that it:

    a. leaves no doubt about the patient's diagnosis.
    b. contains the patient's entire past medical history.
    c. includes only objective findings by the paramedic.
    d. "speaks for itself."

14. The presence of a complete and accurate record is helpful in:

    a. keeping the patient from harm or embarrassment.
    b. ensuring and maintaining patient confidentiality.
    c. averting further legal action during the "discovery phase" of a lawsuit.
    d. developing a plan for definitive treatment.

15. A phrase like _____ is an example of an extraneous or unprofessional statement the paramedic should avoid in documenting the PCR.

    a. "The patient had the beating coming to him."
    b. "The skell just wanted another ride across town."
    c. "She is lonely and is just looking for a little attention."
    d. "The patient stated she vomited four times last night."

16. You are charting a PCR for your last patient and are documenting the intubation you performed. Which of the following aspects of this skill is extraneous information that you need not chart?

    a. the correction of a misplaced tube
    b. the depth of the tube and the method of securing
    c. at least three methods of ensuring correct tube placement
    d. the length and design of stylet used to facilitate the intubation

17. Select the statement that is an example of a pertinent negative the paramedic would document about a patient.

    a. A patient struck his head in an MVC and denies a loss of consciousness.
    b. A patient with dyspnea denies a smoking history of more than ten years.
    c. A patient with a lengthy medical list denies any allergies to medications.
    d. A patient in an MVC has never been involved in a collision until now.

18. _____ findings are information the patient or bystanders tell the paramedic.

    a. Subjective
    b. Neutral
    c. Objective
    d. Biased

19. _____ findings are information the paramedic can measure, such as vital signs.

    a. Subjective
    b. Neutral
    c. Objective
    d. Lawful

20. Patients have a right to have their medical records be:

    a. held from third-party billing agencies.
    b. withheld from medical students.
    c. partially restricted from their HMOs.
    d. held in confidence.

21. You are caring for a patient with acute abdominal pain. He is pale and diaphoretic. During your examination of his abdomen, he tells you he is feeling dizzy and is nauseated. Which of the following will you document as an *objective* finding on the PCR?

    a. nausea
    b. dizziness
    c. pale, diaphoretic skin
    d. acute abdominal pain

22. It is necessary to document multiple sets of vital signs on the PCR:

    a. only when the patient is unstable.
    b. to show trends in the patient's condition.
    c. only when interventions have been applied.
    d. only when the baseline vital signs are abnormal.

23. When documentation is anything less than complete or accurate, the presumption is that the paramedic either did not do the proper care or:

    a. had a bad day.
    b. forgot to include something.
    c. had something to hide.
    d. was not trained properly.

24. You are evaluating a twenty-year-old male with a traumatic injury to the hand and wrist. While at work, his right hand became entangled in equipment, causing it to bend backward in hyperextension. When you document the MOI, which of the following standard terms or planes can you use to describe the injury?

    a. protraction
    b. dorsiflexion
    c. lateral rotation
    d. cephalad extension

25. The documentation for starting IVs in the field should include all the following information, *except*:

    a. size of the angio used.
    b. who started the IV.
    c. who adjusted the drip rate.
    d. the number of attempts if the first was not successful.

26. Most often there is additional documentation associated with the administration of narcotics. Which of the following is not included in that information?

    a. the patient's name
    b. the patient's medical insurance information
    c. the physician who authorized the administration
    d. what effect the medication had on the patient

27. Which of the following is often used as the first line of documentation at an MCI?

    a. donning identification vests
    b. triage tags
    c. labeling sectors
    d. recording transportation destinations

28. You have arrived at the ED with a pediatric patient who you suspect is a victim of child abuse. As this type of call is mandatory reporting in every state, you will:

    a. complete a special incident form.
    b. follow your state and local guidelines.
    c. document your suspicions on the PCR.
    d. provide a written statement to the state police.

29. When making corrections of a recorded error on a PCR, which of the following is the incorrect way to make the change?

    a. Initial and date the mistaken entry.
    b. Draw a single line through the entry.
    c. Write "error" above or next to the entry.
    d. Erase the entry.

30. Which of the following is an example of an unusual situation that the paramedic should record on a PCR?

    a. During the transport, your ambulance passed by a serious MVC.
    b. While immobilizing an extremity that was swollen and deformed, the patient cried out in pain.
    c. Radio failure delayed contact with medical control and subsequent medical orders.
    d. After transferring the patient to a bed in the ED and giving the report, the patient became unresponsive.

31. Documentation of which of the following findings is vital in defending your care of a patient with a suspected fracture or dislocation?

    a. adequacy of the neurovascular supply before and after immobilization
    b. the manner in which the fracture/dislocation was immobilized
    c. the type of splint used
    d. the use of analgesia for pain management

32. If a patient makes statements to questions that do not appear in a check box on the PCR, the paramedic should:

    a. paraphrase the patient's statement into the narrative.
    b. document the statement in "quotes."
    c. use a special incident form for complete accuracy.
    d. write in additional check boxes.

33. The PCR is a legal document in which the paramedic should assure that the expressions and terms used are:

    a. derogatory.
    b. approved by the DOH.
    c. standardized and professional.
    d. judgment biased.

34. When a paramedic documents information about a patient's medication that is being taken "four times a day," which of the following would she use?

    a. q.d.
    b. q.i.d.
    c. t.i.d.
    d. p.r.n.

35. An example of a situation that is not typically documented on a PCR is the:

    a. patient had to be restrained.
    b. patient was hostile or abusive.
    c. patient's marital status.
    d. patient's date of birth.

36. Standardization of the data elements to be included in all PCRs helps to make it easier to:

    a. facilitate corroborating testimony in court.
    b. avoid litigation in the future.
    c. compare data from different agencies.
    d. document the disposition of the call.

37. Which of the following is meant by the document should "stand on its own"?

    a. The record contains everything it should in a clear, legible, and concise fashion.
    b. The record does not contain unprofessional language.
    c. The record does not contain any pertinent negatives.
    d. There are no documented errors.

38. Two types of narrative formats used in documentation of PCRs are:

    a. SOAP and CHART.
    b. CUPS and AVPU.
    c. PMHx and OPQRST.
    d. SAMPLE and APGAR.

39. Ensuring that your documentation is complete, accurate, and legible is one of the _____ of the paramedic.

    a. standing orders
    b. local protocols
    c. professional responsibilities
    d. state DOH regulations

40. Legally, with whom are you not allowed to share a patient's medical information?

    a. the healthcare provider continuing care
    b. a lawyer with a subpoena
    c. a police officer who is a friend of the patient
    d. third-party billing companies

41. Which of the following situations requires extra attention to detail when documenting a PCR?

    a. MCI
    b. Refuse Medical Assistance (RMA)
    c. correcting an error
    d. all of the above

42. When the paramedic documents a call where the patient is refusing care or transport, yet strongly feels that the patient needs medical attention, which of the following should be recorded?

    a. the specific recommendation for care and transport, and consequences of refusing care
    b. a statement that describes your opinion of how difficult and obnoxious the patient was
    c. a subjective reference to how ignorant and indifferent the patient was to your efforts to take care of him
    d. the patient's Social Security number, driver's license number, and insurance information, if possible

43. Ideally, the best time for the paramedic to complete a PCR on a patient is:

    a. en route to the hospital.
    b. while waiting to transfer the patient to a bed.
    c. at the ED, after transfer of the patient to a bed.
    d. after returning to your station from the ED.

44. The part of a PCR that contains the written report that depicts the call is the:

    a. narrative.
    b. addendum.
    c. administrative section.
    d. demographic section.

45. When documenting assessment findings, which of the following is not necessary to record?

    a. pertinent positives
    b. pertinent negatives
    c. normal findings
    d. all findings should be recorded

46. _____ is the writing of false and malicious statements intended to damage a person's character.

    a. Bias
    b. Jargon
    c. Slander
    d. Libel

47. Which of the following statements about documenting PCRs is most correct?

    a. All personnel and resources involved in the call should be recorded.
    b. Using various formats when documenting helps the paramedic to become a proficient narrator.
    c. When documentation is complete, accurate, and legible, there is no chance of becoming involved in litigation.
    d. The discovery phase is the only time a lawyer will be able to gain access to your documentation.

48. Which of the following is a standard term used by the paramedic in documenting something that is situated near the surface of the body?

    a. superior
    b. sagittal
    c. efferent
    d. superficial

49. _____ is a common medical suffix that means stopping or controlling.

    a. -stasis
    b. -stomy
    c. -scopy
    d. -plasty

50. When a paramedic sees the prefix _____, he can recognize that the term is referring to the kidney.

    a. nephr/o-
    b. hepat/o-
    c. gangli/o-
    d. dacry/o-

Exam #20 Answer Form

	A	B	C	D		A	B	C	D
1.	❏	❏	❏	❏	26.	❏	❏	❏	❏
2.	❏	❏	❏	❏	27.	❏	❏	❏	❏
3.	❏	❏	❏	❏	28.	❏	❏	❏	❏
4.	❏	❏	❏	❏	29.	❏	❏	❏	❏
5.	❏	❏	❏	❏	30.	❏	❏	❏	❏
6.	❏	❏	❏	❏	31.	❏	❏	❏	❏
7.	❏	❏	❏	❏	32.	❏	❏	❏	❏
8.	❏	❏	❏	❏	33.	❏	❏	❏	❏
9.	❏	❏	❏	❏	34.	❏	❏	❏	❏
10.	❏	❏	❏	❏	35.	❏	❏	❏	❏
11.	❏	❏	❏	❏	36.	❏	❏	❏	❏
12.	❏	❏	❏	❏	37.	❏	❏	❏	❏
13.	❏	❏	❏	❏	38.	❏	❏	❏	❏
14.	❏	❏	❏	❏	39.	❏	❏	❏	❏
15.	❏	❏	❏	❏	40.	❏	❏	❏	❏
16.	❏	❏	❏	❏	41.	❏	❏	❏	❏
17.	❏	❏	❏	❏	42.	❏	❏	❏	❏
18.	❏	❏	❏	❏	43.	❏	❏	❏	❏
19.	❏	❏	❏	❏	44.	❏	❏	❏	❏
20.	❏	❏	❏	❏	45.	❏	❏	❏	❏
21.	❏	❏	❏	❏	46.	❏	❏	❏	❏
22.	❏	❏	❏	❏	47.	❏	❏	❏	❏
23.	❏	❏	❏	❏	48.	❏	❏	❏	❏
24.	❏	❏	❏	❏	49.	❏	❏	❏	❏
25.	❏	❏	❏	❏	50.	❏	❏	❏	❏

21

Pulmonary and Respiratory

1. The process where oxygenated blood is pumped to the tissues, and waste products returned to the lungs, is called:

   a. respiration.
   b. ventilation.
   c. diffusion.
   d. perfusion.

2. _____ refers specifically to the exchange of carbon dioxide, while _____ refers only to the exchange of oxygen.

   a. Ventilation; oxygenation
   b. Oxygenation; ventilation
   c. Diffusion; oxygenation
   d. Perfusion; ventilation

3. A shift in the oxyhemoglobin saturation curve indicates a change in the affinity of hemoglobin for oxygen. A/an _____ shift decreases it, while a _____ shift of the curve increases the binding (affinity) of oxygen to hemoglobin.

   a. upward; rightward
   b. downward; leftward
   c. rightward; leftward
   d. leftward; rightward

4. When a person develops a fever, the cell's metabolic rate increases and so:

   a. a leftward shift of the oxyhemoglobin saturation curve occurs.
   b. does his oxygen need.
   c. does his hemoglobin need.
   d. a downward shift of the oxyhemoglobin saturation curve occurs.

5. Which of the following factors causes a shift in the oxyhemoglobin curve, decreasing the tissue oxygen delivery?

   a. decreased body temperature
   b. increased body temperature
   c. acidosis
   d. increased metabolic rate

6. The pCO_2 measures ventilation (exchange of carbon dioxide). Normal levels of pCO_2 are _____ mmHg.

   a. 7.35–7.45
   b. 7.40–7.50
   c. 35–40
   d. 40–45

7. pCO_2 is a respiratory:

   a. side-effect.
   b. alkali.
   c. basic.
   d. acid.

8. For every 10 mmHg change of the pCO_2, either up or down, the result is a _____ change in the pH in the opposite direction.

   a. 0.1
   b. 1.0
   c. 1.5
   d. 10.0

9. The pO_2 measures oxygenation at sea level and should normally run greater than _____ mmHg.

   a. 30
   b. 50
   c. 70
   d. 80

10. Which of the following statements about blood gases is correct?

    a. Changes in pO_2 always occur when there is a change in pCO_2.
    b. The only predictable and reproducible relation in blood gases is between the pH and the pCO_2.
    c. Hypoventilation leads to decreased pO_2 and decreased pCO_2.
    d. Hyperventilation raises the pCO_2 and the pO_2.

11. In respiratory acidosis, CO_2 retention leads to increased levels of:

    a. O_2.
    b. pO_2.
    c. pCO_2.
    d. SpO_2.

12. A patient who is hypoventilating, because of a heroin overdose, is most likely experiencing which acid-base disorder?

    a. respiratory acidosis
    b. respiratory alkalosis
    c. metabolic acidosis
    d. metabolic alkalosis

13. Which of the following is a possible cause of an upper airway obstruction?

    a. tonsillitis
    b. pleural effusion
    c. pulmonary embolus
    d. bronchoconstriction

14. Which of the following is not a cause of lower airway obstruction?

    a. empyema
    b. epiglottitis
    c. smooth muscle spasm
    d. obstructive lung disease

15. Which of the following is an example of a perfusion-related factor that may impair gas exchange in the lungs?

    a. FBAO
    b. anemia
    c. epiglottitis
    d. smooth muscle spasm

16. A person with multiple sclerosis or muscular dystrophy may, because of her disease, experience respiratory abnormalities that affect ventilation by:

    a. foreign body obstruction.
    b. impairment of circulatory blood flow.
    c. impairment of chest wall movement.
    d. developing inadequate hemoglobin levels.

17. Audible stridor is a potentially life-threatening sign of respiratory distress that should alert you to the possibility of any of the following, *except*:

    a. asthma.
    b. croup.
    c. epiglottits.
    d. foreign body airway obstruction (FBAO).

18. The presence of grunting is usually a sign of respiratory distress that occurs primarily in infants and small toddlers when the child breathes:

    a. in against a partially closed epiglottis.
    b. in against an airway obstruction.
    c. out against a partially closed epiglottis.
    d. out against an airway obstruction.

19. Which of the following are nonspecific findings associated with respiratory distress?

    a. grunting and wheezing
    b. pallor and diaphoresis
    c. cyanosis and dyspnea
    d. AMS or confusion

20. You are reassessing an adult patient having an asthma attack after administering one nebulized treatment of albuterol and Atrovent. The patient initially was pale and had bilateral wheezing in the apices, and her SpO_2 was in the 90s. She looks no better, and her SpO_2 is now 89, but she is no longer wheezing. Assessment of which of the following can best guide your continued treatment plan with this patient?

    a. pulse rate
    b. mentation
    c. SpO_2 reading
    d. patient's position of comfort

21. When obtaining a focused history from a patient with a pulmonary disease, history of previous intubation is:

    a. an indicator of severe pulmonary disease.
    b. a nonspecific finding associated with respiratory distress.
    c. an indication that you will need to intubate the patient.
    d. not suggestive that intubation may be required again.

22. Certain medications, such as _____, can affect the ability of the sympathetic nervous system to cause bronchodilation and may cause or worsen obstructive lung disease.

    a. antianginals
    b. beta-blockers
    c. inhaled steroids
    d. oral corticosteroids

23. Typical findings associated with _____ include acute chest pain on the affected side, increased respiratory rate, and coughing.

    a. lung cancer
    b. pulmonary edema
    c. upper-respiratory infection
    d. spontaneous pneumothorax

24. The most common cause of spontaneous pneumothorax in an adult is:

    a. COPD.
    b. menstruation.
    c. a congenital bleb.
    d. lung disease involving the connective tissue of the lung.

25. In the face of a respiratory problem, _____ is an ominous sign of severe hypoxemia and suggests imminent cardiac arrest.

    a. a low SpO$_2$ reading
    b. tachypnea
    c. tachycardia
    d. bradycardia

26. The respiratory pattern that is characterized by alternating periods of apnea and deep, rapid breathing is called:

    a. eupnea.
    b. central neurogenic hyperventilation.
    c. Kussmaul.
    d. Cheyne-Stokes.

27. The type of breathing characterized by a series of several short inspirations followed by long, irregular periods of apnea, and associated with increased intracranial pressure, is called:

    a. central neurogen hyperventilation.
    b. ataxic.
    c. apneustic.
    d. Cheyne-Stokes.

28. The most common types of abnormal respiratory patterns seen in the field include tachypnea, bradypnea, apnea, and:

    a. eupnea.
    b. Biot's.
    c. Kussmaul's.
    d. Cheyne-Stokes.

29. Many forms of lung disease cause increased resistance to blood flow in the lungs, causing the right heart to work harder. The heart compensates initially, but later is unable to maintain compensatory efforts, resulting in:

    a. right heart failure.
    b. left heart failure.
    c. pursed-lip breathing.
    d. decreased pulmonary resistance.

30. You have been dispatched to a nursing home for a patient with severe respiratory distress. The patient is a seventy-eight-year-old female with low SpO$_2$ readings (in the 80s). You perform a physical exam and find that the patient has distended neck veins (JVD), wet crackles in the bases of her lungs, peripheral edema, and ascites. Her vital signs are: respiratory rate, 40; pulse rate, 90/irregular; BP, 176/98; and skin CTC is cyanotic, warm, and dry. Based on your findings, what is this patient's primary problem?

    a. pneumonia
    b. lung cancer
    c. right-sided heart failure
    d. obstructive airway disease

31. The _____ deformity seen in some COPD and asthma patients is caused by _____ expiratory resistance to flow and air-trapping.

    a. barrel chest; increased
    b. pigeon chest; increased
    c. barrel chest; decreased
    d. pigeon chest; decreased

32. Crackles heard when breathing result from fluid in the airways, in the interstitial tissue, or in:

    a. both.
    b. a friction rub.
    c. pleurisy.
    d. pericarditis.

33. _____ spasm is a spasmodic contraction of the hands, wrists, feet, and ankles, which is associated with decreased levels of carbon dioxide.

    a. Hypocapopedal
    b. Carbonix
    c. Carpopedal
    d. Carbondorsal

34. Continuous positive airway pressure face masks improve oxygenation in many diseases, including asthma, COPD, and:

    a. sleep apnea.
    b. neoplasm of the lung.
    c. tension pneumothorax.
    d. spontaneous pneumothorax.

35. Capnography measures _____, or how much carbon dioxide is exhaled.

    a. end-tidal CO$_2$
    b. pO$_2$
    c. pCO$_2$
    d. peak flow

36. The most common obstructive airway diseases include asthma and:

    a. URI.
    b. COPD.
    c. cystic fibrosis.
    d. Legionnaires' disease.

37. You have successfully intubated a patient who was in near respiratory arrest as a result of a severe asthma attack. En route to the hospital, the patient is becoming alert and is attempting to pull on the endotracheal tube. Which of the following actions should you take now?

    a. Administer Versed 0.05 mg/kg.
    b. Prepare to extubate the patient.
    c. Administer Solumedrol 125 mg IV.
    d. Administer magnesium 2 grams IV in 50 ml NS over ten minutes.

38. During bronchospasm, the tiny muscle layers surrounding the bronchioles go into spasm and narrow the lumen of the airways. The result is:

    a. irritation.
    b. wheezing.
    c. snoring.
    d. coughing.

39. During an acute asthma attack, mucus production is increased because of _____ in the bronchial airways.

    a. irritation
    b. wheezing
    c. snoring
    d. coughing

40. _____ are the most common asthma triggers.

    a. Chewing tobaccos
    b. Car fumes
    c. Respiratory infections
    d. Flower spores

41. Exercise or fast breathing is a trigger for asthma attacks, especially during _____ weather.

    a. hot
    b. cold
    c. humid
    d. rainy

42. Any condition that leads to _____ may cause carpopedal spasm.

    a. respiratory acidosis
    b. respiratory alkalosis
    c. metabolic acidosis
    d. metabolic alkalosis

43. _____ is a highly specific diagnosis consisting of high permeability pulmonary edema, due to any of several causes, and the inability to adequately oxygenate the blood despite 100% FiO_2.

    a. Status asthmaticus
    b. Ventilation-perfusion mismatch
    c. Adult respiratory distress syndrome
    d. Chronic obstructive pulmonary disease

44. _____ is a severe, prolonged asthma attack that does not respond to standard medications.

    a. Acute bronchial asthma
    b. Status asthmaticus
    c. Allergy-induced asthma
    d. Exercise-induced asthma

45. Death rates from asthma continue to soar despite all of the current knowledge about asthma. Two factors that underlie the fatal trend include decreased airway sensitivity and:

    a. inadequate use of anti-inflammatory medication.
    b. the lack of peak flow meter use.
    c. increased use of antibiotics.
    d. increased exposure to the Lyme-carrying tick.

46. _____ results from overgrowth of the airway mucus glands and excess secretion of mucus that blocks the airway.

    a. Asthma
    b. Chronic bronchitis
    c. Emphysema
    d. Exacerbation

47. _____ results from destruction of the walls of the alveoli, which leads to a decrease in elastic recoil.

    a. Asthma
    b. Chronic bronchitis
    c. Emphysema
    d. Legionnaires' disease

48. Which of the following is the major cause of COPD?

    a. air pollution
    b. cigarette smoking
    c. tuberculosis
    d. asbestos

49. Victims of asthma attacks will have symptoms that _____, as compared with persons with COPD.

    a. are wheezing in nature
    b. are associated with smoking
    c. progressively worsen over several days
    d. come on relatively quickly

50. A young child is presenting with acute respiratory distress and audible wheezing. He has no history of asthma and takes no medications. Which of the following do you attempt to rule out first?

    a. FBAO
    b. COPD
    c. toxic inhalation
    d. asthma

51. Epinephrine, terbutaline, and albuterol all have _____ effects, which are potentially useful in the treatment of obstructive lung disease.

    a. bronchoconstricting
    b. bronchodilating
    c. vasoconstricting
    d. anti-inflammatory

52. Steriods are beneficial in the chronic treatment of nearly all asthma patients and many COPD patients because of the _____ effects.

    a. smooth muscle relaxing
    b. bronchodilating
    c. vasoconstricting
    d. anti-inflammatory

53. The inhaled steroids used in the first line of the treatment of asthma and COPD patients result in _____ side effects than the oral preparations.

    a. more
    b. fewer
    c. the same
    d. different

54. Some EMS systems administer steroids, because these drugs:

    a. take at least one or two hours to work.
    b. work immediately.
    c. are of no benefit after the first thirty minutes of intervention of respiratory distress.
    d. are of minimal benefit after the first thirty minutes of intervention of respiratory distress.

55. _____ is/are one of the major inflammation-causing compounds produced in asthma.

    a. Glucocorticoids
    b. Latex
    c. Leukotrienes
    d. Leukocites

56. Magnesium sulfate has been shown to be of some benefit to some asthmatic patients, primarily because of its _____ effects.

    a. smooth muscle relaxing
    b. bronchodilating
    c. vasoconstricting
    d. anti-inflammatory

57. The accumulation of carbon dioxide in blood is the major stimulus that normally causes:

    a. altered mental status.
    b. hormonal secretions.
    c. us to breathe.
    d. fluid retention.

58. Cigarette smoke directly inhibits the normal:

    a. movement of mucus via bronchial cilia out of the lungs.
    b. response to breathe in teens.
    c. immune response in the elderly.
    d. hormonal response in postmenopausal women.

59. Chronic alcoholics have an increased risk of respiratory infections because of:

    a. decreased thermoregulatory systems.
    b. weakened immune systems caused by ethanol.
    c. increased exposure to hypothermia.
    d. decreased hepatic functions.

60. Which of the following risk factors makes people more likely to get pneumonia?

    a. organ transplant
    b. insulin-dependent diabetes
    c. prolonged acute hypothermia
    d. all of the above

61. Which of the following statements about pneumonia is most correct?

    a. Most pneumonias are caused by viruses.
    b. The clinical approach to viral or bacterial pneumonia is the same.
    c. The clinical approach to viral or bacterial pneumonia is different.
    d. It is possible to tell the difference between viral and bacterial pneumonia in the prehospital setting.

62. A secondary mechanism that stimulates breathing is a lack of oxygen in the blood and is called:

    a. carbon dioxide drive.
    b. hypoxic drive.
    c. bicarboxic force.
    d. bicarbonic influence.

63. Which of the following is an atypical finding associated with pneumonia?

    a. productive cough
    b. pleuritic chest pain
    c. nonproductive cough
    d. decreased breath sounds

64. Atypical symptoms are more common in viral pneumonia, and in the very young or very old. These can include all of the following, *except*:

    a. headache.
    b. muscle aches.
    c. sore throat.
    d. syncope.

65. What should be the primary concern for the paramedic when treating a patient who may have pneumonia?

    a. respiratory distress
    b. respiratory failure
    c. exposure to a contagious patient
    d. severe dehydration

66. Out-of-hospital treatment for respiratory distress with drug therapy of _____ may be helpful, especially if the patient has accompanying obstructive lung disease.

    a. Ventolin
    b. antibiotics
    c. aspirin
    d. calcium

67. Influenza is a specific type of _____ infection that may affect both the upper and lower respiratory tracts.

    a. viral
    b. bacterial
    c. fungal
    d. spore

68. It is impossible to differentiate viral URI from a bacterial URI without:

    a. a good past medical history.
    b. cultures.
    c. the presence of an elevated temperature.
    d. a visit to the emergency department.

69. Most patients with upper respiratory infections (URIs) have spontaneous resolution of their symptoms within seven days:

    a. only when they go to the ED.
    b. only when they see their own MD.
    c. with or without antibiotics.
    d. with or without an underlying disease.

70. Select the statement that is most accurate about URIs.

    a. Some URIs cause bronchoconstriction.
    b. The terms URI and influenza are nearly interchangeable.
    c. URIs are self-limiting and rarely develop into serious complications.
    d. Only people with underlying disease experience two or more URIs a year.

71. A patient who presents with URI and has had his _____ removed is at grave risk for a life-threatening illness.

    a. lung
    b. appendix
    c. spleen
    d. gallbladder

72. The most common cause of primary lung tumors is:

    a. coal miner's lung.
    b. asbestosis.
    c. cigarette smoking.
    d. heredity.

73. Patients with massive pulmonary emboli often suffer a syncopal spell or _____ as the first symptom of the illness.

    a. cardiac arrest
    b. nausea and vomiting
    c. high pressure pulmonary edema
    d. high permeability pulmonary edema

74. A patient who just received treatment with chemotherapy for lung cancer would most likely have which of the following complaints?

    a. nausea, vomiting, and weakness
    b. diaphoresis and shortness of breath
    c. chest pain
    d. vision and equilibrium disturbances

75. A patient who, earlier in the day, received treatment with radiotherapy for lung cancer would most likely experience which of the following symptoms?

    a. fever and chills
    b. dizziness and chest pain
    c. dry cough or shortness of breath
    d. nausea vomiting, and weakness

76. Some lung tumors lead to abnormal production of parathyroid hormone, which causes bone breakdown, _____ serum _____ levels.

    a. lowering; calcium
    b. raising; calcium
    c. lowering; potassium
    d. raising; potassium

77. Persons with acute pulmonary edema caused by _____ have "severe congestive heart failure," but not all patients with "severe congestive heart failure" have pulmonary edema.

    a. ARDS
    b. scorpion bites
    c. pericarditis
    d. cardiac ischemia

78. The primary difference between pulmonary edema and congestive heart failure (CHF) is:

    a. pulmonary edema develops progressively, and CHF does not.
    b. only pulmonary edema is associated with ARDS.
    c. CHF is a spectrum of conditions associated with decreases in cardiac function.
    d. only CHF can be exacerbated by asthma or COPD.

79. Patients with CHF or pulmonary edema may have orthopnea because:

    a. the recumbent position increased venous return to the heart.
    b. the recumbent position decreased venous return to the heart.
    c. these patients have a decreased preload mechanism.
    d. these patients are usually obese, and this increases pulmonary resistance.

80. The role of nitroglycerine in the treatment of patients with acute pulmonary edema is:

    a. to dilate the veins.
    b. to dilate the arteries.
    c. vasodilation of both veins and arteries.
    d. decreasing lymphatic flow from the lungs.

81. Furosemide has all of the following effects in the treatment of acute pulmonary edema, *except*:

    a. vasodilation.
    b. increased lymphatic flow from the lungs.
    c. diuretic effects.
    d. increased cardiac preload.

82. Besides the analgesic effect, morphine sulfate also has which of the following effects on the patient with acute pulmonary edema?

    a. reduces cardiac preload and afterload
    b. increases cardiac preload and afterload
    c. increases cerebral diuresis
    d. has an amnesic affect

83. ACE inhibitors have been used to treat hypertension and CHF for years. The way they work is by blocking:

    a. the hormone aldosterone on the kidneys.
    b. the conversion of angiotensin I to angiotensin II in the lungs.
    c. the collapse of portions of the lung and improving overall ventilation.
    d. vasoconstriction of cardiac arteries.

84. The role of simple positive pressure in the treatment of patients with respiratory distress is to:

    a. decrease intrathoracic pressure.
    b. increase intrathoracic pressure.
    c. regulate pulmonary pressures independently.
    d. regulate pulmonary pressure.

85. A thirty-three-year-old male suddenly develops sharp chest pain and shortness of breath. His wife tells you that the patient has been sick with a cold for a nearly a week. He has been coughing more frequently since the pain began; he states that the pain is stabbing and points to the left chest. Except for smoking, the patient denies any significant past medical history. Vital signs are: respiratory rate, 34/diminished on the right side; pulse rate, 112/regular; BP 140/80; and skin CTC is warm, moist, and good color. What do you suspect is the patient's problem?

    a. pulmonary embolism
    b. acute myocardial infarction
    c. spontaneous pneumothorax
    d. new onset of bronchial asthma

86. Which of the following is not considered a high risk factor for pulmonary embolism?

    a. prolonged bed rest
    b. obesity
    c. pregnancy
    d. IUD contraceptive use

87. The pathology of a pulmonary embolism includes the emboli becoming lodged in:

   a. pulmonary arterial circulation.
   b. pulmonary venous circulation.
   c. deep veins.
   d. the right heart.

88. The occlusion that results from a pulmonary embolism not only results in decreased blood supply to the affected area, but also leads to the release of histamines, which causes _____ in the region of the clot.

   a. bronchospasm
   b. ACS
   c. bronchodilation
   d. tissue necrosis

89. Which of the following conditions can mimic a pulmonary embolism?

   a. hypertensive crisis
   b. ACS
   c. labor
   d. hypoglycemia

90. Which of the following has more significance in the differential diagnosis of a pulmonary embolism than the others?

   a. the presence or absence of pleuritic chest pain
   b. history of a recent URI
   c. use of diuretics
   d. smoking history

91. The most common physical finding associated with pulmonary embolism includes tachypnea and:

   a. cyanosis.
   b. wheezing.
   c. peripheral edema.
   d. tachycardia.

92. Which of the following profiles is most often associated with spontaneous pneumothorax?

   a. elderly, obese, male smoker
   b. elderly, thin, female smoker
   c. young, tall, male smoker
   d. young, petite, female smoker

93. The pathology of hyperventilation results in _____ levels of carbon dioxide and _____ the pH.

   a. low; increases
   b. low; decreases
   c. high; increases
   d. high; decreases

94. What is the major risk in caring for a patient presenting with hyperventilation?

   a. recognizing that the patient is hypoxic
   b. understanding that hyperventilation is caused by many illnesses
   c. assuming that the patient is experiencing a simple anxiety attack
   d. providing high-flow oxygen to a patient in a state of hypocapnea

95. You are treating a patient who is experiencing acute pulmonary edema, but the patient is refusing to wear an oxygen mask. Which of the following is most appropriate for the patient?

   a. Insist that the patient needs the oxygen, and apply the mask anyway.
   b. Offer the patient a nasal cannula.
   c. Consider the need for a ventilator.
   d. Ask medical control for authorization to perform RSI.

96. Your patient is a thirty-six-year-old male who has a c/c of acute non-exertional dyspnea that is getting progressively worse. Wheezing is heard on auscultation, but there is no PMHx of any obstructive respiratory or cardiac diseases. The only medication he takes is O-T-C Motrin® for pain in the leg from a fracture two months ago. Which of the following conditions do you suspect is causing the dyspnea?

   a. pulmonary embolism
   b. spontaneous pneumothorax
   c. hyperventilation syndrome
   d. early CHF

97. When considering the pathology for the cause of the dyspnea described in question 96, which of the following is the most likely cause?

   a. fat embolus from bone marrow
   b. ruptured congenital bleb
   c. anxiety
   d. ACS

98. A slender twenty-four-year-old male is complaining of an acute onset of non-exertional sharp chest pain on the right side and shortness of breath. He is a smoker with a history of a nonproductive cough for two days. Breath sounds are decreased on the right side and vital signs are R/R 36, H/R 116, and B/P 100/80. Which of the following conditions do you suspect?

   a. pneumonia
   b. pulmonary embolus
   c. spontaneous pneumothorax
   d. AMI

99. You are dispatched to an office building for a twenty-eight-year-old female complaining of dizziness and numbness in her hands and legs. Coworkers tell you that the patient has been under a lot of stress, and today she has been especially anxious. The patient denies S.O.B., chest pain, or any recent illnesses, and her vital signs are stable. Based on the initial findings, what do you suspect is the cause of the patient's extremity numbness?

a. CVA
b. TIA
c. psychologic
d. carpopedal spasm

100. Further information about the patient described in question 99 confirms that the patient was hyperventilating prior to EMS arriving. The patient has a PMHx of asthma but has not had an attack in months. Your initial management of this patient includes:

a. providing high-flow oxygen and watching for changes in mental status.
b. withholding oxygen to see if the numbness resolves.
c. beginning an albuterol treatment.
d. calling medical control for advice.

Exam #21 Answer Form

	A	B	C	D			A	B	C	D
1.	❏	❏	❏	❏		26.	❏	❏	❏	❏
2.	❏	❏	❏	❏		27.	❏	❏	❏	❏
3.	❏	❏	❏	❏		28.	❏	❏	❏	❏
4.	❏	❏	❏	❏		29.	❏	❏	❏	❏
5.	❏	❏	❏	❏		30.	❏	❏	❏	❏
6.	❏	❏	❏	❏		31.	❏	❏	❏	❏
7.	❏	❏	❏	❏		32.	❏	❏	❏	❏
8.	❏	❏	❏	❏		33.	❏	❏	❏	❏
9.	❏	❏	❏	❏		34.	❏	❏	❏	❏
10.	❏	❏	❏	❏		35.	❏	❏	❏	❏
11.	❏	❏	❏	❏		36.	❏	❏	❏	❏
12.	❏	❏	❏	❏		37.	❏	❏	❏	❏
13.	❏	❏	❏	❏		38.	❏	❏	❏	❏
14.	❏	❏	❏	❏		39.	❏	❏	❏	❏
15.	❏	❏	❏	❏		40.	❏	❏	❏	❏
16.	❏	❏	❏	❏		41.	❏	❏	❏	❏
17.	❏	❏	❏	❏		42.	❏	❏	❏	❏
18.	❏	❏	❏	❏		43.	❏	❏	❏	❏
19.	❏	❏	❏	❏		44.	❏	❏	❏	❏
20.	❏	❏	❏	❏		45.	❏	❏	❏	❏
21.	❏	❏	❏	❏		46.	❏	❏	❏	❏
22.	❏	❏	❏	❏		47.	❏	❏	❏	❏
23.	❏	❏	❏	❏		48.	❏	❏	❏	❏
24.	❏	❏	❏	❏		49.	❏	❏	❏	❏
25.	❏	❏	❏	❏		50.	❏	❏	❏	❏

	A	B	C	D			A	B	C	D
51.	❏	❏	❏	❏		76.	❏	❏	❏	❏
52.	❏	❏	❏	❏		77.	❏	❏	❏	❏
53.	❏	❏	❏	❏		78.	❏	❏	❏	❏
54.	❏	❏	❏	❏		79.	❏	❏	❏	❏
55.	❏	❏	❏	❏		80.	❏	❏	❏	❏
56.	❏	❏	❏	❏		81.	❏	❏	❏	❏
57.	❏	❏	❏	❏		82.	❏	❏	❏	❏
58.	❏	❏	❏	❏		83.	❏	❏	❏	❏
59.	❏	❏	❏	❏		84.	❏	❏	❏	❏
60.	❏	❏	❏	❏		85.	❏	❏	❏	❏
61.	❏	❏	❏	❏		86.	❏	❏	❏	❏
62.	❏	❏	❏	❏		87.	❏	❏	❏	❏
63.	❏	❏	❏	❏		88.	❏	❏	❏	❏
64.	❏	❏	❏	❏		89.	❏	❏	❏	❏
65.	❏	❏	❏	❏		90.	❏	❏	❏	❏
66.	❏	❏	❏	❏		91.	❏	❏	❏	❏
67.	❏	❏	❏	❏		92.	❏	❏	❏	❏
68.	❏	❏	❏	❏		93.	❏	❏	❏	❏
69.	❏	❏	❏	❏		94.	❏	❏	❏	❏
70.	❏	❏	❏	❏		95.	❏	❏	❏	❏
71.	❏	❏	❏	❏		96.	❏	❏	❏	❏
72.	❏	❏	❏	❏		97.	❏	❏	❏	❏
73.	❏	❏	❏	❏		98.	❏	❏	❏	❏
74.	❏	❏	❏	❏		99.	❏	❏	❏	❏
75.	❏	❏	❏	❏		100.	❏	❏	❏	❏

Cardiology

1. The semilunar valves include the _____ valves.

   a. pulmonic and aortic
   b. pulmonic and mitral
   c. mitral and tricuspid
   d. tricuspid and aortic

2. When one or more valves become narrowed because of congenital damage, the valve is said to be:

   a. stenotic.
   b. murmured.
   c. regurgitant
   d. intrinsic.

3. The coronary sinus, a portion of the coronary circulation, is a large vein that opens into the:

   a. aorta.
   b. right atrium.
   c. vena cava.
   d. left ventricle.

4. While assessing a sixty-five-year-old female with atrial fibrillation, you discover that her radial pulse is less than her apical pulse. This finding is called:

   a. pulsus paradoxus.
   b. pulsus alternans.
   c. pulse deficit.
   d. pulse differential.

5. You are assessing the pulse rate and quality on a twenty-three-year-old male experiencing an asthma attack. You find that the pulse is strong, regular, and tachy; however, the pulse decreases considerably during inspiration. This phenomenon is called:

   a. pulsus paradoxus.
   b. pulsus alternans.
   c. pulse deficit.
   d. pulse differential.

6. The normal heart sound S1 is caused by vibrations caused by the sudden closure of the _____ valves at the start of ventricular systole.

   a. pulmonic and aortic
   b. pulmonic and mitral
   c. mitral and tricuspid
   d. tricuspid and aortic

7. The abnormal heart sound S3, though sometimes present in healthy young persons, most commonly is associated with moderate to severe:

   a. asthma.
   b. pulmonary embolism.
   c. stroke.
   d. heart failure.

8. The abnormal heart sound that occurs when inflammation is present in the parietal and visceral pericardium is a/an:

   a. murmur.
   b. pericardial friction rub.
   c. S4.
   d. S3.

9. The layer of the heart that lines the chambers of the heart and is continuous with the intima is the:

   a. epicardium.
   b. myocardium.
   c. endocardium.
   d. visceral pericardium.

10. Following a severe steering wheel chest impact, the pericardial space rapidly accumulates fluids, resulting in pericardial tamponade. In the average-size adult, tamponade can occur with as little as _____ milliliters of fluid.

    a. 25
    b. 50
    c. 75
    d. 100

11. A potentially fatal bacterial infection commonly affecting heart valves is:

    a. epicarditis.
    b. myocarditis.
    c. endocarditis.
    d. scarlet fever.

12. The majority of coronary artery blood flow and myocardial perfusion occurs during which phase of the cardiac cycle?

    a. systole
    b. diastole
    c. asystole
    d. effusion

13. The relationship between increased stroke volume and increased ventricular end-diastolic volume for a given intrinsic contractility is called:

    a. Beck's triad.
    b. Iowa pressure articulation.
    c. autoregulation.
    d. Starling's law of the heart.

14. When a drug's specific action is a negative chronotropic effect, what effect will it have on the heart?

    a. increased heart rate
    b. decreased heart rate
    c. increased force of muscular contractility
    d. decreased force of muscular contractility

15. When a drug has a positive inotropic effect, the drug will affect the heart in which of the following ways?

    a. increase heart rate
    b. decrease heart rate
    c. increase force of muscular contractility
    d. decrease force of muscular contractility

16. Patients who experience _____ pain most often will be able to localize the pain to a specific area.

    a. somatic
    b. idiopathic
    c. visceral
    d. neurotic

17. A twenty-five-year-old female is complaining of abdominal pain that she describes as intermittent and cramping. What type of pain is the patient most likely experiencing?

    a. somatic
    b. idiopathic
    c. visceral
    d. neurotic

18. Some diabetic patients experience an altered pain perception from a chronic nerve condition called:

    a. dyspepsia.
    b. neuropathy.
    c. parathesia.
    d. ghost pain.

19. People with the preexisting medical condition _____ are more likely to experience a "silent ACS" than those without it.

    a. hypertension
    b. diabetes
    c. Parkinson's
    d. esophageal reflux

20. When there is inadequate blood flow to an organ, such as the heart, _____ occurs initially.

    a. ischemia
    b. infarction
    c. stroke
    d. embolus

21. Fibrinolytics and blood thinners are used to treat occlusions of coronary arteries due to thrombi after an acute MI to restore blood flow. They are also used to treat:

    a. Marfan syndrome.
    b. pulmonary embolism.
    c. congestive heart failure.
    d. abdominal aortic aneurysm.

22. Pain that is felt at a site that is different from that of the injured or diseased part of the body is called:

    a. referred pain.
    b. irritation.
    c. inflammation.
    d. musculoskeletal.

23. The three primary components used for diagnosis of an acute MI include: cardiac enzyme analysis, abnormal ECG and/or ECG changes, and:

    a. vital signs.
    b. daily use of aspirin.
    c. history.
    d. prehospital treatment.

24. An atypical form of chest pain caused by vasospasm of otherwise normal coronary arteries is called _____ angina.

   a. stable
   b. unstable
   c. Wicket's
   d. Prinzmetal's

25. The most frequent cause of acute myocardial infarction (MI) is:

   a. coronary thrombosis.
   b. hypertension.
   c. trauma.
   d. use of recreational drugs.

26. Which of the following symptoms associated with ischemic chest pain is considered atypical for a forty-year-old male?

   a. dyspnea
   b. weakness
   c. diaphoresis
   d. indigestion

27. The ECG wave form that represents the impulse generated as the ventricles depolarize prior to contraction is the:

   a. PR interval.
   b. QRS complex.
   c. J point.
   d. QT interval.

28. ALS was dispatched for an unconscious seventy-two-year-old male. When you arrive, he is conscious, pale, diaphoretic, and supine on the floor. A bystander tells you that he complained of chest pain after waking up. Now the patient describes the pain as 8/10. While your partner administers oxygen, you determine that he is hypotensive, with a BP of 70/34, and has a third-degree heart block with a rate of 38. Which of the following interventions is most appropriate to apply first?

   a. Administer a fluid bolus and aspirin.
   b. Start an IV and administer a dose of atropine.
   c. Sedate the patient and begin transcutaneous pacing.
   d. Administer aspirin and nitroglycerin for the chest pain.

29. ST elevation is usually a sign of severe myocardial injury. However, other common causes of ST elevation that may be confused with ACS are:

   a. myocarditis and gout.
   b. syncope and pluerisy.
   c. acute pericarditis and Prinzmetal's angina.
   d. CHF and pulmonary effusion.

30. Patients with right ventricular infarcts often have problems with hypotension and decreased cardiac output, and are very sensitive to drugs that reduce preload, such as:

   a. nitroglycerine.
   b. aspirin.
   c. dopamine.
   d. morphine.

31. Twelve lead ECG analyses can help to identify the size and location of the infarct that occurs during an ACS, thus helping to guide treatment. A patient experiencing an inferior wall MI of the left ventricle may have abnormalities in which leads?

   a. V_1 and V_2
   b. V_3 and V_4
   c. II, III, and aVF
   d. I, aVL, V_5, and V_6

32. A patient experiencing an acute anterior wall MI of the left ventricle may have abnormalities in which leads?

   a. V_1 and V_2
   b. V_3 and V_4
   c. II, III, and aVF
   d. I, aVL, V_5, and V_6

33. A patient experiencing a septal wall MI may have abnormalities in which leads?

   a. V_1 and V_2
   b. V_3 and V_4
   c. II, III, and aVF
   d. I, aVL, V_5, and V_6

34. The use of drugs, electrolyte imbalances, electrical shock, and trauma are all mechanisms that can produce which of the following conditions?

   a. hypoglycemia
   b. cardiac dysrhythmias
   c. hypertension
   d. Wolff-Parkinson-White syndrome

35. You are interviewing a seventy-four-year-old woman who had a syncopal event while at the market with her daughter. Both the patient and daughter confirm that the patient has a history of periodic loss of consciousness caused by a heart block. They cannot remember what this condition is called, but you suspect which of the following conditions?

   a. unstable syncope
   b. unstable angina
   c. Wolff-Parkinson-White syndrome
   d. Adams-Stokes syndrome

36. Synchronized cardioversion is a timed shock delivered to the heart to convert abnormal rhythms to a normal rhythm. Synchronization is preferred over defibrillation in patients with a pulse because synchronization reduces the energy required to convert and:

    a. reduces the chance of post-shock dysrhythmias.
    b. increases the period of an extra-conduction pathway.
    c. reduces the possibility of pre-excitation syndrome.
    d. increases the stimulation of the relative refractory phase.

37. When injury to the myocardium affects the automaticity and the heart is no longer able to produce the normal pace or rhythm, the treatment of choice in the prehospital setting is:

    a. atropine.
    b. isoproterenol.
    c. external pacing.
    d. defibrillation.

38. When an ECG displays a short PR interval and a wide QRS complex, which characteristically shows early QRS widening referred to as a "delta wave," this is a clue that the patient has:

    a. a hypoxic heart.
    b. myocardial ischemia.
    c. Adams-Stokes syndrome.
    d. Wolff-Parkinson-White syndrome.

39. You are performing a focused history and physical examination for possible ACS on a fifty-five-year-old patient complaining of substernal chest pain and exertional dyspnea. Which of the following pieces of information from the patient's past medical history will rule out this patient as a candidate for reperfusion therapy?

    a. stable angina
    b. kidney disease
    c. mild hypertension
    d. appendectomy eighteen months ago

40. Cardiac muscle tissue has the ability to contract without neural stimulation. This property is called:

    a. self-excitation.
    b. automaticity.
    c. syncytium.
    d. depolarization.

41. Cardiac muscle tissue has the ability to conduct impulses much quicker than regular muscle cells, a property called:

    a. self-excitation.
    b. automaticity.
    c. syncytium.
    d. repolarization.

42. Many patients who take diuretics such as Lasix also take potassium to prevent _____, which is an excessive loss of potassium that occurs with diuresis.

    a. hypokalemia
    b. hyperkalemia
    c. hyponatremia
    d. hypercalcemia

43. When cardiac muscle tissue gets an altered amount of potassium, the effect on the heart is a/an:

    a. increased force of contraction.
    b. decreased force of contraction.
    c. slow heart rate.
    d. fast heart rate.

44. Cardiac muscle tissue uses three primary cations to effect depolarization and repolarization of the heart. These three include potassium, sodium, and:

    a. phosphate.
    b. gluconate.
    c. caitrate.
    d. calcium.

45. While working as part of a medic team standing by at a marathon, you are treating a runner who is exhausted. The patient's vital signs are R/R 16, BP 102/50, and H/R 42. After obtaining a focused history from the patient, which of the following is the most likely cause of the slow heart rate?

    a. use of supplemental salt tablets
    b. dehydration from overexertion
    c. heat stroke
    d. hypoglycemia

46. The pacemaker cells in the _____ of the heart normally initiate the electrical impulses that start the sequence of excitation and conduction through the heart.

    a. SA node
    b. AV node
    c. bundle branches
    d. Purkinje fibers

47. Backup cardiac pacemaker cells are often called _____, meaning that if the normal pacemaker fails, the next one below it will automatically take over stimulation of the entire sequence.

   a. action potential
   b. PVCs
   c. escape foci
   d. discharges

48. Acetylcholine, a neurotransmitter released by parasympathetic motor neurons, has which of the following effects on the heart?

   a. regulates normal contractions
   b. lowers stroke volume
   c. increases heart rate
   d. enhances automaticity

49. The catacholamine _____, released by the adrenal medulla and sympathetic neurons during sympathetic stimulation, increases stroke volume.

   a. dopamine
   b. norepinephrine
   c. epinephrine
   d. adenosine

50. Sympathetic nerves are located throughout the heart. The parasympathetic nerves are located primarily in the:

   a. bundle of His.
   b. Purkinje fibers.
   c. bundle branches.
   d. SA and AV nodes.

51. An irregular connection between the atria and the ventricles that bypasses the AV node is called a/an:

   a. reentry.
   b. aberration.
   c. accessory pathway.
   d. PVC.

52. When conduction of electrical impulses in the heart experiences an alteration of the repolarization wave from its normal direction, which is blocked, to another direction that is not blocked, this is known as:

   a. reentry.
   b. an aberration.
   c. accessory pathway.
   d. PVC.

53. When the heart muscle is injured and the ventricles can no longer pump effectively, the arterial pressures begin to change and:

   a. only the preload is affected.
   b. only the afterload is affected.
   c. the preload and afterload are directly affected.
   d. the preload and afterload are indirectly affected.

54. Hypertension is a devastating disease that places an increased workload on the heart. Specifically, the extra workload causes the left ventricle to:

   a. dystrophy.
   b. myotrophy.
   c. atrophy.
   d. hypertrophy.

55. The primary types of damage that occur with chronic hypertension are aneurysm, stroke, and:

   a. nausea.
   b. deep vein thrombosis.
   c. headache.
   d. renal failure.

56. The treatment plan for hypertensive crisis is to reduce the patient's blood pressure within one or two hours to avoid:

   a. an ACS.
   b. permanent organ damage.
   c. sudden death.
   d. atherosclerosis.

57. A normal defense mechanism designed to maintain cerebral perfusion after an insult such as a stroke or head injury is called:

   a. cerebral autoregulation.
   b. Beck's triad.
   c. hypotension.
   d. hyptertension.

58. A normal property of the brain that maintains cerebral perfusion within a fairly wide range of mean arterial blood pressures is known as:

   a. cerebral autoregulation.
   b. Beck's triad.
   c. Frank-Starling law.
   d. homeostasis.

59. An inflammation of a vein causing pain in the affected part of the body that is accompanied by stiffness and edema is called:

   a. phlebitis.
   b. ascites.
   c. thrombosis.
   d. angioedema.

60. A patient affected with Marfan syndrome may experience sudden death at an early age, usually from which of the following mechanisms?

   a. congestive heart failure
   b. spontaneous papillary rupture
   c. spontaneous pnuemothorax
   d. spontaneous rupture of the aorta

61. You are called to transport a sixty-five-year-old male for evaluation of severe pain in the left calf. The patient tells you the pain began suddenly while he was taking his daily walk, but now that he is sitting, the pain is subsiding. Which of the following conditions do you suspect?

   a. edema
   b. ascites
   c. claudication
   d. muscle cramp

62. In a cardiac contraction, the degree of stretch of the contraction muscle is called the:

   a. atrial pressure point.
   b. ventricular pressure point.
   c. preload.
   d. afterload.

63. The major problems that occur with heart failure are that cardiac output decreases and _____ develop(s).

   a. venous congestion
   b. vasospasms
   c. bradycardia
   d. autoregulation

64. In the early stages of heart failure, the body senses the decrease in cardiac output and attempts to compensate through stimulation of the:

   a. vagus nerve.
   b. sympathetic nervous system.
   c. renal buffer system.
   d. pulmonic system.

65. Left heart failure is more common than right heart failure because the left ventricle is more often affected by:

   a. smoking.
   b. diabetes.
   c. obesity.
   d. chronic hypertension.

66. Prehospital management of cardiogenic shock begins with treating the patient for:

   a. respiratory arrest.
   b. shock.
   c. sepsis infection.
   d. severe dehydration.

67. Chronic right heart failure may present with signs and symptoms of tachycardia, peripheral edema, and:

   a. ascites.
   b. syncope.
   c. back pain.
   d. leg pain.

68. Possible definitive treatment choices for cardiogenic shock may include CABG or catheterization of the blocked coronary artery and:

   a. the use of fibrynolitics.
   b. administration of a Lasix drip.
   c. noninvasive overdrive pacing.
   d. invasive dialysis.

69. You were dispatched to a patient found unresponsive in the park. It is early morning and 25°F. The patient appears to be in his late sixties, smells of urine and alcohol, and is apneic and pulseless. A rapid ECG shows course fibrillation, and you deliver three shocks. There is no change in the rhythm; you continue to work the cardiac arrest. Which of the following factors is most likely the reason the patient's rhythm is resistant to defibrillation?

   a. age
   b. alcohol use
   c. hypothermia
   d. prolonged downtime

70. The goal in the treatment of CHF is to improve oxygenation and ventilation by:

   a. increasing afterload.
   b. decreasing preload.
   c. administering IV fluid therapy.
   d. stopping the possible infarction.

71. When a patient progresses to a state of severe pulmonary edema, more aggressive treatment such as _____ is required to manage the patient.

    a. external pacing
    b. fluid replacement
    c. ventilatory support
    d. obtaining a 12-lead ECG

72. The most severe form of heart failure, resulting in inadequate cardiac output caused by left ventricular malfunction, is called:

    a. cardiogenic shock.
    b. ischemic shock.
    c. sudden death.
    d. cardiomyopathy.

73. To help differentiate between CHF and APE, the paramedic should look for:

    a. shortness of breath.
    b. wet lung sounds.
    c. ECG changes.
    d. past medical history of heart disease.

74. Which of the following is a life-threatening condition with a pathology of an accumulation of fluids into the pericardial sac?

    a. pericarditis
    b. cardiac tamponade
    c. pnuemopericardium
    d. myocarditis

75. You are assessing a fifty-nine-year-old female with a chief complaint of dyspnea. Your initial assessment findings reveal an R/R of 34 and labored, crackles in the bases of the lungs, SpO_2 of 90%, P/R of 112/irregular, and BP of 140/100, and she is afebrile. PMHx includes HTN and COPD. Your first differential diagnosis is:

    a. CHF versus APE.
    b. pneumonia versus URI.
    c. CHF versus pneumonia.
    d. APE versus URI.

76. The initial signs and symptoms of cardiogenic shock are the same as seen with:

    a. neurogenic shock.
    b. ACS.
    c. APE.
    d. CVA.

77. Peripheral edema is more likely to be present with _____ because it takes several hours to days to develop.

    a. chronic CHF
    b. pneumonia
    c. acute myocardial infarction
    d. bronchitis

78. When treating a patient with CHF, which of the following is paramount to improve oxygenation and ventilation?

    a. positioning the patient supine
    b. positioning the patient upright
    c. starting an IV
    d. intubating the patient

79. You have been called to manage a seventy-two-year-old female who awoke suddenly from sleep with shortness of breath and diaphoresis. She tells you that she has a history of heart failure. You suspect that she is presenting with:

    a. anxiety.
    b. exacerbation of COPD.
    c. bronchitis.
    d. paroxysmal nocturnal dyspnea.

80. You are dispatched to the residence of a forty-five-year-old male with seizures. The patient is conscious but confused, and he complains of severe headache and nausea. His family tells you that he had one seizure and was vomiting earlier. You administer oxygen while your partner obtains vital signs: skin CTC is warm, dry, and flushed in the face; respirations 16/nonlabored; pulse 90/irregular; and BP 240/140. Which additional diagnostic information will be most helpful before providing additional treatment?

    a. ECG
    b. SpO_2
    c. temperature
    d. blood glucose

81. Continuing with question 80, you now have the following diagnostic information: ECG is sinus rhythm with PACs; SpO_2 is 97%; temperature is 98.4°F (37.3°C); and blood glucose is 150 mg/dL. This patient is most likely experiencing:

    a. meningitis.
    b. a dysrhythmia.
    c. a diabetic problem.
    d. hypertensive emergency.

82. When cardiac pumping is insufficient to meet the circulatory demand of the body, it is called:

    a. mitral valve prolapse.
    b. heart failure.
    c. ACS.
    d. systemic failure.

83. The _____ is the stretched condition of the heart muscle at the end of diastole, just before contraction.

    a. preload
    b. afterload
    c. refractory period
    d. action potential

84. Aneurysms often go unrecognized until the bulging of the sac grows so large that the pressure it exerts on other structures causes symptoms such as:

    a. pain.
    b. hypotension.
    c. hypertension.
    d. syncope.

85. If an abdominal aortic aneurysm goes unrecognized or untreated it may grow and burst, usually resulting in:

    a. ACS.
    b. CVA.
    c. paralysis.
    d. sudden death.

86. Prehospital management of aortic abdominal aneurysm (AAA) is limited to suspicion or recognition of the condition, supportive care, and:

    a. rapid transport.
    b. stabilization prior to transport.
    c. definitive treatment.
    d. localized treatment.

87. Clinical features associated with hypertensive crisis include:

    a. headache, backache, and dizziness.
    b. headache, vision disturbance, and confusion.
    c. vision disturbance, nausea, and shortness of breath.
    d. chest pain, confusion, and vomiting.

88. Hypertensive emergencies are related to other emergencies such as intracranial hemorrhage, pulmonary edema, ACS, and aortic dissection. When hypertension is associated with these conditions, treatment should be directed at the:

    a. hypertension.
    b. pulmonary edema.
    c. ACS.
    d. primary problem.

89. You are taking care of an elderly female whom you have discovered has accidentally taken an overdose of her potassium medication. Knowing that potassium has important effects on cardiac function, what clinical finding would you expect to be present in this patient?

    a. bradycardia
    b. tachycardia
    c. PVCs
    d. PACs

90. You are evaluating an eighty-two-year-old woman who has had an episode of syncope. She is short of breath, complaining of numbness in both legs and back pain. Her husband tells you that, before passing out, she had complained of lower back pain. She has a history of diabetes and hypertension. Her vitals signs are: skin CTC pale, cool, and dry; respirations 22/shallow; pulse 114/irregular; and BP 78/40. This patient is most likely experiencing:

    a. silent MI.
    b. urinary tract infection.
    c. gastrointestinal bleeding.
    d. dissecting abdominal aortic aneurysm.

91. Aspirin is given to patients with acute chest pain to thin the blood in an effort to:

    a. relieve chest pain.
    b. restore perfusion.
    c. increase myocardial workload.
    d. differentiate angina from ACS.

92. _____ sign is a paradoxical filling of the neck veins during inspiration and suggests a right ventricular infarction, massive pulmonary embolism, or pericarditis.

    a. Beck's
    b. Kussmaul's
    c. Cushing's
    d. Levine's

93. There are several types of pacemakers available for patients with irreversible heart damage. The type of pacemaker a patient receives depends on the:

    a. size of the heart.
    b. sex of the patient.
    c. age of the patient.
    d. location of the damage.

94. While interviewing a patient, she tells you that she has an implanted pacemaker. During your physical examination of the patient, where would you expect to see a scar for the site of the implantation?

    a. left upper back
    b. right lower abdomen
    c. left chest area
    d. right thigh

95. When the heart muscle becomes hypoxic, the myocardium becomes irritable and may cause:

    a. systemic ischemia.
    b. blood loss.
    c. ACS.
    d. dysrhythmias.

96. The clinical manifestation of low arterial pressure, high venous pressure, and quiet heart sounds is referred to as:

    a. Beck's triad.
    b. Cushing's triad.
    c. Trousseau's sign.
    d. Cushing's sign.

97. The definitive treatment of cardiac tamponade is to:

    a. place a chest tube.
    b. relieve cardiac compression.
    c. decompress the chest.
    d. administer IV antibiotic therapy.

98. An irregular connection between the atria and ventricles that bypasses the AV node is called a/an _____ pathway.

    a. reentry
    b. aberration
    c. intrinsic
    d. accessory

99. You are dispatched to a call for severe respiratory distress. Upon arrival, you are brought to a hospice patient with leukemia. A friend called EMS because the patient is too weak to be driven to the hospital. The patient tells you that he becomes short of breath when ambulating, and he denies chest pain. His vital signs are: skin CTC pale, warm, and dry; respirations 22/nonlabored; pulse 56/irregular; and BP 130/76. Your partner administers oxygen while you obtain the ECG. The rhythm is a very narrow complex with a P wave after each QRS complex, and the rate fluctuates between 40 and 60. What is the rhythm?

    a. sinus bradycardia
    b. junctional escape
    c. accelerated junctional
    d. controlled atrial fibrillation

100. Continuing with the patient from question 99, four minutes after you begin transport to the hospital the patient tells you that he now has nausea and chest pain 8/10 that radiates into his neck and back. He states that the pain feels like his angina. His vital signs and ECG are unchanged from the baseline set. What action should you take next?

    a. Obtain a 12-lead ECG.
    b. Administer nitroglycerine and aspirin.
    c. Observe only, since he is a hospice patient.
    d. Administer an antiemetic and call medical control.

Exam #22 Answer Form

	A	B	C	D		A	B	C	D
1.	❏	❏	❏	❏	26.	❏	❏	❏	❏
2.	❏	❏	❏	❏	27.	❏	❏	❏	❏
3.	❏	❏	❏	❏	28.	❏	❏	❏	❏
4.	❏	❏	❏	❏	29.	❏	❏	❏	❏
5.	❏	❏	❏	❏	30.	❏	❏	❏	❏
6.	❏	❏	❏	❏	31.	❏	❏	❏	❏
7.	❏	❏	❏	❏	32.	❏	❏	❏	❏
8.	❏	❏	❏	❏	33.	❏	❏	❏	❏
9.	❏	❏	❏	❏	34.	❏	❏	❏	❏
10.	❏	❏	❏	❏	35.	❏	❏	❏	❏
11.	❏	❏	❏	❏	36.	❏	❏	❏	❏
12.	❏	❏	❏	❏	37.	❏	❏	❏	❏
13.	❏	❏	❏	❏	38.	❏	❏	❏	❏
14.	❏	❏	❏	❏	39.	❏	❏	❏	❏
15.	❏	❏	❏	❏	40.	❏	❏	❏	❏
16.	❏	❏	❏	❏	41.	❏	❏	❏	❏
17.	❏	❏	❏	❏	42.	❏	❏	❏	❏
18.	❏	❏	❏	❏	43.	❏	❏	❏	❏
19.	❏	❏	❏	❏	44.	❏	❏	❏	❏
20.	❏	❏	❏	❏	45.	❏	❏	❏	❏
21.	❏	❏	❏	❏	46.	❏	❏	❏	❏
22.	❏	❏	❏	❏	47.	❏	❏	❏	❏
23.	❏	❏	❏	❏	48.	❏	❏	❏	❏
24.	❏	❏	❏	❏	49.	❏	❏	❏	❏
25.	❏	❏	❏	❏	50.	❏	❏	❏	❏

	A	B	C	D			A	B	C	D
51.	❏	❏	❏	❏	76.	❏	❏	❏	❏
52.	❏	❏	❏	❏	77.	❏	❏	❏	❏
53.	❏	❏	❏	❏	78.	❏	❏	❏	❏
54.	❏	❏	❏	❏	79.	❏	❏	❏	❏
55.	❏	❏	❏	❏	80.	❏	❏	❏	❏
56.	❏	❏	❏	❏	81.	❏	❏	❏	❏
57.	❏	❏	❏	❏	82.	❏	❏	❏	❏
58.	❏	❏	❏	❏	83.	❏	❏	❏	❏
59.	❏	❏	❏	❏	84.	❏	❏	❏	❏
60.	❏	❏	❏	❏	85.	❏	❏	❏	❏
61.	❏	❏	❏	❏	86.	❏	❏	❏	❏
62.	❏	❏	❏	❏	87.	❏	❏	❏	❏
63.	❏	❏	❏	❏	88.	❏	❏	❏	❏
64.	❏	❏	❏	❏	89.	❏	❏	❏	❏
65.	❏	❏	❏	❏	90.	❏	❏	❏	❏
66.	❏	❏	❏	❏	91.	❏	❏	❏	❏
67.	❏	❏	❏	❏	92.	❏	❏	❏	❏
68.	❏	❏	❏	❏	93.	❏	❏	❏	❏
69.	❏	❏	❏	❏	94.	❏	❏	❏	❏
70.	❏	❏	❏	❏	95.	❏	❏	❏	❏
71.	❏	❏	❏	❏	96.	❏	❏	❏	❏
72.	❏	❏	❏	❏	97.	❏	❏	❏	❏
73.	❏	❏	❏	❏	98.	❏	❏	❏	❏
74.	❏	❏	❏	❏	99.	❏	❏	❏	❏
75.	❏	❏	❏	❏	100.	❏	❏	❏	❏

23
Neurology

1. The major function of the nervous system is to:

   a. monitor internal changes of the body.
   b. circulate nutrients to all body cells.
   c. regulate the neurons.
   d. provide support for the body structures.

2. The largest part of the brain is divided into right and left hemisperes and is called the:

   a. cerebellum.
   b. cerebrum.
   c. diencephalon.
   d. brain stem.

3. The _____ is the location in the brain of higher cognitive functions such as learning and language.

   a. corpus callosum
   b. telencephalon
   c. diencephalon
   d. thalamus

4. Blood enters the brain from the two internal carotid arteries and the:

   a. jugular artery.
   b. iliac artery.
   c. basilar artery.
   d. subclavian artery.

5. The structure that forms a circle around the stalk of the pituitary gland and works as a backup mechanism for complications with cerebral blood flow is called the:

   a. foramen magnum.
   b. arch of atlas.
   c. circle of Willis.
   d. cerebral spinal canal.

6. The structures within the brain stem, from top (superior) to bottom (inferior), are the:

   a. pituitary, midbrain, and pons.
   b. midbrain, pons, and medulla oblongata.
   c. pons, midbrain, and medulla oblongata.
   d. medulla oblongata, pituitary, midbrain, and pons.

7. The _____ regulates the biologic clock of the body.

   a. pineal body
   b. medulla
   c. thalamus
   d. optic chiasma

8. The section of the brain responsible for maintaining posture, balance, and voluntary coordination of skilled movements is the:

   a. midbrain.
   b. diencephalon.
   c. cerebellum.
   d. brain stem.

9. Cerebrospinal fluid (CSF) is present in the spinal cord, cavities, and canals of the brain, as well as the:

   a. temporal gap.
   b. parietal shelf.
   c. epidural space.
   d. subarachnoid space.

10. CSF has several functions, one of which is to:

    a. help with coordination and balance.
    b. help regulate the biological clock of the body.
    c. oxygenate tissues in the brain and spinal cord.
    d. help the brain to recognize changes in CO_2 levels.

11. _____ is an increase in the amount of CSF, from either a blockage or decrease in normal reabsorption.

    a. Cerebrosis
    b. Hydrocephalus
    c. Cerebroma
    d. Cephalophoma

12. Which of the meninges is the highly vascular covering of the brain and spinal cord?

    a. dura mater
    b. pia mater
    c. arachnoid membrane
    d. falx cerebelli

13. Meningitis is a potentially life-threatening infection of both the _____ and meninges.

   a. spinal cord
   b. white matter
   c. CSF
   d. gray matter

14. The major difference between gray matter and white matter is that gray matter is:

   a. not covered with myelinated fibers.
   b. covered with myelinated fibers.
   c. ashen colored because of anaerobic metabolism.
   d. there really is no major difference.

15. The fundamental component of the nervous system is the:

   a. myelin.
   b. neuron.
   c. spinal cord.
   d. nerve impulse.

16. All of the following are components of the nerve cell body, *except* the:

   a. soma.
   b. dendrite.
   c. axon.
   d. myelin.

17. Nervous tissue requires a tremendous amount of metabolic energy. For this to occur, it is essential that there be a constant supply of oxygen and:

   a. potassium.
   b. sodium.
   c. glucose.
   d. carbon dioxide.

18. A disease process that destroys the myelin sheath and infects the nerve fibers, impairing nerve function, is called:

   a. multiple sclerosis.
   b. Parkinson's disease.
   c. epilepsy.
   d. Lou Gehrig's disease.

19. Nerve cells communicate with each other primarily through the:

   a. peripheral system.
   b. flowing of acetylcholine.
   c. limbic system.
   d. synapses.

20. High in the brain stem is the _____, which is responsible for maintaining consciousness.

   a. reticular activating system
   b. limbic system
   c. ANS
   d. CNS

21. The twelve pairs of cranial nerves are a component of which part of the nervous system?

   a. autonomic
   b. peripheral
   c. structural
   d. functional

22. _____ is a disorder of the CNS, named after the famous baseball player Lou Gehrig. It has a rapidly progressive deterioration leading to atrophy of all body muscles and death.

   a. Bell's palsy
   b. ALS
   c. Cerebral Palsy
   d. Parkinson's disease

23. A term for a chronic, progressive disease of the CNS characterized by exacerbation and remission of assorted multiple neurologic symptoms is:

   a. epilepsy.
   b. Bell's palsy.
   c. multiple sclerosis.
   d. Parkinson's disease.

24. Which of the following is an abnormal condition related to a structural problem within the brain, rather than an infectious disease of the nervous system?

   a. tetanus
   b. encephalitis
   c. poliomyelitis
   d. hydrocephalus

25. You are assessing a twenty-eight-year-old male complaining of a severe headache. Just before losing consciousness in front of you, he tells you that it came on very suddenly after he experienced a loud sound like a bang in his head. Which of the following conditions do you suspect was the cause of this event?

   a. CVA
   b. TIA
   c. ruptured aneurysm
   d. meningitis

26. You are looking at the chart of an elderly nursing home resident with a diagnosis of dementia. Also included in the history are possible causes of the dementia. Which of the following is most likely the cause of this patient's dementia?

    a. concussion
    b. atherosclerosis
    c. retrograde amnesia
    d. anterograde amnesia

27. Ischemia, ICP, cerebral edema, and brain herniation are all _____ injuries from traumatic brain injury.

    a. primary
    b. secondary
    c. tertiary
    d. irreversible

28. A mild, closed head injury that results in a transient loss of brain function with or without a loss of consciousness is called:

    a. amnesia.
    b. contusion.
    c. concussion.
    d. contra-coup.

29. With the help of the fire department, your patient has been extricated from a vehicle with significant damage following a collision. The patient has been unconscious the entire time, and you strongly suspect that he has a traumatic brain injury. Which of the following can you do to significantly reduce the patient's morbidity?

    a. Administer steroids.
    b. Hyperventilate the patient.
    c. Rapidly transport the patient to a trauma center.
    d. Assess for CSF leakage from the nose and ears.

30. You are assessing a conscious patient with a known condition that causes low levels of dopamine in the parts of the brain that control voluntary movement. Today he has weakness and muscle rigidity in addition to his normal irregular gait and fine resting tremor. What is your impression of this patient?

    a. This is a common neurological emergency.
    b. This is an uncommon neurological emergency.
    c. This is a chronic disorder that does not require emergency care.
    d. This is a chronic disorder that requires prompt emergency care.

31. The major difference between a stroke and a TIA is that:

    a. a TIA always precedes a stroke.
    b. a stroke always precedes a TIA.
    c. the TIA has no lasting effect.
    d. the stroke is considered a warning sign.

32. An undiagnosed TIA is a very high risk factor for:

    a. hypertension.
    b. a major stroke.
    c. new-onset diabetes.
    d. heart disasese

33. A sudden, temporary change in behavior, sensory, or motor activity caused by an excessive or chaotic electrical discharge of one or more groups of neurons in the brain is known as a:

    a. TIA.
    b. CVA.
    c. seizure.
    d. palsy.

34. Which of the following is not a phase of a seizure?

    a. preictal
    b. atonic
    c. ictal
    d. postictal

35. A seizure characterized by impairment of consciousness, including an aura, is a/an _____ seizure.

    a. simple partial
    b. complex partial
    c. absence
    d. complete motor

36. Prolonged or repeated seizures are true emergencies because:

    a. brain damage can occur.
    b. the patient can swallow the tongue.
    c. the patient forgets to breathe.
    d. the acid in the blood decreases.

37. Noncardiac syncope often occurs in patients with no underlying disease, usually from a stressor such as pain, emotion, or:

    a. heat.
    b. cold.
    c. medication.
    d. strobe lights.

38. How is a patient's mental status best assessed?

    a. by speaking with the patient
    b. by assessing the cranial nerves
    c. by checking for symmetry of motor response
    d. by checking for deficits in coordination and reflexes

39. What is the most significant aspect of a neurologic assessment?

   a. performing serial assessments
   b. a positive Babinski sign
   c. absence of seizure activity
   d. medication compliance

40. First developed in 1974, the _____ is an objective measure of the patient's level of consciousness.

   a. GCS
   b. AVPU
   c. Babinski sign
   d. CT scan

41. A respiratory pattern in which an extended inspiratory effort or gasping with a brief expiration, caused by pressure, damage, or surgical removal of the pons in the area of CN IV, is called:

   a. ataxic.
   b. Biot's respiration.
   c. cluster breathing.
   d. apneusis.

42. While assessing an unconscious, head-injured victim of an MVC, you observe the patient's respiratory effort as a pattern of cycles of apnea and hyperventilation. You recognize this pattern as:

   a. autisms.
   b. Kussmaul's breathing.
   c. Cheyne-Stokes respirations.
   d. apneusis.

43. Involuntary neurologic activities such as yawning, hiccupping, coughing, and vomiting are called:

   a. ataxics.
   b. autisms.
   c. clusters.
   d. central neurologic initiations.

44. _____ breathing often precedes agonal breathing and apnea and has no pattern or rhythm with depth or rate.

   a. Biot's
   b. Kussmaul's
   c. Ataxic
   d. Cluster

45. The term for normal visual function of the eyes that depends on the ability of both eyes to fix on the same subject is:

   a. diplopia.
   b. binocular vision.
   c. medial gaze.
   d. vergence reflex.

46. The term _____ refers to the adjustment of the eyes to variations in distance.

   a. accommodation
   b. acuity
   c. conjugate gaze
   d. divergence

47. An involuntary movement of the eyes that can be in any direction, but more often is either verticle or horizontal, is:

   a. doll's eyes.
   b. dysconjugate gaze.
   c. nystagmus.
   d. diplopia.

48. An abnormal constriction of the pupils, caused by certain types of infection and some types of drug overdose, is called:

   a. anisocoria.
   b. glaucoma.
   c. dystonia.
   d. miosis.

49. Nearly ten percent of the population has a congenital inequality of their pupil sizes. The term for this condition is:

   a. anisocoria.
   b. glaucoma.
   c. akinesia.
   d. miosis

50. A brief involuntary movement of distal extremities and facial muscles, which often occurs in Huntington's disease, Parkinson's disease, and thyrotoxosis, is:

   a. chorea.
   b. ballism.
   c. myclonus.
   d. tics.

51. The condition of slow and irregular involuntary winding movements of the extremities, as seen in cerebral palsy, encephalitis, and some drug side effects, is:

   a. akinesia.
   b. athetosis.
   c. dystonia.
   d. dyskinesia.

52. A disorder with characteristics of lack of muscle coordination, involuntary muscle movement, tics, incoherent grunts, barks, and cursing is called:

   a. tremors.
   b. Creutzfeldt-Jakob's disease.
   c. Tourette's syndrome.
   d. Wernicke syndrome.

53. Assessing extraocular movements (EOMs) is the best single method for measuring brain stem integrity. Which of the following is a test for checking EOMs?

   a. Assess for palmar drift.
   b. Assess the patient's gait.
   c. Assess the six cardinal positions of gaze.
   d. Assess discriminative touch, dull versus sharp.

54. While assessing a patient presenting with new stroke symptoms such as dysphasia, difficulty swallowing, and chewing, which cranial nerve do you suspect is being affected?

   a. X
   b. VIII
   c. VI
   d. V

55. _____ is an abnormal gait characterized by unsteady, uncoordinated, wide at the base steps, as seen with drunkenness, heavily medicated persons, or certain medical conditions.

   a. Steppage
   b. Ataxia
   c. Festination
   d. Spastic hemiparesis

56. The loss of sensory and motor function below certain levels of the spine defines a/an:

   a. spinal cord injury.
   b. frontal lobe lesion.
   c. injury to Broca's area.
   d. precursor to ICP.

57. Patients experiencing cerebral vascular accidents including stroke, intracerebral, or subarachnoid hemorrhage can present with typical signs of ____, which can make diagnosis of the underlying problem difficult.

   a. hypothermia
   b. heat stroke
   c. hyperglycemia
   d. memory loss

58. The most common signs of brain dysfunction are AMS and:

   a. hyperglycemia.
   b. loss of motor control.
   c. speech deficits.
   d. behavioral changes.

59. You have been called to care for an unconscious patient with a known brain tumor. The patient presents with the jaws clenched, arms and legs extended. You suspect the lesion is located in the diencephalon, midbrain, or:

   a. pons.
   b. medulla.
   c. thalamus.
   d. insula.

60. _____ posturing, also referred to as flexion, is associated with a lesion at or above the upper brain stem.

   a. Broca's
   b. Wernicke's
   c. Decorticate
   d. Decerebrate

61. Cushing's triad is a/an _____ sign of rising ICP.

   a. early
   b. late
   c. unreliable
   d. insufficient

62. Babinski's reflex is a test to assess for spinal cord dysfunction, specifically in the _____ portion of the motor control system.

   a. pyramidal
   b. extrapyramidal
   c. ipsilateral
   d. lateral

63. Both sides of the brain communicate via _____ to carry out many complex functions.

   a. the corpus callosum
   b. Broca's area
   c. Wernicke's area
   d. the island of Reil

64. The _____ lobe of the brain receives and translates somatic sensations of pain, touch, pressure, heat and cold, and body position.

   a. frontal
   b. parietal
   c. occipital
   d. temporal

65. The _____ links the nervous and endocrine systems, as well as the mind (psyche) and body.

   a. thalamus
   b. insula
   c. pineal body
   d. hypothalamus

66. CSF is produced in the _____ and is completely replaced several times each day.

   a. spine
   b. epidural space
   c. ventricles of the brain
   d. arachnoid space

67. The dura mater has three significant inner extentions: the falx cerebelli, the falx cerebri, and the:

   a. stalk.
   b. soma.
   c. cortex.
   d. tentorium.

68. What type of bleeding occurs in a subdural hematoma?

   a. venous
   b. arterial
   c. systemic
   d. metabolic

69. Of the three types of structural neurons, only the _____ are located only in the brain and spinal cord.

   a. intraneurons
   b. afferent
   c. efferent
   d. interneurons

70. _____ are extensions of the nerve cell body with branches that conduct impulses to the cell body, relaying information to the neuron.

   a. Axons
   b. Dendrites
   c. DNA
   d. RNA

71. The layer or coating around the axon that protects the axon process and increases the conduction of nerve impulses is the:

   a. myelin.
   b. stratum.
   c. swathe.
   d. jacket.

72. The two most common hematomas that may develop within the brain are:

   a. temporal and parietal.
   b. epidural and subdural.
   c. cerebral and epidural.
   d. subdural and cerebral.

73. The most common developmental defect of the CNS occurring while in utero is:

   a. hydrocephalus.
   b. shingles.
   c. spina bifida.
   d. polio.

74. _____ is a viral infection causing inflammation of the gray matter of the spinal cord that may temporarily or permanently affect neurologic functions.

   a. Poliomyelitis
   b. Abscess
   c. Spina bifida
   d. Meningitis

75. Which of the following conditions may be seen with a head CT scan?

   a. concussion
   b. contusion
   c. amnesia
   d. aphasia

76. _____ is the type of amnesia that affects the ability to recall memories from the past.

   a. Aphasic
   b. Non-phasic
   c. Anterograde
   d. Retrograde

77. A forty-eight-year-old male is complaining of a severe headache. He has sinusitis and has had an elevated temperature all day. His vital signs are: skin CTC very warm, flushed, and dry; respirations 20/nonlabored; pulse 88/regular; and BP 142/90. Which of the following is the least likely cause of his headache?

   a. meningitis
   b. encephalitis
   c. brain abscess
   d. subarachnoid hemorrhage

78. _____ stroke is the most common and is caused by a clot that blocks an artery.

   a. Ischemic
   b. Nocturnal
   c. Hemorrhagic
   d. Embolic

79. You are using a thrombolytic checklist on a patient presenting with stroke symptoms. Which of the following is an exclusion criterion for the use of fibryolitics?

   a. alert mental status
   b. able to give consent
   c. uncontrolled hypertension
   d. onset of symptoms <three hours

80. Which of the following medications is made from a plant called belladonna, a drug that causes the pupils to dilate?

   a. atropine
   b. Cardizem
   c. dopamine
   d. Atrovent

81. The _____ test is used in comatose patients to assess for brain stem or oculomotor injury, after neck injury has been ruled out.

    a. accommodation
    b. dolls-eye maneuver
    c. drop-foot
    d. pronator drift

82. The difference of _____ millimeter(s) or more in the size of the pupils is an abnormal finding.

    a. one
    b. two
    c. three
    d. four

83. _____ is the loss of ability to speak because of a defect in or loss of language function.

    a. Ataxia
    b. Aphasia
    c. Dysarthria
    d. Dysphonia

84. All of the following are terms used to describe a patient's muscle tone, *except*:

    a. normal.
    b. rigid.
    c. spastic.
    d. neural.

85. When describing the patient's mental status, avoid terms such as stupor, lethargic, and obtunded because they:

    a. all mean the same thing.
    b. mean different things to different people.
    c. are difficult to spell.
    d. are not real medical terms.

86. An unconscious thirty-six-year-old patient was seen seizing by his family. They tell you that the seizure lasted approximately two minutes, and that he has no history of seizures. You open the airway, administer high-concentration oxygen, complete an initial assessment, and quickly obtain vital signs and a blood glucose reading. Which of the following findings suggests a neurologic deficit?

    a. blood around the mouth
    b. irregular breathing pattern
    c. withdrawing from painful stimulus
    d. blood glucose reading of 180 mg/dl

87. Loss of lateral eye movement is an early sign of:

    a. vision loss.
    b. rising ICP.
    c. decreasing ICP.
    d. an orbital fracture.

88. You are assessing the driver of an automobile that was rear-ended at a moderate speed. The patient is complaining of severe pain in the left leg immediately after the collision, but there is no apparent trauma to the leg. Which of the following do you suspect?

    a. herniated disc
    b. spinal fracture
    c. muscle cramp
    d. faking

89. A functional disorder of the CNS, characterized by unilateral facial paralysis caused by compression of cranial nerve VII (facial nerve), is called:

    a. a brain abscess.
    b. a neoplasm.
    c. Bell's palsy.
    d. ALS.

90. During what part of the day do thrombotic strokes typically occur?

    a. late morning
    b. early afternoon
    c. early evening
    d. during sleep

91. The parents of a six-month-old infant called EMS when the baby had a seizure for the first time. They were extremely upset as they described the baby rolling his eyes back into his head and how it appeared as if he had stopped breathing for a few seconds. Which of the following is the least likely cause of the patient's seizure?

    a. epilepsy
    b. infection
    c. congenital defect
    d. electrolyte abnormality

92. The phase of a seizure characterized by a loss of consciousness with muscle contraction is called:

    a. preictal.
    b. aura.
    c. tonic.
    d. clonic.

93. A _____ event is a transient loss of consciousness caused by a decreased blood supply to the brain.

    a. TIA
    b. CVA
    c. syncopal
    d. seizure

94. The term _____ means new growth and is used synonymously with tumor.

    a. abscess
    b. migraine
    c. neoplasm
    d. foci

95. Which of the following is a possible sign associated with a neurologic disorder, rather than the neurologic disorder itself?

    a. seizures
    b. shingles
    c. hypertension
    d. Alzheimer's

96. Tic douloureux is pain in one or more of the three branches of the _____ cranial nerve that runs along the face.

    a. III
    b. V
    c. VIII
    d. XII

97. Glaucoma can occur as a congenital defect or as a result of another eye disorder, and is associated with:

    a. heredity.
    b. trauma.
    c. hyperthyroidism.
    d. female gender.

98. You are assessing a sixty-two-year-old male who called EMS because he has severe eye pain. The pain came on suddenly while the patient was watching TV. The eye is red, the pupil is dilated, and he tells you his vision is blurred. He also feels nauseated. The patient has no significant medical history and no vision disorders. What could be the cause of his sudden ailment?

    a. stroke
    b. glaucoma
    c. Bell's palsy
    d. trigeminal neuralgia

99. Which part of the neurologic examination is the least exact and informative except in the case of spinal cord injury?

    a. mental status
    b. reflexes
    c. motor function
    d. sensory function

100. The primary motor cortex located in the _____ is connected with the association motor cortex in the basal ganglia and cerebellum.

    a. frontal lobe
    b. occipital lobe
    c. midbrain
    d. parietal lobe

Exam #23 Answer Form

	A	B	C	D		A	B	C	D
1.	❏	❏	❏	❏	26.	❏	❏	❏	❏
2.	❏	❏	❏	❏	27.	❏	❏	❏	❏
3.	❏	❏	❏	❏	28.	❏	❏	❏	❏
4.	❏	❏	❏	❏	29.	❏	❏	❏	❏
5.	❏	❏	❏	❏	30.	❏	❏	❏	❏
6.	❏	❏	❏	❏	31.	❏	❏	❏	❏
7.	❏	❏	❏	❏	32.	❏	❏	❏	❏
8.	❏	❏	❏	❏	33.	❏	❏	❏	❏
9.	❏	❏	❏	❏	34.	❏	❏	❏	❏
10.	❏	❏	❏	❏	35.	❏	❏	❏	❏
11.	❏	❏	❏	❏	36.	❏	❏	❏	❏
12.	❏	❏	❏	❏	37.	❏	❏	❏	❏
13.	❏	❏	❏	❏	38.	❏	❏	❏	❏
14.	❏	❏	❏	❏	39.	❏	❏	❏	❏
15.	❏	❏	❏	❏	40.	❏	❏	❏	❏
16.	❏	❏	❏	❏	41.	❏	❏	❏	❏
17.	❏	❏	❏	❏	42.	❏	❏	❏	❏
18.	❏	❏	❏	❏	43.	❏	❏	❏	❏
19.	❏	❏	❏	❏	44.	❏	❏	❏	❏
20.	❏	❏	❏	❏	45.	❏	❏	❏	❏
21.	❏	❏	❏	❏	46.	❏	❏	❏	❏
22.	❏	❏	❏	❏	47.	❏	❏	❏	❏
23.	❏	❏	❏	❏	48.	❏	❏	❏	❏
24.	❏	❏	❏	❏	49.	❏	❏	❏	❏
25.	❏	❏	❏	❏	50.	❏	❏	❏	❏

	A	B	C	D			A	B	C	D
51.	❏	❏	❏	❏	76.	❏	❏	❏	❏
52.	❏	❏	❏	❏	77.	❏	❏	❏	❏
53.	❏	❏	❏	❏	78.	❏	❏	❏	❏
54.	❏	❏	❏	❏	79.	❏	❏	❏	❏
55.	❏	❏	❏	❏	80.	❏	❏	❏	❏
56.	❏	❏	❏	❏	81.	❏	❏	❏	❏
57.	❏	❏	❏	❏	82.	❏	❏	❏	❏
58.	❏	❏	❏	❏	83.	❏	❏	❏	❏
59.	❏	❏	❏	❏	84.	❏	❏	❏	❏
60.	❏	❏	❏	❏	85.	❏	❏	❏	❏
61.	❏	❏	❏	❏	86.	❏	❏	❏	❏
62.	❏	❏	❏	❏	87.	❏	❏	❏	❏
63.	❏	❏	❏	❏	88.	❏	❏	❏	❏
64.	❏	❏	❏	❏	89.	❏	❏	❏	❏
65.	❏	❏	❏	❏	90.	❏	❏	❏	❏
66.	❏	❏	❏	❏	91.	❏	❏	❏	❏
67.	❏	❏	❏	❏	92.	❏	❏	❏	❏
68.	❏	❏	❏	❏	93.	❏	❏	❏	❏
69.	❏	❏	❏	❏	94.	❏	❏	❏	❏
70.	❏	❏	❏	❏	95.	❏	❏	❏	❏
71.	❏	❏	❏	❏	96.	❏	❏	❏	❏
72.	❏	❏	❏	❏	97.	❏	❏	❏	❏
73.	❏	❏	❏	❏	98.	❏	❏	❏	❏
74.	❏	❏	❏	❏	99.	❏	❏	❏	❏
75.	❏	❏	❏	❏	100.	❏	❏	❏	❏

Endocrinology

1. The most common of the endocrine emergencies is _____, which occurs more frequently than all the rest combined.

   a. fluid imbalance
   b. altered mental status
   c. diabetic problems
   d. respiratory problems

2. Which of the following is not a risk factor predisposing to endocrine disease?

   a. hyperlipidemia
   b. heredity
   c. hypothyroidism
   d. hypopituitarism

3. _____ is the leading cause of adult blindness, end-stage kidney failure, and nontraumatic lower extremity amputations.

   a. Diabetes
   b. Hypopituitarism
   c. Hypothyroidism
   d. Hyperthyroidism

4. The endocrine system is an integrated _____ and co-ordination system enabling reproduction, growth and development, and regulation of energy.

   a. chemical
   b. fluid
   c. muscle
   d. nerve

5. The endocrine system, together with the _____ system, maintains internal homeostasis of the body and coordinates responses to environmental changes and stress.

   a. GI
   b. integumentary
   c. biofeedback
   d. nervous

6. _____ regulate many body functions, such as growth, reproduction, temperature, metabolism, and blood pressure.

   a. Antigens
   b. Hormones
   c. Receptors
   d. Emotions

7. Endocrines are called "ductless glands" because they secrete their chemical hormones directly into the:

   a. brain.
   b. heart.
   c. lungs.
   d. blood.

8. The only known cure for Type I diabetes is:

   a. an adrenal transplant.
   b. a pancreas transplant.
   c. suppression of the adrenals with medication.
   d. suppression of the thyroid gland with medication.

9. The _____ gland, sometimes known as the "master gland," is located at the base of the brain in the cranial cavity.

   a. parathyroid
   b. adrenal
   c. pituitary
   d. gonad

10. Which of the following endocrine glands is responsible for maintaining normal levels of calcium in the blood?

    a. parathyroid
    b. adrenal
    c. pituitary
    d. ovaries

11. The _____ is considered an organ of both the digestive and the endocrine systems.

    a. thyroid
    b. parathyroid
    c. pancreas
    d. testes

12. The _____ gland(s) is/are responsible for secretion of the hormones vital to maintaining the body's water and salt balance.

    a. pancreas
    b. insulin
    c. pituitary
    d. adrenal

13. _____ is one of the major reasons a patient develops an endocrine emergency.

    a. Hyperthermia
    b. Excessive hormone production
    c. Excessive sympathetic stimulation
    d. Disproportionate parasympathetic stimulation

14. In the body's normal regulation of the blood sugar level, insulin is released from the pancreas together with:

    a. epinephrine and glucagon.
    b. glucagon.
    c. amino acids.
    d. fatty acids.

15. Insulin moves sugar molecules from the blood into the cell, where they are:

    a. stored.
    b. bathed.
    c. reconstituted.
    d. broken down.

16. _____ occurs as a result of a viral infection of the pancreas, leading to the formation of antibodies to pancreatic beta-cells that produce insulin.

    a. Type I diabetes
    b. Type II diabetes
    c. Obesity
    d. Insulin receptor resistance

17. Diabetic patients do not always have the classic symptoms of myocardial ischemia, such as crushing substernal chest pain, because:

    a. glucose is the sole source of oxidative metabolism for the CNS.
    b. insulin numbs the pain.
    c. many diabetics have some form of neuropathy.
    d. elevated blood lipid levels alter sensation.

18. Hypoglycemia of more than twenty to thirty minutes' duration results in the production of toxic compounds in the brain that cause:

    a. cardiac arrest.
    b. excessive levels of heat production.
    c. a decrease in the thyroid function.
    d. permanent neuronal damage.

19. Many patients with hyperglycemia are significantly _____; therefore _____ is/are part of the primary treatment.

    a. hyperthermic; cooling
    b. hypothermic; heat
    c. dehydrated; fluids
    d. altered in mental status; insulin

20. Diabetic patients lack the normal effects of insulin; therefore, sugar and other substances such as _____ fail to enter the cells properly.

    a. amino acids
    b. glycogen
    c. proteins
    d. triglycerides

21. Diabetic ketoacidosis (DKA) is a metabolic condition consisting of hyperglycemia, dehydration, and the accumulation of _____ in the body.

    a. ketones and ketoacids
    b. free fatty acids
    c. amino acids
    d. uric acid

22. The effects of osmotic diuresis in diabetic patients cause frequent urination. At times, this can lead to dehydration. Depending on the severity of her condition, the patient may also be deficient in:

    a. ketones and ketoacids.
    b. neurons.
    c. calcium.
    d. total body potassium.

23. The most common reason a diabetic patient develops DKA is because of:

    a. excess glucagon.
    b. infection.
    c. too much insulin.
    d. too little insulin.

24. Which of the following statements about DKA is most accurate?

    a. All patients with hyperglycemia have DKA.
    b. Not every patient with hyperglycemia will have DKA.
    c. Hypoglycemic patients who lapse into a coma will also be in shock.
    d. Distinguishing between hyperglycemia and DKA in the field is relatively easy.

25. During periods of insulin deficiency, _____ is/are broken down to provide energy.

    a. ketones
    b. glucagon
    c. stored fats
    d. epinephrine

26. Ketoacidosis develops when the level of ketones in the _____ is too _____.

    a. blood; high
    b. pancreas; high
    c. blood; low
    d. pancreas; low

27. The diabetic emergency that occurs from a relative insulin deficiency that leads to marked hyperglycemia, but with the absence of ketones and acidosis, is called:

    a. hypoosmolar hyperglycemic nonketotic coma.
    b. hyperosmolar hyperglycemic nonketotic coma.
    c. nonketotic mellitis.
    d. nonketotic osmolitis.

28. Many long-standing diabetic patients remain asymptomatic until their sugar level drops low enough to result in loss of consciousness. This occurs because:

    a. early warning signs from the counter-regulatory hormones fail.
    b. they have aquired dysfunction of the peripheral nervous system.
    c. they develop a tolerance to symptoms.
    d. early warning signs from the beta-cells are inactivated.

29. Which of the following substances can increase a person's sensitivity to hypoglycemia, which may result in a person feeling hypoglycemic symptoms at blood sugar levels not usually associated with causing problems?

    a. poppy seeds
    b. chocolate
    c. peanuts
    d. caffeine

30. The production of glucagons and epinephrine stimulates enzymes that break down glycogen to glucose. This process is called:

    a. homeostasis.
    b. Harada's syndrome.
    c. gluconeogenesis.
    d. glycogenolysis.

31. Hyperglycemia is common in _____ due to insulin resistance and increased glycogenolysis.

    a. massive head trauma
    b. Cushing's sydrome
    c. thyrotoxicosis
    d. myxedema coma

32. Signs and symptoms of new-onset thyrotoxicosis include:

    a. atrial fibrillation and fever.
    b. hypothermia and hypoglycemia.
    c. muscle weakness and hirsuitism.
    d. weight loss and brown pigmentation of the skin.

33. Before the diagnosis of _____ is established, patients often have fatigue, lethargy, and gradual weight gain for years.

    a. hyperthyroidism
    b. hypothyroidism
    c. myxedema coma
    d. Cushing's syndrome

34. The term myxedema generically refers to any and all symptoms of hypothyroidism and may typically include any of the following, *except*:

    a. cool dry skin and slowed reflexes.
    b. hypertension.
    c. coarse, thin hair and brittle nails.
    d. hyperglycemia.

35. You are doing an ALS transfer from one medical facility to another for a patient in full myxedema coma. What dysrhythmia is most common for a patient in this condition?

    a. tachycardia
    b. atrial fibrillation
    c. sinus bradycardia
    d. sick sinus syndrome

36. _____ is a metabolic syndrome resulting from hypersecretion of the glucocorticoid hormone, cortisol, which affects carbohydrate, protein, and lipid metabolism.

    a. Cushing's syndrome
    b. Adrenal insufficiency
    c. Addison's disease
    d. Graves' disease

37. _____ is an endocrine disorder associated with excess growth of body hair, abnormal pattern of fat distribution, adult-onset acne, and purple or dark stretch marks.

a. Thyrotoxicosis
b. Exophthalmus
c. Hypothyroidism
d. Cushing's syndrome

38. Which of the following preexisting conditions would a patient's primary acute complaint not be directly related to?

a. Cushing's syndrome
b. thyroid storm
c. adrenal insuffiency
d. hyperglycemia

39. Autoimmune destruction of the adrenal glands is the most common cause of adrenal insufficiency and is called:

a. Cushing's syndrome.
b. thyroid storm.
c. Addison's disease.
d. Graves' disease.

40. Adrenal insufficiency is inadequate production of adrenal hormones, primarily _____, for any of a number of reasons.

a. adrenocortical
b. cortisol and aldosterone
c. follicle-stimulating hormone (FSH)
d. parathyroid hormone (PTH)

41. The pathophysiology of adrenal insufficiency is that the normal feedback loop between the hypothalamus, pitiuitary gland, and adrenal gland is suppressed because of:

a. the use of oral or inhaled steroids.
b. daily injections of insulin.
c. the use of oral hypoglycemic agents.
d. daily estrogen use.

42. Signs and symptoms of chronic adrenalin sufficiency may include any of the following, *except*:

a. anorexia and weight loss.
b. muscle and joint pain.
c. salt craving and abdominal pain.
d. decreased pigmentation.

43. Acute adrenal insufficiency, sometimes called an Addisonian crisis, presents as hypotension, hypoglycemia, and severe:

a. hypovolemia.
b. hypercarbia.
c. weight loss.
d. muscle and joint pain.

44. Protrusion of the eyeballs (exophthalmus) is a common physical finding in patients with:

a. hyperthyroidism.
b. hypothyroidism.
c. myxedema coma.
d. Cushing's syndrome.

45. Which of the following diabetic medications is an exogenous drug?

a. Novolin
b. Rezulin
c. Glucotrol
d. Glyburide

46. The onset of action is faster and duration is shorter with _____ insulin preparations.

a. beef
b. pork
c. human
d. chicken

47. In addition to $D_{50}W$, thiamine is also considered to be of value in the management of the hypoglycemic diabetic patient who is an alcoholic or:

a. hypothermic.
b. malnourished.
c. hypokalemic.
d. hypotensive.

48. Your patient has a nontraumatic altered mental status. His vital signs are H/R 110, BP 74/44, R/R 20, and his skin is warm and moist. His spouse tells you that he is not diabetic, but he does have asthma and takes steriod inhalers daily. You check his glucose level, and it is 40 mg/dl. After assuring that his airway and breathing are adequate, what would be the next appropriate step in care?

a. administer glucagon
b. give fluid boluses
c. administer dextrose IV
d. administer thiamine

49. As hypoglycemia alone does not typically result in hypotension, which of the following conditions is the patient discussed in question 48 most likely experiencing?

a. acute adrenal insufficiency
b. Cushing's syndrome
c. myxedema
d. thyrotoxicosis

50. Cushing's syndrome is caused by the hypersecretion of glucocorticoids by the _____ gland(s).

a. adrenal
b. thymus
c. reproductive
d. pancreas

51. You are assessing a twenty-two-year-old male with insulin-dependent diabetes mellitus (IDDM) who is having a diabetic event. His girlfriend called because she could not get him up this morning, and says he has been sick with a bad cold for several days. The patient's eyes are open, but he cannot verbalize a response. His breathing is deep and rapid, his skin is warm and dry, and he looks dehydrated. Vital signs are R/R 40, BP 84/50, and P/R 118. While you are checking his glucose level, which diabetic emergency do you suspect?

a. hypoglycemia
b. hyperglycemia
c. HHNC
d. acute adrenal insufficiency

52. What is the significance of the respirations of the patient described in question 51?

a. He is hyperventilating because of dehydration.
b. This is the body's response to hypoosmolarity and high pH.
c. Deep respirations are a response to increased acid levels from ketones.
d. The deep and rapid breathing is caused by the congestion from his cold.

53. Which of the following treatment plans would be the most appropriate for the patient described in question 51?

a. high-flow oxygen, IV fluid boluses, and transport
b. high-flow oxygen, IV dextrose, and fluid boluses
c. IV, $D_{50}W$, and thiamine
d. IV, $D_{50}W$, and IV antibiotics in the hospital

54. The spouse of an unresponsive diabetic male called EMS when she found her husband lying on the kitchen floor in the morning. His initial blood sugar reading was 26 mg/dL, and his vital signs are: skin CTC cool, dry, and pale; respirations 20/puffing and snoring; pulse 70/regular; and BP 110/68. After administer oxygen, starting an IV, and giving 25 grams of dextrose, the patient is still unresponsive and his blood sugar reading is 44 mg/dL. What would be the most appropriate treatment at this point?

a. intubate
b. begin rapid transport
c. administer glucagon IM
d. administer another 25 grams of dextrose

55. You have responded to a suburban residence for a sixty-year-old male with an altered mental status. A neighbor called EMS because the patient is having stroke symptoms and is unable to get out of bed today. The patient is conscious but very confused. His responses are slow, and he feels week. He denies any pain or history of diabetes, his vital signs are R/R 20, BP 100/50, P/R 62, and his skin is warm and dry. Which of the following conditions do you suspect first?

a. CVA
b. diabetic emergency
c. ACS
d. all of the above

56. Further evaluation of the patient described in question 55 reveals that his medications include beta-blocker and antihypertensive meds. His SpO_2 is 99% with oxygen. Before you begin transport, which of the following would be of most value to make a differential diagnosis?

a. 12-lead ECG
b. glucose reading
c. neurologic examination
d. medication changes

57. What is the significance of the medications for the patient described in question 55?

a. Beta-blockers will conceal compensatory signs of shock.
b. Antihypertensives may precipitate hypoglycemia.
c. Antihypertensives may conceal hyperglycemia.
d. Beta-blockers may precipitate a stroke.

58. How fast an injection of glucagon works on a hypoglycemic patient primarily depends on:

    a. the age, gender, and weight of the patient.
    b. the amount of glycogen reserves in the liver.
    c. whether the patient is Type I or Type II diabetic.
    d. the other types of medications the patient is taking.

59. Which of the following hormones produced in the pancreas stimulates an increase in blood sugar?

    a. insulin
    b. glucagon
    c. beta-cell
    d. cortisone

60. Complaints of abdominal pain are associated with which endocrine emergency?

    a. adrenal gland disorders
    b. hypoglycemia
    c. DKA
    d. all of the above

61. You respond to a call for a patient who fell and cannot get up. You find a forty-seven-year-old female who fell while getting out of bed. She has no specific pain, but is c/o increased weakness over the last week. You immediately recognize that she has one of the classic physical findings, the _____ that is associated with Cushing's syndrome.

    a. moon face
    b. bulging eyes
    c. extreme peripheral edema
    d. fruity breath odor

62. You assist the patient described in question 61 to a chair, and she allows you to assess her and take her vital signs. You find that her arms and legs appear to be wasting, compared to the rest of her body. She also has unusual stretch marks on her skin. You attribute these findings to be _____ with Cushing's disease.

    a. typical findings associated
    b. noncompliance of medications associated
    c. side effects of medications associated
    d. none of the findings associated

63. Which of the following conditions is characterized by the body breaking down fat rather than glucose as its energy source?

    a. hypoglycemia
    b. DKA
    c. pancreatitis
    d. insulin shock

64. Which of the following gland(s) is/are the only one(s) with both endocrine and exocrine functions?

    a. thyroid
    b. parathyroids
    c. pancreas
    d. adrenals

65. Which of the following gland(s) is/are responsible for the secretion of antidiuretic hormone?

    a. ovaries
    b. testes
    c. thymus
    d. pituitary

Exam #24 Answer Form

	A	B	C	D		A	B	C	D
1.	❏	❏	❏	❏	27.	❏	❏	❏	❏
2.	❏	❏	❏	❏	28.	❏	❏	❏	❏
3.	❏	❏	❏	❏	29.	❏	❏	❏	❏
4.	❏	❏	❏	❏	30.	❏	❏	❏	❏
5.	❏	❏	❏	❏	31.	❏	❏	❏	❏
6.	❏	❏	❏	❏	32.	❏	❏	❏	❏
7.	❏	❏	❏	❏	33.	❏	❏	❏	❏
8.	❏	❏	❏	❏	34.	❏	❏	❏	❏
9.	❏	❏	❏	❏	35.	❏	❏	❏	❏
10.	❏	❏	❏	❏	36.	❏	❏	❏	❏
11.	❏	❏	❏	❏	37.	❏	❏	❏	❏
12.	❏	❏	❏	❏	38.	❏	❏	❏	❏
13.	❏	❏	❏	❏	39.	❏	❏	❏	❏
14.	❏	❏	❏	❏	40.	❏	❏	❏	❏
15.	❏	❏	❏	❏	41.	❏	❏	❏	❏
16.	❏	❏	❏	❏	42.	❏	❏	❏	❏
17.	❏	❏	❏	❏	43.	❏	❏	❏	❏
18.	❏	❏	❏	❏	44.	❏	❏	❏	❏
19.	❏	❏	❏	❏	45.	❏	❏	❏	❏
20.	❏	❏	❏	❏	46.	❏	❏	❏	❏
21.	❏	❏	❏	❏	47.	❏	❏	❏	❏
22.	❏	❏	❏	❏	48.	❏	❏	❏	❏
23.	❏	❏	❏	❏	49.	❏	❏	❏	❏
24.	❏	❏	❏	❏	50.	❏	❏	❏	❏
25.	❏	❏	❏	❏	51.	❏	❏	❏	❏
26.	❏	❏	❏	❏	52.	❏	❏	❏	❏

	A	B	C	D		A	B	C	D
53.	❏	❏	❏	❏	60.	❏	❏	❏	❏
54.	❏	❏	❏	❏	61.	❏	❏	❏	❏
55.	❏	❏	❏	❏	62.	❏	❏	❏	❏
56.	❏	❏	❏	❏	63.	❏	❏	❏	❏
57.	❏	❏	❏	❏	64.	❏	❏	❏	❏
58.	❏	❏	❏	❏	65.	❏	❏	❏	❏
59.	❏	❏	❏	❏					

25

Allergies and Anaphylaxis

1. When protective cells are able to recognize infections as they enter the body and destroy them prior to causing harm, this is called a/an:

   a. antigen.
   b. antibody.
   c. immune response.
   d. immunity.

2. An _____ is an overreaction by the body's immune response to normally harmless foreign substances, which causes damage to body tissues.

   a. immune response
   b. antibody
   c. allergic reaction
   d. allergy

3. When an antigen and the IgE antibody react, the combination leads to the release of mediators from:

   a. basophils and mast cells.
   b. histamines.
   c. leukotrienes.
   d. antibodies.

4. Swelling of the skin caused by leakage of fluid from the blood vessels into the interstitial and subcutaneous tissues is called:

   a. urticaria.
   b. angioneurotic edema.
   c. angiocerebral edema.
   d. perisacral edema.

5. The most common causes of anaphylaxis include: drugs, insect stings, food, and:

   a. pollen.
   b. animal hair.
   c. animal dander.
   d. blood products.

6. An atypical finding in a patient suspected of a severe allergic reaction is:

   a. dyspnea.
   b. tachycardia.
   c. bradycardia.
   d. hypotension.

7. As anaphylaxis develops, mast cells located in the skin, respiratory tract, and _____ release mediators that are apparent as physical signs and symptoms.

   a. GI tract
   b. nervous system
   c. cardiovascular system
   d. renal system

8. The epinephrine auto-injector contains _____ mg for adults and _____ mg for children.

   a. 0.5; 0:25
   b. 0.5; 0:05
   c. 0.3; 0.33
   d. 0.3; 0.15

9. Besides epinephrine, what other medication classification does the paramedic administer to a patient in anaphylaxis?

   a. beta-blocker
   b. antihistamine
   c. antidiuretic
   d. ACE inhibitor

10. A person who has a latex allergy is likely to have sensitivity to foods such as potatoes, tomatoes, bananas, or apricots because:

    a. latex is used in the pesticides to grow these foods.
    b. farmers and food handlers wear latex during harvesting.
    c. latex sap is chemically related to these fruits and vegetables.
    d. supermarkets wash these foods with equipment that contains latex.

11. When is epinephrine appropriate for IV use over SQ for the patient in anaphylaxis?

    a. when the patient's auto-injector is empty
    b. when the patient has an AMS
    c. when the patient has taken PO Benadryl® prior to EMS arriving
    d. when peripheral circulation is so poor that SQ injections will be ineffective

12. Which of the following would be the most helpful for the paramedic to determine what type of snake or spider bite a patient has sustained?

    a. the size of the bite
    b. the shape of the bite
    c. the markings of the animal
    d. the time of the bite

13. _____ is a natural sap from the rubber tree used to make natural rubber products.

    a. Gum
    b. Latex
    c. Lidocaine
    d. Powder

14. Patients in anaphylaxis may be given corticosteriods that:

    a. slow histamine release.
    b. have a fast-acting effect.
    c. help to produce immunity.
    d. stimulate the antigen effect.

15. The histamine released during anaphylaxis may produce any of the following effects, *except*:

    a. decreased arterial pressure.
    b. increased arterial pressure.
    c. increased capillary permeability.
    d. spasms of the bronchioles.

16. A newborn's immunity is acquired primarily from its mother's antibodies and secondarily:

    a. transferred from breast milk.
    b. through initial immune responses.
    c. through cell-mediated immunity.
    d. from immunoglobulins after fetal circulation stops.

17. Benadryl® is given to patients for allergic reactions because it:

    a. increases heart rate and strength of contractions.
    b. will mediate IgE.
    c. competes with histamine at the receptor sites, blocking the effects of histamine.
    d. stimulates the antigen effect.

18. Anaphylaxis occurs as a result of the release of mediators from mast cells, which are primarily located in the:

    a. endocrine system.
    b. cardiovascular system.
    c. hematopoietic system.
    d. skin, respiratory, and GI tracts.

19. Beta agonists help to reverse some of the _____ associated with anaphylaxis.

    a. edema
    b. bronchospasm
    c. nausea
    d. vasodilation

20. When the body releases histamine in response to exposure to an antigen, the body is trying to:

    a. vasoconstrict bronchial muscles.
    b. increase dilation of the capillaries.
    c. decrease permeability of the arterioles.
    d. minimize exposure to the antigen.

21. Your patient is a six-year-old male who is having an allergic reaction to a known substance (nuts). The exposure occurred thirty minutes ago, and he now has wheezing and hives on his torso. His parents gave him 25 mg of Benadryl® PO just before calling EMS. Your primary concern for this patient is:

    a. the airway.
    b. histamine release.
    c. vasodilation.
    d. IV access.

22. Your management of the patient described in question 21 includes a calm approach with oxygen and:

    a. IV epinephrine 0.1 mg/kg (1:10,000).
    b. IM epinephrine 1.0 mg/kg (1:1,000).
    c. SC epinephrine 0.01 mg/kg (1:1,000).
    d. SC epinephrine 0.1 mg/kg (1:1,000).

23. Which of the following emergency pharmacologic agents is the primary bronchodilator used to treat a patient experiencing an anaphylactic reaction?

    a. albuterol
    b. solumedrol
    c. epinephrine
    d. diphenhydramine

24. The speed of an anaphylactic reaction depends on the route of exposure and the:

    a. degree of sensitivity.
    b. level of consciousness.
    c. patient's age.
    d. preexisting medical conditions.

25. You are halfway through an interfacility transport with a patient on a ventilator and an IV pump when you observe that the patient has developed urticaria around the neck and face. The IV pump has two medications running at a preset rate. When you were given a report prior to transport, you were told that the patient has just started a new IV antibiotic, and the chart indicates the same. You suspect that the patient is having a reaction to the new medication. What action do you take next?

   a. Administer 0.5 mg epinephrine SQ.
   b. Adjust the pump to stop the flow of antibiotic.
   c. Call the origination facility to obtain new orders.
   d. Call ahead to the destination facility to advise them of the problem.

26. The patient you are treating for an anaphylactic reaction is wheezing, hypotensive, and tachycardic five minutes after you have administered epinephrine. Which of the following should the patient receive next?

   a. albuterol
   b. repeat epi and give fluid boluses
   c. Benadryl®
   d. dopamine

27. The patient described in question 26 continues to be hypotensive and tachycardic despite the efforts of your previous treatment. How would you manage the patient en route to the hospital?

   a. Apply MAST/PASG and initiate a rapid transport.
   b. Start administration of a vasopressor.
   c. Prepare for a difficult intubation.
   d. Repeat epi and fluid boluses.

28. Urticaria, or hives, occur as a result of the fluid shift that happens when:

   a. blood vessels dilate and become permeable.
   b. the interstitial spaces overflow into the capillaries.
   c. the intracellular spaces constrict.
   d. antihistamines are no longer effective.

29. What is the mechanism by which Benadryl® helps to clear up hives?

   a. Antihistamines stimulate histamines to withdraw into mast cells.
   b. Antihistamines block H_2 receptors in the skin.
   c. Histamines are destroyed when antihistamines block H_1 receptor sites.
   d. Antihistamines block H_1 receptors in blood vessels.

30. Which of the following effects from the medication dopamine is not desired in anaphylaxis?

   a. increased cardiac contractibility
   b. increased peripheral vasoconstriction
   c. renal and mesentery artery vasodilation
   d. maintenance of systolic pressure

Exam #25 Answer Form

	A	B	C	D		A	B	C	D
1.	❏	❏	❏	❏	16.	❏	❏	❏	❏
2.	❏	❏	❏	❏	17.	❏	❏	❏	❏
3.	❏	❏	❏	❏	18.	❏	❏	❏	❏
4.	❏	❏	❏	❏	19.	❏	❏	❏	❏
5.	❏	❏	❏	❏	20.	❏	❏	❏	❏
6.	❏	❏	❏	❏	21.	❏	❏	❏	❏
7.	❏	❏	❏	❏	22.	❏	❏	❏	❏
8.	❏	❏	❏	❏	23.	❏	❏	❏	❏
9.	❏	❏	❏	❏	24.	❏	❏	❏	❏
10.	❏	❏	❏	❏	25.	❏	❏	❏	❏
11.	❏	❏	❏	❏	26.	❏	❏	❏	❏
12.	❏	❏	❏	❏	27.	❏	❏	❏	❏
13.	❏	❏	❏	❏	28.	❏	❏	❏	❏
14.	❏	❏	❏	❏	29.	❏	❏	❏	❏
15.	❏	❏	❏	❏	30.	❏	❏	❏	❏

26
Gastroenterology and Urology

1. The three major types of acute abdominal pain are visceral, somatic, and:

   a. involuntary.
   b. voluntary.
   c. referred.
   d. diffuse.

2. _____ pain is caused by stimulation of nerve fibers in the parietal peritoneum by chemical or bacterial inflammation.

   a. Visceral
   b. Somatic
   c. Biliary
   d. Radiating

3. _____ pain is caused by sudden stretching or distention of a hollow organ.

   a. Visceral
   b. Somatic
   c. Biliary
   d. Radiating

4. You are assessing a twenty-eight-year-old male complaining of acute abdominal pain radiating around the right side to the back and angle of the scapula. Which of the following is most likely the cause of the pain?

   a. pancreas
   b. gallbladder
   c. kidney stone
   d. duodenal ulcer

5. Possible conditions associated with left lower quadrant pain of the abdomen include:

   a. PID, diverticulitis, and ovarian cyst.
   b. ACS, appendicitis, pancreatitis.
   c. cholecystitis, duodenal ulcer, and bowel obstruction.
   d. gallbladder, lesion, pyelonephritis.

6. A sixty-five-year-old male with cardiac disease is complaining of a sudden onset of pain in his upper thighs and lumbosacral area. You suspect the cause of the pain to be a/an:

   a. ACS.
   b. pulled muscle.
   c. ruptured aneurysm.
   d. appendicitis.

7. Which of the following conditions can mimic a serious GI bleed?

   a. bowel obstruction
   b. ectopic pregnancy
   c. Mallory-Weiss tear
   d. swallowed blood from epistaxis

8. Which of the following conditions is a common cause of upper GI bleeding?

   a. tumors
   b. polyps
   c. fissures
   d. esophageal varices

9. Which of the following conditions is a common cause of lower GI bleeding?

   a. esophagitis
   b. diverticulosis
   c. acute gastritis
   d. peptic ulcer disease

10. You are assessing a thirty-year-old male who is in tears and complaining of acute non-traumatic abdominal pain that radiates into the groin and external genitalia. You suspect the cause of the pain to be:

    a. STD.
    b. renal colic.
    c. appendicitis.
    d. bowel obstruction.

11. While preparing to transport a nursing home resident to the ED for evaluation, the staff reports that the patient has had a melena BM today. What was unusual about the stool?

    a. It appeared tarry and black.
    b. It smelled of vomitus.
    c. Bright red blood was present.
    d. It was yellowish in color.

12. Initial treatment of any patient with GI bleeding, regardless of the location, begins with the administration of high-flow oxygen and:

    a. rapid transport to the ED.
    b. treatment for shock.
    c. treatment for pain control.
    d. nasogastric tube placement.

13. _____ is an acute inflammation of the gallbladder, usually caused by gallstones.

    a. Colitis
    b. Cholecystitis
    c. Crohn's disease
    d. Diverticulitis

14. Your partner is assessing a thirty-five-year-old male with symptoms of malaise, nausea, vomiting, and tenderness on palpation of the upper-right quadrant of the abdomen. After moving the patient to the ambulance, you notice the patient's sclera look yellow. What do you suspect is the patient's problem?

    a. reflux esophagitis
    b. diverticulitis
    c. gastroenteritis
    d. acute hepatitis

15. Orthostasis usually occurs with a _____ % loss of circulating volume.

    a. 5–10
    b. 15–20
    c. 25–30
    d. >35

16. Which of the following causes of abdominal pain is not an immediate life threat?

    a. ACS
    b. ruptured ectopic pregnancy
    c. ruptured viscus
    d. reflux esophagitis

17. The _____ is the most important part of the diagnosis in acute abdominal pain.

    a. blood pressure
    b. history
    c. patient's age
    d. type of pain

18. A slow onset of abdominal pain is more commonly associated with which of the following conditions?

    a. appendicitis
    b. ectopic pregnancy
    c. renal infarction
    d. splenic infarction

19. During the interview with a thirty-eight-year-old female complaining of GI distress, she tells you the pain began shortly after eating lunch. The lunch consisted of fatty food from a fast-food take-out place. Which of the following conditions do you suspect is the cause of the abdominal pain?

    a. cholecystitis
    b. pancreatitis
    c. gastroenteritis
    d. obstruction

20. A forty-year-old male with severe abdominal pain, which began the day before and has progressively worsened, is lying completely still. The patient is very distressed when any attempt is made to move him. What do you suspect is the nature of his distress?

    a. muscle spasms
    b. colic
    c. peritoneal inflammation
    d. obstruction

21. Which of the following characteristics of bowel sounds is the most significant in the field?

    a. decreased sounds
    b. increased sounds
    c. absence of sounds
    d. abnormal sounds

22. The presence of rebound tenderness in the abdomen during the physical examination indicates:

    a. colic.
    b. obstruction.
    c. shock.
    d. peritoneal irritation.

23. In which of the following age groups is a positive tilt test an unreliable finding?

    a. <thirteen
    b. twenty to thirty
    c. thirty to fifty
    d. >sixty-five

24. Probably the most common GI abnormality, which includes symptoms of bloating, pain, and often violent diarrhea, is:

    a. acute gastroenteritis.
    b. acute cholecystitis.
    c. lactose intolerance.
    d. bowel obstruction.

25. A condition that is most frequently found in young adults and is characterized by recurrent abdominal pain, usually crampy in nature, and diarrhea, alternating with periods of constipation, is known as:

    a. acute gastroenteritis.
    b. lactose intolerance.
    c. renal colic.
    d. irritable bowel syndrome.

26. The fluid wave test is performed on the abdomen to assess for the presence of:

    a. tenderness.
    b. ascites.
    c. masses.
    d. edema.

27. Patients that are being treated for acute GI emergencies get nothing by mouth (NPO) because they may need an empty stomach for emergency surgery and:

    a. a full stomach impedes diagnostic testing.
    b. the release of digestive enzymes often worsens the condition.
    c. pain management is contraindicated on a full stomach.
    d. their medication only works on an empty stomach.

28. _____ is a general term for a method, involving a semipermeable membrane, used to separate smaller particles from larger ones in a liquid mixture.

    a. Sifting
    b. DPL
    c. Osmosis
    d. Dialysis

29. A petite twenty-year-old female has abdominal pain with nausea and vomiting. The pain began the day before as cramping in the periumbilical area and has persisted. Today she feels worse, has not eaten, and has been vomiting. The patient has no significant medical history and is currently menstruating. Her vital signs are: skin CTC pale, warm, and dry; respirations 22/nonlabored; pulse 100/regular; and BP 108/60. What initial treatment steps should you begin?

    a. oxygen by cannula, IV fluids, and morphine
    b. oxygen by mask, position of comfort, and IM Phenergan
    c. oxygen as tolerated, IV fluids, IV Phenergan, and morphine
    d. left lateral recumbent with legs flexed, IM morphine and phenergan

30. Continuing with question 29, your physical exam of the patient's abdomen reveals that the pain has radiated to the right lower quadrant. There are no masses or distention, but she has generalized rigidity and tenderness in that area. What do you suspect is the source of her problem?

    a. appendicitis
    b. bowel obstruction
    c. ectopic pregnancy
    d. new onset of Crohn's disease

31. Special considerations for care of the dialysis patient with an acute problem includes:

    a. avoiding taking a BP in any extremity with a fistula.
    b. only taking a BP in the extremity with a graft.
    c. accessing medical control for orders to start an IV.
    d. never asking advice from the dialysis technician.

32. You are transporting a nursing home resident to the hospital for evaluation of dysuria, frequency, urgency, and suprapubic pain. The patient has had the symptoms for two days. What do you suspect is the problem?

    a. kidney stone
    b. UTI
    c. bowel obstruction
    d. bladder obstruction

33. A twenty-year-old female is complaining of abdominal pain and acute urinary retention. Which of the following conditions must be ruled out first?

    a. UTI
    b. ectopic pregnancy
    c. kidney stone
    d. pyelonephritis

34. You are called to a local high school for a male complaining of acute abdominal pain. Upon arrival and initial assessment, you have found that the patient was playing basketball when suddenly he felt severe pain in his left testicle. He denies having abdominal pain but feels nausea. You suspect which of the following?

    a. torsion of the testicle
    b. kidney stone
    c. renal infection
    d. UTI

35. Based on the scenario in question 34, which of the following treatments may be helpful?

    a. ice
    b. oxygen
    c. Trendelenburg position
    d. aspirin

36. One of the functions of the urinary system is:

    a. maintaining proper balance between water and salts in the blood.
    b. to produce aldosterone.
    c. to excrete potassium to solidify waste products.
    d. helping the body eliminate sugar.

37. You are treating a fifty-six-year-old male patient with a complaint of exertional chest pain. Your thorough history taking has revealed that the patient took Viagra® last night. Which of the following treatments would be most appropriate for the relief of this patient's chest pain?

    a. oxygen only
    b. oxygen and nitroglycerin
    c. oxygen and morphine
    d. morphine only

38. The most common STDs in both genders are gonorrhea, syphilis, and:

    a. hepatitis B.
    b. chlamydia.
    c. HIV.
    d. herpes.

39. During your assessment of a thirty-year-old male complaining of acute severe abdominal pain that radiates into the right flank area, you discover that the patient has a history of kidney stones. The patient tells you this pain is just like when he had a kidney stone before. After attention to the ABCs, your management plan for this patient includes:

    a. rapid transport.
    b. pain management.
    c. supportive care only.
    d. treating for shock.

40. Conditions that result in abdominal pain, but do not originate in the abdomen, include all the following, *except*:

    a. pneumonia.
    b. black widow spider bite.
    c. herpes zoster.
    d. Crohn's disease.

41. Which of the following statements about the presence of bright red discoloration in the stool is most correct?

    a. This condition may indicate obstructive jaundice.
    b. This condition only occurs with lower GI bleeding.
    c. This condition may be caused by a malabsorption syndrome.
    d. Bright red blood can occur with bleeding in the lower or upper GI tract.

42. _____ pain is pain from one area that is being sensed in another because of embryologic nerve distribution patterns.

    a. Referred
    b. Acute
    c. Guarded
    d. Reflex

43. A/an _____ GI bleed is bleeding proximal to the duodenojejunal junction.

    a. upper
    b. lower
    c. acute
    d. non-traumatic

44. Which of the following is a definition for the term "hematochezia"?

    a. vomiting bright red blood
    b. bright red blood in the stool
    c. tarry, sticky black stool
    d. vomiting "coffee grounds" digested blood

45. Estimating the amount of blood lost from reports of stool and vomitus, volume is likely to be:

    a. accurate if reported by a paramedic.
    b. candid as reported by the patient.
    c. reliable when reported by a home health aide.
    d. unreliable.

46. Appendicitis is inflammation of the appendix caused by occlusion of the lumen by a:

    a. small tumor.
    b. small piece of stool.
    c. blood clot.
    d. large lesion.

47. Cholecystitis is an acute inflammation of the gallbladder that blocks the lumen, interfering with:

    a. blood flow.
    b. bile flow.
    c. insulin production.
    d. urine production.

48. _____ is a general term indicating inflammation of the colon for any of a number of reasons.

    a. Diverticulitis
    b. Diverticulosis
    c. Colitis
    d. Gastritis

49. Dilations of the veins of the esophagus secondary to increased portal vein pressures result in:

    a. cirrhosis.
    b. peptic ulcer.
    c. gastric ulcer.
    d. varices.

50. Dilations of the veins in the lower portion of the colon result in:

    a. tumors.
    b. hemorrhoids.
    c. colitis.
    d. varices.

Exam #26 Answer Form

	A	B	C	D			A	B	C	D
1.	❏	❏	❏	❏		26.	❏	❏	❏	❏
2.	❏	❏	❏	❏		27.	❏	❏	❏	❏
3.	❏	❏	❏	❏		28.	❏	❏	❏	❏
4.	❏	❏	❏	❏		29.	❏	❏	❏	❏
5.	❏	❏	❏	❏		30.	❏	❏	❏	❏
6.	❏	❏	❏	❏		31.	❏	❏	❏	❏
7.	❏	❏	❏	❏		32.	❏	❏	❏	❏
8.	❏	❏	❏	❏		33.	❏	❏	❏	❏
9.	❏	❏	❏	❏		34.	❏	❏	❏	❏
10.	❏	❏	❏	❏		35.	❏	❏	❏	❏
11.	❏	❏	❏	❏		36.	❏	❏	❏	❏
12.	❏	❏	❏	❏		37.	❏	❏	❏	❏
13.	❏	❏	❏	❏		38.	❏	❏	❏	❏
14.	❏	❏	❏	❏		39.	❏	❏	❏	❏
15.	❏	❏	❏	❏		40.	❏	❏	❏	❏
16.	❏	❏	❏	❏		41.	❏	❏	❏	❏
17.	❏	❏	❏	❏		42.	❏	❏	❏	❏
18.	❏	❏	❏	❏		43.	❏	❏	❏	❏
19.	❏	❏	❏	❏		44.	❏	❏	❏	❏
20.	❏	❏	❏	❏		45.	❏	❏	❏	❏
21.	❏	❏	❏	❏		46.	❏	❏	❏	❏
22.	❏	❏	❏	❏		47.	❏	❏	❏	❏
23.	❏	❏	❏	❏		48.	❏	❏	❏	❏
24.	❏	❏	❏	❏		49.	❏	❏	❏	❏
25.	❏	❏	❏	❏		50.	❏	❏	❏	❏

27
Toxicology

1. The majority of the reported poisoning exposures occur in/on:

   a. the patient's home.
   b. a workplace.
   c. recreational facilities.
   d. the highway.

2. The largest number of poisoning deaths occur in which age group?

   a. one to eight
   b. nine to nineteen
   c. twenty to forty-nine
   d. fifty to seventy

3. Which of the following risk factors most predisposes an individual to a toxic emergency?

   a. gender
   b. unattended children
   c. working at an industrial site
   d. having a known allergic reaction

4. An example of a toxic effect on the respiratory system includes:

   a. the inability of the cells to manufacture ATP.
   b. a slowing of the transmission of nerve impulses.
   c. the development of pulmonary edema.
   d. increased lacrimation.

5. Which of the following is an example of a poison exposure by injection?

   a. insect stinger
   b. poison ivy contact
   c. mushroom digestion
   d. physically handling pesticides

6. When a substance enters the body by passing through the skin, this route of exposure is called:

   a. critical.
   b. absorption.
   c. intermittent.
   d. unpredictable.

7. Once a substance enters the body, the effects it has on the body primarily depend on:

   a. the type of poison.
   b. the patient's past medical history.
   c. the patient's tolerance to the substance.
   d. how many times the patient has been previously exposed.

8. Which of the following sea creatures can inject painful venom into a human's skin?

   a. gar
   b. shark
   c. stingray
   d. sea urchin

9. If a person is exposed to a nerve agent, which of the following signs and symptoms would you expect to find?

   a. salivation and nausea
   b. hallucinations and fever
   c. tachycardia and miosis
   d. euphoria and hyperactivity

10. _____ or syndromes are groupings of drugs that present with similar patterns of toxicity.

    a. Toxidromes
    b. Poisonings
    c. Intoxications
    d. Envenomations

11. The poisoned patient who took a large quantity of _____ may become hyperthermic in normal ambient temperatures.

    a. alcohol
    b. a narcotic
    c. a sedative
    d. aspirin

12. A patient who develops digitalis toxicity is very likely to develop:

    a. tachycardia.
    b. bradycardia.
    c. hypertension.
    d. hyperthermia.

13. _____ cause a person's pupils to become large (mydriasis).

a. Pesticides
b. Cholinergics
c. Anticholinergics
d. Phenothiazines

14. An overdose of narcotics will cause the pupils to be:

a. fixed.
b. dilated.
c. unequal.
d. constricted.

15. _____ is a rare, but potentially deadly, form of food poisoning with serious CNS symptoms.

a. E. coli
b. Botulism
c. Staphylococci
d. Viral food poisoning

16. Common agents that fall into the toxidrome referred to as anticholinergics include:

a. pesticides and nerve agents.
b. LSD, PCP, and mescaline.
c. tricyclic antidepressants and mushrooms.
d. diet pills, caffeine, and cocaine.

17. Euphoria, hypotension, and respiratory depression are most commonly found with which toxidrome?

a. sympathomimetic
b. narcotics
c. anticholinergics
d. hallucinogens

18. Tachycardia, diaphoresis, chest pain, and stroke are most commonly caused by which toxidrome?

a. sympathomimetics
b. anticholinergics
c. cholinergics
d. narcotics

19. What is the most common route of poisoning?

a. absorption
b. inhalation
c. ingestion
d. injection

20. The first cardinal principle of management for all EMS providers when dealing with a toxicologic emergency is to:

a. consider specific antidotes.
b. consider decontamination of the patient.
c. ensure your own safety first.
d. maintain an open airway and breathing.

21. The difference between a poisoning and an overdose is:

a. poisoning involves exposure to a substance that is generally harmful and has no beneficial effects.
b. overdose suggests an excessive exposure to a substance that is not normally used to treat humans.
c. there is no difference between the two terms and they are used interchangeably.
d. all of the above are correct.

22. Inducing vomiting may be part of the appropriate treatment in a patient who has ingested:

a. lye.
b. acid.
c. aspirin.
d. silver nitrate.

23. Vomiting should not be induced if the patient:

a. has taken pills.
b. is over fifty years old.
c. has a decreased mental status.
d. is a known drug abuser.

24. Induced vomiting in a patient who has ingested _____ should be avoided.

a. strychnine
b. an overdose of aspirin
c. an overdose of MAO inhibitors
d. an overdose of acetaminophen

25. Gastric dialysis is a mechanism of poison removal aided by the administration of:

a. activated charcoal.
b. ipecac syrup.
c. tincture of benzene.
d. milk or mild soap.

26. When treating a twenty-seven-year-old male patient who has a history of depression, you determine that the patient may have taken ten to twenty tricyclic antidepressants. His vitals are within normal range, and he is alert at this time. What treatment should be considered?

a. Administer 2 mg Narcan.
b. Transport to the poison control center.
c. Consider administering activated charcoal.
d. Quickly restrain the patient.

27. Exposure to systemic toxins, such as carbon monoxide, often results in:

a. hypoxia.
b. vertigo.
c. diaphoresis.
d. edema.

28. For any patient removed from a fire scene, the paramedic should suspect _____ even when the patient has no burns.

   a. cardiovascular collapse
   b. drug overdose
   c. carbon dioxide exposure
   d. carbon monoxide exposure

29. You have been dispatched to transfer a patient from a medical facility to the ED. The patient has accumulated excessive levels of theophylline. Which of the following effects should you be prepared to manage during the transport?

   a. seizures
   b. metabolic acidosis
   c. malignant hypothermia
   d. acute pulmonary edema

30. A chemical that _____ in the fat of the skin is likely to cause poisoning by absorption.

   a. slowly dissolves
   b. does not dissolve
   c. dissolves easily
   d. traps large particles

31. Symptoms of general toxicity include all the following, *except*:

   a. paralysis.
   b. headache.
   c. AMS.
   d. vomiting.

32. Patients presenting with muscle fasciculation and paralysis may be suffering from:

   a. cholinergic overdose.
   b. CNS toxicity.
   c. aspirin overdose.
   d. narcotic overdose.

33. Your patient is a twenty-two-year-old female who is seven months pregnant. Apparently she took an overdose of over-the-counter medication designed to relieve abdominal cramping. She is alert and oriented, and her vital signs are within normal range. What is your best course of treatment?

   a. Induce vomiting with syrup of ipecac.
   b. Restrain her, as she may become violent.
   c. Monitor her ABCs and administer oxygen.
   d. Administer activated charcoal and rush her to the ED.

34. What does the pathophysiology of poisoning by inhalation involve?

   a. The substance is absorbed into the bloodstream in the intestines.
   b. The substance is absorbed at the alveolar level, leading to systemic toxicity.
   c. The material is absorbed through the skin into the muscles.
   d. The material moves across the blood-brain barrier into the venous system.

35. What desired effect is most helpful to the patient when the paramedic administers Narcan?

   a. immediate withdrawal symptoms from the overdose
   b. reversal of the hypertension
   c. reversal of the respiratory depression
   d. a heightened sensitivity to the surrounding environment

36. Of the following, which substance is not usually absorbed through the skin?

   a. pesticides
   b. nitro
   c. wax
   d. insecticide

37. If your patient was exposed to a herbicide, which antidote may prove useful if authorized by medical control to administer?

   a. Narcan
   b. atropine
   c. Solumedrol
   d. nitrous oxide

38. Your patient is a fifty-two-year-old male who was working in the fields of his farm all day. His wife called the ambulance because he has been acting crazy and very shaky, and has been drooling upon returning home. What could be wrong with him?

   a. He has taken an accidental overdose of beta-blocker.
   b. He had an exposure to lithium.
   c. He had an excessive exposure to insecticide.
   d. He is having a stroke.

39. An acquired resistance to the therapeutic effects of usual doses of a drug is referred to as:

   a. addiction.
   b. tolerance.
   c. dependence.
   d. drug abuse.

40. A psychologic craving for, or reliance on, a chemical agent is referred to as a/an:

    a. addiction.
    b. tolerance.
    c. dependence.
    d. drug abuse.

41. What is the source of most illegal drugs in the United States?

    a. smuggling from Colombia
    b. stolen shipments to hospital pharmacies
    c. artificially manufactured in college labs
    d. they are grown in rural areas

42. A substance that is often abused and called "blow" or "candy" on the street is:

    a. marijuana.
    b. sedative-hypnotics.
    c. cocaine.
    d. opiates.

43. Medications that are often abused, yet are medically prescribed for bed-wetting, seizures, and Tourette's syndrome, include:

    a. narcotics.
    b. tricyclic antidepressants.
    c. cyanide.
    d. sedative-hypnotics.

44. A drug that is frequently abused, which decreases inhibitory synapses in the brain, then excitatory synapses, causing euphoria followed by depression, is called a/an:

    a. opiate.
    b. alcohol.
    c. barbiturate.
    d. mushroom.

45. Which of the following substances has a delayed reaction so that the patient appears fine initially, only to deteriorate later?

    a. cyanide
    b. cocaine
    c. sympathomimetics
    d. tricyclic antidepressants

46. Use of hydrocarbons causing CNS alteration, cardiac dysfunction, and liver dysfunction is often referred to as:

    a. huffing.
    b. freebasing.
    c. snorting.
    d. none of the above.

47. A woman has called EMS because her three-year-old grandson is sick and has been vomiting. She believes he ingested pills from a bottle left out on the table. The child appears inactive but is shivering. He is tachycardic and hypotensive. Which of the following substances did the child most likely ingest?

    a. iron
    b. MAOI
    c. antacid
    d. warfarin

48. When a patient is thought to have sustained carbon monoxide poisoning, his management should include high-concentration oxygen and consideration for:

    a. activated charcoal.
    b. syrup of ipecac.
    c. a hyperbaric chamber.
    d. a large dose of atropine.

49. When a patient with a history of hypertension suddenly stops taking his anti-hypertensive, which of the following emergencies is likely to develop?

    a. acute MI
    b. anxiety and tremors
    c. rebound hypertension
    d. profound hypotension

50. You have been called to a housing project where three preschoolers routinely play in the hallways and basement. The building is old, decaying, and sorely in need of repair. The parent of one child states that her son is complaining of a diffuse crampy abdominal pain and has diarrhea. He has been acting uncoordinated and irritable, and he has memory lapses. What could be the cause of this sickness?

    a. carbon monoxide poisoning.
    b. lead poisoning.
    c. hydrocarbon poisoning.
    d. an overdose of cocaine.

Exam #27 Answer Form

	A	B	C	D		A	B	C	D
1.	❏	❏	❏	❏	26.	❏	❏	❏	❏
2.	❏	❏	❏	❏	27.	❏	❏	❏	❏
3.	❏	❏	❏	❏	28.	❏	❏	❏	❏
4.	❏	❏	❏	❏	29.	❏	❏	❏	❏
5.	❏	❏	❏	❏	30.	❏	❏	❏	❏
6.	❏	❏	❏	❏	31.	❏	❏	❏	❏
7.	❏	❏	❏	❏	32.	❏	❏	❏	❏
8.	❏	❏	❏	❏	33.	❏	❏	❏	❏
9.	❏	❏	❏	❏	34.	❏	❏	❏	❏
10.	❏	❏	❏	❏	35.	❏	❏	❏	❏
11.	❏	❏	❏	❏	36.	❏	❏	❏	❏
12.	❏	❏	❏	❏	37.	❏	❏	❏	❏
13.	❏	❏	❏	❏	38.	❏	❏	❏	❏
14.	❏	❏	❏	❏	39.	❏	❏	❏	❏
15.	❏	❏	❏	❏	40.	❏	❏	❏	❏
16.	❏	❏	❏	❏	41.	❏	❏	❏	❏
17.	❏	❏	❏	❏	42.	❏	❏	❏	❏
18.	❏	❏	❏	❏	43.	❏	❏	❏	❏
19.	❏	❏	❏	❏	44.	❏	❏	❏	❏
20.	❏	❏	❏	❏	45.	❏	❏	❏	❏
21.	❏	❏	❏	❏	46.	❏	❏	❏	❏
22.	❏	❏	❏	❏	47.	❏	❏	❏	❏
23.	❏	❏	❏	❏	48.	❏	❏	❏	❏
24.	❏	❏	❏	❏	49.	❏	❏	❏	❏
25.	❏	❏	❏	❏	50.	❏	❏	❏	❏

28

Environmental Conditions

1. An environmental emergency is a medical condition caused or exacerbated by weather, terrain, or:

   a. age.
   b. health.
   c. medications.
   d. atmospheric pressure.

2. Which of the following age groups are at greater risk for environmental emergencies than others?

   a. teens and geriatrics
   b. middle age and geriatrics
   c. small children and geriatrics
   d. early adult and geriatrics

3. Which of the following general health issues makes a person more susceptible to environmental influences?

   a. obesity
   b. smoking
   c. cancer
   d. hypertension

4. Which of the following medical conditions is a risk factor that predisposes an individual to environmental emergencies?

   a. obesity
   b. diabetes
   c. hypertension
   d. hyperthyroidism

5. Which of the following medications results in an impaired ability to sweat and dissipate heat?

   a. tricyclic antidepressants
   b. antidiabetics
   c. aspirin
   d. diuretics

6. An example of an environmental challenge that involves atmospheric pressure is a _____ accident.

   a. freefalling
   b. diving
   c. caving
   d. skiing

7. Of the following, which is not a principal type of environmental illness?

   a. high-altitude sickness
   b. heat cramps
   c. radiation burns
   d. cold diuresis

8. Which of the following is not a major component of the body's thermoregulatory mechanism?

   a. hypothalamus
   b. metabolic rate
   c. central blood vessels
   d. skin

9. Body heat is generated as a side effect of normal _____ processes.

   a. systemic
   b. cell-mediated
   c. metabolic
   d. neural

10. _____ refers to normal body means of heat loss and gain.

    a. Thermoregulation
    b. Radiation
    c. Conduction
    d. Homeostasis

11. Body heat is gained or dissipated by which of the following mechanisms?

    a. convection
    b. homeostasis
    c. metabolysis
    d. electrolyte balance

12. When a person lays on a cold surface, such as a cold floor, heat is lost from the body by means of:

    a. radiation.
    b. conduction.
    c. convection.
    d. evaporation.

13. When the body is exposed to very high temperatures, _____ becomes the only effective method of heat dissipation.

    a. radiation
    b. conduction
    c. convection
    d. evaporation

14. In heat cramps and heat exhaustion, the underlying problem involves:

    a. dehydration.
    b. exposure.
    c. localized injury.
    d. inadequate thermogenesis.

15. Signs of thermolysis include:

    a. shivering and loss of coordination.
    b. diaphoresis and flushing.
    c. tachypnea and chest pain.
    d. slurred speech and ataxia.

16. A person who is properly acclimatized to warm temperatures is less likely to:

    a. sweat.
    b. disrupt sodium concentrations.
    c. vasodilate.
    d. maintain adequate fluid intake.

17. The primary causes of hypothermia are cold water immersion, cold weather exposure, and _____ hypothermia.

    a. urban
    b. acute
    c. subacute
    d. chronic

18. You are evaluating a fifty-five-year-old female who was outside watching her grandson play ball. She has a c/c of dizziness when she stands up, and a headache. Her clothing is wet with perspiration, but her skin temperature feels normal. Which of the following heat syndromes do you suspect she is experiencing?

    a. cramps
    b. exhaustion
    c. stroke
    d. exertional heat stroke

19. Your management plan for the patient described in question 18 is to cool her off in your ambulance and:

    a. treat for dehydration.
    b. provide high-flow oxygen.
    c. apply ice or ice packs.
    d. administer salt tablets.

20. Severe infection (sepsis) may actually result in _____ when the body's fever-production centers are overwhelmed.

    a. heat exhaustion
    b. heat stroke
    c. hypothermia
    d. exposure

21. The use of which of the following medications can predispose a person to environmental emergencies?

    a. nitrates
    b. estrogens
    c. antihistamines
    d. ACE inhibitors

22. There is a high incidence of heat exhaustion emergencies in individuals who:

    a. take diuretics.
    b. work outside.
    c. exercise routinely.
    d. drink alcohol excessively.

23. Fever is a normal response to the release of chemicals called _____ and usually results from an infection.

    a. pyrogens
    b. pyrexia
    c. pylorus
    d. purines

24. _____ is a normal response to an intact thermoregulatory system, and _____ develops when the thermoregulatory system has failed.

    a. Shivering; hypothermia
    b. Fever; heat stroke
    c. Diaphoresis; heat exhaustion
    d. AMS; heat cramps

25. With the exception of _____, wet clothing loses approximately 90% of its insulating value.

    a. wool
    b. polyester
    c. denim
    d. cotton

26. Conditions that may contribute to hypothermia include all the following, *except*:

    a. hypothyroidism.
    b. brain dysfunction.
    c. hypoglycemia.
    d. hyperglycemia.

27. Which of the following conditions is not usually a predisposing factor for hypothermia?

   a. acute stroke
   b. intoxication
   c. shock
   d. acute MI

28. The severity of hypothermia is determined by the core body temperature (CBT) and the presence of:

   a. frostbite.
   b. signs and symptoms.
   c. frost nip.
   d. cold diuresis

29. A core body temperature (CBT) of less than _____ is suggestive of severe hypothermia.

   a. 95°F
   b. 90°F
   c. 85°F
   d. 80°F

30. A person who has been hiking for several hours in the winter would most likely be at risk for _____ hypothermia.

   a. acute
   b. subacute
   c. chronic
   d. urban

31. An elderly stroke victim who has fallen and is unable to move off a tile floor would most likely be at risk for _____ hypothermia.

   a. acute
   b. subacute
   c. chronic
   d. urban

32. Sometimes hypothermia is a sign of another disease, such as:

   a. stroke.
   b. hypoglycemia.
   c. hyperthyroidism.
   d. hyperplasia.

33. Which of the following cardiac dysrhythmias/disturbances is more common during the rewarming phase rather than the development of hypothermia?

   a. atrial fibrillation (a-fib)
   b. ventricular fibrillation (v-fib)
   c. J waves
   d. long QT

34. Which of the following considerations is most accurate regarding the treatment of severe hypothermia patients?

   a. Cold may affect the potency of first-line cardiac drugs.
   b. The risk of v-fib increases with orotracheal intubation.
   c. The risk of v-fib increases with nasotracheal intubation.
   d. The hypothermic heart is never resistant to defibrillation.

35. The most common dysrhythmias in hypothermia-associated cardiac arrest are:

   a. bradycardia and heart blocks.
   b. v-fib and asystole.
   c. v-tach and a-fib.
   d. bradycardia and asystole.

36. In the management of a cardiac arrest patient with severe hypothermia, the risk of inducing ventricular fibrillation increases when:

   a. the patient is orally intubated.
   b. the patient is nasally intubated.
   c. CPR is administered prior to defibrillation.
   d. the patient is handled roughly during care and transport.

37. During the management of the submersion patient, the paramedic should assume that the patient is _____ until proven otherwise.

   a. brain-dead
   b. hypothermic
   c. in v-fib
   d. experiencing laryngospasm

38. For the paramedic managing the hypothermic patient, the first priority after airway, breathing, and circulation is to:

   a. administer a prophylactic antidysrhythmic.
   b. dress and protect frostbitten extremities.
   c. start an IV lifeline.
   d. stop ongoing heat loss.

39. Frostbite is the formation of _____ within the tissues affected.

   a. hematomas
   b. blood clots
   c. ice crystals
   d. cellulitis

40. The paramedic can differentiate superficial frostbite and deep frostbite in the following way.

   a. Deep frostbitten skin has a white, waxy appearance.
   b. Superficial frostbite feels hard to palpation.
   c. Superficial frostbite only affects small children and the elderly.
   d. Deep frostbite has a temporary decreased loss of sensation.

41. Often, when a frostbitten area is rewarmed, the patient complains of the area feeling numb. This feeling is caused by:

   a. the formation of acute cellulitis.
   b. a lack of oxygen.
   c. the presence of small hematomas.
   d. the formation of blisters.

42. When treating a drowning victim, the paramedic should consider the single most important factor in adult drowning, which is:

   a. the use of alcohol and mind-altering drugs.
   b. associated hypothermia.
   c. an acute medical problem may have precipitated the drowning.
   d. a suicide attempt may have been the cause.

43. When examining victims of submersion, it is important to realize that:

   a. they may appear normal and unaffected.
   b. they are initially going to require hyperventilation.
   c. they must be positioned head down (Trendelenburg position) to facilitate drainage of the lungs.
   d. they may require the Heimlich maneuver, as ingested water may become a foreign-body airway obstruction.

44. Aspiration of either seawater or freshwater decreases pulmonary compliance and results in:

   a. tension pneumothorax.
   b. hypoxia.
   c. pneumonia.
   d. upper respiratory infection.

45. The endpoints in a submersion incident involving saltwater are: pulmonary edema, aspiration injuries, and:

   a. metabolic acidosis.
   b. respiratory acidosis.
   c. metabolic alkalosis.
   d. respiratory alkalosis.

46. The three types of drowning include dry, wet, and:

   a. primary.
   b. secondary.
   c. tertiary.
   d. central.

47. Several complications can occur following submersion incidents, and include all of the following, *except*:

   a. persistent laryngeal spasms.
   b. persistent hypoxemia.
   c. infection.
   d. persistent neurologic deficit.

48. The best predictor of the severity of neurologic deficit following a submersion is the:

   a. type of water the patient aspirated.
   b. time to the first spontaneous gasp following removal from the water.
   c. presence of preexisting medical conditions.
   d. temperature of the water.

49. _____ drowning is defined as the recurrence of respiratory distress after successful recovery from the initial drowning incident, and can occur within a few minutes or up to four days later.

   a. Wet
   b. Primary
   c. Secondary
   d. Central

50. SCUBA is an acronym for:

   a. sealed and condensed underwater breathing apparatus.
   b. self-compressed underwater breathing aperture.
   c. self-contained underwater breathing apparatus.
   d. solid-compact underwater breathing aperture.

51. _____ law states that, in a mixture of gases, the total pressure is equal to the sum of the partial pressures of each gas.

   a. Boyle's
   b. Henry's
   c. Dalton's
   d. George's

52. _____ law states that, at a constant temperature, the volume of a gas varies inversely with the absolute pressure.

   a. Boyle's
   b. Henry's
   c. Dalton's
   d. George's

53. When a diver ascends but forgets to exhale on the way up, the pressure will _____ with ascent, and the volume of gas trapped in the lungs will _____ .

    a. decrease; expand
    b. decrease; shrink
    c. increase; expand
    d. increase; shrink

54. Which of the following injuries will the diver in question 53 most likely experience if the condition persists?

    a. stroke
    b. pericardial tamponade
    c. pneumothorax
    d. loss of consciousness

55. Decompression sickness is an illness during or after a diving ascent, secondary to rapid release of _____ in the blood.

    a. an air embolus
    b. nitrogen bubbles
    c. hydrogen bubbles
    d. subcutaneous air

56. A patient is c/o pain in the legs and shoulders two days after a dive. These symptoms are associated with the:

    a. bends.
    b. staggers.
    c. chokes.
    d. itches.

57. Divers can experience *nitrogen narcosis* at various depths because of the narcotic effect of dissolved nitrogen in the body. The effect is analogous to excessive ethanol levels, and the cause is attributed to _____ law.

    a. Boyle's
    b. Henry's
    c. Dalton's
    d. George's

58. _____ is a preexisting condition that can predispose some divers to the possibility of air embolism during or after a dive.

    a. Age
    b. Asthma
    c. Sinus infection
    d. Being of African American descent

59. Your patient is a thirty-three-year-old male diver who is lying on the pier. He is experiencing stroke-like symptoms immediately after surfacing from an 80-foot dive. He has left-sided motor deficit and is c/o of left-sided numbness and vertigo. Which of the following conditions do you suspect?

    a. air embolism
    b. decompression sickness
    c. nitrogen narcosis
    d. ARDS

60. After managing and supporting the ABCs, how would you manage the patient described in question 59?

    a. Complete a thrombolic checklist.
    b. Consider pain management therapy.
    c. Consider decompression therapy.
    d. Treat for stroke only.

61. When obtaining information about a patient who is experiencing an emergency related to diving, which of the following is not a significant factor?

    a. the number of dives today
    b. the depths of today's dives
    c. the type of gas mixture used
    d. Did the patient fly in an airplane more than twenty-four hours ago?

62. Hyperbaric oxygen is beneficial in both _____ and decompression sickness.

    a. pneumothorax
    b. tamponade
    c. DVT
    d. air embolism

63. Long delays are common for the treatment of decompression sickness in the lay diving populations because:

    a. of the lack of recognition of symptoms.
    b. of the distance to hyperbaric treatment areas.
    c. all diving sites are in foreign countries.
    d. the dive boats rarely have radios.

64. During the predive surface phase of a dive, any of the following potential problems may occur, *except*:

    a. air embolism.
    b. motion sickness.
    c. hyperventilation.
    d. near drowning.

65. During which phase of a dive do squeeze syndromes, involving the ears, most commonly occur?

a. predive surface
b. descent
c. bottom
d. postdive surface

66. Three days into a planned week-long mountain climbing trip in heights reaching 8,000 feet, one of the climbers develops shortness of breath, tachypnea, and cyanosis. What condition is he most likely experiencing?

a. AMS
b. ACS
c. HACE
d. HAPE

67. High-altitude illness occurs as a result of decreased atmospheric pressure, resulting in:

a. hypercarbia.
b. hypoxia.
c. vertigo.
d. dehydration.

68. Which of the following is a highly unlikely cause of altitude sickness?

a. skydiving
b. mountain climbing
c. SCUBA dives at high altitudes
d. flying in an unpressurized aircraft

69. Your patient is a mountain climber who has been sick for two days following an ascent of a mountain in excess of 8,000 feet. He is c/o dizziness, headache, irritability, and exertional SOB. Which of the following conditions do you suspect he has?

a. acute mountain sickness (AMS)
b. high-altitude pulmonary edema (HAPE)
c. high-altitude cerebral edema (HACE)
d. acute flying sickness (AFS)

70. The most important treatment the paramedic can provide for the patient described in question 69 is to:

a. administer high-flow oxygen.
b. administer a diuretic.
c. transport to a hyperbaric therapy center.
d. administer Nifedipine®.

71. You are treating a patient who has suffered first-degree burns that cover 35% of the BSA. You are cooling her with normal saline during the transport. Which of the following mechanisms of heat loss is the patient experiencing?

a. convection
b. radiation
c. evaporation
d. all of the above

72. The patient you are evaluating has frostnip on her fingers and face. While obtaining the focused history on this patient, which of the following are factors that may increase her susceptibility to frostbite?

a. diabetes and smoker
b. headache and sinus infection
c. allergy to PNC
d. hearing deficit

73. A diver has experienced *squeeze* during his last dive. Which body areas can be affected by squeeze?

a. thighs and calves
b. feet and mouth
c. ears and sinuses
d. hands and shoulders

74. For the last two hours, a rescue crew has been carrying a hiker out of the woods. The hiker lost his footing on ice and fractured his femur. The patient is very cold and, within the last ten minutes, has stopped shivering. Why has his shivering stopped?

a. He has gone into shock.
b. His core temperature has reached 92°F.
c. His glucose stores are depleted.
d. He has acute mountain sickness.

75. A diver is experiencing nitrogen narcosis. What is the primary danger for this diver?

a. impaired thinking
b. barotrauma
c. air embolism
d. hypoxia

76. When working in high humidity climates, it is important to recall that sweating becomes ineffective if the relative humidity exceeds _____ %.

a. 15
b. 35
c. 55
d. 75

77. A patient who has generalized hypothermia has been removed from the cold environment. If he is alert, has an open airway, and no nausea, he should be allowed to:

a. refuse medical attention.
b. drink warm fluids.
c. walk around to help warm the body.
d. smoke a cigarette.

78. On the scene at a private residence, you arrive to the backyard to find a small crowd standing around two people doing CPR. The patient is a teenage male who was pulled from the pool. A witness saw the male dive into the pool and then float to the surface, face down. What is the primary concern for this patient?

a. drainage of the lungs
b. correcting hypothermia
c. providing high-quality CPR
d. immobilizing the patient

79. You and your crew take over CPR and continue resuscitative efforts for the patient described in question 78. Initially the patient was easy to ventilate, but now lung compliance is getting hard to bag. What do you suspect is the cause of the increased resistance in ventilation?

a. gastric distention
b. laryngospasm
c. pneumothorax
d. hypercarbia

80. To correct the problem of increased resistance in ventilation of the patient described in question 78, the paramedic would:

a. decompress the stomach.
b. hyperventilate the patient.
c. decompress the chest.
d. intubate the patient.

Exam #28 Answer Form

	A	B	C	D			A	B	C	D
1.	❏	❏	❏	❏		27.	❏	❏	❏	❏
2.	❏	❏	❏	❏		28.	❏	❏	❏	❏
3.	❏	❏	❏	❏		29.	❏	❏	❏	❏
4.	❏	❏	❏	❏		30.	❏	❏	❏	❏
5.	❏	❏	❏	❏		31.	❏	❏	❏	❏
6.	❏	❏	❏	❏		32.	❏	❏	❏	❏
7.	❏	❏	❏	❏		33.	❏	❏	❏	❏
8.	❏	❏	❏	❏		34.	❏	❏	❏	❏
9.	❏	❏	❏	❏		35.	❏	❏	❏	❏
10.	❏	❏	❏	❏		36.	❏	❏	❏	❏
11.	❏	❏	❏	❏		37.	❏	❏	❏	❏
12.	❏	❏	❏	❏		38.	❏	❏	❏	❏
13.	❏	❏	❏	❏		39.	❏	❏	❏	❏
14.	❏	❏	❏	❏		40.	❏	❏	❏	❏
15.	❏	❏	❏	❏		41.	❏	❏	❏	❏
16.	❏	❏	❏	❏		42.	❏	❏	❏	❏
17.	❏	❏	❏	❏		43.	❏	❏	❏	❏
18.	❏	❏	❏	❏		44.	❏	❏	❏	❏
19.	❏	❏	❏	❏		45.	❏	❏	❏	❏
20.	❏	❏	❏	❏		46.	❏	❏	❏	❏
21.	❏	❏	❏	❏		47.	❏	❏	❏	❏
22.	❏	❏	❏	❏		48.	❏	❏	❏	❏
23.	❏	❏	❏	❏		49.	❏	❏	❏	❏
24.	❏	❏	❏	❏		50.	❏	❏	❏	❏
25.	❏	❏	❏	❏		51.	❏	❏	❏	❏
26.	❏	❏	❏	❏		52.	❏	❏	❏	❏

	A	B	C	D			A	B	C	D
53.	❏	❏	❏	❏		67.	❏	❏	❏	❏
54.	❏	❏	❏	❏		68.	❏	❏	❏	❏
55.	❏	❏	❏	❏		69.	❏	❏	❏	❏
56.	❏	❏	❏	❏		70.	❏	❏	❏	❏
57.	❏	❏	❏	❏		71.	❏	❏	❏	❏
58.	❏	❏	❏	❏		72.	❏	❏	❏	❏
59.	❏	❏	❏	❏		73.	❏	❏	❏	❏
60.	❏	❏	❏	❏		74.	❏	❏	❏	❏
61.	❏	❏	❏	❏		75.	❏	❏	❏	❏
62.	❏	❏	❏	❏		76.	❏	❏	❏	❏
63.	❏	❏	❏	❏		77.	❏	❏	❏	❏
64.	❏	❏	❏	❏		78.	❏	❏	❏	❏
65.	❏	❏	❏	❏		79.	❏	❏	❏	❏
66.	❏	❏	❏	❏		80.	❏	❏	❏	❏

29

Infectious and Communicable Diseases

1. A microorganism capable of causing disease is a/an:

   a. host.
   b. pathogen.
   c. parasite.
   d. infectious agent.

2. Nonpathogenic bacteria that live on the human skin, in the GI tract, and in mucous membranes are called:

   a. normal flora.
   b. protozoa.
   c. fungi.
   d. virus.

3. A single-cell microscopic parasitic organism that causes infection is a:

   a. normal flora.
   b. protozoa.
   c. fungus.
   d. virus.

4. A parasitic organism that can only live within a cell of a living animal or plant is a:

   a. helminth.
   b. host.
   c. fungi.
   d. virus.

5. A significant exposure occurs when blood or body fluids come into contact with broken skin, the eyes, parenteral contact, or:

   a. ingestion.
   b. cutaneous contact.
   c. mucous membranes.
   d. transdermal absorption.

6. All of the following can influence an individual's susceptibility to infection, *except*:

   a. age.
   b. gender.
   c. nutrition.
   d. latency period.

7. Which of the following is an example of an external barrier found on the human body?

   a. hair
   b. teeth
   c. skin
   d. earwax

8. The period after an exposure has occurred to a host, when the infection cannot be transmitted to someone else, is the _____ period.

   a. refractory
   b. latency
   c. communicable
   d. disease

9. The duration of time between exposure to a host and the development of signs and symptoms of the disease is the _____ period.

   a. communicable
   b. incubation
   c. immune
   d. inflammatory

10. The duration of time from onset of symptoms to resolution of symptoms or death is called the _____ period.

    a. refractory
    b. resolution
    c. distribution
    d. disease

11. The _____ is responsible for reporting to the county health department communicable diseases seen by prehospital healthcare providers.

    a. paramedic
    b. hospital
    c. patient's personal physician
    d. nursing home

12. The Ryan White Act of 1990 requires that exposure notification to emergency responders must be made within _____ hours.

    a. twelve
    b. twenty-four
    c. forty-eight
    d. seventy-two

13. OSHA is an example of a _____-level agency involved in disease outbreak.

    a. federal
    b. state
    c. local
    d. private sector

14. CDC recommends all of the following immunizations for EMS providers, *except*:

    a. HCV.
    b. HBV.
    c. polio.
    d. MMR.

15. Which of the following infections can be caused by needle stick?

    a. HBV, HCV, and HIV
    b. HBV, HIV, and pneumonia
    c. HIV, UTI, and URI
    d. HIV, TB, and pneumonia

16. The single most important task a healthcare provider can do to reduce the transmission of communicable disease is:

    a. not recap needles.
    b. dispose of all needles into sharps containers.
    c. place biohazards in red bags.
    d. hand washing.

17. Which of the following statements is most accurate about receiving a positive titer for HBV?

    a. Another titer is necessary following an exposure.
    b. Follow-up titers are recommended every five years.
    c. No further titers are necessary, even after an exposure.
    d. Additional boosters are recommended every five years.

18. Which of the following clinical findings would lead you to suspect that a patient is infectious?

    a. shortness of breath
    b. hypertensive teenager
    c. hypothermic geriatric
    d. hypothermic pediatric

19. What is the most common serious infectious disease in the United States?

    a. HIV
    b. AIDS
    c. hepatitis
    d. TB

20. How many types of hepatitis are there?

    a. five
    b. six
    c. seven
    d. eight

21. A person began the series of three hepatitis B vaccinations but failed to receive the last shot. Now, two years later, he wants to complete the vaccination. How should he complete the series?

    a. Restart the entire series.
    b. Repeat only the second dose.
    c. Complete only the third dose.
    d. Completion is no longer recommended.

22. Primary contraction of HCV is through direct contact with blood, such as a needle stick and:

    a. sexual contact.
    b. airborne droplet.
    c. indirect contact with urine.
    d. indirect contact with feces.

23. Which of the following infectious diseases does not have a known vaccine?

    a. HBV
    b. HCV
    c. chicken pox
    d. pneumococcal disease

24. What is the primary mode of transmission for HAV?

    a. needle stick
    b. oral–fecal
    c. airborne droplet
    d. direct contact with blood

25. What is the most common symptom of active TB?

    a. productive cough
    b. shortness of breath
    c. fever
    d. weakness

26. The transmission of _____ occurs from the saliva transferred through animal bites, most commonly by dogs, cats, bats, raccoons, and skunks.

    a. Lyme disease
    b. rabies
    c. arbovirus
    d. West Nile virus

27. Which, of the following, is the cause of most stomach ulcers?

    a. stress
    b. spicy foods
    c. stomach acid
    d. bacteria

28. An acute viral infectious disease of the CNS that causes painful muscle spasms in the throat and interferes with swallowing, leading to dehydration and death, is:

    a. salmonella.
    b. rabies.
    c. AIDS.
    d. arbovirus.

29. _____ is usually transmitted to humans by eating foods contaminated with animal feces.

    a. Salmonella
    b. Rabies
    c. Lyme disease
    d. Arbovirus

30. A person infected with _____ can pass on the disease by touching food after using the toilet and not washing her hands.

    a. salmonella
    b. varicella
    c. Lyme disease
    d. arbovirus

31. Lyme disease is transmitted by a tick bite. The infection does not occur until an infected tick has been attached for _____ hours.

    a. six to twelve
    b. twelve to twenty-four
    c. twenty-four to thirty-six
    d. thirty-six to forty-eight

32. Signs and symptoms of _____ include flu-like symptoms, muscle ache, and joint pain, with or without a rash.

    a. chicken pox
    b. rabies
    c. Lyme disease
    d. pneumonia

33. EMS was called by the husband of a thirty-two-year-old female. He states that his wife has been ill with a cold (sore throat and fever) for three days. Today she complained of a severe headache, has been vomiting, and is now extremely sleepy; he is unable to get her up. She appears dehydrated; her skin is very warm and flushed, with no sign of rash. Vital signs are: respiratory 16/nonlabored; pulse 100/regular; and BP 100/50. Blood sugar is 112 mg/dL, and SpO_2 is 96%. What do you suspect is the cause of her present condition?

    a. influenza
    b. meningitis
    c. Lyme disease
    d. herpes zoster

34. An example of a human internal barrier that protects against infectious diseases is:

    a. normal flora.
    b. an inflammatory response.
    c. Cushing's response.
    d. endorphins.

35. The liaison that is responsible for notification between the hospital and an exposed emergency responder is the EMS agency's:

    a. Medical Director.
    b. designated officer.
    c. chief supervisor.
    d. dispatcher.

36. _____ is an example of a national-level agency involved in disease outbreak.

    a. CDC
    b. NIOSH
    c. U.S. Fire Protection Administration
    d. OSHA

37. _____ is included in the top ten recommended vaccinations for children.

    a. HAV
    b. Varicella
    c. Influenza
    d. HPV

38. _____ is an approach to infection control, which is based on the assumption that all blood and body fluids are potentially infectious.

    a. BSI
    b. PPE
    c. Hand washing
    d. Biohazard labeling

39. The most commonly spread illnesses passed on by touching droplets from sneezing and coughing are influenza, the common cold, and:

    a. TB
    b. HPV
    c. pneumonia
    d. staph

40. Biohazardous wastes are placed in _____ bags that are labeled accordingly for disposal.

    a. clear
    b. yellow
    c. red
    d. green

41. All needles and sharps must be discarded in _____ that are properly labeled.

    a. red bags
    b. puncture-proof containers
    c. red containers
    d. unbreakable glass containers

42. A forty-year-old male is complaining of pain and a rash on his left thoracic area. He states that the pain began two days ago and has persisted. Today the pain is severe and constant. He denies dyspnea, diaphoresis, nausea, or other GI symptoms. When you examine his chest, you see a unilateral rash on the left thoracic area that spreads around to the back. What do you suspect is the cause of his present condition?

    a. ringworm
    b. shingles
    c. trichinosis
    d. tuberculosis

43. A _____ is a test using a sample of blood to measure the amount of antibody against a particular antigen in that blood.

    a. gloucomene
    b. titer
    c. Gram stain
    d. Hemoccult

44. After a paramedic is exposed to HBV while on the job, the _____ must assure and pay for proper medical follow-up.

    a. patient
    b. paramedic
    c. employer
    d. hospital

45. In the United States, _____ is most prevalent in nursing facilities, homeless shelters, prisons, and migrant farm camps.

    a. HBV
    b. HCV
    c. meningitis
    d. tuberculosis

46. _____ is often called the stomach flu. It is incorrectly used to describe many types of infections and irritations of the digestive tract.

    a. Ulcer
    b. Esophageal reflux
    c. Gastroenteritis
    d. *Helicobacteria pylori*

47. Diseases caused by _____ include the West Nile virus, encephalitis, yellow fever, and dengue.

    a. the Lyme tick
    b. arbovirus
    c. meningitis
    d. the plague

48. Advanced clinical features of _____ include AMS, paralysis, parethesia, stiff neck, sensitivity to light, arrhythmias, and chest pain.

    a. varicella
    b. salmonella
    c. Lyme disease
    d. HBV

49. The principal forms of plague are bubonic, septicemic, and:

    a. pneumonic.
    b. pulmonic.
    c. cardiogenic.
    d. enteric.

50. In recent times, the most cases of plague in the United States have been reported in New Mexico, Arizona, California, and:

    a. Alaska.
    b. Colorado.
    c. New York.
    d. Florida.

Exam #29 Answer Form

	A	B	C	D			A	B	C	D
1.	❏	❏	❏	❏	26.	❏	❏	❏	❏
2.	❏	❏	❏	❏	27.	❏	❏	❏	❏
3.	❏	❏	❏	❏	28.	❏	❏	❏	❏
4.	❏	❏	❏	❏	29.	❏	❏	❏	❏
5.	❏	❏	❏	❏	30.	❏	❏	❏	❏
6.	❏	❏	❏	❏	31.	❏	❏	❏	❏
7.	❏	❏	❏	❏	32.	❏	❏	❏	❏
8.	❏	❏	❏	❏	33.	❏	❏	❏	❏
9.	❏	❏	❏	❏	34.	❏	❏	❏	❏
10.	❏	❏	❏	❏	35.	❏	❏	❏	❏
11.	❏	❏	❏	❏	36.	❏	❏	❏	❏
12.	❏	❏	❏	❏	37.	❏	❏	❏	❏
13.	❏	❏	❏	❏	38.	❏	❏	❏	❏
14.	❏	❏	❏	❏	39.	❏	❏	❏	❏
15.	❏	❏	❏	❏	40.	❏	❏	❏	❏
16.	❏	❏	❏	❏	41.	❏	❏	❏	❏
17.	❏	❏	❏	❏	42.	❏	❏	❏	❏
18.	❏	❏	❏	❏	43.	❏	❏	❏	❏
19.	❏	❏	❏	❏	44.	❏	❏	❏	❏
20.	❏	❏	❏	❏	45.	❏	❏	❏	❏
21.	❏	❏	❏	❏	46.	❏	❏	❏	❏
22.	❏	❏	❏	❏	47.	❏	❏	❏	❏
23.	❏	❏	❏	❏	48.	❏	❏	❏	❏
24.	❏	❏	❏	❏	49.	❏	❏	❏	❏
25.	❏	❏	❏	❏	50.	❏	❏	❏	❏

Behavioral and Psychiatric Disorders

1. A/an _____ is a strong feeling, often accompanied by physical signs such as tachycardia and diaphoresis.

   a. disorder
   b. emotion
   c. nightmare
   d. daydream

2. Any disturbance of emotional balance, manifested by maladaptive behavior and impaired function, is called:

   a. insanity.
   b. mental disorder.
   c. normalcy.
   d. malfunction.

3. Which of the following statements about mental illness is true?

   a. In the United States, behavioral and psychiatric disorders incapacitate more people than all other health problems combined.
   b. Mental disorders are most often incurable.
   c. Studies have shown that most mentally disabled patients are unstable and dangerous.
   d. Abnormal behavior is always bizarre.

4. Which of the following statements about mental illness is false?

   a. In many cases, psychiatric illness has an organic basis.
   b. Many patients with mental illness are calm and never present a danger.
   c. Having a mental disorder is cause for embarrassment and shame.
   d. Modern medical and psychotherapeutic techniques can provide stabilized treatment for most mental disorders.

5. Intermittent explosive disorder is an impulse-control disorder in which a person has an impulse to:

   a. pull his own hair out.
   b. defecate in unusual places.
   c. set fires with the use of pyrotechnics.
   d. lose control and become aggressive.

6. Delirium and dementia are examples of _____ disorders.

   a. cognitive
   b. psychotic
   c. mood
   d. somatoform

7. _____ is a type of disorder that involves gross distortions of reality.

   a. Anxiety
   b. Schizophrenia
   c. Substance-related
   d. Somatoform

8. A mood disorder consisting of alternating periods of depression and mania is called:

   a. dementia.
   b. psychosis.
   c. hallucinations.
   d. bipolar.

9. Panic disorders, phobias, and post-traumatic syndromes are all examples of _____ disorders.

   a. insanity
   b. mood
   c. anxiety
   d. paranoia

10. Dependence is a _____ craving for a chemical agent, resulting from abuse or addiction.

    a. psychologic
    b. physical
    c. neural
    d. spiritual

11. _____ disorders are a group of neurotic disorders with symptoms suggesting physical disease, but with no demonstrable organic causes.

    a. Dissociative
    b. Somatoform
    c. Eating
    d. Factitious

12. A type of neurosis in which emotions are so repressed that a split occurs in the personality is what type of disorder?

    a. dissociative
    b. somatoform
    c. insanity
    d. factitious

13. _____ disorders are a large category of mental disorders characterized by inflexible and maladaptive behavior that impairs a person's ability to function in society.

    a. Dissociative
    b. Impulsive
    c. Personality
    d. Schizophrenic

14. Select the statement that is most correct about psychological behavior.

    a. Mental disorders are incurable.
    b. Abnormal behavior is always bizarre.
    c. All mental patients are unstable and dangerous.
    d. Some type of psychological aspect accompanies every illness and injury.

15. With respect to medical legal concerns, the paramedic should be aware of local facilities and procedures for:

    a. alcohol ingestion.
    b. registration of sexual predators.
    c. crisis intervention.
    d. definitive care.

16. The paramedic is responsible for knowing both local protocols and _____ regarding treatment of persons with mental illnesses.

    a. family wishes
    b. state laws
    c. advanced directives
    d. federal briefs

17. Many mental illnesses have been shown to occur from a chemical alteration in the brain. These chemicals are called:

    a. neurons.
    b. antidepressants.
    c. neurotransmitters.
    d. neuters.

18. Just because a person is on a "psych" drug does not mean that he has an emotional illness, as several of these agents are useful in other conditions, such as:

    a. diabetes.
    b. toothaches.
    c. acne.
    d. migraine headaches.

19. When a paramedic is assessing a patient displaying abnormal motor activity, she should always consider the possibility of hypoxia, drug intoxification, blood sugar abnormality, and:

    a. pain.
    b. abnormal thought content.
    c. stimulated intellectual function.
    d. mood disorders.

20. During the assessment of a patient, the paramedic should be alert for examples of overt behaviors associated with behavioral and psychiatric disorders, such as:

    a. poor hygiene.
    b. hypoglycemia.
    c. a lack of family support.
    d. multiple pets.

21. _____ are irrational, intense, and obsessive fears of specific things, such as an object or a physical situation.

    a. Hysterias
    b. Impulses
    c. Anxieties
    d. Phobias

22. Which of the following is an example of when the paramedic may need to transport a patient against his will?

    a. when the patient has no available transportation
    b. when the patient exhibits a danger to others
    c. when emergency dental care is needed
    d. after the patient falls and needs assistance getting up

23. Most people have fears and concerns. However, these fears become _____ when they significantly interfere with normal daily activities.

   a. phobias
   b. addictions
   c. impulses
   d. nightmares

24. The state of incoherent excitement, confused speech, restlessness, and sometimes hallucinations often caused by acute illness or drug intoxication is referred to as:

   a. depression.
   b. delirium.
   c. dementia.
   d. paranoia.

25. The police have just turned a patient over to you after an apparent attempt to harm herself. She is sixteen years old, with a history of depression. Today she used a razor blade to make numerous superficial cuts on her arms and thighs. Which of the following approaches should be avoided with this patient?

   a. Ask the patient if she intended to kill herself today.
   b. Ask the patient is she has any specific plans to kill herself.
   c. Ask the patient is there is anyone else she would like to harm.
   d. Assume the patient's actions were not an actual suicide attempt.

26. A _____ is something done by a person intending to ask for help rather than die.

   a. homicide attempt
   b. homicide gesture
   c. suicide attempt
   d. suicide gesture

27. A behavioral emergency only occurs when a person is:

   a. insane.
   b. neurotic.
   c. unable to cope.
   d. experiencing a loss.

28. _____ is when a patient has no conception whatsoever of reality.

   a. Psychosis
   b. Neurosis
   c. Anxiety
   d. Phobia

29. The best way to deal with a patient experiencing hallucinations is:

   a. to use a chemical restraint.
   b. the "talk-down" technique.
   c. to use physical restraint.
   d. to shout at the patient.

30. Which of the following is an atypical sign or symptom suggesting that a person may be depressed?

   a. paranoia
   b. sleep disturbances
   c. decreased appetite
   d. significant weight loss

31. The most common organic cause of apparent emotional and psychiatric illness in the elderly population is:

   a. inactivity.
   b. alcoholism.
   c. medication.
   d. seasonal weather changes.

32. Mania, or excessive hyperactivity, is an example of a/an _____ disorder.

   a. impulsive control
   b. eating
   c. personality
   d. mood

33. _____ is a condition characterized by an overwhelming desire to continue taking a drug on which one has become "hooked" through repeated consumption.

   a. Dependence
   b. Intoxication
   c. Addiction
   d. Abuse

34. _____ relates to acute effects of taking a substance and may or may not be related to dependence.

   a. Alcoholism
   b. Intoxication
   c. Addiction
   d. Abuse

35. True _____ is both a psychologic and physical event, whereby the patient has both a physical and psychologic craving for the drug, as well as for the effect.

   a. dependence
   b. intoxication
   c. addiction
   d. neurosis

36. As a rule, if a person has a psychiatric disorder and then develops a drug addition or alcoholism, the underlying psychiatric condition:

    a. improves.
    b. worsens.
    c. is cured.
    d. shows no change.

37. With respect to emotional illness, the term for assuming a certain body–language position suggestive of a particular emotion is:

    a. affect.
    b. fear.
    c. mental status.
    d. posture.

38. The term _____ refers to a state of mind in which one is uncertain of the present time, place, or self-identity.

    a. anger
    b. delirium
    c. confusion
    d. bipolar

39. The term _____ refers to the emotional tone behind an expressed emotion or behavior.

    a. fear
    b. anxiety
    c. affect
    d. mental status

40. While interviewing an emotionally disturbed patient, which of the following is a positive therapeutic interview technique the paramedic might use?

    a. Look directly into the patient's eyes.
    b. Promptly interrupt the patient when she becomes too talkative.
    c. Avoid asking questions about the immediate problem.
    d. Engage in active listening.

41. Management of behavioral emergencies begins with maintaining scene and personal safety, and then the paramedic should:

    a. begin the physical exam.
    b. attempt to build a good rapport with the patient.
    c. wait until the crisis team arrives before beginning care.
    d. have the police stand over the patient.

42. If a situation escalates and you become trapped by the patient, what should you do until help arrives?

    a. Scream for help.
    b. Do not say anything.
    c. Keep talking to the patient.
    d. Threaten the patient with bodily harm.

43. All of the following are factors that increase the risk that a person is suicidal, *except*:

    a. no prior history of suicide attempts.
    b. male gender.
    c. excessive alcohol or drug use.
    d. a person who is divorced.

44. Studies report that the risk of suicide in men is double that of women after experiencing a divorce or marital separation primarily because:

    a. men are mentally weaker than women.
    b. women have better support systems.
    c. men lack certain female hormones.
    d. women tend to remarry more quickly than men.

45. The term _____ refers specifically to physical problems brought about by underlying emotional problems.

    a. somatogenesis
    b. pseudopsychosis
    c. psychosomatic illness
    d. psychogenic disease

46. You are on the scene with police for an "emotionally disturbed person." A twenty-year-old female is pacing back and forth in her backyard, bragging about how tough she is, despite just being assaulted by her boyfriend. This patient is exhibiting clues that she:

    a. is bipolar.
    b. may attempt suicide.
    c. may develop violent behavior.
    d. has ingested excessive alcohol.

47. Which of the following statements about neurotic fear is true:

    a. A person with neurosis is probably insane.
    b. People with neurosis are not crazy.
    c. Most people with neurosis cannot cope with their fears.
    d. Neurosis is a normal anxiety reaction to a perceived fear.

48. Elderly persons commonly appear to have organic illnesses such as cardiac conditions when, in reality, they are:

    a. severely depressed.
    b. lonely.
    c. overmedicated.
    d. undermedicated.

49. Which of the following statements best describes how phobias can be unhealthy?

    a. Phobias can cause AMS.
    b. People with phobias are prone to ACS.
    c. Phobias are not unhealthy.
    d. Phobias can interfere with daily living activities.

50. Which of the following statements about the use of "open-ended" questions with behavioral patients is most accurate?

    a. They are used to encourage better patient responses.
    b. They do not tend to lead the patient to a specific answer.
    c. They are more likely to provoke an untoward emotional response.
    d. They do not give the patient the opportunity to express his anger verbally.

Exam #30 Answer Form

	A	B	C	D		A	B	C	D
1.	❏	❏	❏	❏	26.	❏	❏	❏	❏
2.	❏	❏	❏	❏	27.	❏	❏	❏	❏
3.	❏	❏	❏	❏	28.	❏	❏	❏	❏
4.	❏	❏	❏	❏	29.	❏	❏	❏	❏
5.	❏	❏	❏	❏	30.	❏	❏	❏	❏
6.	❏	❏	❏	❏	31.	❏	❏	❏	❏
7.	❏	❏	❏	❏	32.	❏	❏	❏	❏
8.	❏	❏	❏	❏	33.	❏	❏	❏	❏
9.	❏	❏	❏	❏	34.	❏	❏	❏	❏
10.	❏	❏	❏	❏	35.	❏	❏	❏	❏
11.	❏	❏	❏	❏	36.	❏	❏	❏	❏
12.	❏	❏	❏	❏	37.	❏	❏	❏	❏
13.	❏	❏	❏	❏	38.	❏	❏	❏	❏
14.	❏	❏	❏	❏	39.	❏	❏	❏	❏
15.	❏	❏	❏	❏	40.	❏	❏	❏	❏
16.	❏	❏	❏	❏	41.	❏	❏	❏	❏
17.	❏	❏	❏	❏	42.	❏	❏	❏	❏
18.	❏	❏	❏	❏	43.	❏	❏	❏	❏
19.	❏	❏	❏	❏	44.	❏	❏	❏	❏
20.	❏	❏	❏	❏	45.	❏	❏	❏	❏
21.	❏	❏	❏	❏	46.	❏	❏	❏	❏
22.	❏	❏	❏	❏	47.	❏	❏	❏	❏
23.	❏	❏	❏	❏	48.	❏	❏	❏	❏
24.	❏	❏	❏	❏	49.	❏	❏	❏	❏
25.	❏	❏	❏	❏	50.	❏	❏	❏	❏

31

Hematology

1. What is the name of the body system that produces blood cells?

   a. hepatic
   b. hemophilic
   c. hematopoietic
   d. uremic

2. The key components of the body system described in question 1 include the liver, spleen, and:

   a. kidneys.
   b. bone marrow.
   c. gray matter.
   d. CFS.

3. The majority of the blood cells are formed in the:

   a. spleen.
   b. liver.
   c. lungs.
   d. bone marrow.

4. The average pH of the blood is:

   a. 7.30
   b. 7.35
   c. 7.40
   d. 7.45

5. Men have approximately _____ cc of blood per kg of body weight.

   a. 60
   b. 70
   c. 80
   d. 90

6. During fetal development, red blood cells are produced in the:

   a. lungs.
   b. kidneys.
   c. umbilical cord.
   d. spleen.

7. All the elements in the red cells, white cells, and platelets are derived from the:

   a. leukocytes.
   b. stem cell.
   c. monocytes.
   d. erythrocytes.

8. How many days do mature red blood cells normally circulate in the blood?

   a. 30
   b. 60
   c. 120
   d. 240

9. Hemoglobin byproducts are excreted by the body in the form of:

   a. bilirubin.
   b. hemotoxins.
   c. urine.
   d. cytokines.

10. The measure of the number of red blood cells per unit of blood volume is called the:

    a. pulse oximetry.
    b. end tidal CO_2.
    c. hematocrit.
    d. hematacult.

11. When a patient has a low number of red blood cells, this chronic condition is called:

    a. hematuria.
    b. polycythemia.
    c. hypocythemia.
    d. anemia.

12. The normal range of hematocrit for women is:

    a. 36–46.
    b. 44–49.
    c. 50–54.
    d. 55–60.

13. The normal range of hematocrit for men is:

    a. 36–42.
    b. 40–45.
    c. 41–53.
    d. 50–55.

14. Neutrophils, eosinophils, and basophils are different types of:

    a. platelets.
    b. granulocytes.
    c. leukocytes.
    d. hemoglobins.

15. Cells without intracellular granules are called:

    a. neutrophils.
    b. monocytes.
    c. exudates.
    d. hemocells.

16. The main function of a leukocyte is to:

    a. carry oxygen to body cells.
    b. provide the color for the blood.
    c. maintain host defenses against infection.
    d. keep the blood clean of byproducts.

17. When the body's volume feedback systems sense a low number of circulating red and white blood cells and platelets, the _____ stimulate(s) the _____ to manufacture additional cells.

    a. kidneys and spleen; SCF
    b. spleen and liver; kidneys
    c. kidneys and liver; bone marrow
    d. liver; kidneys and bone marrow

18. Antibody-mediated immunity is also called:

    a. humoral immunity.
    b. anemia.
    c. cellular immunity.
    d. leukemia.

19. When a patient has a low number of white blood cells (WBCs), this is called:

    a. leukopenia.
    b. leukocytosis.
    c. leukemia.
    d. anemia.

20. Platelets circulate in the blood for an average of _____ days before being removed by the spleen.

    a. two to five
    b. seven to ten
    c. twenty to twenty-eight
    d. thirty to forty-five

21. The aggregation of platelets may be decreased by:

    a. high cholesterol in foods.
    b. polycythemia.
    c. anti-inflammatory drugs.
    d. chronic anemia.

22. Immediately following a vascular injury, which of the following inflammatory responses occurs first?

    a. Tissues swell and become edematous.
    b. Protein-rich fluid leaks out from the vessels.
    c. Blood vessels dilate and develop increased permeability.
    d. WBCs line up along the inside of the blood vessels walls.

23. The substance that is the final "glue" that completes the blood clot is:

    a. hemoglobin.
    b. epithelium.
    c. fibrin.
    d. elastin.

24. Human blood groups are determined by the presence or absence of two antigens, A and B, on the surface of _____ cells.

    a. platelet
    b. red blood
    c. white blood
    d. stem

25. The universal blood recipients with type _____ blood have no antibodies.

    a. A
    b. B
    c. AB
    d. O

26. People with type _____ have no antigens and are considered universal donors.

    a. A
    b. B
    c. AB
    d. O

27. Which of the following hematologic conditions is associated with shortness of breath and severe abdominal pain?

    a. anemia
    b. sickle cell crisis
    c. leukemia
    d. myeloma

28. The hematologic condition that rarely affects females but is sex-linked by transmission from a mother to a son, and is characterized by excessive bleeding after minor wounds, is:

    a. anemia.
    b. sickle cell disease.
    c. hemophilia.
    d. leukemia.

29. _____ results from a malignant tumor of blood-forming tissues, and is characterized by abnormalities of the bone marrow, spleen, lymph nodes, and liver.

    a. Polycythemia
    b. Sickle cell disease
    c. Hemophilia
    d. Leukemia

30. Which of the following drugs or herbs does not decrease the aggregation of platelets?

    a. thyme
    b. aspirin
    c. ibuprofen
    d. ginseng

31. _____ is the body's natural and normal way of preventing excess blood clot formation.

    a. Fibrinolysis
    b. Electrolysis
    c. Plasminolysis
    d. Neutrolysis

32. Leukemia is a form of cancer that causes which of the following leukocyte disorders?

    a. leukopenia
    b. leukocytosis
    c. abnormal WBC function
    d. abnormal WBC destruction

33. Which of the following granulocytes in the blood are important in fighting allergic reactions?

    a. neutrophils and eosinophils
    b. neutrophils and basophils
    c. eosinophils and basophils
    d. all of the above

34. When a clinician refers to a patient's H & H, she is referring to the patient's hematocrit and:

    a. hypoxia.
    b. hemoglobin.
    c. hematology.
    d. hematuria.

35. Which of the following conditions, when severe, is characterized by fatigue, dyspnea, chest pain, or syncopy?

    a. anemia
    b. leukemia
    c. lymphomas
    d. hemophilia

Exam #31 Answer Form

	A	B	C	D			A	B	C	D
1.	❏	❏	❏	❏		19.	❏	❏	❏	❏
2.	❏	❏	❏	❏		20.	❏	❏	❏	❏
3.	❏	❏	❏	❏		21.	❏	❏	❏	❏
4.	❏	❏	❏	❏		22.	❏	❏	❏	❏
5.	❏	❏	❏	❏		23.	❏	❏	❏	❏
6.	❏	❏	❏	❏		24.	❏	❏	❏	❏
7.	❏	❏	❏	❏		25.	❏	❏	❏	❏
8.	❏	❏	❏	❏		26.	❏	❏	❏	❏
9.	❏	❏	❏	❏		27.	❏	❏	❏	❏
10.	❏	❏	❏	❏		28.	❏	❏	❏	❏
11.	❏	❏	❏	❏		29.	❏	❏	❏	❏
12.	❏	❏	❏	❏		30.	❏	❏	❏	❏
13.	❏	❏	❏	❏		31.	❏	❏	❏	❏
14.	❏	❏	❏	❏		32.	❏	❏	❏	❏
15.	❏	❏	❏	❏		33.	❏	❏	❏	❏
16.	❏	❏	❏	❏		34.	❏	❏	❏	❏
17.	❏	❏	❏	❏		35.	❏	❏	❏	❏
18.	❏	❏	❏	❏						

32

Gynecology and Obstetrics

1. Which of the following structures does not form the female external genitalia?

   a. mons pubis
   b. urethra
   c. perineum
   d. urinary meatus

2. Which of the following structures of the female genitalia is responsible for sexual hormone secretion?

   a. ovaries
   b. fallopian tubes
   c. myometrium
   d. fimbriae

3. Which of the following statements about the fallopian tubes and their functions is most correct?

   a. Ova take twenty-one days to travel through the fallopian tubes.
   b. The fimbriae at the ends of the tubes are connected to the ovaries.
   c. Fertilization of the ovum usually occurs in one of the fallopian tubes.
   d. The fallopian tubes produce hormones that regulate female reproduction.

4. The base of the uterus is called the:

   a. fundus.
   b. cervix.
   c. uterine cavity.
   d. endometrium.

5. A developing child in utero under eights weeks gestation is called a/an:

   a. fetus.
   b. embryo.
   c. ova.
   d. oocyte.

6. The umbilical vein is responsible for:

   a. the production of amniotic fluid.
   b. carrying fetal blood to the placenta.
   c. returning oxygenated blood from the fetus to the placenta.
   d. returning oxygenated blood from the placenta to the fetus.

7. Endometrial cells can sometimes migrate to an area in the body other than the uterus. This condition is called:

   a. cystitis.
   b. endometritis.
   c. endometriosis.
   d. ectopic pregnancy.

8. The normal menstrual cycle is twenty-eight days and can be divided into three phases: menses, the proliferative phase, and:

   a. the secretory phase.
   b. the sloughing phase.
   c. PMS.
   d. post-capillary washout.

9. _____ is a condition that involves both physical and emotional symptoms that occur regularly in many women during the premenstrual phase of their reproductive cycle.

   a. Meiosis
   b. Amenorrhea
   c. Mittelschmerz
   d. Premenstrual dysphoric disorder

10. Some women experience intense feelings of depression, irritability, anxiety, or withdrawal prior to each menses. These women may also feel fatigued and experience temporary weight gain during the same time frame. The treatment for this condition is:

    a. supplemental iron therapy.
    b. estrogen hormone therapy.
    c. testosterone hormone therapy.
    d. aimed at relieving the symptoms.

11. The hormone _____ is responsible for stimulating bone and muscle growth.

    a. estrogen
    b. progesterone
    c. actin
    d. testosterone

12. The hormone responsible for restoring and preparing the uterus for pregnancy after menses is:

   a. estrogen.
   b. progesterone.
   c. oxytocin.
   d. pitocin.

13. Fertilization is the union of the egg and sperm, which forms the:

   a. zygote.
   b. ovum.
   c. fetus.
   d. corpus luteum.

14. Amenorrhea in the adult female is considered abnormal in which of the following circumstances?

   a. pregnancy
   b. malnutrition
   c. syphilis infection
   d. extreme and prolonged exercise

15. _____ is/are the leading cause of female infertility and ectopic pregnancy.

   a. Peritonitis
   b. Genital warts
   c. Vaginal yeast infections
   d. PID

16. What is the most common bacterial STD?

   a. syphilis
   b. gonorrhea
   c. pubic lice
   d. chlamydia

17. Of the following conditions, which one does not produce vaginal bleeding?

   a. labor
   b. sexual abuse
   c. urinary tract infection
   d. pelvic inflammatory disease

18. Cystitis is a/an _____ infection, which often occurs secondary to a urinary tract infection (UTI).

   a. kidney
   b. bladder
   c. urethra
   d. ovarian

19. You are assessing a twenty-six-year-old female who is twenty-four weeks pregnant. She is complaining of acute abdominal pain that is constant and severe. The pregnancy has been normal, and she has prenatal care. She feels the baby moving. However, she is having a small amount of bloody discharge that just began. You suspect which of the following?

   a. ectopic pregnancy
   b. abruptio placenta
   c. placenta previa
   d. spontaneous abortion

20. How do you manage the patient described in question 19?

   a. Administer high-flow oxygen and begin transport.
   b. Treat for shock and begin transport.
   c. Have the patient call her gynecologist, because delivery is imminent.
   d. Prepare the patient mentally for a spontaneous abortion.

21. Pregnant women with a negative Rh factor may become sensitized if the fetus has a positive Rh factor. If a fetus in any subsequent pregnancies has a positive Rh factor, Rh antibodies may cross the placenta and:

   a. suppress the immune response.
   b. destroy fetal cells.
   c. cause gestational diabetes.
   d. precipitate preclampsia.

22. You are dispatched to a call for respiratory distress. Upon arrival, you find a thirty-six-year-old female who is thirty-eight weeks pregnant. She is having severe difficulty breathing that began one hour ago and is getting progressively worse. She has no history of asthma, COPD, or cardiac problems, and her pregnancy has been normal with regular prenatal care. What do you suspect is the problem?

   a. heart attack
   b. hyperventilation
   c. pulmonary embolism
   d. pneumothrorax

23. Your management plan for the patient in question 22 includes:

   a. nitrates and Lasix.
   b. nebulized albuterol treatment.
   c. assisted breathing with CPAP.
   d. rapid transport for a life-threatening condition.

24. Which of the following is an abnormal condition during pregnancy that needs to be managed promptly?

    a. hypertension
    b. increased cardiac output
    c. increased resting heart rate
    d. decreased blood pressure during second trimester

25. Women in third trimester pregnancy are at increased risk of vomiting during injury and illness because of:

    a. a decreased tidal volume.
    b. slowed peristalsis.
    c. increased appetite.
    d. nausea from morning sickness.

26. Palpation of the fundus during active labor is performed to determine all the following, *except*:

    a. size of the baby's head.
    b. duration of contraction.
    c. to estimate gestational age.
    d. strength of contraction.

27. Back labor is back pain caused by the fetus pressing against the _____ during labor.

    a. spine
    b. kidneys
    c. bladder
    d. vena cava

28. The hormone _____ secreted by the pituitary gland stimulates the uterus to produce stronger contractions.

    a. estrogen
    b. progesterone
    c. oxytocin
    d. epinephrine

29. In which of the following cases would it be appropriate not to start an IV on a woman in active labor?

    a. Contractions are abnormal.
    b. Labor is two weeks early, but the mother is mentally competent and refuses.
    c. Postpartum hemorrhage began before delivery of the placenta.
    d. The mother is full term with twins.

30. While assisting the mother during delivery, the paramedic prepares to prevent an explosive delivery by:

    a. coaching the mother to breathe deeply.
    b. coaching the mother to pant during contractions.
    c. having the mother raise her hips when the head delivers.
    d. holding one hand on the baby's head while the mother is pushing.

31. Once the baby's head delivers, the paramedic should:

    a. inspect the head for trauma.
    b. inspect for a nuchal cord.
    c. perform the first APGAR score.
    d. dry the head and face.

32. Once the baby's head is out, the natural progression is for the baby's face to turn:

    a. laterally.
    b. superiorly.
    c. purple.
    d. inferiorly.

33. The APGAR score is a well-accepted assessment score chart for evaluating infants by rating the muscle tone, heart rate, respirations, and:

    a. reflex and color.
    b. color and weight.
    c. BP and reflex.
    d. BP and color.

34. In the field, the primary reason to cut the cord soon after the birth is that:

    a. the baby will suckle quicker.
    b. stage III of labor will progress quicker.
    c. the baby will be easier to manage and assess.
    d. the mother will not tear the cord.

35. When the cord is not cut immediately, the infant should be placed _____ to prevent placental transfusion.

    a. at a higher level than the placenta
    b. at a lower level than the placenta
    c. in an incubator
    d. in an infant swaddler

36. When access for medication is needed in the newborn, which of the following is preferred?

    a. IO
    b. ET
    c. umbilical vein cannulation
    d. umbilical artery cannulation

37. You have arrived at the scene of a serious MVC and find an unconscious young woman, who is obviously pregnant, behind the wheel. She is breathing agonal respirations as you approach. You assist her ventilations while your crew quickly extricates her from the vehicle. You advise your crew to position her on a long board with:

    a. her legs elevated.
    b. her head elevated.
    c. the right side of the board elevated slightly.
    d. the left side of the board elevated slightly.

38. You continue to aggressively treat the patient in question 37 by intubating her, while your crew obtains vital signs. Her pulse is 110, and BP is 80/40. Your management plan en route includes:

    a. aggressive fluid replacement.
    b. the application of MAST/PASG.
    c. the use of vasopressors.
    d. rapid transport to the nearest ED.

39. Listening for fetal heart tones is the standard of care:

    a. for distressed fetuses in the prehospital setting.
    b. only when a Doppler is available.
    c. only in third trimester pregnancies.
    d. in the clinical setting and not in the field.

40. Which of the following facts about Braxton Hicks contractions is least correct?

    a. They can be relieved by drinking milk.
    b. They are often relieved with mild exercise.
    c. They are relatively short-lived and benign.
    d. They are practice contractions to prepare for actual labor.

41. The primary impact on the fetus from a state of shock in the mother includes:

    a. increased risk of hypothermia.
    b. hypoglycemic environment for the fetus.
    c. decreased liver function for the fetus.
    d. shunting of blood from the fetus.

42. Which of the following is a secondary injury from a sexual assault?

    a. lacerations to the external genitalia
    b. STDs
    c. bruising on the mons pubis
    d. rectal tears

43. You and your partner are caring for the victim of a rape. As your partner assesses her wounds and obtains baseline vital signs, you consider how to preserve evidence and take which of the following actions?

    a. Place any items removed from the patient into separate bags.
    b. Place any items removed from the patient into a plastic bag.
    c. Allow the patient to void and change her clothes prior to transport.
    d. Place all of the items belonging to the patient together in the same bag.

44. After assessing and addressing any life-threatening conditions, the management of the victim of a sexual assault is focused on:

    a. preserving evidence of the crime.
    b. providing emotional support.
    c. cleaning superficial wounds.
    d. reporting the crime to the appropriate person.

45. Sexual assault is a crime of violence and can occur in any age group. It is estimated that _____ females is raped during her lifetime.

    a. one in three
    b. one in five
    c. one in ten
    d. one in twenty

46. _____ is the cessation of ovarian function and menstrual activity.

    a. Menarche
    b. Menopause
    c. Amenorrhea
    d. Mittelschmerz

47. Which of the following is an example of a gynecological emergency?

    a. UTI
    b. gallstones
    c. gestational diabetes
    d. ruptured ovarian cyst

48. _____ is characterized by lower abdominal pain experienced by some women at the time of ovulation.

    a. Menarche
    b. Menopause
    c. Amenorrhea
    d. Mittelschmerz

49. _____ is an acute or chronic inflammation of the endometrium caused by bacterial infection.

    a. Endometriosis
    b. Endometritis
    c. Cystitis
    d. Oophritis

50. The complications of vaginal bleeding include:

    a. infection.
    b. tissue scarring.
    c. shock and death.
    d. infertility.

51. You have been called to a multiparous woman who is having contractions and is at thirty-four weeks gestation. She tells you that the baby has not yet moved into a head-down position. Her labor is very active, and she feels like the baby is coming. You move the patient to your stretcher and prepare for transport. What is your management plan for this patient?

    a. Begin rapid transport to the hospital.
    b. Prepare for imminent delivery.
    c. Administer Pitocin®, as the fetus is premature.
    d. Position the mother in the Trendelenburg position.

52. How would you assess the woman in question 51 for signs of imminent delivery?

    a. Measure the height of her fundus.
    b. Count her contractions.
    c. Observe the birth canal for crowning.
    d. Palpate the fundus for strength of contractions.

53. Next, how would you continue to manage the patient in question 52?

    a. Start an IV and prepare an OB delivery kit.
    b. Monitor, reassess, and continue rapid transport.
    c. Titrate the Pitocin® drip until desired effect is obtained.
    d. Call ahead to the ED to advise of cesarean section delivery.

54. As your partner backs into the ED, the baby's feet and buttocks present. How would you continue?

    a. Ask the patient to stop pushing.
    b. Quickly move her into the ED before the head delivers.
    c. Allow the cord to deliver and support the body.
    d. Place a gloved hand in the birth canal to hold the fetus.

55. You are dispatched to a residence for postpartum hemorrhage. You arrive and find that a thirty-two-year-old woman has given birth to a healthy baby with the help of a certified midwife. The pregnancy and birth were normal; however, after the delivery of the placenta, the patient has had heavy blood loss, despite uterine massage. What is your management plan for this patient?

    a. Assist the midwife with direct pressure on the uterus.
    b. Treat for shock and begin transport.
    c. Encourage the mother to have the baby nurse during transport.
    d. Insert trauma dressings in the birth canal, apply MAST/PASG, and begin transport.

56. Before you began transport for the patient in question 55, the midwife showed you that the placenta was whole, and, during your assessment of the patient, you do not observe any peritoneal tears. You suspect the cause of the heavy bleeding may be all the following, *except*:

    a. lack of uterine tone.
    b. a vaginal or cervical tear.
    c. a clotting disorder.
    d. the presence of an undelivered fetus.

57. Despite all your treatment on-scene and en route to the hospital, the patient continues to hemorrhage and is dropping her blood pressure steadily. You call medical control and give a report. The doctor gives you an order to:

    a. administer an additional fluid bolus of up to 2 liters.
    b. begin a Pitocin® drip.
    c. stop uterine massage and inflate MAST/PASG.
    d. begin a dopamine drip.

58. When placed in the position of having to assist with the delivery of multiple fetuses, such as twins, which of the following should be considered?

    a. One of the twins will always be born breech.
    b. Nearly 40% of twin deliveries are premature.
    c. Delivery of multiples is never the same as a single delivery.
    d. The mother will always know how many fetuses she is carrying.

59. It is rare that the paramedic would ever have to place a gloved hand into the birth canal to manage the delivery. These rare occurrences include an umbilical cord presentation and a:

    a. complicated breech delivery.
    b. shoulder dystocia presentation.
    c. nuchal cord presentation.
    d. cephalopelvic disproportion.

60. After assisting with the normal delivery of a healthy baby, the patient suddenly complains of severe lower abdominal pain. She does not deliver the placenta but begins heavy bleeding, and the uterus is presenting from the vagina. You immediately recognize this as uterine inversion. Your management plan for this patient is to:

    a. attempt to deliver the placenta to control the bleeding.
    b. cover the protruding tissue with moist, sterile dressings.
    c. prepare to intubate the patient, as she will probably develop a pulmonary embolus.
    d. start an IV, apply MAST/PASG, and begin a rapid transport.

Exam #32 Answer Form

	A	B	C	D		A	B	C	D
1.	❑	❑	❑	❑	27.	❑	❑	❑	❑
2.	❑	❑	❑	❑	28.	❑	❑	❑	❑
3.	❑	❑	❑	❑	29.	❑	❑	❑	❑
4.	❑	❑	❑	❑	30.	❑	❑	❑	❑
5.	❑	❑	❑	❑	31.	❑	❑	❑	❑
6.	❑	❑	❑	❑	32.	❑	❑	❑	❑
7.	❑	❑	❑	❑	33.	❑	❑	❑	❑
8.	❑	❑	❑	❑	34.	❑	❑	❑	❑
9.	❑	❑	❑	❑	35.	❑	❑	❑	❑
10.	❑	❑	❑	❑	36.	❑	❑	❑	❑
11.	❑	❑	❑	❑	37.	❑	❑	❑	❑
12.	❑	❑	❑	❑	38.	❑	❑	❑	❑
13.	❑	❑	❑	❑	39.	❑	❑	❑	❑
14.	❑	❑	❑	❑	40.	❑	❑	❑	❑
15.	❑	❑	❑	❑	41.	❑	❑	❑	❑
16.	❑	❑	❑	❑	42.	❑	❑	❑	❑
17.	❑	❑	❑	❑	43.	❑	❑	❑	❑
18.	❑	❑	❑	❑	44.	❑	❑	❑	❑
19.	❑	❑	❑	❑	45.	❑	❑	❑	❑
20.	❑	❑	❑	❑	46.	❑	❑	❑	❑
21.	❑	❑	❑	❑	47.	❑	❑	❑	❑
22.	❑	❑	❑	❑	48.	❑	❑	❑	❑
23.	❑	❑	❑	❑	49.	❑	❑	❑	❑
24.	❑	❑	❑	❑	50.	❑	❑	❑	❑
25.	❑	❑	❑	❑	51.	❑	❑	❑	❑
26.	❑	❑	❑	❑	52.	❑	❑	❑	❑

	A	B	C	D			A	B	C	D
53.	❏	❏	❏	❏		57.	❏	❏	❏	❏
54.	❏	❏	❏	❏		58.	❏	❏	❏	❏
55.	❏	❏	❏	❏		59.	❏	❏	❏	❏
56.	❏	❏	❏	❏		60.	❏	❏	❏	❏

33

Trauma Systems and Mechanisms of Injury

1. The leading cause of work-related fatal injuries in the United States is:

   a. falls.
   b. fires and explosions.
   c. transportation incidents.
   d. exposure to harmful substances.

2. The top three causes of trauma death, in order of most to least, are:

   a. MVCs, poisonings, and falls.
   b. MVCs, homicides, and suicides.
   c. falls, poisonings, and homicides.
   d. falls, drownings, and suicides.

3. Getting a complete and accurate account of the MOI can help emergency care providers identify nearly 95% of the possible injuries sustained in most cases, because:

   a. the patient will not know the extent of his own injuries.
   b. many MOIs have predictable patterns for specific injuries.
   c. serious and life-threatening injuries can always be identified early.
   d. early recognition of possible injuries by the paramedic can save the patient from needing rehabilitation.

4. What percent of trauma is life threatening?

   a. >1%
   b. 5%
   c. 10%
   d. 15%

5. The two major factors for the extent of traumatic injury are the amount of energy exchanges to the body and:

   a. the patient's age.
   b. anatomic structures that are involved.
   c. past medical history (PMH).
   d. the use of any safety restraints.

6. The three phases of trauma care include preincident, postincident, and:

   a. golden hour.
   b. incident.
   c. platinum ten minutes.
   d. physical therapy.

7. After personal safety and management of the patient's ABCs, _____ is the most important information to obtain about any trauma victim.

   a. MOI
   b. past medical history (PMH)
   c. organ donor status
   d. DNAR status

8. Paramedics can make a big difference in trauma prevention by doing all the following, *except*:

   a. assisting in public education of seat belt use.
   b. setting the example.
   c. promoting legislation to reduce the use of weapons.
   d. filling out an organ donor card.

9. The paramedic can make a significant impact on the life or death of a trauma victim by:

   a. wearing the appropriate PPE.
   b. stabilizing the patient prior to transport.
   c. minimizing scene time when appropriate.
   d. transporting the trauma patient to the nearest facility.

10. The paper entitled "Accidental Death and Disability: The Neglected Disease of Modern Society" is also known as the:

    a. Ryan White Act.
    b. Highway Safety Act of 1966.
    c. Trauma Prevention Act.
    d. White Paper.

11. The components of a trauma system include all of the following, *except*:

    a. injury prevention programs.
    b. hospice care.
    c. definitive care.
    d. trauma critical care.

12. A trauma _____ is a reporting system designed to collect trauma-related data in an effort to improve the quality and cost-effectiveness of care and to aid in outcomes of research.

    a. registry
    b. chronicle
    c. journal
    d. catalog

13. Which of the following statements about trauma centers is not correct?

    a. Trauma centers must meet strict criteria to be designated a trauma center.
    b. A delineated criterion for a trauma center includes personnel.
    c. A delineated criterion for a trauma center includes use of air–medical transport.
    d. Not all hospitals that care for acutely injured patients are trauma centers.

14. In which of the following patient scenarios should the paramedic transport the patient to the nearest hospital, even if it is not a trauma center?

    a. critical burns
    b. multiple system trauma
    c. traumatic cardiac arrest
    d. pregnant patient involved in a significant MOI

15. Which of the following patient situations is an indication for the use of air-medical transport?

    a. access to a remote area
    b. extremely combative patient
    c. patient with injuries induced by barotrauma
    d. inclement weather too severe for ground ambulance transport

16. Which of the following patient situations is a contraindication for the use of air-medical transport?

    a. traumatic cardiac arrest
    b. patient requires a surgical airway
    c. patient with spinal cord injury from a diving accident
    d. ground transport poses a threat to the patient's survival

17. _____ means that energy cannot be created or destroyed, only transferred or exchanged.

    a. Kinetic energy
    b. Force
    c. Newton's first law of motion
    d. Conservation of energy

18. The concept "An object in motion tends to stay in motion, and an object at rest tends to stay at rest" describes:

    a. kinetic energy.
    b. force.
    c. Newton's first law of motion.
    d. conservation of energy.

19. _____ means that the more speed that is involved, the more energy there is.

    a. Kinetic energy
    b. Force
    c. Newton's first law of motion
    d. Conservation of energy

20. _____ is the creation of a cavity in an object that can be permanent or temporary.

    a. Energy
    b. Force
    c. Cavitation
    d. Puncture

21. Which of the following components of kinetic energy makes the greatest impact on a trauma victim?

    a. mass
    b. velocity
    c. acceleration
    d. deceleration

22. Which of the following are the actual units for kinetic energy?

    a. foot-pounds
    b. mile-grams
    c. meter-liters
    d. inch-ounces

23. When does the golden hour for the trauma victim begin?

    a. when the first responder arrives at the patient's side
    b. when the paramedic arrives on the scene
    c. immediately after the injury is sustained
    d. immediately upon arriving at the ED

24. What is meant by the third collision in the MOI of a trauma victim?

   a. Third collision is the internal organs striking against the body.
   b. This is a triad of injuries involving the head, neck, and spine.
   c. Third collision refers to multiple injuries.
   d. Third collision pertains to children involved in motor vehicle collisions.

25. Why are some bullets designed to tumble when fired from a gun?

   a. Tumbling bullets are faster.
   b. Tumbling decreases the force of impact.
   c. Penetration is streamlined with tumbling.
   d. Tumbling creates greater tissue damage.

26. You are sizing up the scene at an MVC, and you see that the vehicle with the only patient involved was rear-ended, which resulted in her vehicle being pushed off the road and into a ditch. What type of force(s) has this patient experienced in this MOI?

   a. blunt penetrating
   b. rapid acceleration
   c. rapid deceleration
   d. rapid acceleration and deceleration

27. Which of the following MOIs is not usually associated with predictable injury patterns?

   a. motorcycle collisions
   b. auto–pedestrian collisions
   c. falls
   d. GSWs

28. The three phases associated with the blast effect are the primary phase, the secondary phase, and the _____ phase.

   a. late
   b. triage
   c. tertiary
   d. end-stage

29. During the secondary phase of the blast effect, the potential for injury comes from:

   a. the heat wave.
   b. flying articles.
   c. pressure waves.
   d. the patient striking an object.

30. Which of the following penetrating MOIs has the greatest potential for energy exchange?

   a. high-power rifle
   b. knife
   c. shotgun
   d. hanging

31. Which of the following will generate the greatest amount of kinetic energy?

   a. 90 kg patient traveling at 30 mph
   b. 80 kg patient traveling at 40 mph
   c. 70 kg patient traveling at 50 mph
   d. 60 kg patient traveling at 60 mph

32. You are assessing a patient who was a victim of a significant blast injury. He has the clinical findings of a closed pneumothorax. Which of the following is the most likely cause of his injury?

   a. heat wave
   b. compression
   c. flying article
   d. sound wave

33. During the _____ phase of the blast effect, injuries can result from the patient becoming a flying object and striking other objects.

   a. end-stage
   b. secondary
   c. late
   d. tertiary

34. Your patient is the victim of a motorcycle collision and has bilateral femur fractures. What type of impact did the patient most likely sustain?

   a. frontal
   b. rear-end
   c. side
   d. rotational

35. Cervical spine injuries are most common with what type of collision?

   a. frontal
   b. rear-end
   c. primary
   d. secondary

36. Your patient was assisted out of a house fire by a fireman who found him lying on the bedroom floor unconscious. Which of the following pieces of information about the MOI is the most significant for this patient?

   a. cause of the fire
   b. when the fire was started
   c. smoke condition in the room in which the patient was found
   d. presence of a carbon monoxide detector in the house

37. What is the most likely cause of the unconsciousness in the patient described in question 36?

    a. airway burns
    b. super-heated air
    c. CO_2 inhalation
    d. shock

38. The patient you are assessing fell from a tall ladder while at work. Which of the following aspects of the MOI should the paramedic focus on?

    a. point of impact of the body
    b. the distance of the fall
    c. the type of surface of the impact
    d. the combination of forces involved

39. When a projectile such as a bullet passes through the body, it creates a wave of pressure that can compress organs and tissue, causing:

    a. contusion, fracture, or rupture.
    b. liquidation.
    c. collapse and disintegration.
    d. spontaneous combustion.

40. Which of the following aspects of a GSW should the paramedic focus on?

    a. the gender of the shooter
    b. the wind speed at the time of the shooting
    c. the level of gravity at the time of the shooting
    d. the type of empty shell casings

41. Your patient is the victim of a motorcycle collision where he was T-boned at an intersection by a car. Which of the following injury patterns are most associated with lateral impact motorcycle collisions?

    a. bilateral femur fractures
    b. crush injuries
    c. pelvis dislocation
    d. pneumothorax

42. Which of the following is an injury associated with third collision MOI?

    a. brain contusion
    b. fractured pelvis
    c. dislocated knee
    d. neck injury

43. By performing a rapid assessment and life-saving procedures, minimizing scene time to _____ minutes and transporting the patient to an appropriate facility, the paramedic makes the difference between life or death for a trauma patient.

    a. ten
    b. fifteen
    c. thirty
    d. sixty

44. As a general rule, the entrance wound of a GSW is usually smaller than the exit wound because of:

    a. proximity of the shooter.
    b. positioning of the patient.
    c. cavitation.
    d. dissection.

45. During the primary phase of the blast effect, there is a pressure wave that can cause major damage to the:

    a. eyes and skin.
    b. lungs and GI tract.
    c. head and neck.
    d. hearing.

46. The pathologic effects of the pressure wave during the blast effect include:

    a. lacerations and bruising.
    b. rupture of an organ or air embolism.
    c. whiplash and sprains.
    d. shattering.

47. During the third phase of an auto–pedestrian collision, the patient can sustain injuries from:

    a. the impact of the vehicle.
    b. the fall onto the hood of the vehicle.
    c. going into the vehicle.
    d. being run over by the vehicle.

48. The victim of a motorcycle collision who does not wear a helmet has a _____ % increased risk of brain injury.

    a. 30
    b. 50
    c. 300
    d. 500

49. Which of the following statements about air bags in motor vehicles is most correct?

    a. Air bags do not work without the use of seat belts.

    b. Air bags may produce minor facial and forearm abrasions.

    c. The smoke associated with the discharge of the air bag is noxious.

    d. There is no risk of injury from the protective cover over the air bag upon discharge.

50. Which of the following statements about shoulder restraints is correct?

    a. They prevent hyperflexion of the upper torso.

    b. The do not prevent forward motion of the upper torso in frontal impact collisions.

    c. Neck injuries can still be prevented, even without the use of a lap restraint.

    d. Shoulder restraints provide more benefit when the seat is very close to the dashboard.

Exam #33 Answer Form

	A	B	C	D			A	B	C	D
1.	❏	❏	❏	❏		26.	❏	❏	❏	❏
2.	❏	❏	❏	❏		27.	❏	❏	❏	❏
3.	❏	❏	❏	❏		28.	❏	❏	❏	❏
4.	❏	❏	❏	❏		29.	❏	❏	❏	❏
5.	❏	❏	❏	❏		30.	❏	❏	❏	❏
6.	❏	❏	❏	❏		31.	❏	❏	❏	❏
7.	❏	❏	❏	❏		32.	❏	❏	❏	❏
8.	❏	❏	❏	❏		33.	❏	❏	❏	❏
9.	❏	❏	❏	❏		34.	❏	❏	❏	❏
10.	❏	❏	❏	❏		35.	❏	❏	❏	❏
11.	❏	❏	❏	❏		36.	❏	❏	❏	❏
12.	❏	❏	❏	❏		37.	❏	❏	❏	❏
13.	❏	❏	❏	❏		38.	❏	❏	❏	❏
14.	❏	❏	❏	❏		39.	❏	❏	❏	❏
15.	❏	❏	❏	❏		40.	❏	❏	❏	❏
16.	❏	❏	❏	❏		41.	❏	❏	❏	❏
17.	❏	❏	❏	❏		42.	❏	❏	❏	❏
18.	❏	❏	❏	❏		43.	❏	❏	❏	❏
19.	❏	❏	❏	❏		44.	❏	❏	❏	❏
20.	❏	❏	❏	❏		45.	❏	❏	❏	❏
21.	❏	❏	❏	❏		46.	❏	❏	❏	❏
22.	❏	❏	❏	❏		47.	❏	❏	❏	❏
23.	❏	❏	❏	❏		48.	❏	❏	❏	❏
24.	❏	❏	❏	❏		49.	❏	❏	❏	❏
25.	❏	❏	❏	❏		50.	❏	❏	❏	❏

34

Hemorrhage and Shock

1. The two general locations of severe hemorrhage are:

   a. head and neck.
   b. extremities and back.
   c. internal and external.
   d. chest and pelvis.

2. When a patient has signs of hypovolemia and there are no external reasons, the paramedic should consider:

   a. esophageal varices.
   b. occult GI bleeding.
   c. dehydration.
   d. head trauma.

3. Bleeding described as spurting bright red is usually from a/an:

   a. vein.
   b. artery.
   c. capillary.
   d. vesicle.

4. A patient was shot in the stomach. Upon arrival, after assuring that the police have secured the scene, the paramedic is able to talk directly to the patient, who is alert and complaining of severe pain. The paramedic is unable to obtain a radial pulse. What grade/stage of hemorrhage would you suspect the patient is in?

   a. one
   b. two
   c. three
   d. four

5. Based on the scenario in question 4, approximately how much blood has the patient lost up to the point of initial assessment by the paramedic?

   a. up to 15%
   b. 15 to 25%
   c. 25 to 35%
   d. >35%

6. What treatment would be appropriate for this patient?

   a. sedate and intubate on-scene
   b. two large bore IVs en route
   c. vasopressors
   d. two large bore IVs on-scene

7. When the systolic BP drops from a hemorrhage, it is referred to as _____ shock.

   a. hypervolemic
   b. decompensated
   c. irreversible
   d. compensated

8. In the formula CO = HR x SV, the SV is usually approximately _____ per heartbeat in an adult.

   a. 25 cc
   b. 50 cc
   c. 70 cc
   d. 120 cc

9. The body's compensatory mechanism for blood loss in the short term is to increase the cardiac output by:

   a. peripheral vasodilation.
   b. increasing the heart rate.
   c. increasing the stroke volume.
   d. decreasing vascular resistance.

10. What is the objective measure of vasoconstriction during hemorrhage?

    a. increase in systolic pressure
    b. increase in diastolic pressure
    c. decrease in systolic pressure
    d. decrease in diastolic pressure

11. For the long term, how can you increase your SV?

    a. weight loss through healthy diet
    b. take medication to slow the heart rate
    c. aerobic exercise on a regular basis
    d. lift weights on a regular basis

12. When the body's compensatory system signals the sympathetic nervous system to release epinephrine, the alpha-1 effects will cause:

    a. bronchodilation.
    b. vasoconstriction.
    c. positive inotropic effects.
    d. positive chronotropic effects.

13. When the body's compensatory system signals the sympathetic nervous system to release epinephrine, the beta-1 effects will cause:

    a. bronchodilation.
    b. vasoconstriction.
    c. positive dromotropic effects.
    d. smooth muscle dilation in the GI tract.

14. The chemical that is released during shock, which starts to act as an antidiuretic, is called:

    a. insulin.
    b. aldosterone.
    c. arginine vasopressin.
    d. glucagon.

15. A potent vasoconstrictor that promotes sodium reabsorption and decreases urine output in shock states is:

    a. insulin.
    b. aldosterone.
    c. arginine vasopressin.
    d. angiotensin II.

16. Following injury and volume loss, the patient is often:

    a. hypoglycemic.
    b. hyperglycemic.
    c. flushed and warm.
    d. depleted of urine.

17. When the compensatory mechanisms are overwhelmed, all of the following occur, *except*:

    a. preload decreases.
    b. cardiac output decreases.
    c. myocardial blood supply increases.
    d. capillary and cellular changes.

18. At the cellular level, during low perfusion states when the post-capillary sphincter relaxes, this is called the _____ phase.

    a. ischemia
    b. washout
    c. stagnation
    d. final

19. During low perfusion states, the pre-capillary sphincters relax in response to lactic acid and:

    a. decreased carbon dioxide.
    b. vasomotor center failure.
    c. hypothermia.
    d. aerobic metabolism.

20. _____ shock is characterized by signs and symptoms of late shock, but is refractory to treatment.

    a. Hypovolemic
    b. Distributive
    c. Irreversible
    d. Obstructive

21. Which one of the following signs or symptoms may differentiate cardiogenic shock from hypovolemic shock?

    a. chief complaint of chest pain
    b. presence of tachycardia
    c. absence of diaphoresis
    d. poor CTC

22. Which of the following signs may differentiate distributed shock from hypovolemic shock?

    a. chief complaint of dyspnea
    b. presence of tachycardia
    c. absence of diaphoresis
    d. flushed skin

23. Which of the following signs may differentiate obstructive shock from hypovolemic shock?

    a. chief complaint of abdominal pain
    b. presence of JVD
    c. presence of tachycardia
    d. poor CTC

24. Intravenous volume expanders that have the same tonicity as plasma are the _____ solutions.

    a. isotonic
    b. hypertonic
    c. hypotonic
    d. synthetic

25. When using intravenous volume expanders, it is important to recall that only about _____ of the fluid infused stays in the intravascular space.

    a. 1/4
    b. 1/3
    c. 1/2
    d. 2/3

26. When a crystalloid IV volume expander such as normal saline is used, the amount that shifts out of the intravascular space moves into the _____ within approximately one hour.

    a. interstitial space
    b. lungs
    c. intracellular compartment
    d. kidneys

27. Which of the following statements is most correct about intravenous volume expanders?

    a. They should only be used en route to the ED.
    b. Hypertonic solutions are best in the prehospital setting.
    c. Isotonic solutions are not routinely used in or out of the ED.
    d. They do not carry hemoglobin.

28. You are assessing an eighteen-year-old male who crashed his dirt bike. He has an obvious closed femur fracture and abdominal pain. His mental status is alert, but initially he had a brief loss of consciousness, and his vital signs are R/R 30 and shallow, P/R 110, and BP 116/56. His skin is warm and moist. Which stage of shock is indicated by the pulse and blood pressure?

    a. compensated
    b. decompensated
    c. distributive
    d. obstructive

29. Based on the scenario in question 28, the most likely cause of the shock is:

    a. head injury.
    b. internal bleeding.
    c. substantial vasodilation.
    d. loss of venous capacitance.

30. Baroreceptors located in the carotid sinuses and _____ are stimulated by decreased blood flow.

    a. intestines
    b. aortic arch
    c. cerebellum
    d. medulla

31. When baroreceptors sense decreased blood flow and activate the vasomotor center, as a result there is:

    a. vasodilation of the peripheral vessels.
    b. vasodilation of the great vessels.
    c. vasoconstriction of the peripheral vessels.
    d. vasoconstriction of the central organs.

32. When the sympathetic nervous system is stimulated in response to shock, epinephrine and norepinephrine are secreted from the:

    a. thalamus.
    b. hypothalamus.
    c. adrenal gland.
    d. pituitary gland.

33. Which of the following is an early sign of hypovolemic shock?

    a. narrowing pulse pressure
    b. increased peripheral vascular resistance
    c. increased stroke volume
    d. loss of vasomotor tone

34. When the body senses hypovolemia, several regulatory systems are put into play to try to compensate. These include sympathetic responses, vasoconstriction, and:

    a. endocrine responses.
    b. CO_2 elimination.
    c. metabolic purging.
    d. osmotic channeling.

35. The maximum amount of intravenous volume expanders prudent for field administration is about _____ liters so as to avoid reducing hematocrit from being effective.

    a. 1–2
    b. 2–3
    c. 4–5
    d. 5–6

36. The indication for the use of PASG/MAST in _____ is still relatively unchanged.

    a. chest trauma
    b. abdominal hemorrhage
    c. stabilization of pelvic fractures
    d. pregnancy

37. Despite the controversies in the use of PASG/MAST, the _____ still recommends that the suit be available for immediate use in hospital emergency departments.

   a. National Registry
   b. ACEP
   c. JEMS
   d. NHTSA

38. Decreased perfusion can be caused by an event resulting in blood loss, kinking of the great vessels (i.e., tension pneumo), or:

   a. by release of antidiuretic hormone.
   b. an allergic reaction.
   c. a failure in the buffer system.
   d. loss of vasomotor tone.

39. _____ defends the fluid volume and reduces urine output by promoting sodium reabsorption and water retention in the kidney.

   a. ACTH
   b. Angiotensin I
   c. Aldosterone
   d. Glucagon

40. Renin is released by _____ and catalyzes the conversion of angiotensinogen to angiotensin I.

   a. arterioles in the kidney.
   b. transfer of fatty acids into mitochondria.
   c. cells in the adrenal cortex.
   d. circulating epinephrine.

Exam #34 Answer Form

	A	B	C	D		A	B	C	D
1.	❏	❏	❏	❏	21.	❏	❏	❏	❏
2.	❏	❏	❏	❏	22.	❏	❏	❏	❏
3.	❏	❏	❏	❏	23.	❏	❏	❏	❏
4.	❏	❏	❏	❏	24.	❏	❏	❏	❏
5.	❏	❏	❏	❏	25.	❏	❏	❏	❏
6.	❏	❏	❏	❏	26.	❏	❏	❏	❏
7.	❏	❏	❏	❏	27.	❏	❏	❏	❏
8.	❏	❏	❏	❏	28.	❏	❏	❏	❏
9.	❏	❏	❏	❏	29.	❏	❏	❏	❏
10.	❏	❏	❏	❏	30.	❏	❏	❏	❏
11.	❏	❏	❏	❏	31.	❏	❏	❏	❏
12.	❏	❏	❏	❏	32.	❏	❏	❏	❏
13.	❏	❏	❏	❏	33.	❏	❏	❏	❏
14.	❏	❏	❏	❏	34.	❏	❏	❏	❏
15.	❏	❏	❏	❏	35.	❏	❏	❏	❏
16.	❏	❏	❏	❏	36.	❏	❏	❏	❏
17.	❏	❏	❏	❏	37.	❏	❏	❏	❏
18.	❏	❏	❏	❏	38.	❏	❏	❏	❏
19.	❏	❏	❏	❏	39.	❏	❏	❏	❏
20.	❏	❏	❏	❏	40.	❏	❏	❏	❏

35

Soft Tissue Trauma

1. An example of a closed soft tissue injury that may produce cardiac dysrhythmia is a/an:

   a. crushing injury.
   b. epidural hematoma.
   c. subdural hematoma.
   d. hematoma from a failed IV access attempt.

2. Two common examples of soft tissue trauma that may be fatal are hematomas and:

   a. secondary infections.
   b. abrasions.
   c. genital warts.
   d. insect bites.

3. Any physical activity that increases the exposure of the skin to the environment and _____ will increase the risk of a soft tissue injury.

   a. sea/saltwater
   b. physical forces
   c. blood-borne pathogens
   d. airborne pathogens

4. Which of the following is not a layer of the skin?

   a. cutaneous
   b. subcutaneous
   c. superficial lesion
   d. deep fascia

5. Which section of skin contains the stratum germinativum or basal layer?

   a. dermis
   b. epidermis
   c. subcutaneous lesion
   d. deep fascia

6. Fibroblasts, macrophages, and MAST cells are located in the:

   a. dermis.
   b. epidermis.
   c. superficial fascia.
   d. deep fascia.

7. The _____ is a thick, dense layer of fibrous tissue that provides support and protection for the underlying structures.

   a. dermis
   b. epidermis
   c. superficial fascia
   d. deep fascia

8. The skin follows the contours of the underlying structures, creating a natural stretch in the skin called:

   a. tension lines.
   b. stretch marks.
   c. relief stretch.
   d. strain outlines.

9. _____ is the phase of normal wound healing where clotting begins.

   a. Hemostasis
   b. Epithelialization
   c. Collagen synthesis
   d. Neurovascularization

10. The phase of normal healing that involves fibroblast-forming scar tissue that holds the wound edges together tightly is called:

    a. epithelialization.
    b. collagen synthesis.
    c. stretch marks.
    d. tension lines.

11. _____ is the phase of wound healing through reestablishment of skin layers in the first twelve hours.

    a. Epithelialization
    b. Collagen synthesis
    c. Inflammation
    d. Fibroblast formation

12. Normal wound healing can be altered by which of the following factors?

    a. skin temperature
    b. ambient temperature
    c. body region
    d. dry skin

13. Which of the following medications is known to interfere with the normal wound-healing process?

   a. nitrates
   b. laxatives
   c. corticosteroids
   d. anticonvulsives

14. Which of the following medical conditions does not typically affect normal wound healing?

   a. severe alcoholism
   b. diabetes
   c. acne
   d. cardiovascular disease

15. What types of wounds are considered high risk for healing problems and infections?

   a. slivers
   b. abrasions
   c. human bites
   d. insect stings or bites

16. Excessive accumulation of scar tissue that extends beyond the original wound borders is called a:

   a. keloid scar.
   b. stretch mark.
   c. suture over-healing.
   d. hypertrophic scar.

17. Plastic surgery is often requested for wound closures for the purpose of:

   a. minimizing the number of stitches used.
   b. cosmetically acceptable healing.
   c. closing gaps that are too large for sutures.
   d. closing gaps that are too small for sutures.

18. Which of the following soft tissue injuries often requires sutures?

   a. degloving
   b. abrasions
   c. ulcers
   d. abscesses

19. The most common and dangerous infectious disease that EMS providers are at risk for exposure to when treating patients with external bleeding is:

   a. AIDS
   b. hepatitis
   c. meningitis
   d. tuberculosis

20. In a/an _____, the epidermis remains intact when cells are damaged and the blood vessels in the dermis are torn, causing swelling and pain. The pain can be delayed for up to twenty-four to forty-eight hours after the injury.

   a. contusion
   b. laceration
   c. abrasion
   d. ulcer

21. A/An _____ is a break in the skin of varying depth usually caused by very sharp objects, such as a knife.

   a. abrasion
   b. laceration
   c. incision
   d. avulsion

22. A flap of torn, loose tissue that may not be viable for reimplantation is called an:

   a. abrasion.
   b. amputation.
   c. impalement.
   d. avulsion.

23. A jagged wound caused by forceful impact with a sharp object, which may cause the ends to bleed freely, is called a/an:

   a. laceration.
   b. amputation.
   c. evisceration.
   d. puncture.

24. Which of the following is not a type of amputation?

   a. degloving injury
   b. ring injury
   c. complete
   d. partial

25. During which phase(s) of a blast injury would open soft tissue trauma most likely occur?

   a. primary and secondary
   b. primary and tertiary
   c. secondary only
   d. primary only

26. A/An _____ injury is an injury from a compressive force sufficient to interfere with the normal metabolic function of the involved tissue.

   a. puncture
   b. crush
   c. impaled
   d. blast

27. Field management for the patient with crush syndrome is focused on aggressive fluid therapy and the administration of:

a. oxygen to restore hypoxic tissue.
b. epinephrine to dilate the vessels.
c. glucagon to metabolize stores of needed glucose.
d. sodium bicarbonate to neutralize the buildup of acids.

28. While on vacation, a twenty-year-old male broke his arm skiing and subsequently had a cast applied. The next day, the patient awoke to find his fingers swollen and cyanotic. What type of soft tissue injury is associated with an improperly applied cast and has likely occurred with this patient?

a. puncture
b. contusion
c. hematoma
d. crush injury

29. In a crush syndrome injury, after the initial damage to soft tissue, the cells in the crushed area become starved for oxygen and _____ occurs.

a. compartment syndrome
b. anaerobic metabolism
c. unconsciousness
d. respiratory acidosis

30. Your patient was involved in a work-related accident that required extrication and disentanglement from machinery. He is alert and has a closed femur fracture. He is complaining of pain and paresthesia in the affected leg, and you cannot palpate a distal pulse. You suspect he is developing compartment syndrome in the thigh. Without proper intervention, how long does the patient have before cell death can occur?

a. ninety minutes
b. two to four hours
c. four to six hours
d. six to eight hours

31. In the pathophysiology of compartment syndrome, the tissue pressure rises above the _____ pressure, resulting in ischemia to muscle.

a. venous
b. arterial
c. osmotic
d. capillary hydrostatic

32. A patient who is developing compartment syndrome is likely to complain of _____ in the affected extremity.

a. pulselessness
b. nothing unusual
c. weakness and pain
d. a burning sensation

33. The "Ps" of compartment syndrome include all of the following, *except*:

a. palpation.
b. pain.
c. paresis.
d. pulselessness.

34. Blast injuries can occur from any explosion, but they are often more serious when they occur:

a. in a shopping mall.
b. at a fire scene.
c. inside a confined space.
d. in a railroad yard.

35. Initial treatment priorities for soft tissue injuries caused by blasts include:

a. observing for signs of compartment syndrome.
b. flushing the patient of combustible materials.
c. considering that both internal and external injuries are possible.
d. copious amounts of fluid administration.

36. Which of the following is not a method of hemorrhage control?

a. direct pressure
b. pressure dressing
c. pressure points
d. indirect pressure

37. _____ is the quickest and most efficient means of bleeding control.

a. Direct pressure
b. Elevation
c. Tourniquet application
d. Pressure points

38. The purpose of controlling a hemorrhage by direct pressure is to limit additional significant blood loss and to:

a. limit exposure to communicable disease.
b. promote localized clotting.
c. stop the arterial blood flow.
d. avoid the use of indirect pressure.

39. Your patient is a twenty-three-year-old male who has a tree branch six inches in diameter impaled through the left thigh. You are trying to control bleeding at the site of the wound. Which of the following methods of bleeding control should you avoid with this type of injury?

a. direct pressure
b. elevation
c. pressure dressing
d. pressure point

40. Which of the following is incorrect about the use of pressure dressings?

    a. They provide a continuous mechanical pressure on the wound site.

    b. A circumferential bandage should not be used on the neck.

    c. The bandage should not occlude or impede venous blood flow.

    d. The bandage should not occlude or impede arterial blood flow.

41. In which of the following situations would the use of a pressure dressing be most appropriate?

    a. open wound on the neck

    b. open head wound over a skull depression

    c. pregnant trauma patient with an abdominal evisceration

    d. a wound in which applying a pressure point has not slowed the bleeding

42. A pressure point is a location where a/an:

    a. artery runs over a bone and close to the skin.

    b. artery runs under a vein and close to the skin.

    c. vein runs over a bone and close to the heart.

    d. paramedic can reach with a venous tourniquet.

43. The use of a pressure point to control hemorrhage is indicated in situations where bleeding is not controlled by:

    a. direct pressure.

    b. the application of ice.

    c. an occlusive dressing.

    d. tourniquet.

44. Do not apply a tourniquet directly around a knee or elbow, as _____ in that area, and it will not adequately control the bleeding.

    a. serious nerve damage will result

    b. it may cut the skin or tissue

    c. there is too much bone

    d. there is no artery

45. Once a tourniquet is applied, the decision implies that you will:

    a. take if off once bleeding has been controlled.

    b. lose the limb to save the life.

    c. replace it with an air splint when one is available.

    d. loosen it when the patient experiences paresthesia.

46. The difference between a sterile and non-sterile dressing is that a sterile dressing has gone through:

    a. the process to eliminate bacteria from the dressing material.

    b. hermetically sealed packaging.

    c. special quality control regiments.

    d. a process to apply a residue to the gauze.

47. An occlusive dressing does not allow _____ through the dressing.

    a. passage of air

    b. passage of blood

    c. surfactant

    d. embolism to develop

48. The type of dressing that has been designed not to damage the surface of the wound when it is removed is a/an _____ dressing.

    a. occlusive

    b. sterile

    c. non-sterile

    d. non-adherent

49. The type of dressing that is designed to stick onto a wound surface by incorporating wound exudates into the dressing mesh is called a/an _____ dressing.

    a. occlusive

    b. adhesive

    c. improperly applied

    d. sterile wrap

50. A properly applied dressing may result in which of the following?

    a. increased tissue damage

    b. ineffective bleeding control

    c. unnecessary patient discomfort

    d. decreased risk of wound infection

51. You are at the residence of a patient who cut herself with a box cutter. The wound is deep in the palm, but you have controlled the bleeding with direct pressure and a pressure dressing. She is refusing transport because she does not have insurance. What can you say to the patient to help persuade her to receive further medical attention right away?

    a. Tell her that having medical insurance is not important.

    b. Explain that a tetanus shot and sutures are necessary.

    c. Explain that the bleeding may resume and become life threatening.

    d. Tell her that cosmetic surgery will be necessary because of the location of the injury.

52. Continuing with question 51, despite all of your efforts to convince the patient to go to the hospital, she still refuses. She says that she will go to her own physician later. What instructions can you give her to help minimize the risk of infection until she receives further medical attention?

    a. Change the dressing frequently.
    b. Take aspirin as needed for the pain.
    c. Do not allow the dressing to get wet.
    d. Clean the wound and apply a topical ointment.

53. How often is the immunization for tetanus recommended?

    a. every year
    b. every five years
    c. every ten years
    d. every twelve years

54. The paramedic can minimize the risk of infection for a patient with an open wound by:

    a. covering the wound with a dry, sterile dressing.
    b. covering the wound with a wet, sterile dressing.
    c. cleansing and debriding the wound as needed.
    d. placing an occlusive dressing.

55. Considerations for the treatment of an amputated part include that the amputated part should:

    a. be wrapped in dry, sterile dressing.
    b. be wrapped in a sterile, moist gauze pad.
    c. be placed in a bag with ice.
    d. always be transported with the patient.

56. Hyperbaric oxygen treatment is sometimes recommended to prevent _____ and improve healing in crush injuries.

    a. respiratory acidosis
    b. pulmonary embolus
    c. gangrene
    d. deep vein thrombosis

57. After the ABCs, the most important treatment in the patient with a crush injury is:

    a. the observation of the presence of ECG changes or dysrhythmias.
    b. to administer 20% solution of mannitol.
    c. transport to a hyperbaric treatment facility.
    d. to administer IV fluid therapy using the Parkland formula.

58. The _____, also called the superficial fascia, contains loose connective tissue and fat that provides both insulation and protection from trauma.

    a. cutaneous layer
    b. subcutaneous layer
    c. basal layer
    d. reticular dermis

59. During the _____ phase of normal wound healing, special cells "invade" the blood clot and release mediators that help fight local infections, as well as initiate the healing process.

    a. hemostasis
    b. inflammation
    c. epithelialization
    d. neovascularization

60. _____ is/are an excessive accumulation of scar tissue confined within the original wound borders and is common in areas of high tissue stress, such as flexion creases across joints.

    a. Hypertrophic scar
    b. Keloid scar
    c. Stretch marks
    d. Inflammation

Exam #35 Answer Form

	A	B	C	D			A	B	C	D
1.	❏	❏	❏	❏		27.	❏	❏	❏	❏
2.	❏	❏	❏	❏		28.	❏	❏	❏	❏
3.	❏	❏	❏	❏		29.	❏	❏	❏	❏
4.	❏	❏	❏	❏		30.	❏	❏	❏	❏
5.	❏	❏	❏	❏		31.	❏	❏	❏	❏
6.	❏	❏	❏	❏		32.	❏	❏	❏	❏
7.	❏	❏	❏	❏		33.	❏	❏	❏	❏
8.	❏	❏	❏	❏		34.	❏	❏	❏	❏
9.	❏	❏	❏	❏		35.	❏	❏	❏	❏
10.	❏	❏	❏	❏		36.	❏	❏	❏	❏
11.	❏	❏	❏	❏		37.	❏	❏	❏	❏
12.	❏	❏	❏	❏		38.	❏	❏	❏	❏
13.	❏	❏	❏	❏		39.	❏	❏	❏	❏
14.	❏	❏	❏	❏		40.	❏	❏	❏	❏
15.	❏	❏	❏	❏		41.	❏	❏	❏	❏
16.	❏	❏	❏	❏		42.	❏	❏	❏	❏
17.	❏	❏	❏	❏		43.	❏	❏	❏	❏
18.	❏	❏	❏	❏		44.	❏	❏	❏	❏
19.	❏	❏	❏	❏		45.	❏	❏	❏	❏
20.	❏	❏	❏	❏		46.	❏	❏	❏	❏
21.	❏	❏	❏	❏		47.	❏	❏	❏	❏
22.	❏	❏	❏	❏		48.	❏	❏	❏	❏
23.	❏	❏	❏	❏		49.	❏	❏	❏	❏
24.	❏	❏	❏	❏		50.	❏	❏	❏	❏
25.	❏	❏	❏	❏		51.	❏	❏	❏	❏
26.	❏	❏	❏	❏		52.	❏	❏	❏	❏

	A	B	C	D		A	B	C	D
53.	❑	❑	❑	❑	57.	❑	❑	❑	❑
54.	❑	❑	❑	❑	58.	❑	❑	❑	❑
55.	❑	❑	❑	❑	59.	❑	❑	❑	❑
56.	❑	❑	❑	❑	60.	❑	❑	❑	❑

36

Burns

1. Approximately 80% of the fire- and burn-related deaths that occur in the United States are a result of a/an _____ fire.

   a. house
   b. automobile
   c. camp
   d. brush

2. Burns are the leading cause of trauma in the _____ age group.

   a. newborn
   b. toddler and preschool
   c. teenage
   d. elderly

3. The elderly are in a high-risk group for burns primarily because of:

   a. forgetting to change batteries in smoke detectors.
   b. elder abuse.
   c. smoking in bed.
   d. impairment of mobility or sensation.

4. Prevention strategies to decrease the number of scalding injuries in children include all the following, *except*:

   a. never drinking hot liquids while holding a child.
   b. cooking on backburners whenever possible.
   c. turning down the thermostat on the hot water heater to 120 degrees.
   d. testing the water temperature of a bath before allowing the child to enter.

5. Which of the following is not a pathophysiologic or system complication of a burn injury?

   a. decreased catecholamine release
   b. fluid and electrolyte loss
   c. renal, liver, and heart failure
   d. hypothermia

6. A burn classified as _____ is one that extends to the fascia.

   a. superficial
   b. deep fascia
   c. full thickness
   d. partial thickness

7. Which of the following is not a classification of a burn injury?

   a. superficial
   b. deep fascia
   c. partial thickness
   d. full thickness

8. A _____-degree burn involves the outermost layer of skin, the epidermis, as well as the dermal layer.

   a. first
   b. second
   c. third
   d. fourth

9. The three classifications of burn severity do not include:

   a. minor.
   b. moderate.
   c. eschar.
   d. severe.

10. The "rule of nines" is a method of determining:

    a. body surface area burned.
    b. severity of burn.
    c. classification of burn.
    d. type and degree of burn.

11. Burns on the hands or feet, inhalation burns, and electrical burns are all examples of burn injuries that:

    a. are associated with shock from blood loss.
    b. require transport to the nearest hospital.
    c. require transport to a burn specialty center.
    d. do not have a good prognosis for full recovery.

12. Which of the following does not have a significant impact on the management and prognosis of the burn-injured patient?

    a. the patient's age
    b. the patient's gender
    c. preexisiting medical problems
    d. associated trauma injury

13. Preexisting medical problems with _____ can make it very difficult for the burn patient to handle the tremendous movement of body fluids that occurs with a burn injury.

    a. seizures
    b. allergies
    c. the kidneys
    d. hypertension

14. Using the pediatric "rule of nines," estimate the percentage of BSA for a scald burn involving both lower legs, up to the knees.

    a. 12%
    b. 18%
    c. 20%
    d. 24%

15. The phases of "burn" shock include all the following, *except* the _____ phase.

    a. fluid shift
    b. compensation
    c. resolution
    d. hypermetabolic

16. During the body's initial response to a burn, there is a _____ in response to the pain from the burn.

    a. fluid shift
    b. release of catecholamines
    c. burst of energy
    d. decrease in cardiac output

17. During the _____ phase of a burn injury, there is a release of vasoactive substances from the burned tissues causing wound edema, fluid loss, and hypovolemia.

    a. emergent
    b. compensation
    c. fluid shift
    d. resolution

18. The _____ phase of burn shock usually occurs within 24 hours of the burn injury. In this phase, the scar tissue is laid down and healing occurs.

    a. emergent
    b. fluid shift
    c. resolution
    d. hypermetabolic

19. In 60–70% of all thermal burn patients who die, there is an associated inhalation injury when these patients either have cyanide intoxication or:

    a. carbon monoxide poisoning.
    b. asbestosis.
    c. nitrogen narcosis.
    d. thermal inhalation.

20. _____ is the thick and nonelastic scab or immediate scar that forms on the skin following a burn.

    a. Epithelialization
    b. Collagen synthesis
    c. Coagulation synthesis
    d. Eschar

21. When a circumferential scar forms around an extremity, _____ can be the resulting complication.

    a. circulatory compromise
    b. severe fluid loss
    c. rebound acidosis
    d. cosmetic uncertainty

22. When obtaining assessment findings of the patient with a thermal burn, which of the following is least significant?

    a. the specific MOI
    b. fluid replacement amounts
    c. preexisting medical conditions
    d. the classification and severity of the burn

23. *After* managing the ABCs on the patient with a thermal burn, which of the following is appropriate treatment?

    a. Maintain body heat.
    b. Apply topical analgesia.
    c. Remove the patient to a safe area.
    d. Stop the burning process.

24. The Parkland formula is used by many burn centers to _____ for the burn patient.

    a. measure scar formation
    b. determine fluid replacement
    c. determine the prognosis
    d. measure circulatory compromise

25. Which of the following factors can reduce the risk of inhalation injury for the victim involved in a house fire?

    a. screaming for help
    b. standing in a room with flames
    c. crawling on the floor in a room with flames
    d. being within an enclosed area involving a fire

26. Which of the following signs or conditions may indicate that a patient has an inhalation injury?

    a. hoarseness
    b. peripheral edema
    c. pain or paresthesia
    d. skin sloughing on the anterior chest

27. Regardless of the cause, _____ therapy for carbon monoxide inhalation is beneficial as it helps decrease the time it takes for the hemoglobin to become saturated with oxygen instead of CO.

    a. endotracheal intubation
    b. hyperbaric nitrogen
    c. hyperbaric oxygen
    d. positive pressure ventilation

28. Which of the following products will produce the most severe burn?

    a. cement
    b. hot tar
    c. hot grease
    d. pepper spray

29. When a patient has been burned with a dry powder, special considerations include:

    a. washing it off, then determining what it is.
    b. brushing it off and calling the poison control center for decon procedures.
    c. avoiding exposure to the chemical.
    d. waiting for the fire department to do the decon.

30. Which of the following is appropriate management of a chemical injury to the eye?

    a. continuous irrigation
    b. cover the affected eye with a dressing
    c. allow the patient to rub his eyes to facilitate drainage
    d. never remove contact lenses

31. The burning sensation of tear gas lasts for about _____ hour(s), while pepper gas lasts about _____ hours.

    a. one; two
    b. four; two
    c. five; four
    d. six; four

32. To minimize the effects of tear gas or pepper spray, the paramedic can:

    a. get the patient to blow her nose and spit out any residue.
    b. instruct the patient to rub her eyes.
    c. use circular strokes to sponge off any residue.
    d. avoid using water to flush the skin.

33. When a patient with contact lenses has an eye injury or burn from a chemical agent, the paramedic should:

    a. use the Morgan lens® on the unaffected eye and allow it to drain into the affected eye.
    b. remove the lenses with a gloved hand or assist the patient in doing so.
    c. place the Morgan lens® over the contact and irrigate with normal saline.
    d. never use a Morgan lens® on an eye injury caused by a chemical burn.

34. Select the statement that is most accurate about the severity of electrical burns.

    a. The entrance wound will always be more critical than the exit wound.
    b. The exit wound will always be more critical than the entrance wound.
    c. An electric burn that causes internal injury may eventually cause cancer.
    d. The path of electricity through the body may cause serious complications.

35. In the United States, about _____ people die from electrical shock each year.

    a. 100
    b. 1,000
    c. 10,000
    d. 100,000

36. The very first action to take when responding to a call for an electrocution is to:

    a. determine if there were any witnesses to the electrocution.
    b. determine if the unresponsive patient is in ventricular fibrillation.
    c. identify the source of the electricity prior to approaching the patient.
    d. wait for the fire department or power company to determine if the scene is safe to enter.

37. Direct current (DC), which has zero frequency but may be intermittent or pulsating, is:

    a. more dangerous then alternating current (AC).
    b. less dangerous than AC.
    c. the cause of circumferential burns more often than AC.
    d. the cause of circumferential burns less often than AC.

38. Alternating current at _____ Hz, which is household current, produces muscle tetany and tends to "freeze" the patient to the current source.

    a. 20
    b. 40
    c. 60
    d. 120

39. _____ is a lifesaving or limb-saving procedure used to allow expansion of the chest or restore circulation to an extremity in which the scar has formed a tight circumferential band.

    a. Circumcision
    b. Escharotomy
    c. Mesopexy
    d. Lyophilization

40. Which of the following skin conditions has the least resistance to electrical voltage?

    a. dry, intact skin
    b. wet, intact skin
    c. a thickly calloused palm or sole
    d. moist mucous membrane (mouth)

41. When assessing the victim of an electrical burn, the paramedic should look for an entry and exit point of the current, because:

    a. anything in the path is "fair game" for injury.
    b. both sites are always easy to find.
    c. the exit wound will indicate how much internal damage is present.
    d. the entry wound will indicate how much internal damage is present.

42. Which of the following signs or symptoms is not commonly found in a person who has sustained an electrical burn?

    a. trauma from falling
    b. hearing impairment or vision loss
    c. malocclusion
    d. muscle contractions or pain

43. Your patient is a forty-year-old male who was taken to the first-aid room by his coworkers after he suffered an accidental exposure to superheated gases. He is alert and shows signs of respiratory distress. He is wheezing, complains of difficulty swallowing, and is cyanotic. You suspect that his upper airway is swelling. What can you do to keep his airway from swelling any further?

    a. There is nothing you can do.
    b. Administer humidified oxygen.
    c. Endotracheally intubate the patient.
    d. Administer high-concentration oxygen.

44. Which of the following electrical burns is least likely to produce both an entry and exit wound?

    a. lightning strike
    b. arc injury
    c. direct contact with an electrical source
    d. indirect contact with an electrical source

45. All of the following statements about the management of the patient with an electrical injury are correct, *except*:

    a. do not touch the patient until you are sure that the power is turned off.
    b. treatment of an electric injury is the same as for a thermal injury.
    c. the potential for internal injury is less than a thermal injury.
    d. monitor the patient's ECG to identify hyperkalemia and cell death.

46. The most common entry point for an electrical burn is the:

    a. head.
    b. heart.
    c. hands.
    d. feet.

47. Which of the following is not a common physiologic dysfunction associated with electrical burns?

    a. involuntary muscular contractions
    b. singed nasal hairs
    c. seizures
    d. respiratory arrest

48. The _____ is/are the most common exit point for an electrical burn.

    a. head
    b. eyes
    c. rectum
    d. feet

49. Ionizing radiation produces immediate chemical effects, known as _____, on human tissue.

    a. ionization
    b. particle density
    c. radionization
    d. micronization

50. In which of the following circumstances should the paramedic suspect that a burn injury is a possible result of child abuse?

    a. when the history is inconsistent with the injuries
    b. when the burns are located on the front of the body
    c. when the burns are located on the back of the body
    d. when the body surface area of the burn is more than 30%

51. _____ is/are one type of ionizing radiation that can cause a burn injury.

   a. Radar
   b. Neutrons
   c. Radio waves
   d. Microwaves

52. _____ are small particles that are high in energy and can be dangerous if inhaled or ingested.

   a. Alpha particles
   b. Beta particles
   c. Geiger rays
   d. Microwaves

53. The most penetrating particles are _____, for which exposure causes direct tissue damage.

   a. alpha particles
   b. beta particles
   c. gamma rays
   d. neutrons

54. _____ are slow moving and contain low energy, so objects such as newspaper or clothing can stop them.

   a. Alpha particles
   b. Beta particles
   c. Geiger rays
   d. Gamma rays

55. A gauge of the likely injury to an irradiated part of an organism is called the:

   a. whole body exposure.
   b. comparable radiation sickness.
   c. radiation absorbed dose (RAD).
   d. roentgen equivalent in man (REM).

56. Radiation sickness results when humans or animals are exposed to excessive doses of _____ radiation.

   a. radio wave
   b. microwave
   c. ionizing
   d. nonionizing

57. How can the paramedic determine the severity of radiation illness following an exposure?

   a. by the severity of symptoms
   b. by obtaining a Geiger counter reading
   c. by the changes in the white blood cells
   d. by determining the length of exposure

58. _____ is/are very sensitive to radiation, and the higher the absorbed dose, the more depressed the count will be.

   a. Red blood cells
   b. White blood cells
   c. Platelets
   d. Hemoglobin

59. You are going to be transporting a patient who has just received radiation therapy as part of her cancer treatment and is experiencing complications. Which of the following signs or symptoms can you expect the patient to be experiencing?

   a. dysrhythmia
   b. pulmonary edema
   c. difficulty swallowing
   d. nausea and vomiting

60. What is the difference between a clean and a dirty radiation accident?

   a. In a clean accident, the patient has external exposure but not internal.
   b. In a clean accident, the patient has internal exposure but not external.
   c. In a dirty accident, the patient continues to be a hazard of exposure to responders.
   d. In a dirty accident, the patient is exposed to an ionizing source but is not radioactive.

Exam #36 Answer Form

	A	B	C	D		A	B	C	D
1.	❏	❏	❏	❏	27.	❏	❏	❏	❏
2.	❏	❏	❏	❏	28.	❏	❏	❏	❏
3.	❏	❏	❏	❏	29.	❏	❏	❏	❏
4.	❏	❏	❏	❏	30.	❏	❏	❏	❏
5.	❏	❏	❏	❏	31.	❏	❏	❏	❏
6.	❏	❏	❏	❏	32.	❏	❏	❏	❏
7.	❏	❏	❏	❏	33.	❏	❏	❏	❏
8.	❏	❏	❏	❏	34.	❏	❏	❏	❏
9.	❏	❏	❏	❏	35.	❏	❏	❏	❏
10.	❏	❏	❏	❏	36.	❏	❏	❏	❏
11.	❏	❏	❏	❏	37.	❏	❏	❏	❏
12.	❏	❏	❏	❏	38.	❏	❏	❏	❏
13.	❏	❏	❏	❏	39.	❏	❏	❏	❏
14.	❏	❏	❏	❏	40.	❏	❏	❏	❏
15.	❏	❏	❏	❏	41.	❏	❏	❏	❏
16.	❏	❏	❏	❏	42.	❏	❏	❏	❏
17.	❏	❏	❏	❏	43.	❏	❏	❏	❏
18.	❏	❏	❏	❏	44.	❏	❏	❏	❏
19.	❏	❏	❏	❏	45.	❏	❏	❏	❏
20.	❏	❏	❏	❏	46.	❏	❏	❏	❏
21.	❏	❏	❏	❏	47.	❏	❏	❏	❏
22.	❏	❏	❏	❏	48.	❏	❏	❏	❏
23.	❏	❏	❏	❏	49.	❏	❏	❏	❏
24.	❏	❏	❏	❏	50.	❏	❏	❏	❏
25.	❏	❏	❏	❏	51.	❏	❏	❏	❏
26.	❏	❏	❏	❏	52.	❏	❏	❏	❏

	A	B	C	D		A	B	C	D
53.	❏	❏	❏	❏	57.	❏	❏	❏	❏
54.	❏	❏	❏	❏	58.	❏	❏	❏	❏
55.	❏	❏	❏	❏	59.	❏	❏	❏	❏
56.	❏	❏	❏	❏	60.	❏	❏	❏	❏

Head and Facial Trauma

1. The primary problem for paramedics managing a patient with blunt force trauma to the face or head is:

   a. spinal shock.
   b. blowout fractures.
   c. airway compromise.
   d. traumatic brain injury (TBI).

2. Common MOIs for penetrating injuries to the face or head include:

   a. MVCs.
   b. sticks or clubs.
   c. body-to-body contact.
   d. GSWs.

3. A patient who has suffered blunt force trauma to the face and head is most likely to have which of the following associated injuries?

   a. blindness
   b. hearing loss
   c. hoarseness
   d. cervical spine injury

4. Injuries to the throat can be fatal when:

   a. the patient has a very short neck.
   b. the patient is very young or elderly.
   c. there is an associated cervical spine injury.
   d. there is an associated injury to the major blood vessels.

5. A _____ is a hemorrhage in the anterior chamber of the eye.

   a. conjunctival hemorrhage
   b. detached retina
   c. blowout fracture
   d. hyphema

6. When traumatic pressure is transmitted through the eyeball to the relatively thin bone in the medial and inferior portions of the orbit, causing it to break, this is called a:

   a. posterior chamber divide.
   b. detached retina.
   c. blowout fracture.
   d. hyphema.

7. Isolated injuries to the mouth, such as from a _____, are very common, accounting for as much as 50% of facial trauma.

   a. punch
   b. MVC
   c. penetrating trauma
   d. fishhook

8. The LeFort classifications categorize facial fractures into three types. The higher the number, the more significant the damage, and the more potential there is for a:

   a. complicated airway.
   b. brain injury.
   c. spinal cord injury.
   d. vision disturbance.

9. LeFort fractures are based on:

   a. clinical impression.
   b. history of MOI.
   c. X-ray or CT scan findings.
   d. a combination of all of these.

10. The critical structures in the neck include all of the following, *except*:

    a. larynx and trachea.
    b. carotid arteries.
    c. vertebral arteries.
    d. cranial nerves one to five.

11. The _____ ear canal is considered a mucous membrane that secretes wax for protection.

    a. pinna
    b. outer
    c. external
    d. inner

12. The middle ear is separated from the external canal by the:

    a. pinna.
    b. eardrum.
    c. cartilage.
    d. inner ear.

13. Light receptors to color vision, which are located in the posterior chamber of the eye, are called:

    a. optic nerves.
    b. retinas.
    c. rods.
    d. cones.

14. The _____ is the transparent covering of the iris and pupil, which admits light into the eye.

    a. conjuctiva
    b. lens
    c. sclera
    d. cornea

15. _____ provide protection for the eye and help to lubricate the surface.

    a. Lens
    b. Eyelids
    c. Lacrimal apparatus
    d. Conjuctiva

16. The _____ are responsible for peripheral vision and low light, night sight conditions.

    a. pupils
    b. rods
    c. cones
    d. retinas

17. Which of the following is not a major muscle of the mouth?

    a. hypoglossal
    b. tongue
    c. orbicular oris
    d. masseter muscle

18. The bones of the mouth include the palate, jawbone, and:

    a. hyoid.
    b. teeth.
    c. zygomatic.
    d. mastoid process.

19. When the paramedic examines the patient's face and the jaws, and notes that the teeth do not meet as they should, this is called:

    a. diplopia.
    b. malocclusion.
    c. a depressed zygoma.
    d. tetany.

20. When a patient has sustained an eye injury, often the recommendation is to cover both eyes to limit or prevent:

    a. the onset of dysconjugate gaze in the unaffected eye.
    b. the onset of dysconjugate gaze in the affected eye.
    c. movement from conjugate gaze of the uninjured eye.
    d. movement from conjugate gaze of the injured eye.

21. In the United States, approximately four _____ people sustain a head injury each year.

    a. out of a thousand
    b. thousand
    c. million
    d. billion

22. The highest risk of head injury occurs in _____ between _____ years of age.

    a. males; two and twelve
    b. males; fifteen and twenty-four
    c. females; fifteen and twenty-four
    d. females; sixty-five and eighty-five

23. The most common cause of head trauma and subdural hematoma is:

    a. MVC.
    b. falls in the elderly.
    c. sports.
    d. falls in the presence of alcohol abuse.

24. The scalp has an important freely moveable sheet of connective tissue called the _____ that helps to deflect blows.

    a. parietal fold
    b. mastoid sheath
    c. emissary
    d. galea

25. The actual bones that comprise the skull are double-layered with a spongy middle layer, allowing them to:

    a. facilitate drainage in the event of a hemorrhage.
    b. aerate the meninges.
    c. be strong yet light in weight.
    d. recycle cerebrospinal fluid.

26. Trauma to the _____ may cause disruption of the voluntary skeletal movement and may result in extremity paralysis, paresthesia, or weakness.

    a. medulla
    b. cerebrum
    c. brain stem
    d. occiput

27. When a person is struck in the _____ lobe, it may cause the patient to see "stars," have blurred vision, or experience other visual disturbances.

    a. temporal
    b. parietal
    c. occipital
    d. frontal

28. The cranial nerves (CN) that can be affected in head injury are the oculomotor nerve CN _____ and the vagus nerve CN _____.

    a. II; X
    b. III; V
    c. III; X
    d. IV; XII

29. The _____ controls the degree of activity of the central nervous system (e.g., maintaining sleep and wakefulness).

    a. vagus nerve
    b. hypothalamus
    c. foramen magnum
    d. reticular activating system

30. The arachnoid membrane, which appears to look like a web of blood vessels, is actually composed of:

    a. venous blood vessels that reabsorb CSF.
    b. venous blood vessels that drain the cerebral sinuses.
    c. arteries that stimulate cerebral function.
    d. arteries that manufacture CSF.

31. The brain has a very high metabolic rate and consumes _____% of the body's oxygen supply.

    a. 5
    b. 10
    c. 20
    d. 50

32. A mechanism called _____ is responsible for regulating the body's blood pressure to maintain the cerebral perfusion pressure (CPP).

    a. intercerebral pressure
    b. intracerebral pressure
    c. autoregulation
    d. mean arterial force

33. A twenty-year-old male fell off a ladder at work. He landed on his back, struck his head, and experienced a brief loss of consciousness. Upon awakening, he is confused and does not remember how he fell. He remains conscious for the entire time you are attending to him. What type of head injury has this patient experienced?

    a. coup
    b. contra coup
    c. linear skull fracture
    d. basilar skull fracture

34. Continuing with question 33, what type of brain injury has the patient most likely experienced?

    a. contusion
    b. concussion
    c. epidural hematoma
    d. subarachnoid hematoma

35. Cerebral contusion, intracranial hemorrhage, and epidural hematoma are all examples of _____ brain injuries.

    a. peripheral
    b. focal
    c. subarachnoid
    d. diffuse axonal

36. _____ is the effect of acceleration or deceleration on the brain.

    a. Coup
    b. Contra coup
    c. Focal
    d. Diffuse axonal injury

37. A/an _____ is a mild diffuse axonal injury, which results in a transient episode of neuronal dysfunction with rapid return to normal neurologic activity.

    a. subarachnoid injury
    b. concussion
    c. epidural hematoma
    d. contusion

38. Which of the following is not a type of skull fracture that can be determined by an X-ray?

    a. linear
    b. depressed
    c. Battle's sign
    d. basilar

39. The most common type of skull fracture, which may or may not result in leaking of CSF, is a _____ fracture.

    a. linear
    b. depressed
    c. basilar
    d. penetrating

40. _____ hematomas are bleeds that are more common in elderly and alcoholic patients who fall down and hit their heads often.

a. Acute subdural
b. Chronic subdural
c. Acute epidural
d. Chronic epidural

41. When intracranial pressure (ICP) in the brain rises due to a hemorrhage, it can cause the brain to shift downward, resulting in any of the following assessment findings, *except*:

a. vomiting.
b. tachycardia.
c. irregular respirations.
d. unequal or nonreactive pupils.

42. The "Cushing" response in brain herniation with hypotension and bradycardia is a late response and usually precedes death by only _____ minutes.

a. four to six
b. ten
c. fifteen
d. twenty

43. Which of the following assessment findings will initially be present when a patient experiences a loss of cerebral autoregulation?

a. seizures
b. Cushing's reflex
c. a drop in blood pressure
d. elevated blood pressure

44. You are transporting an unconscious patient with a massive head injury as a result of a serious MVC. You have intubated her and have two IVs in place. The patient's initial GCS was 6, and her vital signs were: respiratory 16/irregular; pulse 50/regular; and BP 170/100. Her pupils are still reactive, and she withdraws with flexion to pain stimuli. What part of the brain is the increasing ICP impacting at this point?

a. lower brain stem
b. middle brain stem
c. upper brain stem
d. cerebral cortex and upper brain stem

45. Which of the following statements is incorrect regarding the impact of increasing ICP on the lower brain stem or medulla?

a. Vegetative functions are temporarily impaired because of the pressure.
b. The patient's injury is not considered survivable.
c. The respirations are ataxic or absent.
d. The ECG will have QRS, ST segment, and T wave changes.

46. With GCS being an objective measure of eye opening, verbal response, and motor response in a numerical score, a moderate head injury would be:

a. 13 to 15.
b. 8 to 12.
c. 5 to 8.
d. <8.

47. Intracranial bleeding from a/an _____ hematoma results in the presence of blood in the CSF.

a. epidural
b. subdural
c. subarachnoid
d. intracerebral

48. When assessing a patient's head for possible depressed and open skull fractures, the paramedic should be careful to use the _____ to palpate and not "poke" into the fracture site.

a. pads of the fingers
b. flat side of a tongue depressor
c. stethoscope with a sterile gauze
d. palm of the hand

49. Which of the following signs and symptoms are atypical for a patient with an expanding intracranial hematoma?

a. nausea and vomiting
b. changes in mental status
c. tachycardia and tachypnea
d. headache with increasing severity

50. You are interviewing a medical patient who had a seizure. When you inquire about his past medical history, he tells you that two years ago he suffered a traumatic brain injury. As a result of the injury, he experienced changes in his personality as well as seizures. What part of his brain did he injure?

a. frontal lobe
b. parietal lobe
c. occipital lobe
d. temporal lobe

51. The appropriate management of a head injury by the paramedic includes all the following, *except*:

a. assuring an adequate airway, ventilation, and oxygenation.
b. aggressive hyperventilation.
c. assuring adequate circulation.
d. conducting serial neurologic assessments.

52. If hypotension develops in the patient with a head injury, it is most likely caused by bleeding from:

a. another organ or injuries besides the brain.
b. the middle meningeal artery.
c. a subarachnoid hemorrhage.
d. the circle of Willis.

53. Studies have shown that _____ improves outcomes in combative head trauma patients.

    a. the use of steroids
    b. osmotic diuretics given in the field
    c. aggressive hyperventilation
    d. paralysis prior to intubation

54. In the patient with a head injury, the use of glucose is recommended:

    a. after intubation of a combative patient.
    b. only when hypoglycemia is confirmed.
    c. only when given simultaneously with steroids.
    d. prior to sedation for intubation.

55. When treating a patient with signs and symptoms of increasing ICP, the paramedic should first:

    a. paralyze then intubate the patient.
    b. assure adequate tidal volume.
    c. hyperventilate the patient.
    d. administer an osmotic diuretic.

56. In the management of a head injury patient, the paramedic should assure that the cerebral perfusion pressure is maintained by making sure to keep the _____ BP over _____ mmHg.

    a. systolic; 70
    b. systolic; 100
    c. diastolic; 50
    d. diastolic; 70

57. While assuring a patent airway in the patient with head trauma, the paramedic should avoid _____ as it may increase the ICP.

    a. inserting an OPA
    b. using a water-soluble jelly
    c. nasal intubation
    d. oral-tracheal intubation

58. When assessing a patient suspected of having an expanding intracranial hematoma, which of the following is the most important finding?

    a. the history of the MOI
    b. the past medical history
    c. the patient's current medications
    d. when the patient ate last

59. An unconscious patient with an open head injury has nonreactive pupils and shows abnormal flexion when pain is applied. What is this patient's GCS?

    a. 3
    b. 4
    c. 5
    d. 6

60. Which of the following types of skull fractures is easily missed in the absence of symptoms developing from an underlying hematoma?

    a. linear
    b. depressed
    c. Battle's sign
    d. basilar

Exam #37 Answer Form

	A	B	C	D		A	B	C	D
1.	❏	❏	❏	❏	27.	❏	❏	❏	❏
2.	❏	❏	❏	❏	28.	❏	❏	❏	❏
3.	❏	❏	❏	❏	29.	❏	❏	❏	❏
4.	❏	❏	❏	❏	30.	❏	❏	❏	❏
5.	❏	❏	❏	❏	31.	❏	❏	❏	❏
6.	❏	❏	❏	❏	32.	❏	❏	❏	❏
7.	❏	❏	❏	❏	33.	❏	❏	❏	❏
8.	❏	❏	❏	❏	34.	❏	❏	❏	❏
9.	❏	❏	❏	❏	35.	❏	❏	❏	❏
10.	❏	❏	❏	❏	36.	❏	❏	❏	❏
11.	❏	❏	❏	❏	37.	❏	❏	❏	❏
12.	❏	❏	❏	❏	38.	❏	❏	❏	❏
13.	❏	❏	❏	❏	39.	❏	❏	❏	❏
14.	❏	❏	❏	❏	40.	❏	❏	❏	❏
15.	❏	❏	❏	❏	41.	❏	❏	❏	❏
16.	❏	❏	❏	❏	42.	❏	❏	❏	❏
17.	❏	❏	❏	❏	43.	❏	❏	❏	❏
18.	❏	❏	❏	❏	44.	❏	❏	❏	❏
19.	❏	❏	❏	❏	45.	❏	❏	❏	❏
20.	❏	❏	❏	❏	46.	❏	❏	❏	❏
21.	❏	❏	❏	❏	47.	❏	❏	❏	❏
22.	❏	❏	❏	❏	48.	❏	❏	❏	❏
23.	❏	❏	❏	❏	49.	❏	❏	❏	❏
24.	❏	❏	❏	❏	50.	❏	❏	❏	❏
25.	❏	❏	❏	❏	51.	❏	❏	❏	❏
26.	❏	❏	❏	❏	52.	❏	❏	❏	❏

	A	B	C	D			A	B	C	D
53.	❏	❏	❏	❏		57.	❏	❏	❏	❏
54.	❏	❏	❏	❏		58.	❏	❏	❏	❏
55.	❏	❏	❏	❏		59.	❏	❏	❏	❏
56.	❏	❏	❏	❏		60.	❏	❏	❏	❏

38

Spinal Trauma

1. Which age group has the highest incidence of spinal cord injury?

    a. men, thirty-one to fifty
    b. men, sixteen to thirty
    c. women, thirty-one to fifty
    d. women, sixteen to thirty

2. It is estimated that _____ % of spinal cord injury is caused by improper handling of the patient.

    a. 5
    b. 10
    c. 25
    d. 35

3. The spine consists of interconnected bone and:

    a. ligaments.
    b. muscles.
    c. tendons.
    d. all of the above.

4. The ligament that prevents hyperflexion in the spine is the:

    a. anterior longitudinal.
    b. posterior longitudinal.
    c. cruciform.
    d. atlantoaxial.

5. A ligament that is shaped like a cross and supports the atlas vertebrae is the:

    a. anterior longitudinal.
    b. posterior longitudinal.
    c. cruciform.
    d. atlantoaxial.

6. The second cervical vertebrae is also called the:

    a. cribiform.
    b. atlas.
    c. axis.
    d. pivotal.

7. The ligament that serves to hold the odontoid process close to the anterior arch is the:

    a. anterior longitudinal.
    b. transverse.
    c. cruciform.
    d. atlantoaxial.

8. The atlas pivots on the _____ or odontoid process of the axis, which permits rotation of the head.

    a. dens
    b. cribiform
    c. foramen
    d. cruciform

9. The area of the spine that is the most protected from injury is the:

    a. cervical.
    b. thoracic.
    c. lumbar.
    d. abdominal.

10. There are _____ pair of spinal nerves that are responsible for the sensory and motor function of the body below the head.

    a. twenty-four
    b. twenty-seven
    c. thirty-one
    d. thirty-eight

11. The _____, which is a fusion of three to five bones, is commonly referred to as the tailbone.

    a. coccyx
    b. sacrum
    c. cauda equina
    d. spinous process

12. The vertebrae consist of the body, the vertebral arch, and the:

    a. foramen magnum.
    b. transverse process.
    c. spina bifida.
    d. spinous foramen.

13. The posterior aspect of the vertebrae that projects back from the junction of two lamina is called the:

    a. vertebral arch.
    b. spinous process.
    c. intercerebral disk.
    d. transverse process.

14. The relatively soft, gel-like internal portion of the disk is called the:

    a. annulus fibrosis.
    b. lamina.
    c. odontoid.
    d. nucleus pulposus.

15. Where does the spinal cord end?

    a. C-6
    b. T-5
    c. L-2
    d. L-6

16. Where does cerebral spinal fluid come from?

    a. The intervertebral disks.
    b. It is manufactured in the ventricles of the brain.
    c. It is manufactured in the pancreas.
    d. It is stored in the bile duct.

17. The material that is located in the anatomical spinal tracts is called:

    a. white matter.
    b. melanin.
    c. myelin sheath.
    d. gray matter.

18. The _____ carries impulses from body parts and sensory information to the brain.

    a. sensory system
    b. ascending nerve tracts
    c. descending nerve tracts
    d. parasympathetic nervous system

19. Corticospinal and reticulospinal are two types of:

    a. sensory system nerves.
    b. ascending nerve tracts.
    c. descending nerve tracts.
    d. parasympathetic NS.

20. What is a funiculus?

    a. a group of nerve fibers with a similar function
    b. a ligament found in the spinal column
    c. the key to the corticospinal tract
    d. the center of the reticulospinal tract

21. The lateral spinothalamic tracts:

    a. conduct sensory impulses of touch and pressure to the brain.
    b. send muscular impulses from the brain to muscle.
    c. conduct impulses of pain and temperature to the brain.
    d. coordinate impulses necessary for muscular movements.

22. A particular area where the spinal nerve provides either motor stimulation, sensations, or both is called a/an:

    a. ganglion.
    b. dermatome.
    c. axon.
    d. nerve band.

23. Following a significant MOI, a patient experiences loss of motor and sensory function from the nipple line, down. What is the highest level of the spine that has been affected?

    a. C-3
    b. C-5
    c. C-7
    d. T-4

24. Following a significant MOI, a patient experiences loss of movement of the diaphragm and loss of sensory function below the shoulder. What is the highest level of the spine that may have been affected?

    a. C-3
    b. C-4
    c. C-5
    d. C-6

25. One of the few exceptions for immobilizing a patient's neck in the position discovered, rather than the normal anatomical position is:

    a. level of consciousness.
    b. resistance to movement.
    c. uncontrolled bleeding from the scalp.
    d. the need to manage the airway with an advanced airway.

26. Your patient has experienced a significant MOI, which you believe requires spinal immobilization. The patient is not willing to have a rigid collar placed on her neck because it will make her feel restricted. She is, however, willing to lie down on a backboard. What is the most appropriate way to proceed with this patient?

    a. Do nothing but transport the patient.
    b. Insist on the rigid collar and immobilize the patient.
    c. Refuse to transport the patient unless she cooperates fully.
    d. Have the patient sign a refusal for the collar, and immobilize her without it.

27. You are assessing a female who was a passenger involved in an MVC. She is complaining of neck, back, and chest pain. When you are listening for breathing sounds, you see that she has lipstick on her shirt as if someone kissed her upper chest. You also see that she is wearing the same color lipstick. How does this finding relate to the MOI?

    a. The patient suffered a rotational MOI.
    b. The patient experienced hyperflexion.
    c. The patient experienced hyperextension.
    d. The MOI was severe enough to have caused a loss of consciousness.

28. When the spinal cord is transected at the _____ level, the result is permanent paraplegia.

    a. cervical
    b. thoracic
    c. sacral
    d. coccyx

29. Which of the following statements about spinal injuries is most correct?

    a. Spinal cord injuries always have accompanying soft tissue injuries.
    b. All spinal cord injuries can be detected by X-ray, MRI, or CT scan.
    c. The spinal cord may be injured without accompanying bone or soft tissue injury.
    d. The patient with a spinal cord injury has sharp pain over the injury site, with or without palpation.

30. When is partial spinal immobilization used in the field?

    a. when the distance a patient fell is <30 feet
    b. when the MOI is not severe
    c. if the patient prefers not to lie down
    d. it should not be used at all

31. You are treating a toddler who fell out of a shopping cart and lacerated his head. He was initially unconscious, but now is crying and covered with blood. How should he be managed?

    a. cervical collar application and hemorrhage control
    b. full spinal immobilization with the parent providing support
    c. hemorrhage control and transport in a child car seat
    d. backboard and manual head stabilization by the parent

32. Your adult patient is refusing spinal immobilization following a minor MVC, even though she has new tenderness in her neck, shoulders, and lower back. You are making the decision as to whether the patient is reliable to refuse treatment or not. What factor is most significant in making this determination?

    a. the patient's age
    b. vital signs
    c. mental status
    d. positive pain on palpation of the spine

33. If a patient with an "uncertain MOI" complains of having some minor neck pain upon moving his head, you should:

    a. determine the range of motion.
    b. continue your assessment and document the complaint.
    c. fully immobilize the spine.
    d. call medical control for permission to clear the c-spine.

34. Why should you palpate the spinous process if you suspect a neck injury?

    a. This will rule out neck injury.
    b. Tender areas may not hurt unless palpated.
    c. Patients appreciate the extra care.
    d. The vertebrae may be dislocated even though there is still movement.

35. You have assessed a patient's upper and lower extremities before and after immobilizing her to a long backboard. Which of the following findings is most significant?

    a. pain in both arms before and after immobilization
    b. parathesia in the left leg after, not before, immobilization
    c. weakness in the right arm before, not after, immobilization
    d. weakness in the right arm before and after immobilization

36. You are treating a construction worker who did not have a helmet on while he was walking under a platform and was struck on the head by a large falling brick. Which of the following MOIs most likely occurred?

    a. vertical compression of the spine
    b. hyperflexion of the head and neck
    c. hyperextension of the head and neck
    d. distraction of the neck

37. You and your partner are immobilizing a patient who attempted to hang himself. Which of the following injuries do you associate with a hanging?

   a. rotational neck injury
   b. flexion of the neck
   c. vertical compression of the neck
   d. distraction of the neck

38. You arrive at the scene of a vehicle that was T-boned in an intersection. The EMT–Bs are short-boarding the driver who is complaining of neck and back pain. Which of the following injuries do you suspect?

   a. rotational neck injury
   b. flexion of the neck
   c. vertical compression of the neck
   d. distraction of the neck

39. The type of spinal cord injury that is characterized by a temporary disruption of cord-mediated functions is a cord:

   a. concussion.
   b. contusion.
   c. compression.
   d. transection.

40. The type of spinal cord injury that is characterized by hypotension and vasodilation, loss of bladder and bowel control, and priaprism in male patients is:

   a. spinal hemorrhage.
   b. spinal shock.
   c. neurogenic shock.
   d. cord laceration.

41. You are called to assist a patient who has fallen but has no complaint of injury. The patient has a preexisting spinal cord injury, which has left him with a loss of motor function and pain sensation, but only on the left side of his body. Which of the following conditions does this patient have?

   a. anterior cord syndrome
   b. central cord syndrome
   c. incomplete spinal cord transection
   d. Brown–Sequard syndrome

42. Degenerative disc disease is caused by a narrowing of the intervertebral disc, which results in:

   a. epidural abscess.
   b. spinal cord tumors.
   c. variable segment instability.
   d. a structural defect in the lamina or vertebral arch.

43. It is estimated that _____ % of the population experience some degree of low back pain during their lifetime.

   a. 20–30
   b. 40–50
   c. 60–90
   d. 80–100

44. When making a decision about immobilizing a patient wearing a helmet, which of the following criteria would be a reason to remove the helmet?

   a. The helmet is the proper size.
   b. The head moves around inside the helmet.
   c. The helmet does not interfere with airway management.
   d. The helmet interferes with the application of a cervical collar.

45. In which of the following spinal disorders is heredity considered to be a significant factor?

   a. degenerative disc
   b. spondylolysis
   c. low back pain syndrome
   d. spinal cord tumors

46. What is the primary management of a patient with severe low back pain?

   a. palliative care
   b. full spinal immobilization
   c. partial spinal immobilization
   d. rapid transport to an ED

47. What is the most common cause of spinal cord tumors?

   a. trauma
   b. heredity
   c. metastasis
   d. PCBs

48. The diameter of the spinal cord is approximately _____ mm, and the diameter of the spinal column is approximately _____ mm.

   a. 5; 10
   b. 10; 15
   c. 15; 20
   d. 20; 25

49. Which of the following statements is not correct about rigid cervical collars?

   a. They are also referred to as extrication collars.
   b. They limit movement of the neck.
   c. They totally eliminate neck movement.
   d. They are the standard for cervical immobilization.

50. Which of the following is the primary reason for removing a helmet from a patient with a suspected SCI?

    a. the paramedic is trained to do it
    b. airway management
    c. the patient needs to be immobilized
    d. ED staff does not have sufficient training to do it

51. Which of the following is not an indication for rapid extrication?

    a. compensating shock
    b. decompensating shock
    c. penetrating chest wound
    d. penetrating abdominal wound

52. For which of the following adult ambulatory patients is a standing takedown indicated?

    a. fall from a standing position with two possible fractured wrists, and no LOC
    b. female who tripped and fell, breaking her nose, yet she denies pain on palpation of her neck and back
    c. passenger involved in a high-speed MVC complaining of a headache after the collision
    d. driver with an MOI that involved airbag deployment, seat belt use, no LOC, and no complaint of injury

53. When should a child be removed from a car seat to immobilize the spine?

    a. when the child is crying
    b. when the parents are distressed
    c. when it is necessary for the patient to be supine
    d. when you cannot palpate the child's back

54. Patients are immobilized in the neutral, in-line anatomic position for all of the following reasons, *except* that this:

    a. position allows for the most space for the cord.
    b. position is the most comfortable for the patient.
    c. is the most stable position for the spinal column.
    d. position will help to reduce cord hypoxia.

55. Which of the following is a principle of spinal immobilization?

    a. The goal is to prevent further injury.
    b. Fifteen percent of secondary spinal injuries are preventable with immobilization.
    c. Spinal immobilization should begin after the initial assessment.
    d. Spinal immobilization should be applied to any patient with back pain.

56. Patients with herniated intervertebral disks are commonly affected in which two areas of the spine?

    a. cervical and thoracic
    b. thoracic and lumbar
    c. lumbar and sacral
    d. lumbar and cervical

57. What is the preferred method for assessing a patient for spinal tenderness?

    a. Palpate over each of the spinal processes.
    b. Palpate over each of the vertebral bodies.
    c. Ask the patient to move all four extremities.
    d. Ask the patient if he has any back pain.

58. The evaluation of motor function of the lower extremities includes assessment of plantar flexion and:

    a. great toe flexion.
    b. foot dorsiflexion.
    c. Babinski's reflex.
    d. plantar reflex.

59. The causes of traumatic spinal cord injury include direct trauma, excessive movement, and:

    a. directions of force.
    b. degeneration.
    c. Achilles' heel.
    d. blight reflexes.

60. You are assessing a conscious twenty-year-old male who was removed from a pool on a backboard by lifeguards on the scene. Your assessment findings include hypotension, bradycardia, and skin that is pink and warm. He is flaccid from the waist down. What do you suspect with these findings?

    a. spinal shock
    b. neurogenic shock
    c. spinal cord compression
    d. disk prolapse

Exam #38 Answer Form

	A	B	C	D		A	B	C	D
1.	❏	❏	❏	❏	27.	❏	❏	❏	❏
2.	❏	❏	❏	❏	28.	❏	❏	❏	❏
3.	❏	❏	❏	❏	29.	❏	❏	❏	❏
4.	❏	❏	❏	❏	30.	❏	❏	❏	❏
5.	❏	❏	❏	❏	31.	❏	❏	❏	❏
6.	❏	❏	❏	❏	32.	❏	❏	❏	❏
7.	❏	❏	❏	❏	33.	❏	❏	❏	❏
8.	❏	❏	❏	❏	34.	❏	❏	❏	❏
9.	❏	❏	❏	❏	35.	❏	❏	❏	❏
10.	❏	❏	❏	❏	36.	❏	❏	❏	❏
11.	❏	❏	❏	❏	37.	❏	❏	❏	❏
12.	❏	❏	❏	❏	38.	❏	❏	❏	❏
13.	❏	❏	❏	❏	39.	❏	❏	❏	❏
14.	❏	❏	❏	❏	40.	❏	❏	❏	❏
15.	❏	❏	❏	❏	41.	❏	❏	❏	❏
16.	❏	❏	❏	❏	42.	❏	❏	❏	❏
17.	❏	❏	❏	❏	43.	❏	❏	❏	❏
18.	❏	❏	❏	❏	44.	❏	❏	❏	❏
19.	❏	❏	❏	❏	45.	❏	❏	❏	❏
20.	❏	❏	❏	❏	46.	❏	❏	❏	❏
21.	❏	❏	❏	❏	47.	❏	❏	❏	❏
22.	❏	❏	❏	❏	48.	❏	❏	❏	❏
23.	❏	❏	❏	❏	49.	❏	❏	❏	❏
24.	❏	❏	❏	❏	50.	❏	❏	❏	❏
25.	❏	❏	❏	❏	51.	❏	❏	❏	❏
26.	❏	❏	❏	❏	52.	❏	❏	❏	❏

	A	B	C	D			A	B	C	D
53.	❏	❏	❏	❏		57.	❏	❏	❏	❏
54.	❏	❏	❏	❏		58.	❏	❏	❏	❏
55.	❏	❏	❏	❏		59.	❏	❏	❏	❏
56.	❏	❏	❏	❏		60.	❏	❏	❏	❏

39

Thoracic Trauma

1. Chest injuries are the _____ leading cause of trauma deaths each year in the United States.

   a. primary
   b. second
   c. third
   d. fifth

2. Thoracic trauma can impair ventilation in many ways, such as:

   a. collapsing of alveoli.
   b. bruising of lung tissue.
   c. laceration of the trachea.
   d. disruption of the bellows action.

3. The major problem with the injury to the mediastinum is:

   a. tearing of a great vessel.
   b. contusion of the heart.
   c. esophageal spasm.
   d. aortic seizure.

4. An esophageal injury such as a _____ may occur to the esophagus when the throat or upper chest is perforated.

   a. spasm
   b. tear
   c. flare-up
   d. fracture

5. When an explosion occurs within a confined space, the pressure injures the lung tissue, causing:

   a. necrosis.
   b. petechial impressions.
   c. massive lung contusions to develop.
   d. tears.

6. The presence of subcutaneous emphysema on the closed anterior chest of a patient, as a result of a significant MOI, is suggestive of what type of internal injury?

   a. aortic rupture
   b. ruptured diaphragm
   c. perforated lung tissue
   d. perforated esophagus

7. Which of the following is not a muscle of the thorax?

   a. external intercostals
   b. mesotendons
   c. internal intercostals
   d. trapezius

8. _____ is/are a major muscle that moves the head and is also an accessory muscle of breathing, as it helps to lift the chest cage.

   a. Sternocleidomastoid
   b. Rhomboids
   c. Pectoralis major
   d. Latissimus dorsi

9. The muscle that originates in the occipital bone and inserts into the clavicle, with its function being to raise and lower the shoulders, is called the:

   a. rhomboid.
   b. trapezius.
   c. external costals.
   d. sternocleidomastoid.

10. The trachea extends from the anterior throat into the chest cavity and then bifurcates at the carina into the:

    a. parenchyma.
    b. anterior rhomboid major.
    c. distal rhomboid minor.
    d. mainstem bronchi.

11. _____ is the lung tissue itself rather than all the supporting connective tissues.

    a. Parenchyma
    b. Bronchi
    c. Alveoli
    d. Pleura

12. All of the following are major arteries of the chest, *except* the:

    a. aorta.
    b. internal mammary artery.
    c. carotid artery.
    d. inferior vena cava.

13. Which of the following is not a major vein of the chest?

    a. aorta
    b. internal jugular
    c. external jugular
    d. subclavian

14. The _____ is/are located in the mediastinum, or center of the chest.

    a. diaphragm
    b. trachea
    c. abdominal aorta
    d. lungs

15. The mechanical process of ventilation involves all of the following, *except*:

    a. during inspiration, the diaphragm and intercostal muscles contract.
    b. diaphragmatic contraction creates a vacuum in the chest cavity.
    c. positive intrathoracic pressure pushes air out of the lungs.
    d. negative intrathoracic pressure "sucks" air into the lungs, expanding them.

16. Any injury that affects the diaphragm, intercostal muscles, or _____ can severely affect the mechanics of ventilation.

    a. vagus nerve
    b. accessory muscles of breathing
    c. aortic arch
    d. sacral spine

17. The ability to exchange gas during respiration is a function of all of the following elements, *except*:

    a. serous pleural fluid.
    b. alveolar capillary interface.
    c. pulmonary circulation.
    d. acid-base balance.

18. Chemoreceptors, located in the aortic arch and _____, measure carbon dioxide levels in the blood.

    a. capillary beds
    b. carotid sinus
    c. parenchyma
    d. alveoli

19. Impairment of gas exchange as a result of chest trauma occurs in which of the following mechanisms?

    a. contusions on the lung tissue
    b. disruption of the bellows action
    c. ineffective diaphragmatic contraction
    d. disassociation of the alveoli from the parenchyma

20. Assessment findings of the patient who has experienced thoracic trauma may include a pulse that is:

    a. tachycardic from shock.
    b. bradycardic from a conduction problem.
    c. in deficit from damage to a great vessel.
    d. all of the above.

21. Fractures of the left lower ribs are often associated with:

    a. splenic rupture.
    b. pneumothorax.
    c. renal contusions.
    d. perforated bowels.

22. When managing a patient with suspected rib fractures, it is important to encourage the patient to cough and take frequent deep breaths in order to:

    a. expand all of the air sacs.
    b. assess the effectiveness of the splint.
    c. fully evaluate the patient's level of discomfort.
    d. prevent the patient from developing hypotension.

23. Ribs _____ are most often fractured because they are thin and poorly protected.

    a. one to three
    b. four to nine
    c. ten to twelve
    d. none of the above

24. Fractures of the first and second ribs indicate _____ and may also involve a rupture of the aorta, tracheobronchial tree injury, or a vascular injury.

    a. mild trauma
    b. moderate trauma
    c. severe trauma
    d. all of the above

25. A flail segment is a very serious chest injury and has mortality rates of _____% because of the associated injuries and impact on ventilations.

    a. 5–10
    b. 10–20
    c. 20–40
    d. 40–50

26. Which of the following statements about the pathology of a flail segment is incorrect?

    a. If the flail segment is small, the paradoxical movement is minimal because of muscle spasm.
    b. Pain is a contributing factor to the severity of this injury.
    c. Pain can reduce thoracic expansion and decrease ventilation.
    d. The arterial blood flow is impaired, resulting in a ventilation–perfusion mismatch.

27. Which of the following is the most common associated complication of a flail segment?

    a. pulmonary contusion
    b. subcutaneous emphysema
    c. pericardial effusion
    d. pulmonary edema

28. The most common cause of a sternal fracture is a/an _____ injury caused by an MVC.

    a. penetrating
    b. blunt blow to the chest
    c. acceleration
    d. deceleration compression

29. The main reason why a sternal fracture has such a high mortality rate is:

    a. because of the high incidence of vomiting.
    b. that nearly all of these patients lose consciousness.
    c. because of the associated injuries.
    d. that these patients are often given too much fluid prehospitally.

30. When assessing the patient with a simple pneumothorax, the patient may have decreased chest wall movement and slight pleuritic chest pain, which may be referred to the:

    a. shoulder or arm on the unaffected side.
    b. shoulder or arm on the affected side.
    c. abdomen and upper thighs.
    d. neck.

31. A patient with an open pneumothorax can develop a ventilation–perfusion mismatch as a result of:

    a. atelectasis.
    b. extreme pain.
    c. hypoventilation.
    d. subcutaneous emphysema.

32. When dealing with a developing open pneumothorax, if the resistance to air flow through the respiratory tract is greater than resistance through the open hole, the:

    a. respiratory effort is effective.
    b. respiratory effort is ineffective.
    c. one-way flap will develop over the opening.
    d. mediastinum will move in the direction of the injured lung.

33. The pathophysiology of a tension pneumothorax includes:

    a. lung collapse with mediastinal shift to the lateral side.
    b. fluid backup in the unaffected lung as a result of shunting.
    c. collapse of the lung causes left-to-right intrapulmonary shunting and hypercarbia.
    d. a serious reduction in cardiac output caused by deformation of the vena cava, reducing preload.

34. Which of the following assessment findings will most likely be atypical in a patient with a tension pneumothorax?

    a. unilateral decreased or absent breath sounds
    b. hyporesonance and mediastinal shift to the ipsilateral side
    c. tachypnea, cyanosis, and extreme anxiety
    d. narrow pulse pressure and JVD

35. It is not uncommon for an intercostal artery to bleed as much as _____ cc per minute into the chest.

    a. 10
    b. 20
    c. 40
    d. 50

36. Bleeding from a pulmonary contusion generally causes 1,000 to 1,500 cc of blood loss, although the chest cavity can hold some _____ cc of blood.

    a. 2,000 to 3,000
    b. 3,000 to 4,000
    c. 4,000 to 5,000
    d. 5,000 to 6,000

37. Intrapulmonary hemorrhage occurs in either the bronchus or the:

    a. alveoli.
    b. aorta.
    c. parenchyma.
    d. pleural space.

38. When evaluating the patient with a developing hemothorax, you can expect to find the signs and symptoms of shock as well as:

    a. subcutaneous emphysema.
    b. respiratory distress.
    c. hyper resonance.
    d. signs of acute MI.

39. The out-of-hospital management of a hemopneumothorax includes:

    a. the use of vasopressors.
    b. positive pressure ventilation.
    c. aggressive fluid replacement.
    d. aggressive fluid evacuation by chest decompression.

40. Pulmonary contusions are very common with blunt thoracic trauma, but are often missed on evaluation because of:

    a. an overexpansion effect.
    b. an inertial effect.
    c. the high incidence of other associated injuries.
    d. the Spalding effect.

41. Which of the following assessment findings is atypical of a patient who has a lung contusion?

    a. decreased SpO_2
    b. tachypnea and dyspnea
    c. coughing and hemoptysis
    d. cyanosis to the face and neck

42. Patients with pulmonary contusions also tend to have other severe thoracic and _____ injuries, so always assume multiple potential injuries are present.

    a. head
    b. neck
    c. spinal cord
    d. abdominal

43. The purpose of the pericardium is to anchor the heart and restrict excess movement, as well as:

    a. prevent the kinking of the great vessels.
    b. facilitate right-to-left pulmonary shunting.
    c. link the lymphatic system.
    d. conduct electrical impulses.

44. The major problem in pericardial tamponade is the impairment of _____, which significantly decreases the amount of blood the heart is able to pump out.

    a. pulmonic systolic filling
    b. ventricular diastolic filling
    c. pulmonic diastolic emptying
    d. ventricular diastolic emptying

45. You suspect that a patient is in cardiac tamponade, but there is too much ambient noise to hear the classic "muffled heart sounds" that you are supposed to listen for. Instead, you look for other clues, such as:

    a. a cough and hemoptysis.
    b. subcutaneous emphysema.
    c. JVD and narrow pulse pressure.
    d. retrosternal and interscapular pain.

46. A victim of an assault states that he was struck in the chest with a pipe. Your physical exam reveals sternal crepitus, and crepitus over the left fifth and six ribs and the sternum. His lung sounds are clear, but he is guarded and says it hurts to take a breath. His pulse rate is 118/regular, BP is 134/80, and skin CTC is pale, warm, and dry, with no JVD. In addition to the fractures, what internal injury is the patient likely to have?

    a. aortic dissection
    b. myocardial contusion
    c. tension pneumothorax
    d. pericardial tamponade

47. Many patients with myocardial contusion are relatively asymptomatic initially in the absence of associated injuries. Helpful signs include ECG changes, if present, and persistent:

    a. sinus tachycardia without obvious hypovolemia.
    b. right bundle branch block.
    c. atrial flutter.
    d. atrial fibrillation.

48. The management of the patient with a myocardial contusion after airway and ventilation control includes:

    a. administration of fluids.
    b. considering antidysrhythmics.
    c. considering vasopressor agents.
    d. all of the above.

49. The management of a patient with a myocardial rupture includes supportive care of the ABCs and observing for the onset of _____ following trauma.

    a. severe headache
    b. abdominal distention
    c. CHF or pulmonary edema
    d. neurologic deficits

50. The primary causes of aortic dissection/rupture are MVCs and:

    a. GSWs.
    b. falls.
    c. rib fractures.
    d. associated diaphragmatic rupture.

51. Aortic dissection/rupture is a very critical injury where ____% of the patients die instantaneously.

    a. 10–20
    b. 40–60
    c. 60–80
    d. 85–95

52. When examining a patient who is suspected of having an aortic dissection/rupture, any of the following findings may be present, *except*:

    a. a different BP on each arm.
    b. retrosternal or interscapular pain.
    c. pleuritic pain in the neck.
    d. ischemic pain of the extremities.

53. Which of the following treatment options should be avoided in the patient with a suspected ruptured diaphragm who is experiencing respiratory distress?

    a. IV fluids
    b. antiemetics
    c. Trendelenburg position
    d. positive pressure ventilation

54. Upon examination of the patient with an esophageal injury, the paramedic may find that the patient is having symptoms and signs of a:

    a. cardiac event.
    b. CVA.
    c. seizure.
    d. tension pneumothorax.

55. All of the following are typical assessment findings in a patient with traumatic asphyxia, *except*:

    a. cyanosis to the face and upper neck.
    b. JVD.
    c. the skin below the crush area is cyanotic.
    d. petechia in the upper chest, neck, and face.

56. The management of the patient with traumatic asphyxia includes:

    a. IV fluids for hypotension.
    b. needle decompression prior to the release of compression.
    c. needle decompression after the release of compression.
    d. MAST/PASG.

57. Tracheobronchial injury is rare and occurs in:

    a. blunt chest trauma.
    b. penetrating chest trauma.
    c. both blunt and penetrating chest trauma.
    d. high incidents in COPD patients.

58. Which of the following is an atypical assessment finding in a patient with a tracheobronchial injury?

    a. the patient is difficult to intubate
    b. signs of tension pneumothorax that do not respond to a needle decompression
    c. dyspnea and hemoptysis
    d. tachy-brady dysrhythmias

59. The most frequent cause of an esophageal injury is from:

    a. a Mallory-Weiss tear.
    b. blunt trauma.
    c. penetrating trauma.
    d. acceleration forces.

60. You are assessing a thirty-three-year-old female who was the driver of a vehicle involved in a moderate-speed rear-end MVC. She is complaining of increased difficulty breathing, and pain in the lower chest and upper abdomen. She has the presence of a scaffold abdomen, there are bowel sounds in the lower right chest, and the area is dull to percussion. You suspect:

    a. diaphragmatic injury.
    b. tension pneumothorax.
    c. ectopic pregnancy.
    d. aortic dissection.

Exam #39 Answer Form

	A	B	C	D		A	B	C	D
1.	❏	❏	❏	❏	27.	❏	❏	❏	❏
2.	❏	❏	❏	❏	28.	❏	❏	❏	❏
3.	❏	❏	❏	❏	29.	❏	❏	❏	❏
4.	❏	❏	❏	❏	30.	❏	❏	❏	❏
5.	❏	❏	❏	❏	31.	❏	❏	❏	❏
6.	❏	❏	❏	❏	32.	❏	❏	❏	❏
7.	❏	❏	❏	❏	33.	❏	❏	❏	❏
8.	❏	❏	❏	❏	34.	❏	❏	❏	❏
9.	❏	❏	❏	❏	35.	❏	❏	❏	❏
10.	❏	❏	❏	❏	36.	❏	❏	❏	❏
11.	❏	❏	❏	❏	37.	❏	❏	❏	❏
12.	❏	❏	❏	❏	38.	❏	❏	❏	❏
13.	❏	❏	❏	❏	39.	❏	❏	❏	❏
14.	❏	❏	❏	❏	40.	❏	❏	❏	❏
15.	❏	❏	❏	❏	41.	❏	❏	❏	❏
16.	❏	❏	❏	❏	42.	❏	❏	❏	❏
17.	❏	❏	❏	❏	43.	❏	❏	❏	❏
18.	❏	❏	❏	❏	44.	❏	❏	❏	❏
19.	❏	❏	❏	❏	45.	❏	❏	❏	❏
20.	❏	❏	❏	❏	46.	❏	❏	❏	❏
21.	❏	❏	❏	❏	47.	❏	❏	❏	❏
22.	❏	❏	❏	❏	48.	❏	❏	❏	❏
23.	❏	❏	❏	❏	49.	❏	❏	❏	❏
24.	❏	❏	❏	❏	50.	❏	❏	❏	❏
25.	❏	❏	❏	❏	51.	❏	❏	❏	❏
26.	❏	❏	❏	❏	52.	❏	❏	❏	❏

	A	B	C	D			A	B	C	D
53.	❑	❑	❑	❑		57.	❑	❑	❑	❑
54.	❑	❑	❑	❑		58.	❑	❑	❑	❑
55.	❑	❑	❑	❑		59.	❑	❑	❑	❑
56.	❑	❑	❑	❑		60.	❑	❑	❑	❑

40

Abdominal Trauma

1. Abdominal trauma is the _____ leading cause of preventable trauma death.

   a. second
   b. third
   c. fourth
   d. fifth

2. The abdominal cavity can hide significant blood loss. As much as _____ liter(s) can be lost before any signs of distention are apparent.

   a. 1
   b. 1.5
   c. 2
   d. 2.5

3. Immediate concerns, after the ABCs, in the management of the patient with abdominal trauma are hemorrhage, major organ damage, and:

   a. the possibility of peritonitis.
   b. the possible use of vasopressors.
   c. IV fluid replacement.
   d. associated chest injuries.

4. Abdominal trauma often goes unrecognized because the _____ is/are often unrecognized.

   a. signs of shock
   b. golden hour
   c. MOI
   d. platinum ten minutes

5. Motor vehicle crashes often involve _____ forces that compress internal organs and cause shearing of organs that are suspended by ligaments.

   a. rapid acceleration
   b. twisting
   c. rapid deceleration
   d. sublexation

6. The _____ is the section of the small intestine that is approximately 8 feet in length, absorbing the majority of the food we eat.

   a. duodenum
   b. jejunum
   c. ileum
   d. colon

7. The _____ is the last section of the small intestine and varies in length from 15 to 25 feet.

   a. duodenum
   b. jejunum
   c. ileum
   d. colon

8. You are assessing the abdomen of a young adult male with a complaint of abdominal pain. You see that he has an old scar in the midline and ask him about it. He tells you that he had a hernioplasty two years ago. What procedure did he have?

   a. aortic graph
   b. hernia repair
   c. removal of the spleen
   d. removal of the appendix

9. The _____ is the largest organ in the body and often sustains injuries during rapid deceleration forces.

   a. liver
   b. kidney
   c. heart
   d. lung

10. _____ pain is caused by irritation of the peritoneum and is more commonly described as diffuse rather than localized.

    a. Visceral
    b. Somatic
    c. Obstructive
    d. Muscle spasm

11. You have just finished a light palpation of all four quadrants of a patient with an MOI suggestive of possible internal injury. You discovered that the patient had pain on palpation in the ULQ without rebound tenderness. What type of pain does the examination reflect?

    a. somatic
    b. visceral
    c. guarded
    d. obstructive

12. What organ(s) may be injured in the patient described in question 11?

    a. appendix and small intestine
    b. liver and stomach
    c. stomach and spleen
    d. liver and gallbladder

13. Kehr's sign is an assessment finding of pain in the abdomen that radiates to the left shoulder. This finding indicates:

    a. acute bowel obstruction.
    b. intraperitoneal bleeding and/or irritation.
    c. aortic aneurysm.
    d. ileus.

14. When a patient has ecchymosis in the umbilical area caused by peritoneal bleeding, this is known as:

    a. Cullen's sign.
    b. Grey–Turner's sign.
    c. periumbilical guarding.
    d. peritoneal's sign.

15. You and your crew have been dispatched to a football game at a local high school for a traumatic injury. Upon arrival you find a diaphoretic twenty-nine-year-old male who is doubled over in severe pain. He tells you that suddenly, without warning, while he was sitting on the bench, he started having excruciating pain in his left testicle. He also says he feels like he is going to vomit. What do you suspect is the cause of his pain?

    a. kidney stone
    b. renal colic
    c. testicular torsion
    d. intra-abdominal bleeding

16. Continuing with question 15, what is the most appropriate initial management plan for this patient?

    a. Provide oxygen by cannula and administer IM morphine.
    b. Secure the patient to a long spine board with legs flexed.
    c. Move the patient into his position of comfort, and then administer analgesia and an antiemetic.
    d. Administer high-flow oxygen, start two large bore IVs, and give a fluid bolus.

17. How would you treat the patient described in question 15?

    a. Treat for shock and begin a rapid transport.
    b. Administer oxygen and transport on a backboard.
    c. Manage his pain and transport gently.
    d. Apply ice and place him in the Trendelenburg position.

18. The definitive treatment for his condition in most cases is:

    a. prompt surgery.
    b. pain management and bed rest.
    c. manual repositioning in the ED.
    d. rest, abundant hydration, and pain management.

19. After arriving on the scene of a possible assault, you find a twenty-six-year-old male who denies being assaulted but confesses that he has a large foreign body stuck in his anus. He is bleeding from the rectum, has acute abdominal pain, and is tachycardic. The immediate complications associated with this type of emergency include:

    a. perforations and hemorrhage.
    b. traumatic peristalsis.
    c. alimentary spasms.
    d. hematuria.

20. What do you suspect is the cause of the abdominal pain and tachycardia in the patient described in question 19?

    a. the patient is unable to pass gas
    b. contamination from fecal matter
    c. peritonitis from blood loss
    d. ischemia from bowel strangulation

21. What is your management plan for the patient described in question 19?

    a. Keep the patient in a position of comfort.
    b. Attempt to remove the foreign object and control bleeding.
    c. Keep the patient supine with knees flexed.
    d. Apply ice and elevate the legs.

22. Associated signs and symptoms that should be anticipated by the paramedic for the patient described in question 19 include:

    a. dysrhythmias.
    b. narrowed pulse pressure.
    c. widening pulse pressure.
    d. nausea and vomiting.

23. You are on the scene of an MVC and find that the driver was apparently ejected from the vehicle after it crashed into a guardrail. The patient looks about fifty years old, is unconscious, and has no outward signs of trauma. Her breathing is shallow, clear, and equal, 16 bpm; pulse is 130 and weak; BP is 76/24 mmHg. The most likely cause of hypotension is:

    a. head injury.
    b. aortic aneurysm.
    c. intra-abdominal bleeding.
    d. spinal cord injury.

24. Initial treatment for the patient in question 23 includes all of the following, *except*:

    a. airway management.
    b. spinal immobilization.
    c. IV fluid replacement.
    d. rapid transport to a trauma center.

25. Primary traumatic injuries associated with consensual sex include all of the following, *except*:

    a. restraint injuries.
    b. tears from body jewelry.
    c. fractured penis.
    d. peritonitis.

26. During your assessment of a third-trimester female who was the driver of a vehicle involved in a moderate-speed collision, you recall that the patient can lose up to _____ of her blood volume before signs of shock are evident.

    a. 15%
    b. 25%
    c. 35%
    d. 45%

27. Direct trauma to the abdomen of the pregnant patient may result in all of the following conditions, *except*:

    a. uterine inversion.
    b. premature labor.
    c. abruptio placenta.
    d. uterine rupture.

28. During the assessment of a patient who has pain from irritation of the diaphragm, to what area would you expect the patient's pain to radiate?

    a. back
    b. shoulder
    c. lower abdomen
    d. it will not radiate anywhere

29. Besides the kidneys and spleen, which of the following organs is partially located within the retroperitoneal cavity?

    a. liver
    b. gallbladder
    c. pancreas
    d. duodenum

30. _____ is the term for decreased motility of the intestine.

    a. Alimentary
    b. Viscus
    c. Excursion
    d. Ileus

Exam #40 Answer Form

	A	B	C	D		A	B	C	D
1.	❑	❑	❑	❑	16.	❑	❑	❑	❑
2.	❑	❑	❑	❑	17.	❑	❑	❑	❑
3.	❑	❑	❑	❑	18.	❑	❑	❑	❑
4.	❑	❑	❑	❑	19.	❑	❑	❑	❑
5.	❑	❑	❑	❑	20.	❑	❑	❑	❑
6.	❑	❑	❑	❑	21.	❑	❑	❑	❑
7.	❑	❑	❑	❑	22.	❑	❑	❑	❑
8.	❑	❑	❑	❑	23.	❑	❑	❑	❑
9.	❑	❑	❑	❑	24.	❑	❑	❑	❑
10.	❑	❑	❑	❑	25.	❑	❑	❑	❑
11.	❑	❑	❑	❑	26.	❑	❑	❑	❑
12.	❑	❑	❑	❑	27.	❑	❑	❑	❑
13.	❑	❑	❑	❑	28.	❑	❑	❑	❑
14.	❑	❑	❑	❑	29.	❑	❑	❑	❑
15.	❑	❑	❑	❑	30.	❑	❑	❑	❑

41

Musculoskeletal Trauma

1. As we get older, our bones become more prone to fracture because they:

   a. become denser.
   b. become more porous.
   c. are subjected to more stress.
   d. can no longer utilize calcium.

2. The axial skeleton consists of the skull, vertebral column, and:

   a. bony thorax.
   b. pelvis.
   c. rhomboids.
   d. soleus.

3. The pectoral girdle is composed of the:

   a. scapula and manubrium.
   b. latissimus dorsi.
   c. pubis.
   d. clavicle and scapula.

4. When muscles contract, they pull the _____, which then cause(s) the bones to move at the joints.

   a. tendons
   b. ligaments
   c. marrow
   d. Haversian canals

5. The three structural classifications of joints are:

   a. fusion, synovial, and skeletal.
   b. fibrous, cartilaginous, and synovial.
   c. named for the specific location in the body.
   d. named for the bones that make up the joint.

6. In addition to providing support and protection for internal organs, bones are also responsible for:

   a. homeostasis.
   b. range of motion.
   c. fighting infection.
   d. producing red blood cells.

7. The diaphysis, epiphysis, and periosteum are specific:

   a. parts of a long bone.
   b. types of smooth muscle.
   c. injuries associated with fractures.
   d. causes of pathological fractures.

8. _____ is the area between the epiphysis and diaphysis.

   a. Metaphysis
   b. Periosteum
   c. Haversian canals
   d. Bone marrow sheds

9. Which of the following is not a part of the humerus?

   a. the neck and shaft
   b. medial and lateral condyle
   c. the olecranon
   d. the elbow

10. The _____ is located on the little finger side of the lower arm and is part of the wrist joint.

    a. radius head
    b. radius shaft
    c. ulna head
    d. ulna shaft

11. You have been called to transport a football player who has separated his shoulder. This injury is actually a dislocation of the:

    a. acromioclavicular joint.
    b. sternoclavicular joint.
    c. metaphysis.
    d. olecranon.

12. A patient with a _____ fracture can easily go into decompensated shock from the 2,000 cc blood loss that can occur over the first two hours following the fracture.

    a. femur
    b. pelvis
    c. spinal
    d. tibula

13. Of the following components, which is not part of the pelvis?

    a. ilium
    b. ischium
    c. acetabulum
    d. femur

14. A _____ is a rounded protuberance at the articulation of a bone, similar to a knuckle.

    a. trochanter
    b. condyle
    c. phalange
    d. fossa

15. The tibia, located in the _____ lower leg, is made up of the tibia plateau, the shaft, and the _____

    a. anterior; medial malleolus
    b. anterior; lateral condyle
    c. posterior; medial malleolus
    d. posterior; lateral condyle

16. Along with muscles and tendons, the long bones are involved in:

    a. flexion.
    b. extension.
    c. rotation.
    d. all of the above.

17. The fibula, which is located in the _____ leg, is made up of the head, the shaft, and the _____ malleolus.

    a. upper; medial
    b. lower; lateral
    c. anterior; medial
    d. posterior; lateral

18. Which of the following is not a type of muscle?

    a. smooth
    b. skeletal
    c. axial
    d. cardiac

19. _____ muscle is found in the lower airways, blood vessels, and intestines.

    a. Smooth
    b. Skeletal
    c. Axial
    d. Cardiac

20. Connective tissue covering the epiphysis, which acts as a surface for articulation, is called:

    a. tendon.
    b. cartilage.
    c. ligament.
    d. muscle.

21. _____ is/are connective tissue that support the joints and allow(s) for range of motion.

    a. Tendons
    b. Cartilage
    c. Ligaments
    d. Muscles

22. _____ can relax or contract to alter the inner lumen diameter of vessels.

    a. Gomphoses
    b. Smooth muscle
    c. Tendons
    d. Cardiac muscle

23. Bones articulate at joints where they are:

    a. opposed.
    b. unopposed.
    c. padded by cartilage.
    d. at a diagonal direction from one another.

24. The attribute of a muscle being able to generate an impulse is referred to as:

    a. automaticity.
    b. excitability.
    c. conduction.
    d. rhythm.

25. _____ is/are under conscious control, include(s) the major muscle mass of the body, and allow(s) for mobility.

    a. Smooth muscle
    b. Skeletal muscle
    c. Cartilage
    d. Ligaments

26. The two major hinged joints in the body are the:

    a. jaw and digits.
    b. elbow and wrist.
    c. elbow and knee.
    d. hip and shoulder.

27. A _____ is a line of fusion between two bones that are separate in early development.

    a. symphysis
    b. gomphosis
    c. syndesmosis
    d. condyloid

28. Immovable joints, where one bone is fitted into a socket of another that is not intended for movements, such as a tooth, are:

   a. symphyses.
   b. gomphoses.
   c. syndesmoses.
   d. condyloids.

29. _____ are articulations in which the bones are united by ligaments.

   a. Fusions
   b. Cartilage
   c. Syndesmoses
   d. Condyloids

30. A _____ joint is a joint filled with fluid, which lubricates the articulated surfaces.

   a. cartilaginous
   b. synchondrosis
   c. symphysis
   d. synovial

31. A/an _____ fracture is a fracture that tears away the outer covering of the bone, often involving most of the length of the bone.

   a. spiral
   b. comminuted
   c. greenstick
   d. oblique

32. Flexion, extension, abduction, and circumduction are all movements allowed by what type of joint?

   a. sychondrosis
   b. gomphosis
   c. transvere
   d. synovial

33. A fracture where the break is at a right angle to the axis of the long bone is called a/an _____ fracture.

   a. epiphyseal
   b. transverse
   c. oblique
   d. comminuted

34. An uncomplicated tibia/fibula fracture can bleed about _____ cc over the first two hours.

   a. 500
   b. 1,000
   c. 1,500
   d. 2,000

35. A partial dislocation of a joint is called a:

   a. subluxation.
   b. luxation.
   c. sprain.
   d. stress fracture.

36. A complete disruption of the integrity of a joint is called a:

   a. sprain.
   b. dislocation.
   c. fracture.
   d. subluxation.

37. All of the following are typical causes of pathologic fractures, *except*:

   a. osteoporosis.
   b. metastasis from cancer.
   c. cancer of the bone.
   d. occupational repetitive motions.

38. The knee dislocation can completely disrupt the blood supply to the lower leg when the _____ is displaced to the _____, compressing the posterior tibial artery.

   a. tibia; anterior
   b. tibia; posterior
   c. fibula; anterior
   d. fibula; posterior

39. The elbow, when dislocated, is very serious and can threaten the:

   a. brachial plexus, causing paralysis.
   b. radial plexus, causing paralysis.
   c. brachial artery and blood supply to the arm.
   d. radial artery and blood supply to the arm.

40. A fracture is considered complicated if it involves any one or more of the following conditions, *except*:

   a. a crushing injury.
   b. painful, swollen deformity.
   c. decreased distal pulse.
   d. diminished distal sensory or motor function.

41. Non-traumatic causes of inflammation and degeneration of the joints include:

   a. diabetes and stress.
   b. bursitis and gouty arthritis.
   c. obesity and Crohn's disease.
   d. stroke and coronary artery disease.

42. The principal use of a traction splint on a femur fracture is to:

   a. keep the patient from moving the injured extremity.
   b. provide complete pain relief.
   c. prevent swelling and blood loss.
   d. relieve the muscle spasms that can worsen the injury.

43. Realignment of dislocations should be considered if distal circulation is impaired or:

   a. if the patient is in pain.
   b. when the deformity is gross.
   c. when the patient signs a release first.
   d. transportation is long or delayed.

44. The difference between a knee dislocation and a patella dislocation is that:

   a. a knee dislocation involves the tibia popping out of the knee joint.
   b. a patella dislocation is much more dangerous than a knee dislocation.
   c. the knee dislocation requires surgery and the patella dislocation does not.
   d. the patella dislocation should never be manipulated in the field.

45. The combination of a long board and PASG/MAST may be used for a _____ fracture, because of the normal blood loss accompanying this type of fracture.

   a. pelvic
   b. mid-shaft femur
   c. proximal femur
   d. tibia/fibula

46. Prior to splinting a patient who had dislocated his left shoulder, you assessed positive distal pulse, motor, and sensation in the extremity. After the application of a sling and swathe, the patient complains of paresthesia and numbness in the arm and fingers. What action should you now take?

   a. Apply ice and administer morphine IM or IV.
   b. Loosen the sling and swathe, and reassess.
   c. Remove the splint and pull traction on the arm, and resplint.
   d. Give early notification to the ED that the patient has a new deficit.

47. Cold is used initially to reduce the swelling and pain of a fracture. Heat can be useful to improve circulation, but only after the:

   a. initial swelling has gone down.
   b. first hour.
   c. first twelve hours.
   d. first twenty-four hours.

48. A Colles' fracture is a common fracture of the:

   a. shoulder.
   b. hand.
   c. wrist.
   d. forearm.

49. The key objective in the management of a closed long bone fracture is to carefully splint the long bone in a straight position without:

   a. causing the patient any pain.
   b. the use of analgesics.
   c. allowing the bone to protrude through the skin.
   d. forgetting to assess for DCAP-BTLS.

50. Which of the following is not a typical finding at the site of a musculoskeletal injury?

   a. pain or tenderness
   b. crepitation
   c. diaphoresis
   d. capillary refilling

Exam #41 Answer Form

	A	B	C	D		A	B	C	D
1.	❏	❏	❏	❏	26.	❏	❏	❏	❏
2.	❏	❏	❏	❏	27.	❏	❏	❏	❏
3.	❏	❏	❏	❏	28.	❏	❏	❏	❏
4.	❏	❏	❏	❏	29.	❏	❏	❏	❏
5.	❏	❏	❏	❏	30.	❏	❏	❏	❏
6.	❏	❏	❏	❏	31.	❏	❏	❏	❏
7.	❏	❏	❏	❏	32.	❏	❏	❏	❏
8.	❏	❏	❏	❏	33.	❏	❏	❏	❏
9.	❏	❏	❏	❏	34.	❏	❏	❏	❏
10.	❏	❏	❏	❏	35.	❏	❏	❏	❏
11.	❏	❏	❏	❏	36.	❏	❏	❏	❏
12.	❏	❏	❏	❏	37.	❏	❏	❏	❏
13.	❏	❏	❏	❏	38.	❏	❏	❏	❏
14.	❏	❏	❏	❏	39.	❏	❏	❏	❏
15.	❏	❏	❏	❏	40.	❏	❏	❏	❏
16.	❏	❏	❏	❏	41.	❏	❏	❏	❏
17.	❏	❏	❏	❏	42.	❏	❏	❏	❏
18.	❏	❏	❏	❏	43.	❏	❏	❏	❏
19.	❏	❏	❏	❏	44.	❏	❏	❏	❏
20.	❏	❏	❏	❏	45.	❏	❏	❏	❏
21.	❏	❏	❏	❏	46.	❏	❏	❏	❏
22.	❏	❏	❏	❏	47.	❏	❏	❏	❏
23.	❏	❏	❏	❏	48.	❏	❏	❏	❏
24.	❏	❏	❏	❏	49.	❏	❏	❏	❏
25.	❏	❏	❏	❏	50.	❏	❏	❏	❏

42
Neonatology

1. Vessels of fetal circulation include all of the following, *except*:

   a. umbilical arteries.
   b. umbilical vein.
   c. ductus venosus.
   d. foramen arteriosus.

2. After birth, fetal circulation changes and the _____ turn(s) into a fibrous cord that serves as a ligament.

   a. umbilical arteries
   b. umbilical vein
   c. ductus venosus
   d. foramen arteriosus

3. After the baby takes its first breath, the _____ closes and shunts blood to the lungs.

   a. foramen ovale
   b. ductus venosus
   c. ductus arteriosus
   d. foramen arteriosus

4. Newborns are very sensitive to hypoxia, and, if they experience hypoxia or severe acidosis, a serious condition called _____ may occur.

   a. persistent fetal circulation
   b. hypoxic apnea
   c. neonatal pulmonary syndrome
   d. hypoxic drive syndrome

5. The condition described in question 4 can be corrected or avoided by:

   a. performing CPR as needed.
   b. intubating the newborn after birth.
   c. stimulating the newborn to breathe.
   d. administering epinephrine.

6. When apnea occurs in infants that were born full term where no cause for the apnea can be determined, this condition is called:

   a. primary apnea.
   b. secondary apnea.
   c. apparent life-threatening event (ALTE).
   d. apnea of infancy.

7. There are three causes of infant apnea: central, obstructive, and:

   a. anomaly.
   b. mixed.
   c. complete.
   d. incomplete.

8. The most common cause of Down syndrome occurs when a baby is born with _____ rather than two copies of chromosome 21.

   a. one
   b. three
   c. four
   d. five

9. The paramedic can recognize a newborn that is born with Down syndrome by which of the following characteristics?

   a. large ears with an abnormal shape
   b. overall muscle tone that is rigid and spastic
   c. small tongue in relation to the size of the mouth
   d. flat facial profile with a small nose and depressed nasal bridge

10. Other distinguishing characteristics of Down syndrome include:

    a. joint contraction.
    b. excessively large fontanels.
    c. a downward slant of the eyes.
    d. an excessive space between the large and second toe.

11. The paramedic can recognize a newborn that is born with the birth defect spina bifida because the infant will have:

    a. overall weak body muscle tone.
    b. exposed spinal structures.
    c. excessively large fontanels.
    d. exceedingly small fontanels.

12. Of the following, which is an avoidable antepartum factor that can affect childbirth?

    a. multiple fetuses
    b. no prenatal care
    c. gestational diabetes
    d. hypertension syndromes

13. Of the following, which is a significant antepartum factor that classifies the newborn as "high risk"?

    a. pyloric stenosis
    b. prolonged labor
    c. lactose intolerance
    d. feeding problems

14. _____ account(s) for 20% of infant deaths, more than from any other single cause.

    a. Birth defects
    b. Premature labor
    c. Meconium aspiration
    d. Placenta previa

15. Factors that are associated with low birth weights include all of the following, *except*:

    a. gestational diabetes.
    b. prolonged labor.
    c. the mother's use of alcohol.
    d. multiple fetuses.

16. Babies born with a low birth weight range from _____ grams.

    a. 500–2,500
    b. 1,000–3,500
    c. 1,500–4,500
    d. 2,000–5,000

17. Which of the following is not a risk factor associated with crack/cocaine use by a pregnant woman?

    a. miscarriage
    b. premature labor
    c. placenta previa
    d. abruptio placenta

18. Immediately after birth, the paramedic evaluates:

    a. for aspiration syndrome.
    b. approximate weight and length.
    c. for meconium staining and nuchal cord.
    d. respiratory effort, pulse rate, and skin color.

19. At one minute after birth, the paramedic evaluates and scores:

    a. birth weight and length.
    b. best eye opening, verbal, and motor response.
    c. appearance, pulse, grimace, activity, and reflex.
    d. blood pressure, pulse oximetry, and blood glucose.

20. In the clinical setting, newborns are screened for genetic and _____ disorders, shortly after birth.

    a. teratogenic
    b. cardiovascular
    c. infectious
    d. metabolic

21. When a baby is born without enough thyroid hormone (congenital hypothyroidism), this condition can lead to:

    a. myxedema.
    b. poor growth and mental retardation.
    c. abnormal protrusion of the eyes.
    d. goiter.

22. The newborn that is born with fetal alcohol syndrome (FAS) can be distinguished by which of the following characteristics?

    a. low birth weight, small head, and small eye openings
    b. low birth weight, large head, and thick upper lip
    c. upward slant of eyes and small head
    d. protruding upper jaw and thinned lips

23. Which of the following statements about FAS is not correct?

    a. FAS does not occur with consumption of very small amounts of alcohol during pregnancy.
    b. FAS is distinguished by developmental disabilities.
    c. FAS can result in infant and fetal death.
    d. Cardiovascular defects are associated with FAS.

24. Your patient is a twenty-three-year-old female who is in custody of the police. She is in active labor. The police state that she is high on heroin. Which of the following complications can you expect with this delivery?

    a. prolonged labor and fetal distress
    b. prolapsed cord
    c. decreased mental status of the newborn
    d. breech presentation and delivery

25. How would you manage the delivery for the patient described in question 24?

  a. Monitor, transport, and consider administration of Pitocin®.
  b. Attempt to prevent delivery and begin a rapid transport.
  c. Administer oxygen, assist ventilations, and administer Narcan®.
  d. Assist with the delivery of the breech baby.

26. Common traumatic injuries to the newborn associated with childbirth include all of the following, *except*:

  a. barotrauma.
  b. CVA.
  c. spinal cord injury.
  d. forceps trauma to the head.

27. Which of the following birth-related injuries is associated with shoulder dystocia?

  a. spinal cord injury
  b. fractured clavicle
  c. brachial plexus injury
  d. hypothermia

28. Your partner has just assisted with the delivery of a thirty-eight-week gestation newborn. You have assessed the infant after one minute and have determined that the infant's heart rate is 60 bpm even after you have warmed, dried, stimulated, and provided blow-by oxygen. What would you do next?

  a. Suction for meconium.
  b. Assist with ventilations by bag mask.
  c. Intubate the newborn.
  d. Start CPR.

29. In continuing with the care of the newborn in question 28, after thirty seconds you assess the heart rate, which has not increased from 60 bpm. What would you do next?

  a. Administer high-flow oxygen.
  b. Assist with ventilations by bag mask.
  c. Intubate the newborn.
  d. Start CPR.

30. The initial steps of postarrest stabilization for the neonate include:

  a. keeping the baby warm and continuing oxygen delivery.
  b. starting an IV drip of lidocaine.
  c. administering an epinephrine bolus every five minutes.
  d. placing a nasogastric tube.

31. Major risk factors associated with premature birth include all of the following, *except*:

  a. hypoxia.
  b. hypothermia.
  c. hypoglycemia.
  d. hyperglycemia.

32. The out-of-hospital delivery puts the premature infant at an increased risk for problems associated with:

  a. hypoxia.
  b. vomiting.
  c. jaundice.
  d. hyperglycemia.

33. Neonates can lose body heat rapidly for all of the following reasons, *except* that they have:

  a. excessive heat loss through breathing.
  b. a larger body surface area.
  c. smaller amounts of subcutaneous fat.
  d. temperature regulation mechanisms that are immature.

34. The most common causes of neonatal seizures are hypoxia, fever, infection, and:

  a. hypoglycemia.
  b. alcohol.
  c. drugs.
  d. genetic disorders.

35. Any fever in neonates is serious and requires evaluation because of their:

  a. immature lungs.
  b. immature thermoregulatory system.
  c. high risk of seizures from fever.
  d. high risk of aspiration.

36. The neonate can develop infection from the mother _____ birth.

  a. before and during
  b. during
  c. during and after
  d. before, during, and after

37. Jaundice occurs when a baby's immature liver cannot dispose of excess:

  a. insulin.
  b. glycogen.
  c. bilirubin.
  d. urine.

38. Approximately 60% of full-term infants and 80% of premature infants develop jaundice in the first _____ of life.

    a. two to three minutes
    b. two to three hours
    c. two to three days
    d. two to three weeks

39. The most common causes of vomiting in the neonate include: infections, increased ICP, and:

    a. drug withdrawal.
    b. genetic disorders.
    c. metabolic disorders.
    d. pyloric stenosis.

40. Complications from vomiting in the neonate include: aspiration, dehydration, and:

    a. seizures.
    b. lactose intolerance.
    c. increased ICP.
    d. electrolyte imbalance.

41. Diarrhea in neonates is difficult to assess because:

    a. of residual meconium.
    b. all stools are loose.
    c. diapers can change stool consistency.
    d. of the large amount of bile excretion.

42. Neonates are prone to abdominal distention because of gastric and fluid distention caused by immature digestive systems. Other causes of distention include:

    a. drug or alcohol withdrawal.
    b. hernias.
    c. hypoglycemia.
    d. neurologic abnormalities.

43. ALS transport has been requested for a twenty-day-old baby, from a pediatrician's office to the hospital. The baby is crying persistently and the transport is for severe distention of the abdomen caused by a possible bowel obstruction. Your primary concern during the transport is:

    a. to prevent infectious exposure.
    b. to watch the baby's airway.
    c. to stop the baby's crying.
    d. to infuse at least 20 cc saline per kg.

44. During an emergency involving a neonate, medication administration via the _____ route can lead to low plasma levels and should be the last choice.

    a. ETT
    b. IV
    c. IO
    d. rectal

45. Which of the following complications is not associated with providing positive pressure ventilations to the neonate?

    a. barotrauma
    b. pneumothorax
    c. distended abdomen
    d. diaphragmatic herniation

46. The most common type of hernia associated with neonates is a/an _____ hernia.

    a. diaphragmatic
    b. inguinal
    c. umbilical
    d. hiatal

47. Using the inverted pyramid of newborn resuscitation, ALS interventions are begun only after airway, ventilation, and _____ are performed.

    a. suction
    b. oxygenation
    c. CPR
    d. initial transport

48. Besides airway problems, _____ problems are the most common potentially life-threatening disorder that affects neonates.

    a. hypoglycemia
    b. hypothermia
    c. fluid imbalance
    d. congenital heart

49. Of the following list of drugs or substances, which is not a teratogen?

    a. alcohol
    b. lithium
    c. concentrated lemon juice
    d. vitamin A and its derivatives

50. During the delivery of twins, the paramedic can tell if the babies are fraternal or identical because fraternal twins:

    a. develop from the same zygote.
    b. always have their own placenta.
    c. (one) will present as a breech.
    d. have their own umbilical cords.

Exam #42 Answer Form

	A	B	C	D		A	B	C	D
1.	❑	❑	❑	❑	26.	❑	❑	❑	❑
2.	❑	❑	❑	❑	27.	❑	❑	❑	❑
3.	❑	❑	❑	❑	28.	❑	❑	❑	❑
4.	❑	❑	❑	❑	29.	❑	❑	❑	❑
5.	❑	❑	❑	❑	30.	❑	❑	❑	❑
6.	❑	❑	❑	❑	31.	❑	❑	❑	❑
7.	❑	❑	❑	❑	32.	❑	❑	❑	❑
8.	❑	❑	❑	❑	33.	❑	❑	❑	❑
9.	❑	❑	❑	❑	34.	❑	❑	❑	❑
10.	❑	❑	❑	❑	35.	❑	❑	❑	❑
11.	❑	❑	❑	❑	36.	❑	❑	❑	❑
12.	❑	❑	❑	❑	37.	❑	❑	❑	❑
13.	❑	❑	❑	❑	38.	❑	❑	❑	❑
14.	❑	❑	❑	❑	39.	❑	❑	❑	❑
15.	❑	❑	❑	❑	40.	❑	❑	❑	❑
16.	❑	❑	❑	❑	41.	❑	❑	❑	❑
17.	❑	❑	❑	❑	42.	❑	❑	❑	❑
18.	❑	❑	❑	❑	43.	❑	❑	❑	❑
19.	❑	❑	❑	❑	44.	❑	❑	❑	❑
20.	❑	❑	❑	❑	45.	❑	❑	❑	❑
21.	❑	❑	❑	❑	46.	❑	❑	❑	❑
22.	❑	❑	❑	❑	47.	❑	❑	❑	❑
23.	❑	❑	❑	❑	48.	❑	❑	❑	❑
24.	❑	❑	❑	❑	49.	❑	❑	❑	❑
25.	❑	❑	❑	❑	50.	❑	❑	❑	❑

Pediatrics

1. Because of the child's stage of emotional development in the _____ age group, this group is the most difficult to evaluate.

   a. neonate
   b. infant
   c. toddler
   d. adolescent

2. In the _____ age group, feelings of guilt and fear of pain often dominate the thinking of these children.

   a. infant
   b. toddler
   c. preschool
   d. school-age

3. Children in the _____ age group are extremely concerned about modesty and are terrified of disfigurement and death.

   a. toddler
   b. preschool
   c. school-age
   d. adolescent

4. Which of the following statements about an infant's airway is incorrect?

   a. The infant's tongue is very large in relation to the size of the mouth.
   b. The small trachea of an infant is more anterior than in an adult's airway.
   c. The smallest diameter of the airway in an infant is at the cricoid ring.
   d. The largest diameter of the airway in an infant is at the cricoid ring.

5. Infants are obligate nose breathers until _____ months of age, and they might not open their mouths to breathe even when their nose becomes obstructed from a cold, creating periods of apnea.

   a. three
   b. six
   c. nine
   d. twelve

6. In the infant, the fontanels are used as a diagnostic aid in assessing for shock, dehydration, and:

   a. head injury.
   b. hypoglycemia.
   c. hyperthermia.
   d. hypothermia.

7. Which of the following is a unique characteristic of an infant's chest?

   a. Sternal retractions are normal in this age group.
   b. Abdominal or "belly breathing" is normal in this age group.
   c. The respiratory muscles are exceptionally well developed.
   d. Infants have the ability to compensate for long periods of time when in respiratory distress.

8. Which of the following is correct about the infant's thermoregulatory system?

   a. Infants do not have the ability to shiver to create body heat.
   b. Skin color is a poor indicator of hyperthermia.
   c. Skin color is a poor indicator of hypothermia.
   d. Full-term infants are born with a mature temperature regulation.

9. _____ is the number one cause of death in children over one year of age.

   a. sudden infant death syndrome (SIDS)
   b. Abuse
   c. Infection
   d. Trauma

10. Which of the following is the immediate concern for the paramedic when treating a child who has a poisoning or drug overdose?

    a. respiratory depression
    b. anaphylaxis
    c. vomiting and aspiration
    d. shock

11. Which of the following statements about pediatric trauma is most correct?

    a. Pneumothorax and hemothorax are injuries that do not occur in small children.
    b. Injuries to the head, face, and neck occur with more frequency in children than in adults.
    c. Pediatric trauma care for EMS providers is more intensive than adult trauma care.
    d. Injuries to the chest and abdomen occur infrequently and are of little concern for the paramedic.

12. The greatest incidence of SIDS occurs:

    a. during the winter months.
    b. more often with females.
    c. during the summer months.
    d. when the infant sleeps on its back.

13. Risk factors for pediatric suicide that are generally out of the child's control include all of the following, *except*:

    a. access to alcohol and drugs.
    b. inadequate support system.
    c. exposure to domestic violence.
    d. family history of depression.

14. The most common triggers of asthma in children are:

    a. seizures.
    b. viral infections.
    c. cold temperatures.
    d. very warm temperatures.

15. Physical complaints associated with depression in children include:

    a. headache and muscle ache.
    b. nausea and vomiting.
    c. dizziness.
    d. delay in puberty.

16. A child abuse or neglect injury can be physical, sexual, or _____ in nature.

    a. emotional
    b. financial
    c. self-destructive
    d. congenital

17. When a paramedic notes the presence of multiple bruises of various ages on a child during a physical examination, she should document the findings by noting:

    a. the estimated age of each bruise.
    b. the location and color of each bruise.
    c. who she suspects caused the bruising.
    d. the detailed story behind every bruise.

18. Which of the following is an example of child neglect?

    a. burns on the genitalia
    b. signs of malnourishment
    c. signs of shaken baby syndrome
    d. a central nervous system injury

19. Shaken baby syndrome is a group of signs and symptoms associated with:

    a. severe head trauma.
    b. paralyzing spinal injury.
    c. a long history of child abuse.
    d. intra-abdominal hemorrhage.

20. Evidence shows that most children with shaken baby syndrome are:

    a. also victims of sexual abuse.
    b. under one year old when trauma is inflicted.
    c. between the ages of eighteen months and two years.
    d. predominantly from homes in the middle to upper class.

21. Signs and symptoms of stroke are _____ in a child as in an adult.

    a. the same
    b. less severe
    c. more severe
    d. completely different

22. Which one of the following childhood infectious diseases is still not preventable?

    a. tetanus
    b. rubeola
    c. meningitis
    d. poliomyelitis

23. Your patient is a seven-year-old with Coxsackie virus (hand, foot, and mouth syndrome). You are aware that this condition is highly contagious, so you don gloves and avoid contact with:

    a. rashes and feces.
    b. discharge from the eyes.
    c. cuts or open wounds.
    d. respiratory secretions.

24. Dispatched to a local high school, you have been asked to transport a teenager with infectious mononucleosis. The nurse tells you that this condition is mildly contagious, and to wear gloves and avoid contact with:

    a. urine or feces.
    b. discharge from blisters.
    c. saliva or blood.
    d. rash or hives.

25. Which of the following conditions requires isolation technique for PPE?

    a. whooping cough (pertussis)
    b. viral meningitis
    c. meningococcemia meningitis
    d. impetigo

26. Which of the following statements about febrile seizures is most correct?

    a. Febrile seizures have no lasting neurological effects.
    b. Febrile seizures are associated with physical abuse.
    c. Febrile seizures often have lasting neurological effects.
    d. Most febrile seizures are focal and last several minutes.

27. _____ is/are the number one reason for children missing school and the number one reason for pediatric ED visits caused by chronic illness.

    a. Allergies
    b. Diabetes
    c. Croup
    d. Asthma

28. Your patient is a five-year-old male with symptoms of an upper respiratory infection, nausea, vomiting, and confusion. The parents tell you that the child has been sick with the flu, but the confusion is new. The child's medications include nebulized Albuterol® as needed for the last week and over-the-counter Bayer® Children's aspirin as needed for fevers. You suspect the child:

    a. is developing pneumonia.
    b. is presenting with Reye's syndrome.
    c. is having an AMS caused by dehydration.
    d. may have had a seizure.

29. Your management of the patient discussed in question 28 will include support and care of the ABCs and:

    a. administration of Ventolin and Solu-Medrol®.
    b. IV fluids and seizure precautions.
    c. considering the use of acetaminophen.
    d. administration of prophylactic rectal diazepam.

30. When asthma is triggered, changes in the airways occur. Which of the following is the correct sequence of airway changes?

    a. bronchoconstriction, inflammation, and excess mucus production
    b. wheezing, excess mucus production, and bronchoconstriction
    c. inflammation, excess mucus production, and bronchoconstriction
    d. mucus production, wheezing, and bronchoconstriction

31. _____ is a condition characterized by infections of the bronchioles that results in swelling of the lower airways and tachypnea, retractions, and cyanosis.

    a. Epiglottitis
    b. Croup
    c. Bronchiolitis
    d. Pneumonia

32. Your patient is a five-year-old who is having difficulty breathing. The patient has difficulty exhaling, the SpO_2 is 94% with oxygen, and there are decreased breath sounds bilaterally with no wheezing. Which of the following conditions do you suspect?

    a. allergic reaction
    b. bronchiolitis
    c. foreign body airway obstruction
    d. asthma attack

33. Your management plan for the patient discussed in question 32 includes continued oxygenation and:

    a. supportive care and reassessment.
    b. gentle transport with a parent close by.
    c. nebulized Ventolin.
    d. epinephrine and Benadryl®.

34. _____ is a condition precipitated by a viral or bacterial infection and is characterized by fever, tachypnea, rales, consolidation in one or more lobes, and cough.

    a. Asthma
    b. Croup
    c. Bronchiolitis
    d. Pneumonia

35. Croup causes the tissue _____ the glottal opening to swell compared to epiglottitis, which causes the tissue _____ the glottal opening to swell, resulting in a higher risk of complete airway obstruction.

    a. under; above
    b. above; under
    c. lateral to; under
    d. lateral to; above

36. Why does the prevalence of asthma decrease as children get older?

    a. As the immune system matures, some children outgrow the condition.
    b. Some children outgrow the condition with the use of steroids.
    c. Natural antibodies develop with the use of steroids.
    d. As airways enlarge, some children outgrow the condition.

37. The most prominent indicator of respiratory failure in children is:

  a. increased use of accessory muscles.
  b. low SpO₂ levels.
  c. decreased level of consciousness.
  d. decreased capillary filling.

38. Besides cool or cold temperatures, hypothermia in children can be caused by:

  a. prolonged infection.
  b. diarrhea.
  c. vomiting.
  d. seizures.

39. Children who are diagnosed with a new onset of diabetes mellitus will usually present to the paramedic as being:

  a. hyperactive.
  b. hypothermic.
  c. hyperglycemic.
  d. hypoglycemic.

40. Congenital heart defects are deformities of the structures of the heart that occur:

  a. after the first month of life.
  b. after six months of life.
  c. only when the mother has used drugs during pregnancy.
  d. while the fetus is developing in utero.

41. The significant problem associated with heart defects is that they:

  a. disrupt normal blood flow.
  b. cause murmurs.
  c. cause dysrhythmias.
  d. cause arrhythmias.

42. A defect of the heart that is characterized by valves that are absent, too small, or do not close completely is called:

  a. stenosis.
  b. coarctation.
  c. truncus.
  d. valvulitis.

43. The most common cardiac dysrhythmias seen in children are tachycardias, bradycardias, and:

  a. ventricular fibrillation.
  b. bundle branch blocks.
  c. heart blocks.
  d. asystole.

44. Always consider _____ to be the underlying cause of cardiac dysrhythmias in children until proven otherwise.

  a. hypoglycemia
  b. hypothermia
  c. hypoxia
  d. heredity

45. A highly contagious bacterial or viral disease in children that is characterized by discharge from the eyes is:

  a. impetigo.
  b. conjunctivitis.
  c. Lyme disease.
  d. German measles.

46. The pediatric patient who presents with sunken eyes, recent weight loss, and tachycardia should be evaluated to rule out:

  a. polio.
  b. pertussis.
  c. naphylaxis.
  d. dehydration.

47. You are transporting an infant to the ED for evaluation of a URI. The child has been sick with fever, decreased PO intake, and vomiting. During the transport, the child experiences a febrile seizure. Which of the following is the most appropriate treatment for the child?

  a. Apply ice packs to the torso and head.
  b. Administer IV fluids.
  c. Administer Valium®.
  d. Use gentle cooling measures.

48. You are dispatched at 3:00 a.m. for a four-year-old sick child. Upon arrival at the residence, the parents tell you that the child has been sick with a cold, but tonight it suddenly got worse when the child spiked a temperature. The child is having difficulty breathing, and has a sore throat and difficulty swallowing. You suspect the child has:

  a. croup.
  b. bronchiolitis.
  c. epiglottitis.
  d. a partial obstruction.

49. Which of the following is inappropriate management for the patient discussed in question 48?

  a. Keep a parent with the child at all times.
  b. Visualize the airway for an obstruction.
  c. Permit the child to sit up.
  d. Minimize handling and examining to prevent agitation.

50. While attempting to apply an oxygen mask to the patient discussed in question 48, the child resists. How should you proceed next?

    a. Consider the use of blow-by oxygen.
    b. Insist that the parent hold the mask in place.
    c. Turn up the liter flow so it feels like a fan.
    d. Consider RSI.

51. Transportation considerations for the patient discussed in question 48 should include:

    a. immediate, but calm, transport.
    b. rapid transport with lights only.
    c. laying the child down on the stretcher with the parent nearby.
    d. strapping the parent to the stretcher with the child in his lap.

52. Police have called you to care for a teenager who has overdosed on methadone. The fourteen-year-old is unconscious with shallow respirations and no signs of outward trauma. After managing the ABCs, your primary concern is:

    a. to begin a rapid transport.
    b. the patient's mental status.
    c. to be prepared for seizures.
    d. to administer IV fluids.

53. Appropriate ALS management for the patient described in question 52 includes administering:

    a. 5 mg Valium®.
    b. 2–4 ml/kg D-50 W.
    c. 0.1 mg/kg naloxone.
    d. atropine 0.5–1.0 mg.

54. You arrive at the scene of a motor vehicle collision to find an unconscious six-year-old male lying supine on the pavement. A witness tells you the child ran out in front of a moving car and was struck. What type of injuries do you suspect?

    a. head, chest, and upper extremities
    b. head, chest, and lower extremities
    c. chest, abdomen, and upper extremities
    d. chest, abdomen, and lower extremities

55. The injury pattern for the patient described in question 54 is common and is also described as:

    a. Cushing's triad.
    b. Waddell's triad.
    c. Hendrick's triage.
    d. greenstick pattern.

Exam #43 Answer Form

	A	B	C	D		A	B	C	D
1.	❏	❏	❏	❏	26.	❏	❏	❏	❏
2.	❏	❏	❏	❏	27.	❏	❏	❏	❏
3.	❏	❏	❏	❏	28.	❏	❏	❏	❏
4.	❏	❏	❏	❏	29.	❏	❏	❏	❏
5.	❏	❏	❏	❏	30.	❏	❏	❏	❏
6.	❏	❏	❏	❏	31.	❏	❏	❏	❏
7.	❏	❏	❏	❏	32.	❏	❏	❏	❏
8.	❏	❏	❏	❏	33.	❏	❏	❏	❏
9.	❏	❏	❏	❏	34.	❏	❏	❏	❏
10.	❏	❏	❏	❏	35.	❏	❏	❏	❏
11.	❏	❏	❏	❏	36.	❏	❏	❏	❏
12.	❏	❏	❏	❏	37.	❏	❏	❏	❏
13.	❏	❏	❏	❏	38.	❏	❏	❏	❏
14.	❏	❏	❏	❏	39.	❏	❏	❏	❏
15.	❏	❏	❏	❏	40.	❏	❏	❏	❏
16.	❏	❏	❏	❏	41.	❏	❏	❏	❏
17.	❏	❏	❏	❏	42.	❏	❏	❏	❏
18.	❏	❏	❏	❏	43.	❏	❏	❏	❏
19.	❏	❏	❏	❏	44.	❏	❏	❏	❏
20.	❏	❏	❏	❏	45.	❏	❏	❏	❏
21.	❏	❏	❏	❏	46.	❏	❏	❏	❏
22.	❏	❏	❏	❏	47.	❏	❏	❏	❏
23.	❏	❏	❏	❏	48.	❏	❏	❏	❏
24.	❏	❏	❏	❏	49.	❏	❏	❏	❏
25.	❏	❏	❏	❏	50.	❏	❏	❏	❏

	A	B	C	D			A	B	C	D
51.	❏	❏	❏	❏		54.	❏	❏	❏	❏
52.	❏	❏	❏	❏		55.	❏	❏	❏	❏
53.	❏	❏	❏	❏						

Geriatrics

1. _____ is the study of the problems of all aspects of aging.

   a. Oldentology
   b. Agentology
   c. Genealogy
   d. Gerontology

2. As the body ages, the skin begins to sag and wrinkles develop because of the:

   a. increased vascularity in the skin.
   b. loss of elastic fiber.
   c. loss of T-cell function.
   d. loss of sebaceous glands.

3. With aging, the musculoskeletal system is affected by:

   a. the forming of opacities.
   b. decreased muscle and bone mass.
   c. hypertrophy of muscles.
   d. increasing bone marrow production.

4. Changes in the respiratory system caused by the effects of aging include all of the following, *except*:

   a. a decreased gag reflex increases the risk of aspiration.
   b. lung capacity diminishes with the loss of elasticity.
   c. the chest wall becomes stiff and rigid, increasing the risk for fractures.
   d. decreased cilia increase the risk of infectious pulmonary diseases.

5. With aging comes a decreased _____ response, which affects the ability to increase the heart rate in response to stress and exercise.

   a. estrogen
   b. catecholamine
   c. androgen
   d. progesterone

6. Which of the following is a psychologic change associated with aging?

   a. loss of support system
   b. increased isolation
   c. increased depression
   d. decreased depression

7. The changes in the endocrine system caused by aging include decreased reproductive functions and:

   a. decrease in thyroid function.
   b. atrophy of hormone receptors.
   c. surgical removal of the pancreas.
   d. excessive sympathetic stimulation.

8. During perimenopause (the years before menopause), about 90% of women experience irregular menses and begin to experience the symptoms of menopause. This is caused by:

   a. excessive hormone production.
   b. the drop in sexual hormone levels.
   c. increased release of catecholamines.
   d. decreased release of catecholamines.

9. In addition to the classic symptoms of hot flashes and irregular menstrual periods, nearly 80% of menopausal women experience other symptoms that are collectively called:

   a. post-maternal pattern.
   b. menacing disorder.
   c. menopausal syndrome.
   d. PMS.

10. In the year 2030, it is projected that one in _____ people will be age sixty-five or older in the United States.

    a. three
    b. five
    c. ten
    d. twenty-five

11. Which of the following groups are living longer?

    a. married people
    b. cohabiting people
    c. people who have attained higher education
    d. all of the above

12. As the baby boomers grow older, it is estimated that treating psychiatric illnesses will become a crisis in the United States, with the numbers of mentally ill seniors expected to _____ by the year 2030.

    a. double
    b. triple
    c. quadruple
    d. increase tenfold

13. The actual number of people dying from _____ has risen 37% since 1950 and remains the number one cause of death in the United States.

    a. heart disease
    b. cancer
    c. COPD
    d. diabetes

14. The elderly are highly susceptible to head injuries from falling because:

    a. the frequency of falling on the head increases with age.
    b. medications they take often include blood thinners.
    c. thinning hair does not protect the scalp as well as thick hair.
    d. the brain and vessels tear on the sharp, bony edges inside the skull.

15. What is the difference in the pathology of cardiovascular emergencies in older adults compared to that of younger adults?

    a. The catecholamine response in cardiac emergencies increases with age.
    b. Younger adults tend to die from ACS rather than heart failure.
    c. Coronary artery disease predisposes the elderly to superior outcomes.
    d. There is really no difference when an older or younger adult experiences an ACS.

16. The elderly patient often has atypical cardiac pain, which may be as subtle as a new onset of weakness or dyspnea. One of the reasons this occurs is:

    a. diminished pain perception.
    b. depression of the central nervous system.
    c. suppression of the inflammatory response.
    d. due to changes experienced during menopause.

17. Currently the single greatest health problem in the United States, it is estimated that nearly 55% of all Americans will have _____ by age sixty.

    a. a stroke
    b. diabetes
    c. hypertension
    d. cancer

18. You are assessing a sixty-four-year-old female with a chief complaint of difficulty breathing, which has been getting worse over the past two days. She is overweight and has a history of congestive heart failure. She does not move much from her recliner except to use the bathroom. She also has new pleuritic chest pain and describes chronic pain in her lower left leg. Which of the following conditions should you suspect first?

    a. pneumonia
    b. emphysema
    c. chronic bronchitis
    d. pulmonary embolism

19. Continuing with the patient in question 18, your partner administers oxygen and obtains vital signs while you obtain an ECG. Her vitals signs are: skin CTC warm, moist, and pale; respirations 28/shallow and lung sounds clear; pulse 70/irregular; BP 168/110; and ECG is controlled atrial fibrillation. Your treatment plan now includes:

    a. IV access only.
    b. nitrates and Lasix.
    c. IV fluids and analgesia.
    d. nebulized bronchodilators.

20. Emergencies with Alzheimer's patients fall into three categories. Which of the following is not one of those categories?

    a. behavioral
    b. psychiatric
    c. metabolic
    d. neurologic

21. A common emergency that occurs with patients who have Parkinson's is:

    a. hypoglycemia.
    b. injuries from falling.
    c. transient ischemic attack (TIA).
    d. recurrent thoughts of death.

22. _____ is a chronic and progressive neurologic condition that robs memory and intellect.

    a. Parkinson's
    b. Alzheimer's
    c. Hypothyroidism
    d. Hyperthyroidism

23. _____ is/are an important indicator of the general well-being and mental health of older Americans.

    a. Age and gender
    b. Height and weight
    c. Depressive symptoms
    d. The use of multiple medications

24. Thyroid disease, such as hypothyroidism, in elders can predispose them to risks such as:

    a. hypothermia.
    b. cholecystitis.
    c. diverticulitis.
    d. malnutrition.

25. Special considerations for diabetes in the elderly include all of the following, *except*:

    a. cognitive impairments may hinder an older person from preparing meals.
    b. the elderly have decreased susceptibility to certain infections.
    c. neuropathy is more prevalent in the elderly.
    d. slower metabolism affects carbohydrate absorption.

26. The most common causes of minor GI bleeds in the elderly are:

    a. peptic ulcer and angiodysplasia.
    b. diverticular diseases.
    c. hemorrhoids and colorectal cancer.
    d. bowel obstruction.

27. Common GI problems in the elderly, such as _____, are most often caused by cancer, adhesions, or hernias.

    a. bowel obstructions
    b. hemorrhoids
    c. gastritis
    d. peptic ulcers

28. You are dispatched to the residence of a patient with abdominal pain. The patient is an eighty-four-year-old female who is alert and complaining of abdominal pain of 8/10. She has had the pain for nearly four hours and describes it as "cramping." She also has nausea and has vomited twice. The patient denies dyspnea, chest pain, or weakness. Vital signs are: skin CTC is warm and dry, with good color; respiratory rate 22/nonlabored; pulse rate 70/regular; and BP 140/100. What is your first impression of this patient?

    a. unstable with a GI bleed
    b. stable with a bowel obstruction
    c. stable with a urinary tract infection
    d. unstable with a possible cardiac event

29. Continuing with the patient in question 28, the patient's ECG is sinus with a first-degree AV block, SpO_2 is 98%, and blood sugar is 110 mg/dL. She is taking atenolol for hypertension, Nexium for her stomach, miacalcin for osteoporosis, and hydrocodone for back pain. The patient's last bowel movement was two days ago, and she feels distended. Which of the patient's medications is most likely contributing to her chief complaint?

    a. atenolol
    b. miacalcin
    c. Nexium
    d. hydrocodone

30. _____ is a chronic inflammatory disease of the bones that results in thickening, softening, and eventual bowing of the bone.

    a. Osteoporosis
    b. Paget's disease
    c. Osteoarthritis
    d. Gout

31. You are obtaining a focused history from a seventy-six-year-old female with a new GI bleed. Which of her medications could be the cause of the GI bleed?

    a. Colace
    b. codeine
    c. ibuprofen
    d. oxycodone

32. Elderly patients with slowed metabolism can get increased amounts of medications in the body from normal doses that can reach lethal levels. This is commonly referred to as:

    a. concurrent disease overdose.
    b. altered hepatic function.
    c. depressed renal function.
    d. drug toxicity.

33. Which of the following is not a type of nursing home regulated by state and federal standards?

    a. intermediate care facilities
    b. residential care facilities
    c. skilled nursing facilities
    d. senior retirement facilities

34. Independent living with limited nursing care, social, recreation, and rehabilitation activities is an example of a/an _____ nursing home.

    a. intermediate care facility
    b. residential care facility
    c. skilled nursing facility
    d. senior retirement facility

35. Which of the following statements about "falls" that occur among elderly people is least accurate?

   a. Injuries resulting from falls are the sixth leading cause of death in those over sixty-five.
   b. In the elderly, falling is widely recognized as a major life- and health-threatening problem.
   c. Fractures from falls cost an estimated one billion dollars annually in the United States.
   d. Common injuries from falls include hip and upper limb fractures.

36. Affective disorders increase the risk of injury in the elderly by interfering with:

   a. thermoregulation.
   b. the tasks of daily living.
   c. the immune response.
   d. cardiac output.

37. Because the elderly are susceptible to problems with metabolizing medications, the paramedic should assume that the patient's medications could be contributing to nearly any health problem. Which type of medication requires frequent monitoring by testing the levels in the blood?

   a. digitalis
   b. ramipril
   c. amoxicillin
   d. furosemide

38. _____ is/are ischemic and sometimes necrotic damage to the skin, subcutaneous tissue, and often muscle caused by prolonged periods of immobilization.

   a. Folliculitis
   b. Ulcers
   c. Pressure sores
   d. Abscesses

39. Your patient's nephew called EMS because, when he stopped in to check on his uncle as he does each day, he found him acting confused. He describes finding his uncle sitting in a very warm room, wearing several layers of clothing, but still shivering and cold to the touch. When there is no obvious environmental explanation, the paramedic should assume that hypothermia in the elderly is caused by:

   a. hypoglycemia.
   b. hypothyroidism.
   c. severe infection.
   d. adverse medication reaction.

40. Any older person can become a victim of abuse, with the most common abusers being:

   a. landlords.
   b. neighbors.
   c. friends.
   d. family members.

41. Which of the following is not typically considered a form of abuse in the elderly?

   a. financial abuse
   b. emotional neglect
   c. resistance abuse
   d. institutional abuse

42. Physiologic changes in the respiratory system that occur with aging include a decrease in airway cilia and diminished cough and gag reflexes. These changes increase the risk of:

   a. sustaining rib fractures with coughing.
   b. obtaining infectious pulmonary diseases.
   c. diminishing the inflammatory response.
   d. lung shrinkage (atrophy) and compliance.

43. During the physical examination, the older patient must be handled gently so as not to:

   a. cause any additional injury.
   b. confuse the patient with your specialized equipment.
   c. overwhelm the caretaker with your techniques.
   d. force the patient to receive unwanted care.

44. Unless there is an obvious environmental explanation, assume that hypothermia in the elderly is caused by _____ until proven otherwise.

   a. severe infection
   b. hypothyroidism
   c. osmotic diuresis
   d. hypoglycemia

45. The most common complications that result from osteoporosis include hip fractures and:

   a. sepsis.
   b. vertebral fractures.
   c. deep vein thrombosis.
   d. pulmonary embolism.

46. Select the physiologic change that is abnormal or inconsistent with the aging process.

   a. developing dementia
   b. decreased brain mass
   c. altered pain perception
   d. conduction system abnormalities

47. When formulating a field impression for the patient with diseases of the nervous system, the paramedic should always consider _____ early on, as a potential cause of AMS.

   a. hypothyroidism
   b. hypothermia
   c. hypoglycemia
   d. dementia

48. Non-acute causes of confusion in the elderly include:

   a. dementia.
   b. delirium.
   c. depression.
   d. all of the above.

49. _____ is the leading cause of new-onset blindness and end-stage renal disease in the elderly.

   a. Stroke
   b. Diabetes
   c. Hypertension
   d. Adverse medication reaction

50. _____ is/are a service for home care patients who require palliative and supportive care for terminal illnesses.

   a. Mental health day care
   b. Case management
   c. Hospice programs
   d. Day hospitals

Exam #44 Answer Form

	A	B	C	D		A	B	C	D
1.	❏	❏	❏	❏	26.	❏	❏	❏	❏
2.	❏	❏	❏	❏	27.	❏	❏	❏	❏
3.	❏	❏	❏	❏	28.	❏	❏	❏	❏
4.	❏	❏	❏	❏	29.	❏	❏	❏	❏
5.	❏	❏	❏	❏	30.	❏	❏	❏	❏
6.	❏	❏	❏	❏	31.	❏	❏	❏	❏
7.	❏	❏	❏	❏	32.	❏	❏	❏	❏
8.	❏	❏	❏	❏	33.	❏	❏	❏	❏
9.	❏	❏	❏	❏	34.	❏	❏	❏	❏
10.	❏	❏	❏	❏	35.	❏	❏	❏	❏
11.	❏	❏	❏	❏	36.	❏	❏	❏	❏
12.	❏	❏	❏	❏	37.	❏	❏	❏	❏
13.	❏	❏	❏	❏	38.	❏	❏	❏	❏
14.	❏	❏	❏	❏	39.	❏	❏	❏	❏
15.	❏	❏	❏	❏	40.	❏	❏	❏	❏
16.	❏	❏	❏	❏	41.	❏	❏	❏	❏
17.	❏	❏	❏	❏	42.	❏	❏	❏	❏
18.	❏	❏	❏	❏	43.	❏	❏	❏	❏
19.	❏	❏	❏	❏	44.	❏	❏	❏	❏
20.	❏	❏	❏	❏	45.	❏	❏	❏	❏
21.	❏	❏	❏	❏	46.	❏	❏	❏	❏
22.	❏	❏	❏	❏	47.	❏	❏	❏	❏
23.	❏	❏	❏	❏	48.	❏	❏	❏	❏
24.	❏	❏	❏	❏	49.	❏	❏	❏	❏
25.	❏	❏	❏	❏	50.	❏	❏	❏	❏

The Challenged Patient

1. You are assessing a patient who has a hearing impairment. The patient tells you that he lost part of his hearing when he had meningitis as a child. What type of deafness do you suspect he has?

   a. conductive
   b. pagetoid
   c. sensorineural
   d. paradoxic

2. One clue that a patient has a hearing impairment is a patient's inability to respond to verbal communication:

   a. even when you shout.
   b. even when you are extra nice.
   c. unless you are direct and forceful.
   d. unless you are making direct eye contact.

3. Which of the following actions is inappropriate when communicating with a deaf patient who reads lips?

   a. making eye contact prior to speaking
   b. speaking slowly with exaggerated lip movement
   c. speaking slowly without exaggerated lip movement
   d. speaking normally without exaggerated lip movement

4. Acute causes of visual impairment include:

   a. optic neuritis or neurosis.
   b. cataracts and glaucoma.
   c. strokes and CNS infections.
   d. diabetic retinopathy or MS.

5. Which of the following conditions may result in a transient blindness for the patient?

   a. acute head injury
   b. near drowning
   c. TIA
   d. acute hypothermia

6. Stuttering is a/an _____ disorder, which is one of the four types of speech impairments.

   a. fluency
   b. language
   c. articulation
   d. voice production

7. The group of speech disorders that affects understanding of language, forming language, or expressing language is collectively referred to as:

   a. aphasia.
   b. dysarthria.
   c. fluency disorders.
   d. amentia.

8. When a patient is able to understand language and form speech patterns but is unable to express them properly because of physical impairment of the speech pathways, this condition is called:

   a. aphasia.
   b. dysarthria.
   c. fluency disorder.
   d. amentia.

9. Patients with a/an _____ disorder may exhibit hoarseness, an inappropriate pitch, or an abnormal nasal resonance.

   a. fluency
   b. language
   c. articulation
   d. voice production

10. Which of the following is the most significant finding of a speech impairment for a patient in the emergency setting?

    a. hearing loss with an acute onset
    b. hearing loss with a slow onset
    c. a possible associated psychiatric disorder
    d. chronic slurred speech

11. Etiologies of obesity in humans have been associated with:

    a. a low metabolic rate.
    b. a high basal metabolic rate.
    c. decreased insulin production.
    d. the use of stimulant agents.

12. The patient you are assessing states that he is hearing voices, and his caretaker confirms that the patient has no concept of reality. Which of the following conditions does the patient have?

    a. hyalosis
    b. telepathy
    c. psychoses
    d. neuroses

13. When dealing with a patient who is experiencing hallucinations, the best management is to gently calm and reassure the patient that everything is all right using a technique called "_____ down."

    a. stand
    b. talk
    c. take
    d. show

14. Developmental disability refers to an impaired or insufficient development of

    a. speech.
    b. the brain.
    c. sensory function.
    d. motor coordination.

15. When managing patients with Down syndrome, the paramedic should keep in mind all of the following, *except*:

    a. these patients have a below-average IQ.
    b. that many have a congenital heart defect.
    c. they have a unique airway anatomy.
    d. they have abnormal intestines.

16. Psychoses are often associated with an underlying biochemical brain disease, such as:

    a. brainwashing.
    b. TIA.
    c. stroke.
    d. deficiency of neurotransmitters.

17. The more practical and current term for emotional or mental impairment is:

    a. maladaptive behavior.
    b. misunderstood manners.
    c. cerebrally challenged.
    d. comprehension deficit.

18. When treating a patient with a history of chronic arthritis, the paramedic may have to accommodate the patient in which of the following ways?

    a. Decreased range of motion may limit the physical exam.
    b. Speak slowly, because the patient may not understand everything you say.
    c. Paralysis of respiratory muscles may require ventilatory support.
    d. Obtaining a complete list of medications may be challenging and take more time than usual.

19. While performing a physical examination on a cancer patient, it would not be uncommon to find:

    a. transdermal pain medications.
    b. a medical alert tag with cancer information.
    c. spastic paralysis of extremities.
    d. multiple lesions on the torso.

20. When caring for a patient with cerebral palsy, the paramedic should anticipate that the patient:

    a. will be unable to ambulate.
    b. may require respiratory support.
    c. will understand everything you say and do.
    d. will typically have mild to severe retardation.

21. When caring for a patient with multiple sclerosis, it is not uncommon for the patient to be unpleasant, angry, hostile, or mean. This is normal and occurs because the patient:

    a. is seeking attention.
    b. is prone to mood disorders.
    c. has an expressive speech disorder.
    d. is taking medications that produce these emotions.

22. You are assessing a patient who is hypertensive and complaining of weakness. The patient has a history of myasthenia gravis, so you contact medical control before administering medication because:

    a. many common medications may worsen an exacerbation.
    b. the patient will probably refuse any treatment.
    c. these symptoms require treatment that is different from other patients.
    d. you may have to give the patient additional doses of her own medication.

23. A patient with spina bifida may require special attention to _____, which are often present with these patients.

    a. catheters
    b. open sores
    c. contractures
    d. muscle spasms

24. For the paramedic, the phrase "terminally ill" usually means that the patient has a condition that will result in his or her death within the next:

    a. six to twelve months.
    b. twelve to eighteen months.
    c. one to two years.
    d. five years.

25. When caring for the patient with a terminal illness such as cancer, a major issue for the paramedic is:

    a. DNAR status.
    b. pain control.
    c. "end of life" priorities.
    d. living will status.

26. The patient you are caring for is competent but very sick. He states that he is going to refuse transport because he cannot afford to pay. To get him to go to the hospital, you should:

    a. tell him that the care will be free this time.
    b. tell him that his bill will be reduced.
    c. try to convince him that his health should be the first priority.
    d. tell him that he will die if he does not come with you.

27. If the patient described in question 26 still refuses to go to the hospital despite all of your efforts, what should you do next?

    a. Call the police and ask for restraints.
    b. Acknowledge that the competent patient has a right to refuse care.
    c. Force him to go anyway.
    d. Call medical control for consent to restrain the patient.

28. Common causes of conductive hearing loss include:

    a. injury or earwax.
    b. birth defects and aging.
    c. medications and tumors.
    d. mumps or measles.

29. Approximately 80% of hearing loss is related to the loss of _____ sounds.

    a. low-pitched
    b. high-pitched
    c. distant
    d. isolated

30. Which of the following is an example of a degenerative disease that causes chronic progressive vision loss?

    a. stroke
    b. multiple sclerosis
    c. congenital cataracts
    d. central nervous system infection

31. A nursing home resident requires transport for evaluation of a possible UTI. You observe that the patient's extremities are grossly contracted and that she will not fit on your stretcher like most patients. Which of the following would be appropriate for this patient?

    a. Only force the extremities to move enough to fit the patient on the stretcher.
    b. Refuse to transport the patient.
    c. Pad the contractures and use extra care during the move.
    d. Consider administering a muscle relaxant prior to moving the patient.

32. Transport of the patient with cystic fibrosis may require which of the following accommodations by the paramedic?

    a. respiratory support
    b. management of catheters
    c. padding of contractures
    d. medical consent by a caregiver

33. Cultural differences in patients vary. The paramedic should be aware of each patient's private/personal space needs. Assessment is best initiated by:

    a. examining the patient with no one else present.
    b. pointing to an area of the body before touching it.
    c. asking the patient's spouse for permission to examine.
    d. only performing the physical exam while in the ambulance.

34. When caring for patients with cultural backgrounds that differ from your own, the most important concept for the paramedic is that:

    a. language barriers will never compound cultural differences.
    b. cultural differences will limit the paramedic's judgment.
    c. patients with cultural differences have different needs and wants.
    d. cultural-based preferences may conflict with a paramedic's learned medical practice.

35. Which of the following statements about cultural diversity is incorrect?

    a. All people share common problems or situations.
    b. People identify with their ethnic cultural background.
    c. The paramedic should respect the integrity of cultural beliefs.
    d. Different individuals within the same family may have different sets of beliefs.

36. When caring for an obese patient, additional manpower may be required as well as:

    a. specialized assessment skills.
    b. extra PPE for unique physical ailments.
    c. specialized management skills.
    d. appropriately sized diagnostic devices.

37. When caring for a patient who speaks a different language, which of the following should the paramedic do first?

    a. Use a phrase or picture book.
    b. Speak in English first to determine if the patient can understand even a little of the language.
    c. Let the patient put on your stethoscope and speak into the bell.
    d. Give the patient a paper and pen, and encourage him to draw a picture.

38. When caring for a patient with a visual impairment, to lessen the patient's fear or anxiety the paramedic should:

    a. describe everything she is going to do before actually doing it.
    b. not ask the patient about her visual impairment.
    c. leave her leader dogs at the residence, because the ambulance is unsafe.
    d. avoid explaining what care may be in store for her.

39. A patient with stroke-like symptoms is unable to say what he means. What type of speech disorder is the patient most likely experiencing?

    a. expressive aphasia
    b. receptive aphasia
    c. dysarthria
    d. fluency disorder

40. You are assessing a patient who awoke with stroke symptoms approximately twenty minutes ago. The patient is conscious but unable to speak. What is most significant about this finding?

    a. The patient is most likely very alert and frustrated by this deficit.
    b. The patient will not likely be able to recover from this deficit.
    c. The patient is very likely to have airway problems associated with this deficit.
    d. The patient is most likely experiencing cognitive deficits and does not understand what is happening.

41. The most common cause of either para- or quadriplegia is:

    a. muscular dystrophy.
    b. multiple sclerosis.
    c. trauma.
    d. birth defect.

42. Special accommodations for the care of a patient with a preexisting quadriplegia include:

    a. involving the alert and oriented patient in any decisions regarding movement and transport.
    b. obtaining consent for treatment from the patient's caregiver.
    c. full spinal immobilization.
    d. complete neurologic assessment and documentation.

43. Which of the following patients is most likely to develop hyperactivity or become dangerous while in the care of EMS?

    a. psychotic person
    b. neurotic person
    c. homeless person
    d. financially impaired person

44. Obesity is defined as being _____ above ideal body weight.

    a. 5–10%
    b. 10–20%
    c. 20–30%
    d. 30–40%

45. It is estimated that one in _____ Americans meets the definition for obesity.

    a. two
    b. three
    c. four
    d. five

46. For the paramedic, the most dangerous patients with communicable diseases are those with:

    a. cancer.
    b. minor symptoms.
    c. mental impairments.
    d. emotional impairments.

47. _____ is the most common cause of impaired vision in the field.

    a. Stroke
    b. Traumatic injury
    c. Complications of diabetes
    d. Not wearing prescribed corrective lenses

48. Classic signs and symptoms of myasthenia gravis include:

    a. chest pain and shortness of breath.
    b. drooping eyelids and difficulty swallowing.
    c. headache and hypertension.
    d. memory loss and cognitive dysfunction.

49. In most cases, prehospital care of the patient with myasthenia gravis will include:

    a. oxygen and nitroglycerin.
    b. supportive care and transport.
    c. oxygen and Lopressor.
    d. reorientation to time and place.

50. When caring for a patient with a previous head injury that resulted in a permanent cognitive deficit, which of the following pieces of information from the family or caretaker is the most significant to you?

    a. The patient also has motor and neurologic deficits.
    b. The patient functions in the upper range of retardation.
    c. There has been a recent change in the patient's behavior.
    d. The patient is not legally able to sign for treatment or billing.

Exam #45 Answer Form

	A	B	C	D		A	B	C	D
1.	❏	❏	❏	❏	26.	❏	❏	❏	❏
2.	❏	❏	❏	❏	27.	❏	❏	❏	❏
3.	❏	❏	❏	❏	28.	❏	❏	❏	❏
4.	❏	❏	❏	❏	29.	❏	❏	❏	❏
5.	❏	❏	❏	❏	30.	❏	❏	❏	❏
6.	❏	❏	❏	❏	31.	❏	❏	❏	❏
7.	❏	❏	❏	❏	32.	❏	❏	❏	❏
8.	❏	❏	❏	❏	33.	❏	❏	❏	❏
9.	❏	❏	❏	❏	34.	❏	❏	❏	❏
10.	❏	❏	❏	❏	35.	❏	❏	❏	❏
11.	❏	❏	❏	❏	36.	❏	❏	❏	❏
12.	❏	❏	❏	❏	37.	❏	❏	❏	❏
13.	❏	❏	❏	❏	38.	❏	❏	❏	❏
14.	❏	❏	❏	❏	39.	❏	❏	❏	❏
15.	❏	❏	❏	❏	40.	❏	❏	❏	❏
16.	❏	❏	❏	❏	41.	❏	❏	❏	❏
17.	❏	❏	❏	❏	42.	❏	❏	❏	❏
18.	❏	❏	❏	❏	43.	❏	❏	❏	❏
19.	❏	❏	❏	❏	44.	❏	❏	❏	❏
20.	❏	❏	❏	❏	45.	❏	❏	❏	❏
21.	❏	❏	❏	❏	46.	❏	❏	❏	❏
22.	❏	❏	❏	❏	47.	❏	❏	❏	❏
23.	❏	❏	❏	❏	48.	❏	❏	❏	❏
24.	❏	❏	❏	❏	49.	❏	❏	❏	❏
25.	❏	❏	❏	❏	50.	❏	❏	❏	❏

46

Acute Interventions in the Home Care Patient

1. The roles of the home care professional and the paramedic are similar in that they both:

   a. offer supportive healthcare of the patient living at home.
   b. can provide emergency advance cardiac life support.
   c. offer palliative care.
   d. offer routine monitoring at home.

2. The roles of the home care professional and the paramedic are different in that only the paramedic can:

   a. offer supportive healthcare of the patient living at home.
   b. provide emergency advanced cardiac life support.
   c. offer palliative care.
   d. offer routine monitoring at home.

3. A typical example of a patient requiring home health services is a/an:

   a. diabetic.
   b. post MI.
   c. asthma.
   d. cerebral palsy.

4. Examples of diseases or conditions typical to the home care patient include:

   a. complications from infections.
   b. arthritis.
   c. gout.
   d. pregnancy.

5. _____ is intended to maximize the quality of a chronically ill patient's life.

   a. Acute care
   b. Palliative care
   c. Meals on Wheels
   d. A neighborhood health center

6. Which of the following home health services is not a skilled service?

   a. shopping service
   b. infant care
   c. case management
   d. nursing

7. Home health services that are considered support services include all the following, *except*:

   a. housekeeping.
   b. dental care.
   c. companions.
   d. personal care for grooming and dressing.

8. Palliative and support services for the terminally ill patient under medical supervision are provided by:

   a. hospice programs.
   b. church groups.
   c. HMOs.
   d. community centers.

9. Emergency problems related to circulatory pathologies that are typical to the home care patient include:

   a. wound care.
   b. sleep apnea.
   c. obstructed shunts.
   d. sepsis.

10. Why are home healthcare services becoming the preference for patients and their families?

    a. These services help to reduce expensive inpatient stays.
    b. The HMOs are quicker to pay for these services than hospitalizations.
    c. There is no room left in the nursing homes.
    d. Nursing facilities are too expensive.

11. Hospice care emphasizes comfort measures and counseling to provide for physical, spiritual, social, and _____ needs.

    a. financial
    b. long-distance
    c. long-term
    d. economic

12. _____ care provides supportive care, comfort care, and referral for patient conditions such as chemotherapy, pain management, or daily activities.

    a. Acute
    b. Home
    c. Hospice
    d. HMO

13. _____ care provides services such as help with DNARs, advanced directives, and bereavement care.

    a. Acute
    b. Home
    c. Hospice
    d. HMO

14. Any home care patient who _____ has the potential to receive care, or a lack of care, that can become detrimental to him or her.

    a. is not ambulatory
    b. has an infectious disease
    c. requires high maintenance
    d. does not have life insurance

15. Which of the following is an example of a complication of in-home care that would result in the patient having to be hospitalized?

    a. bed-wetting
    b. anxiety
    c. sleeplessness
    d. infections

16. _____ care is the work toward the relief of pain and suffering, and provision of care for chronically ill patients and their family and friends.

    a. Palliative
    b. Modified
    c. Advanced
    d. Progressive

17. Which of the following situations with airway devices in the home would EMS most likely be called to assist?

    a. discontinued use
    b. obstructed tubing
    c. replacing existing tubing
    d. routine suctioning

18. Which of the following devices is an example of an enhanced alveolar ventilation device found in the home?

    a. nasal canula
    b. simple face mask
    c. pulmonary function meter
    d. oxygen purifier

19. Which of the following is not a modification of traditional positive pressure ventilation?

    a. BiPAP
    b. CPAP
    c. PPEK
    d. PEEP

20. Which of the following is considered noninvasive ventilation?

    a. ETT
    b. EOA
    c. BiPAP
    d. PEEP

21. A home monitoring device that detects changes in thoracic or abdominal movement and heart rate is called a/an:

    a. apnea monitor.
    b. nebulizer.
    c. ventilator.
    d. pulmonary function meter.

22. While caring for a patient with a vascular access device (VAD), which of the following complications would not be a reason to transport the patient to the hospital?

    a. dislodgement
    b. discomfort
    c. embolism
    d. extravastion

23. Which of the following is not a common VAD found in the home care setting?

    a. Port-A-Cath®
    b. Hickman®
    c. Groshon®
    d. Extracath®

24. Your patient is having an acute onset of respiratory distress. She is tachypnic, cyanotic, and diaphoretic, and states the symptoms came on suddenly. Your assessment reveals that the patient has a VAD in place because she is a cancer patient who is receiving chemotherapy. Which of the following complications do you suspect?

    a. embolism
    b. ACS
    c. infection
    d. sepsis

25. After providing high-flow oxygen, your management plan for the patient described in question 24 should include:

    a. ventilatory support as needed and rapid transport.
    b. IV fluid challenge, aspirin, and morphine.
    c. nitro, aspirin, and morphine.
    d. nitro, Lasix, and rapid transport.

26. All of the following are devices for the GU tract that are commonly found in home care settings, *except*:

    a. Canadian catheter®.
    b. suprapubic catheters.
    c. Condom catheter®.
    d. Foley catheter®.

27. Which of the following GI tract devices is not commonly found in the home care setting?

    a. colostomy bags
    b. J-tubes
    c. G-tubes
    d. P-tubes

28. The primary reasons patients are sent home with urinary catheters include:

    a. trauma and paralysis.
    b. UTI and urinary retention.
    c. immobilization and sedation.
    d. pregnancy and postoperative care.

29. When a patient in the home care setting experiences failure of a GU device, the paramedic is likely to find which problem associated with the failure of that device during her assessment?

    a. hematuria
    b. dark urine
    c. leaking catheter
    d. full bladder bag

30. The terminally ill patient has several rights, one of which includes the right to:

    a. free institutional care.
    b. home healthcare with charge.
    c. choose the place to die and time of death.
    d. unlimited resources for pain management.

31. There are _____ stages a dying person typically goes through, much like the stages in the grieving process following a death.

    a. four
    b. five
    c. six
    d. seven

32. During the first stage of dying, a person experiences "shock and disbelief" and finally acceptance. This first stage can take moments or months before moving on to the second stage, which is:

    a. bargaining.
    b. anger.
    c. depression.
    d. detachment.

33. For the dying person, acquiescence is achieved in the final stage of:

    a. bargaining.
    b. anger.
    c. depression.
    d. detachment.

34. Examples of wound closure techniques that the paramedic may be called to assess in the home care patient include all the following, *except*:

    a. squamous.
    b. sutures.
    c. wires.
    d. staples.

35. Which of the following is not a gastric emptying or feeding device?

    a. NG tube
    b. colostomy
    c. urostomy
    d. Peg tube

36. The general term for an operation in which an artificial opening in the body is formed is:

    a. incisure.
    b. ostomy.
    c. ectomy.
    d. intomy.

37. When assessing a patient in the home care setting who receives dialysis regularly, which of the following devices would you expect to find?

    a. VAD
    b. feeding tube
    c. pulmonary function meter
    d. suprapubic catheter

38. A home health aide has called you to transport a home resident with chronic MS who has a urostomy and a feeding tube. The patient is tachypnic, febrile, and tachycardic. The aide tells you the urine output is decreased and the feeding schedule has been normal. Which of the following complications do you suspect first?

    a. local infection of the urostomy
    b. local infection of the feeding tube
    c. systemic infection
    d. respiratory infection

39. Your patient is a sixty-six-year-old male terminal cancer patient at home complaining of abdominal pain with a slow and progressive onset over two days. His vital signs, including temperature, are normal. He denies any chest pain or shortness of breath. PO intake has been normal. What other information from the patient would be pertinent now?

    a. any changes in bowels
    b. any changes in medications
    c. any nausea or vomiting
    d. all of the above

40. A physical examination of the patient described in question 39 reveals a distended abdomen with diffuse pain on palpation. The patient has had no nausea or vomiting, but has not had a bowel movement in two days. What do you suspect is the cause of his abdominal pain?

    a. GI bleed
    b. hemorrhoids
    c. obstruction
    d. diverticulitis

41. Your management plan for the patient described in question 39 includes:

    a. oxygen, IV fluids, and rapid transport.
    b. oxygen and pain management.
    c. position of comfort and supportive care.
    d. suppository and transport.

42. You have been called to evaluate a bedridden home care patient. The visiting nurse discovered that the patient had hematuria this morning when she was checking the patient's Foley catheter®. Which of the following might be the cause of the hematuria?

    a. cystitis
    b. infection
    c. urethritis
    d. any of the above

43. Your management plan for the patient described in question 42 includes:

    a. oxygen, IV fluids, and rapid transport.
    b. supportive care and routine transport.
    c. changing the catheter and return to service.
    d. treating for shock.

44. The paramedic should respectfully interact with family members of the home care patient when present, because:

    a. they often know more about the patient's special needs than anyone else.
    b. they have the patient's advanced directives.
    c. most often they will not let the patient speak for herself.
    d. you are required to do so.

45. You have been called to a residence for a respiratory distress call. Upon arrival, the family tells you that the patient does not want to be transported because the patient has an end-stage terminal illness. They allow you in to assess, but state, "Hospice is on the way and we made a mistake by calling EMS." What would be appropriate management for this patient?

    a. Wait for hospice to arrive and then leave.
    b. Insist to the family that the patient should be transported.
    c. Call for police assistance.
    d. Offer assistance to the patient and then insist on transport.

Exam #46 Answer Form

	A	B	C	D			A	B	C	D
1.	❏	❏	❏	❏		24.	❏	❏	❏	❏
2.	❏	❏	❏	❏		25.	❏	❏	❏	❏
3.	❏	❏	❏	❏		26.	❏	❏	❏	❏
4.	❏	❏	❏	❏		27.	❏	❏	❏	❏
5.	❏	❏	❏	❏		28.	❏	❏	❏	❏
6.	❏	❏	❏	❏		29.	❏	❏	❏	❏
7.	❏	❏	❏	❏		30.	❏	❏	❏	❏
8.	❏	❏	❏	❏		31.	❏	❏	❏	❏
9.	❏	❏	❏	❏		32.	❏	❏	❏	❏
10.	❏	❏	❏	❏		33.	❏	❏	❏	❏
11.	❏	❏	❏	❏		34.	❏	❏	❏	❏
12.	❏	❏	❏	❏		35.	❏	❏	❏	❏
13.	❏	❏	❏	❏		36.	❏	❏	❏	❏
14.	❏	❏	❏	❏		37.	❏	❏	❏	❏
15.	❏	❏	❏	❏		38.	❏	❏	❏	❏
16.	❏	❏	❏	❏		39.	❏	❏	❏	❏
17.	❏	❏	❏	❏		40.	❏	❏	❏	❏
18.	❏	❏	❏	❏		41.	❏	❏	❏	❏
19.	❏	❏	❏	❏		42.	❏	❏	❏	❏
20.	❏	❏	❏	❏		43.	❏	❏	❏	❏
21.	❏	❏	❏	❏		44.	❏	❏	❏	❏
22.	❏	❏	❏	❏		45.	❏	❏	❏	❏
23.	❏	❏	❏	❏						

47
Ambulance Operations and Medical Incident Command

1. _____ standards are minimum standards and are not considered the "gold standard."

   a. National
   b. State
   c. Local
   d. Regional

2. The U.S. General Services Administration's Automotive Commodity Center issues the federal regulations specifying:

   a. the required response times for high-rise buildings.
   b. BLS equipment that is mandatory on all ambulances.
   c. ALS equipment that is required on ambulances.
   d. ambulance design and manufacturing requirements.

3. Documented check sheets for ambulances are mandatory both for good practice and:

   a. for OSHA.
   b. for NIOSH.
   c. as a risk management tool.
   d. for professional services only.

4. Which of the following is not typically found on a vehicle/equipment checklist?

   a. oxygen therapy and suction equipment
   b. supplies for childbirth
   c. restock items to be obtained from the hospital
   d. equipment for the transfer of the patient

5. Special considerations for EMS providers who carry medications on their vehicles include:

   a. routinely checking expiration dates.
   b. having the junior EMS provider restock.
   c. getting the Medical Director to authorize medication purchases.
   d. billing the patients to recoup the cost of the medications.

6. OSHA requires that the ambulance be properly disinfected:

   a. once every twenty-four hours.
   b. on a weekly basis, even if there were no transports that week.
   c. after the transport of any patient with a potentially communicable disease.
   d. after the transport of any patient.

7. Each service is required, by OSHA or the state equivalent of OSHA, to have an exposure control plan that specifies:

   a. which mask to place on a TB patient.
   b. cleaning requirements.
   c. when to open vents in the ambulance.
   d. how to transfer potentially communicable patients.

8. The strategy used by an EMS agency to maneuver its ambulances and crews in an effort to reduce response times is referred to as:

   a. line of response.
   b. ambulance deployment.
   c. ambulance stratagem.
   d. zoning.

9. _____ is the ability to muster additional crews, should all the regularly staffed ambulances be on calls or a multiple casualty incident overtaxes the system's resources.

   a. Standards of reliability
   b. System status management
   c. Peak-load backup
   d. Reserve capacity

10. A computerized personnel and ambulance deployment system designed to meet service demands with fewer resources, and to ensure appropriate response time and vehicle locations is called:

   a. standards of reliability.
   b. system status management.
   c. peak-load backup.
   d. reserve capacity.

11. Appropriate response time has to be determined by each community based on:

   a. its resources.
   b. ACLS standards.
   c. American Heart Association standards.
   d. national standards.

12. The number one rule of medicine, "Do no harm!" relates to all of the following people, *except* the:

   a. ambulance operator.
   b. EMT–B.
   c. paramedic.
   d. patient.

13. In addition to personal injury and vehicle repair or replacement, the costs of ambulance collisions include:

   a. increased insurance premiums.
   b. downtime.
   c. lawsuits.
   d. all of the above.

14. One concept that appears in most laws in statutes that deal with emergency vehicle operation is the concept of:

   a. res ipsa locquitor.
   b. negligence.
   c. due regard.
   d. causation.

15. The language described in the concept in question 14 sets up a _____ standard for the operator of an emergency vehicle than for any other driver on the road.

   a. safer
   b. higher
   c. lower
   d. liberal

16. Typical laws allow the operator of an ambulance, while in emergency operation, to be exempt from:

   a. passing over railroad crossings with the gates down.
   b. passing a school bus operator with the blinking red lights on.
   c. the posted parking regulations.
   d. none of the above.

17. Studies have shown that most other motorists do not see or hear your ambulance until it is within _____ feet of their vehicles.

   a. 10 to 25
   b. 25 to 50
   c. 50 to 100
   d. 100 to 200

18. All of the following are recommended guidelines for the proper use of a siren, *except*:

   a. do not pull up close to a vehicle and then sound your siren.
   b. use the siren sparingly and only when you must.
   c. use the siren at all times while the lights are on.
   d. never assume all motorists will hear your siren.

19. Whenever the ambulance is on the road, day or night, the headlights should be turned on to:

   a. increase its visibility.
   b. comply with insurance stipulations.
   c. receive lower insurance premiums.
   d. annoy other motorists.

20. When your ambulance is the first to arrive at the scene of a highway incident and no potential hazards are apparent, you should park your emergency vehicle at least _____ the wreckage.

   a. 50 feet in front of
   b. 100 feet in front of
   c. 50 feet behind
   d. 100 feet behind

21. In 1969, R. Adams Cowley, MD, convinced the _____ state legislature to fund the first statewide state police "medevac" program.

   a. New York
   b. California
   c. Florida
   d. Maryland

22. An MCI is a _____, which results in casualties severely burdening or exceeding the normal EMS resources of an agency in whose area the event occurs.

   a. mass casualty incident
   b. multiple casualty incident
   c. many citizens injured
   d. mixed community incident

23. When you are the first to arrive at the scene of an MCI, the first size-up radio report to the dispatcher is very important and should include:

    a. specific location of the incident.
    b. location of the triage sector.
    c. the time of arrival.
    d. the exact number of patients.

24. A _____ incident is one where the patients need rescue or extrication to gain access to them.

    a. dangerous
    b. safe
    c. continued
    d. closed

25. Though originally developed for fire services, the incident command system (ICS) has been adopted to serve all emergency response disciplines and consists of procedures for controlling:

    a. the media.
    b. equipment and facilities.
    c. critical incident stress.
    d. post-incident stress.

26. ICS is designed to begin developing from the time an incident occurs until:

    a. all victims are safely away from the incident.
    b. the fire or hazard is extinguished or contained.
    c. the requirement for management and operations no longer exists.
    d. all emergency medical responders are safely away.

27. _____ is the functional component of an IMS, which is responsible for obtaining information about the use of technical specialists.

    a. Operations
    b. Planning
    c. Logistics
    d. Finance

28. A key component of ICS is _____, which is the desired number of subordinates that one supervisor can manage effectively at an incident.

    a. consolidated action plan
    b. span of control
    c. singular command
    d. unified command

29. The incident commander is the individual with overall responsibility for managing the incident, which includes:

    a. prioritizing training efforts.
    b. assessing overhaul costs.
    c. designating hospital bed priorities.
    d. developing the incident action plan.

30. While working in an MCI, the use of bibs and vests serves a value in:

    a. making it easy to identify the command officers.
    b. making the command officers safer, with better visibility.
    c. keeping order and avoiding chaos.
    d. identifying the priority of the patients.

31. It is not uncommon for physicians and nurses to stop at the scene of an MCI and offer assistance. Besides utilizing them in the treatment sector, what other area may be appropriate for their expertise?

    a. safety
    b. communications
    c. triage
    d. rescue

32. A very useful aspect to the use of triage tags at an MCI is that:

    a. patients can fill them out themselves.
    b. they do not take any training to use.
    c. they are inexpensive.
    d. they help to eliminate the need to reassess each patient over and over again.

33. Performing a post-incident critique is commonly done after an MCI because:

    a. it serves the same function as a CISD.
    b. every incident has something to teach.
    c. it may involve media coverage.
    d. commanders can critique without the fear of offending anyone.

34. Because there may be units from many different jurisdictions at an MCI, it is easier to use simple sector titles based on:

    a. preference of the incident commander.
    b. geographic location.
    c. available resources.
    d. the function they serve.

35. What is the role of the EMS command or medical command at an MCI?

   a. to be involved in drilling
   b. to be involved in planning and education
   c. to work cooperatively with other emergency commanders
   d. to establish a command post and designate another to stay there

36. An incident involving a residential house fire where all the patients are out on the front lawn of the home is an example of a/an _____ incident.

   a. open
   b. closed
   c. continuing
   d. dangerous

37. The _____ section at an MCI is responsible for providing services and materials, such as the communications unit, medical unit, or food unit, for the incident.

   a. operations
   b. planning
   c. logistics
   d. command

38. When all of the involved agencies at an MCI contribute to the command process by determining the overall goals and objects, and use joint planning for tactical activities, they are working under:

   a. OHSA CFR 29.
   b. NFPA standard 1500.
   c. singular command.
   d. unified command.

39. During an MCI, a consolidated action plan should be developed at the:

   a. dispatch center.
   b. unified command post.
   c. first arriving emergency vehicle.
   d. discretion of the incident commander.

40. START is an acronym for:

   a. simple triage and rapid transport.
   b. standardized triage on rapid timetable.
   c. short triage, alert by radio, and treat.
   d. stage, triage, assess, rate, and transport.

41. At an MCI, triage is done on all patients in an effort to assure that:

   a. the most serious patients are treated and transported first.
   b. all the critical patients go to the best hospitals.
   c. the most important patients get the ALS care.
   d. all low-priority patients receive a different standard of care.

42. One of the most helpful tips that can smooth out operations at an MCI is:

   a. to never let the driver, keys, or stretcher get separated from their ambulance.
   b. to use multiple radios with multiple channels to avoid confusion at the scene.
   c. to drive directly into the incident and look around to see where you are needed.
   d. to talk to the media and keep them advised of the evolving events.

43. Each corner of the ambulance should have flashers that are large and blinking in tandem or unison to help oncoming vehicles:

   a. identify the name of the EMS service.
   b. identify the location and size of the ambulance.
   c. know where the EMS personnel are going to place the cones.
   d. anticipate the placement of flares.

44. While working at the scene of a highway incident, beware that the _____ of the ambulance often obstruct(s) the view of the warning lights to other motorists.

   a. lighted flares
   b. reflector tape
   c. open rear doors
   d. inexperienced driver

45. Fixed-wing aircraft are used as the primary means of emergency transport in:

   a. remote regions, such as parts of Alaska.
   b. missions under fifty miles from a hospital facility.
   c. search and rescue missions.
   d. access to remote areas.

46. Special consideration for aeromedical transport includes the need to intubate the patient prior to flight because of:

   a. the pressure changes during ascent and decent.
   b. limited treatment area in the aircraft.
   c. the temperature changes during the flight.
   d. the various altitudes that the helicopter flies.

47. A helicopter requires a landing zone of approximately _____ feet on relatively level ground.

    a. 50 × 50
    b. 50 × 100
    c. 100 × 100
    d. 100 × 200

48. Which of the following is a special treatment consideration if a patient is going to be transported by helicopter?

    a. Convert IV bags over to pressure infuser bags.
    b. Stay clear of the tail rotor wash only when moving the patient.
    c. Allow the flight crew to direct and maintain a safe landing zone.
    d. Keep all traffic and vehicles 100 feet or more from the helicopter.

49. The Commission of Accreditation of Air Medical Services (CAAMS) was developed as a voluntary process for aeromedical services to:

    a. enforce the FAA standards for air travel.
    b. enforce standards for worker safety.
    c. help communities obtain funding for aeromedical programs.
    d. strengthen the safety of the aviation transport environment.

50. One major disadvantage of aeromedical evacuation is:

    a. cabin size.
    b. the need for special fuel.
    c. rapid access to remote areas.
    d. the need for technical training.

Exam #47 Answer Form

	A	B	C	D		A	B	C	D
1.	❏	❏	❏	❏	26.	❏	❏	❏	❏
2.	❏	❏	❏	❏	27.	❏	❏	❏	❏
3.	❏	❏	❏	❏	28.	❏	❏	❏	❏
4.	❏	❏	❏	❏	29.	❏	❏	❏	❏
5.	❏	❏	❏	❏	30.	❏	❏	❏	❏
6.	❏	❏	❏	❏	31.	❏	❏	❏	❏
7.	❏	❏	❏	❏	32.	❏	❏	❏	❏
8.	❏	❏	❏	❏	33.	❏	❏	❏	❏
9.	❏	❏	❏	❏	34.	❏	❏	❏	❏
10.	❏	❏	❏	❏	35.	❏	❏	❏	❏
11.	❏	❏	❏	❏	36.	❏	❏	❏	❏
12.	❏	❏	❏	❏	37.	❏	❏	❏	❏
13.	❏	❏	❏	❏	38.	❏	❏	❏	❏
14.	❏	❏	❏	❏	39.	❏	❏	❏	❏
15.	❏	❏	❏	❏	40.	❏	❏	❏	❏
16.	❏	❏	❏	❏	41.	❏	❏	❏	❏
17.	❏	❏	❏	❏	42.	❏	❏	❏	❏
18.	❏	❏	❏	❏	43.	❏	❏	❏	❏
19.	❏	❏	❏	❏	44.	❏	❏	❏	❏
20.	❏	❏	❏	❏	45.	❏	❏	❏	❏
21.	❏	❏	❏	❏	46.	❏	❏	❏	❏
22.	❏	❏	❏	❏	47.	❏	❏	❏	❏
23.	❏	❏	❏	❏	48.	❏	❏	❏	❏
24.	❏	❏	❏	❏	49.	❏	❏	❏	❏
25.	❏	❏	❏	❏	50.	❏	❏	❏	❏

Rescue Awareness and Operations

1. The level of rescue training that all paramedics should be trained in is the _____ level.

   a. technical
   b. command
   c. awareness
   d. operations

2. What should set the priority of each rescue?

   a. The time police are able to hold back traffic.
   b. The abilities of the heavy rescue team.
   c. The patient's medical condition.
   d. The EMS providers' need to return to service.

3. Awareness-level training involves the ability to:

   a. comprehend the hazards.
   b. command the incident.
   c. mitigate all hazards.
   d. discern the causes of the reactions.

4. A successful rescue requires:

   a. medical training.
   b. mechanical training.
   c. a combination of a & b.
   d. a patient with minor injuries.

5. In general, all paramedics should have the proper training and PPE to:

   a. allow them to access the patient.
   b. provide assessment of the patient.
   c. provide management of the patient at the scene.
   d. all of the above.

6. It is essential that the paramedic know:

   a. when to enter an unstable situation.
   b. when it is or is not safe to gain access.
   c. how to stabilize a toxic atmosphere.
   d. how to enter a below-grade rescue.

7. What PPE should be immediately available to all the paramedics?

   a. helmets and eye protection
   b. turnout gear and lights
   c. SCBA
   d. back-country survival gear

8. Why are construction hard hats inappropriate for rescue work?

   a. Their duckbill brim is removable.
   b. They do not withstand severe impact.
   c. They are not warm enough.
   d. They have no ANSI rating.

9. What type of helmets are often used in confined space rescue?

   a. standard type fire helmets
   b. kayaking helmets
   c. leather fire helmets
   d. climbing helmets

10. Eye protection should be approved by:

    a. ANSI.
    b. EPA.
    c. NFPA.
    d. EDNA.

11. Eye protection is best provided by:

    a. regular glasses.
    b. a fire helmet face shield.
    c. contact lenses.
    d. industrial safety glasses.

12. The best gloves for rescue work by paramedics are:

    a. latex.
    b. rubber.
    c. leather work gloves.
    d. heavy gauntlet-style firefighting gloves.

13. Nomex®, PBI®, or flame-retardant cotton may be utilized by EMS providers as part of their turnout gear because these materials:

    a. provide limited flash protection.
    b. provide complete flash protection.
    c. are inexpensive and readily available.
    d. provide protection against sharp, jagged metal or glass.

14. What is the best blanket to use for patient protection from heat and glass dust?

    a. inexpensive vinyl tarps
    b. aluminized rescue blankets
    c. wool blankets
    d. plastic sheeting

15. What should be used to shield the patient from sharp-edged objects or glass during a rescue?

    a. plastic sheeting
    b. sheets
    c. backboards
    d. vinyl tarps

16. What type of respiratory protection is considered adequate for most rescues?

    a. N-95
    b. HEPA mask
    c. surgical mask
    d. non-rebreather mask

17. Which is the last technique to employ in a water rescue?

    a. reach
    b. row
    c. throw
    d. go

18. The most common associated problem in water rescue is:

    a. strainers.
    b. hydraulics.
    c. eddies.
    d. hypothermia.

19. Another name for written safety procedures used by rescue teams is:

    a. protocols.
    b. regulations.
    c. SOPs.
    d. bylaws.

20. The first three phases of a rescue operation are:

    a. hazard control, disentanglement, and gaining access.
    b. hazard control, gaining access, and medical treatment.
    c. arrival and size-up, gaining access, and disentanglement.
    d. arrival and size-up, hazard control, and gaining access.

21. The person responsible for making the "go/no go" decision for a rescue operation is called the:

    a. incident commander.
    b. lead medic.
    c. team leader.
    d. safety officer.

22. For the patient who is entrapped for a considerable amount of time, the paramedic must be prepared to:

    a. rise above swift running waters.
    b. provide immense psychological support.
    c. overcome life-threatening atmospheres.
    d. develop the plan for, and lead in, the disentanglement.

23. What is the value of a rescue plan?

    a. It describes how to respond to every incident.
    b. Improvement of personnel safety and operational success.
    c. There are fewer rescuers needed at incidents.
    d. The location to which units respond is specified.

24. Rescues that will take an extended amount of time may require:

    a. staging with protection from weather.
    b. food and hydration for personnel.
    c. rotation of personnel.
    d. all of the above.

25. Fluid for rehydration of personnel should consist of any of the following, *except*:

    a. water.
    b. Gatorade®.
    c. coffee.
    d. POWERade®.

26. Upon arrival at the rescue incident, the EMS crew should:

    a. conduct a scene size-up.
    b. determine the hospital destination.
    c. disentangle the patient.
    d. set out flares on the roadway.

27. Upon arrival at a rescue search, what is the purpose of doing a risk versus benefit analysis?

   a. to determine the cause of the incident
   b. to determine if it is a body recovery
   c. to determine the full damage of the incident
   d. to be eligible for federal funding

28. Examples of on-scene hazards that need to be controlled by the paramedic upon arrival at the scene include:

   a. a car fire.
   b. chemical spills.
   c. creating a safe perimeter.
   d. downed electrical wires.

29. _____ in an example of a safety precaution to be taken at every rescue.

   a. Utilizing triage tags
   b. Establishing EMS command
   c. Wearing the appropriate PPE
   d. Performing an initial assessment on each patient

30. _____ is an example of a potential hazard that may exist at the scene of a rescue.

   a. A confined space
   b. More than two patients
   c. More than one EMS service
   d. More than one emergency service

31. When a rescue situation involves a hidden patient, the paramedic should consider requesting:

   a. a surgeon to the scene.
   b. a helicopter to the scene.
   c. an on-scene SAF specialist.
   d. medical control to the scene.

32. In what phase of a rescue is the first patient contact typically made by EMS?

   a. after gaining access
   b. arrival and size-up
   c. after hazard control
   d. after disentanglement

33. Paramedics should not enter an area to provide patient care unless they are:

   a. trained in all aspects of rescue.
   b. authorized by medical control to do so.
   c. protected from hazards with PPE.
   d. responding in a two-medic unit.

34. The rescue term that means to remove the debris or parts of the vehicle from around the patient(s) so the patient may be freed for removal is:

   a. evacuation.
   b. extrication.
   c. disentanglement.
   d. gaining access.

35. The initial ALS interventions may be held off and only BLS provided when patients are found in any of the following situations, *except*:

   a. stranded in swift moving water.
   b. entrapped in vehicles with a fire.
   c. just removed from a pool.
   d. overcome by life-threatening atmospheres.

36. In the situations listed in question 35, rapid transport of a non-stabilized patient to a safer location is justified based on the:

   a. high volume of patients.
   b. risk of injury to the rescuers.
   c. expense of the cost of care.
   d. age of the patient involved.

37. The most technical and time-consuming part of a rescue is the _____ phase.

   a. hazard control
   b. extrication
   c. disentanglement
   d. removal

38. The patient packaging should take into consideration the:

   a. distance the ambulance will travel to the hospital.
   b. means of egress.
   c. duration of disentanglement.
   d. age of the patient.

39. If it is necessary to lift a patient vertically out of a narrow hole, the best device to consider using is a:

   a. scoop stretcher.
   b. SKED.
   c. KED.
   d. Stokes® basket.

40. Paramedics should consider which of the following to prepare for a water rescue incident?

   a. Learn dive rescue.
   b. Wear a PFD around water or ice.
   c. Take a boating course.
   d. Learn scuba.

41. With the exception of hot tubs, most bodies of water are considered cold water. What is the problem with being immersed in cold water?

    a. The patient inhales water faster.
    b. The patient loses salts and electrolytes rapidly.
    c. The patient's body is less buoyant.
    d. Hypothermia can rapidly set in.

42. Humans cannot maintain body temperature in water that is less than _____ °F.

    a. 98
    b. 96
    c. 94
    d. 92

43. Compared to the air, water causes heat _____ at a rate _____ times faster.

    a. loss; five
    b. loss; twenty-five
    c. gain; ten
    d. gain; fifteen

44. Why should hypothermic patients be removed from water in a horizontal position?

    a. They may have too much blood in the periphery.
    b. They may be dehydrated from cold diuresis.
    c. They do not tolerate the vagal stimuli.
    d. They cannot tolerate the increased ICP.

45. When suddenly submerged while waiting for rescue, you should assume the _____ position.

    a. sniffing
    b. heat escape lessening position (HELP)
    c. tripod
    d. floating

46. A survivability estimate should be done quickly after arriving at the scene of a water rescue incident. Of the following, which is not relevant to the estimate?

    a. number of trained and equipped rescuers
    b. past history of submersion
    c. any known trauma to the patient
    d. age of the patient

47. What is the primary danger of a low head dam?

    a. The water can rise above the dam.
    b. The water tends to throw objects clear.
    c. It is easy to get stuck on large rocks or boulders.
    d. Recirculating water is difficult to get out of.

48. If you accidentally fall into a body of swiftly moving water, what should you do?

    a. float downstream feet first
    b. assume the HELP position
    c. attempt to walk out
    d. float downstream head and hands first

49. Water moving through obstructions is sometimes called a "strainer." Examples include each of the following, *except*:

    a. a large boulder in the water.
    b. downed trees.
    c. grating over a pipe entry.
    d. wire rebar.

50. When water turns a bend in the river, the _____ of the curve moves _____ of the curve.

    a. inside; faster than the outside
    b. inside; slower than the outside
    c. outside; slower than the inside
    d. outside; faster than the inside

51. Alcohol is a contributory factor to as many as _____ % of boating fatalities.

    a. 10
    b. 30
    c. 50
    d. 75

52. What is the most effective strategy of preventing deaths from boating accidents?

    a. requiring boating education
    b. enforcing anti-drinking laws
    c. carrying a PFD for each boater
    d. each boater wearing a PFD

53. The protective response of the human body to cold water submersion is called the:

    a. mainstream reflex.
    b. mammalian diving reflex.
    c. immersion factor.
    d. HELP response.

54. Upon arrival at a water rescue, the focus of what the paramedic should ask the bystanders is:

    a. the precise location where the patient went under.
    b. how long the patient was in the water.
    c. if the patient seemed intoxicated.
    d. what the patient was wearing.

55. When a patient is found in a pool and is suspected to have a neck injury, to properly apply a backboard in the pool takes at least _____ rescuers in the water.

    a. one
    b. two
    c. three
    d. four

56. According to NIOSH, it is estimated that _____ % of the fatalities associated with confined spaces are people attempting to rescue the patient.

    a. 10
    b. 20
    c. 40
    d. 60

57. What is the biggest problem with confined spaces?

    a. They are oxygen deficient.
    b. They are difficult to crawl through.
    c. They are not well lit.
    d. They contain hazardous materials.

58. Which statement is most accurate about an employer's responsibility in regard to confined work spaces?

    a. All confined work spaces must have the appropriate permit.
    b. Non-permitted work sites are unlikely locations for emergencies.
    c. All employers are required to develop a confined space rescue program.
    d. Most employers are required to develop a confined space rescue program.

59. What is the hazard associated with dust?

    a. It has a terrible odor.
    b. It can damage emergency equipment.
    c. It can create an explosive hazard.
    d. It is difficult to see.

60. Water seepage, ground vibrations, and disregarding safety regulations are some of the reasons for:

    a. structural collapse.
    b. vehicle rescue.
    c. a trench cave-in.
    d. a confined space rescue.

61. The initial response of the EMS provider to a cave-in should include size-up and:

    a. stabilization of the scene.
    b. establishing a perimeter.
    c. access to the patients.
    d. initiating extrication.

62. The trench rescue team should make access to the cave-in only after:

    a. shoring is in place.
    b. the patient has been located.
    c. all the dirt has been removed.
    d. ropes have been properly placed.

63. What is the greatest hazard when working a highway operation?

    a. broken glass
    b. crowds
    c. fire hazards
    d. traffic

64. When working at the scene of a highway rescue that involves a vehicle with an alternative fuel source, one potential danger is:

    a. the risk of fire or explosion.
    b. not being able to turn off the vehicle.
    c. not being able to stabilize the vehicle.
    d. not being able to disconnect the battery.

65. The ambulance loading area at a highway operation should:

    a. be used as a point to congregate.
    b. not be directly exposed to traffic.
    c. rely on the rear blinking lights to stop cars.
    d. be off the side of the road.

66. When parked at the scene of a highway operation, the ambulance should:

    a. shut off all the lights.
    b. turn on only a minimum of warning lights.
    c. keep on the alternating head lights.
    d. turn on all the emergency lights.

67. When using flares at a highway operation, they should:

    a. direct the flow of traffic away from emergency workers.
    b. only be placed by law enforcement personnel.
    c. be used when the ground is wet.
    d. not be used if there is snow on the road.

68. Why should the paramedic be especially concerned when a vehicle has gone off the road into tall grass?

    a. The potential for a fire hazard is increased.
    b. It will be difficult to find the vehicle.
    c. The potential for an electric hazard is greater.
    d. Patients may wander away from the scene.

69. Why can an energy-absorbing bumper be a hazard to EMS personnel?

    a. The fluid they leak is highly toxic.
    b. If loaded, they may release when unexpected.
    c. They can hide the true damage to the vehicle.
    d. They have been known to explode.

70. A supplemental restraint system may be a potential hazard to rescue personnel because:

    a. the straps can get in the way.
    b. the straps are difficult to cut.
    c. it can be difficult to remove from the patient.
    d. it can inflate when not expected.

71. If, upon arrival at the scene of a car crash, the vehicle is on its side, off the road on an embankment, it will be necessary to rapidly:

    a. gain access.
    b. stabilize the vehicle.
    c. disentangle the patient.
    d. extricate the patient.

72. After assuring that the vehicle's ignition has been turned off, what can the paramedic do to prepare to gain access?

    a. Tell the patient to try to crawl out.
    b. Attempt to climb up on the car and open the door.
    c. Stabilize the vehicle with cribbing.
    d. Break both the front and rear windows.

73. The part of an auto's anatomy that separates the engine compartment from the occupant compartment is called the:

    a. rocker panel.
    b. firewall.
    c. Nader pin.
    d. "A" post.

74. The reason why the doors do not fly open when a car is involved in a collision is because of the:

    a. firewall.
    b. tempered glass.
    c. Nader pin.
    d. roof support posts.

75. The windshield in vehicles is made of _____ glass.

    a. unbreakable
    b. safety
    c. tempered
    d. plastic

76. Glass that has a plastic laminate layer, which limits how it breaks, is called _____ glass.

    a. Nader
    b. tempered
    c. safety
    d. UV shield

77. The easiest way to break the _____ glass in the rear window is with a _____ object.

    a. tempered; sharp
    b. safety; sharp
    c. tempered; blunt
    d. safety; blunt

78. Unless the hydraulic spreader is used for accessing a crushed car door, the _____ must be disengaged prior to manually prying the door open.

    a. key
    b. door reinforcement bar
    c. battery cable
    d. Nader pin

79. The first step in accessing a car with a crushed door that has no safety hazards and is stabilized is to:

    a. break the glass in the rear window.
    b. remove the Nader pin.
    c. remove the roof.
    d. try to open all four doors first.

80. After taking the first step as described in question 79, the paramedic should next consider the need to:

    a. cut off the door at the hinges.
    b. pull the steering wheel through the windshield.
    c. gain access through the window farthest away from the patient.
    d. remove the roof of the vehicle.

81. The area at a collision scene where the rescue takes place is called the:

    a. outer circle.
    b. inner circle.
    c. command post.
    d. hot zone.

82. A steep slope that, in good weather, is capable of being walked up without using your hands is called:

    a. high angle.
    b. low angle.
    c. flat terrain.
    d. limited access terrain.

83. When transporting a patient over rough terrain, it is recommended that a _____ stretcher be used.

    a. folding
    b. Stokes®
    c. wheeled
    d. limited access

84. The strongest basket stretchers are made of:

    a. wire and tubular metal.
    b. aluminum and plastic.
    c. enduro-plastic.
    d. polycarbonate.

85. Of the following preparations for transporting a patient over rough terrain, which is not necessary?

    a. A harness should be applied to the patient.
    b. A litter should be used to protect the patient's face.
    c. Leg stirrups should be applied to the patient.
    d. The patient should be restrained in a body bag.

86. A team of rescuers to carry out a Stokes® and patient over rough terrain consists of _____ rescuers and extra teams if the personnel are available.

    a. four
    b. five
    c. six
    d. eight

87. Even though you may not be trained in high-angle rescue, there will be a need for helpers at the scene to:

    a. haul on the lines as instructed.
    b. rappel down to the patient.
    c. set up the rigging.
    d. coil the rope.

88. When an aerial ladder is used to remove a Stokes® basket from a building's roof, it is necessary to:

    a. belay the basket with a rope.
    b. use the ladder like a crane.
    c. strap the basket to the end of the ladder.
    d. slide the basket down the top of the ladder.

89. When a helicopter is used to pick up a Stokes® and move it to another nearby location, this is called a:

    a. flying Baker maneuver.
    b. rappel-based rescue.
    c. one-skid rescue.
    d. short haul.

90. A patient who has fallen off a cliff, who is still alive and will need a lengthy litter carryout, could benefit from a paramedic being trained to:

    a. cleanse wounds.
    b. reposition dislocations.
    c. manage hyperthermia.
    d. assess a 12-lead ECG.

Exam #48 Answer Form

	A	B	C	D		A	B	C	D
1.	❏	❏	❏	❏	27.	❏	❏	❏	❏
2.	❏	❏	❏	❏	28.	❏	❏	❏	❏
3.	❏	❏	❏	❏	29.	❏	❏	❏	❏
4.	❏	❏	❏	❏	30.	❏	❏	❏	❏
5.	❏	❏	❏	❏	31.	❏	❏	❏	❏
6.	❏	❏	❏	❏	32.	❏	❏	❏	❏
7.	❏	❏	❏	❏	33.	❏	❏	❏	❏
8.	❏	❏	❏	❏	34.	❏	❏	❏	❏
9.	❏	❏	❏	❏	35.	❏	❏	❏	❏
10.	❏	❏	❏	❏	36.	❏	❏	❏	❏
11.	❏	❏	❏	❏	37.	❏	❏	❏	❏
12.	❏	❏	❏	❏	38.	❏	❏	❏	❏
13.	❏	❏	❏	❏	39.	❏	❏	❏	❏
14.	❏	❏	❏	❏	40.	❏	❏	❏	❏
15.	❏	❏	❏	❏	41.	❏	❏	❏	❏
16.	❏	❏	❏	❏	42.	❏	❏	❏	❏
17.	❏	❏	❏	❏	43.	❏	❏	❏	❏
18.	❏	❏	❏	❏	44.	❏	❏	❏	❏
19.	❏	❏	❏	❏	45.	❏	❏	❏	❏
20.	❏	❏	❏	❏	46.	❏	❏	❏	❏
21.	❏	❏	❏	❏	47.	❏	❏	❏	❏
22.	❏	❏	❏	❏	48.	❏	❏	❏	❏
23.	❏	❏	❏	❏	49.	❏	❏	❏	❏
24.	❏	❏	❏	❏	50.	❏	❏	❏	❏
25.	❏	❏	❏	❏	51.	❏	❏	❏	❏
26.	❏	❏	❏	❏	52.	❏	❏	❏	❏

	A	B	C	D			A	B	C	D
53.	❏	❏	❏	❏	72.	❏	❏	❏	❏
54.	❏	❏	❏	❏	73.	❏	❏	❏	❏
55.	❏	❏	❏	❏	74.	❏	❏	❏	❏
56.	❏	❏	❏	❏	75.	❏	❏	❏	❏
57.	❏	❏	❏	❏	76.	❏	❏	❏	❏
58.	❏	❏	❏	❏	77.	❏	❏	❏	❏
59.	❏	❏	❏	❏	78.	❏	❏	❏	❏
60.	❏	❏	❏	❏	79.	❏	❏	❏	❏
61.	❏	❏	❏	❏	80.	❏	❏	❏	❏
62.	❏	❏	❏	❏	81.	❏	❏	❏	❏
63.	❏	❏	❏	❏	82.	❏	❏	❏	❏
64.	❏	❏	❏	❏	83.	❏	❏	❏	❏
65.	❏	❏	❏	❏	84.	❏	❏	❏	❏
66.	❏	❏	❏	❏	85.	❏	❏	❏	❏
67.	❏	❏	❏	❏	86.	❏	❏	❏	❏
68.	❏	❏	❏	❏	87.	❏	❏	❏	❏
69.	❏	❏	❏	❏	88.	❏	❏	❏	❏
70.	❏	❏	❏	❏	89.	❏	❏	❏	❏
71.	❏	❏	❏	❏	90.	❏	❏	❏	❏

Hazardous Material Awareness and Operations

1. The first standard to guide hazardous material (haz-mat) operations specifically for EMS workers was NFPA:

   a. 472
   b. 473
   c. 704
   d. 1500

2. NFPA standard _____ established a system of placarding and labeling fixed facilities for hazardous materials.

   a. 472
   b. 473
   c. 704
   d. 1500

3. _____ is the minimal level of hazmat training at which the responder can perform risk assessment procedures and conduct basic control, containment, and confinement operations.

   a. First responder awareness
   b. First responder operations
   c. Hazardous material technician
   d. Hazardous material specialist

4. Which of the following is not a typical method for identifying hazardous materials?

   a. NFPA 472
   b. dispatcher-obtained information
   c. material safety data sheets (MSDS)
   d. Department of Transportation (DOT) placards

5. There are _____ levels of hazmat training required by the Occupational Safety and Health Administration (OSHA) regulations.

   a. four
   b. five
   c. six
   d. ten

6. The _____ provides written information about the names of substance, UN numbers, placard facsimiles, emergency action guides, and evacuation and isolation information.

   a. *North American Emergency Response Guidebook*
   b. MSDS
   c. CHEMTREC
   d. bill of lading

7. DOT placards classify gases into the following categories: corrosive, flammable, poison A, and:

   a. poison B.
   b. combustible.
   c. noncorrosive.
   d. nonflammable.

8. _____ are used throughout the industry as a means of identifying chemicals and complying with the employee's Right to Know.

   a. Shipping papers
   b. Bills of lading
   c. MSDS
   d. Waybills

9. The stages of metabolism of a poison are the same as with any drug and include all of the following, *except*:

   a. absorption.
   b. distribution
   c. elimination.
   d. adaptation.

10. _____ is/are how and what a poison does to the body.

    a. Poison actions
    b. Poison adaptations
    c. Degradation
    d. Absorption

11. Decontamination is the physical or _____ process of removing hazardous material from exposed persons or equipment.

   a. mechanical
   b. chemical
   c. filtration
   d. biodegradable

12. The procedure for the decontamination (decon) of a critical patient is a _____-step process.

   a. two
   b. four
   c. seven
   d. eight

13. The decon corridor, which consists of _____ stages, is the method used for decontamination of noncritical patients and rescuers.

   a. five
   b. six
   c. seven
   d. eight

14. Water is a universal decon solution that dilutes and reduces _____ absorption.

   a. metabolic
   b. topical
   c. enteral
   d. parenteral

15. Which of the following is not a common solution used by EMS providers for decon?

   a. tincture of green soap
   b. isopropyl alcohol
   c. vegetable oil
   d. milk

16. The properties of potential hazards for chemical substances, which are listed on 704 placards and other references, include flammability, health hazards, and:

   a. reliability.
   b. toxicity.
   c. relativity.
   d. reactivity.

17. Prior to working at an incident where hazmat is present, _____ is/are established to prevent injury and unnecessary exposure to the substance.

   a. officers
   b. zones
   c. quarters
   d. precedence

18. A paramedic with first responder awareness training can take which of the following actions at the scene of a hazmat exposure?

   a. Don level 1 and 2 PPE.
   b. Participate in containment.
   c. Collect a sample of the material for the ED.
   d. Instruct the patient to remove contaminated shoes and clothing.

19. _____ is how much substance it takes to cause a physiologic response.

   a. Dose response
   b. Route of exposure
   c. Synergistic effect
   d. Toxicity

20. One factor that can make field decontamination of a patient difficult is:

   a. having an MSDS available.
   b. unlimited level of training.
   c. wearing PPE that is compatible with all chemicals.
   d. critical patient condition.

21. The maximum concentration to which a healthy adult can be exposed to a hazardous material without risk of injury is called the:

   a. ceiling level.
   b. flash point.
   c. permissible exposure limit.
   d. threshold limit value-ceiling.

22. _____ is a time-weighted average concentration that must not be exceeded during any eight-hour work shift or forty-hour workweek.

   a. Ceiling level
   b. Short-term exposure limit
   c. Permissible exposure limit
   d. Threshold limit value

23. The reference book *North American Emergency Response Guidebook* gives the paramedic three methods to reference a substance, leading to a guide that provides all of the following information, *except*:

   a. potential hazards.
   b. access to MSDS.
   c. first aid treatment.
   d. safety precautions.

24. The Occupational Health and Safety Administration (OSHA) regulations are published in the:

    a. product packaging labels.
    b. MSDS
    c. *North American Emergency Response Guidebook*
    d. Code of Federal Regulations (CFR)

25. CHEMTREC is an information resource service operated by the _____ and is available by an 800 phone number for detailed information on the chemicals involved and the manufacturer of the chemical.

    a. Centers for Disease Control (CDC)
    b. Federal Regulatory Commission
    c. DOT
    d. Chemical Manufacturers Association

Exam #49 Answer Form

	A	B	C	D			A	B	C	D
1.	❏	❏	❏	❏		14.	❏	❏	❏	❏
2.	❏	❏	❏	❏		15.	❏	❏	❏	❏
3.	❏	❏	❏	❏		16.	❏	❏	❏	❏
4.	❏	❏	❏	❏		17.	❏	❏	❏	❏
5.	❏	❏	❏	❏		18.	❏	❏	❏	❏
6.	❏	❏	❏	❏		19.	❏	❏	❏	❏
7.	❏	❏	❏	❏		20.	❏	❏	❏	❏
8.	❏	❏	❏	❏		21.	❏	❏	❏	❏
9.	❏	❏	❏	❏		22.	❏	❏	❏	❏
10.	❏	❏	❏	❏		23.	❏	❏	❏	❏
11.	❏	❏	❏	❏		24.	❏	❏	❏	❏
12.	❏	❏	❏	❏		25.	❏	❏	❏	❏
13.	❏	❏	❏	❏						

50

Crime Scene Awareness

1. _____ is one type of violence that threatens citizens and government.
   a. Suicide
   b. Homicide
   c. Terrorism
   d. Domestic violence

2. As part of the hazard awareness in the scene size-up, the paramedic's safety concerns should begin:
   a. in the classroom.
   b. with information obtained from dispatch.
   c. as soon as you enter the neighborhood.
   d. when you arrive at the call address.

3. If, while on the scene, the paramedic becomes aware of a potential threat, weapons, or any violent or abusive action towards him, the paramedic should:
   a. look for a second exit.
   b. retreat right away.
   c. intercede with pepper spray.
   d. wait for police before further intervention.

4. _____ is an example of a nonviolent danger that may pose a threat to the paramedic responding to an emergency.
   a. A vicious pet
   b. A downed power line
   c. Carbon monoxide poisoning
   d. A crowd in front of a residence

5. Why might the paramedic be mistaken for a police officer and thus put himself in danger?
   a. Paramedics arrive in vehicles with lights and sirens.
   b. Some paramedics wear a badge and holsters with medical equipment in them.
   c. Some EMS agencies wear uniforms that resemble the police uniforms in their neighborhood.
   d. Any of the above could cause the paramedic to be mistaken for law enforcement.

6. When dispatched to a known violent scene, the paramedic should stage the vehicle:
   a. at least 50 feet from the scene.
   b. at least 100 feet from the scene.
   c. out of sight of the scene.
   d. directly behind a police vehicle.

7. One strategy to practice, in an effort to avoid injury to yourself and your crew, is to:
   a. stand to the side of the door before ringing or knocking.
   b. backlight your partner while he rings or knocks on the front door.
   c. broadcast your approach with lights and sirens, right up to the residence.
   d. announce your presence, then knock or ring, and listen for signs of danger.

8. When approaching a vehicle that is at the side of the road, clues that typically indicate there may be a dangerous condition include all of the following, *except*:
   a. signs of alcohol or drug use.
   b. arguing between the occupants of the vehicle.
   c. any open or unlatched hood or trunk.
   d. all the doors are locked.

9. Before getting out of the ambulance to approach a vehicle on the highway, it is a good idea to notify the dispatcher of the situation and the:
   a. exact location.
   b. color of the vehicle.
   c. number of occupants.
   d. lack of activity where activity is likely.

10. The paramedic should initially approach the vehicle from the passenger side because the:
    a. posts of the vehicle will keep the paramedic safe from a gunshot.
    b. driver would normally expect the police to approach on the driver's side.
    c. paramedic will have a better view of a dangerous situation.
    d. traffic side is usually inaccessible.

11. While approaching a vehicle on the highway, one partner initially remains in the ambulance to watch for hazards, while the other paramedic who is going to approach the vehicle should:

a. chock the wheels of the vehicle.
b. copy the license plate number and state.
c. have a portable radio in hand.
d. set up a safety zone.

12. In a number of communities, the medical personnel wear white shirts and bright colored jackets with retro-reflective stripes and large clear lettering that says "EMS" because:

a. this is a great public relations tactic.
b. it keeps them from looking like police officers.
c. it makes them more visible in traffic.
d. it is the boss's idea.

13. The Crips, Bloods, Latin Kings, and the Banditos are all names of:

a. rock bands.
b. schools.
c. street gangs.
d. rap groups.

14. EMS providers may be called to respond to a clandestine drug lab for:

a. injuries from an explosion.
b. monitoring suspicious patients.
c. assisting the DEA with moving chemicals.
d. assistance in breaking down the cookers.

15. A clandestine drug lab is designed to do chemical:

a. synthesis and create drugs.
b. conversion of drugs.
c. extraction and prepare tablets.
d. any of the above.

16. It is not uncommon for _____ in or near a clandestine drug lab to warn the criminals of the approach of intruders.

a. undercover FBI to be
b. snipers to be staged
c. booby traps to be set
d. children

17. The presence of a street gang in a community increases the:

a. value of the properties.
b. awareness for graffiti.
c. potential for street violence.
d. Good Samaritan effort.

18. Street gangs often have unique clothing that they call their _____ , which are an identifier of the group and may represent the member's status within the group.

a. leathers
b. rags
c. colors
d. stripes

19. If you believe that you have arrived at the scene of a clandestine drug lab, the safest action for you is to:

a. not move, but call for police.
b. act as if you do not know that it is a drug lab.
c. care for the patient but watch out for chemical exposure.
d. leave immediately and call law enforcement.

20. Who is considered the best personnel to manage an incident at a clandestine drug lab?

a. the fire department
b. the DEA
c. a chemical specialist from the nearest college
d. the hazmat team

21. The victim of domestic violence may be a male or female who is experiencing physical, emotional, sexual, verbal, or _____ violence.

a. critical
b. accusing
c. economic
d. judgmental

22. Which of the following clues might cause you to suspect that a patient is a victim of domestic violence?

a. The patient has very poor hygiene.
b. The patient fears her next-door neighbor.
c. The living conditions are extremely unsanitary.
d. The patient has injuries that do not match her story.

23. Which of the following actions should the paramedic avoid if she suspects domestic violence?

a. Treat the patient.
b. Provide a phone number for a domestic violence hotline or shelter.
c. Protect the victim by getting between the victim and the abuser.
d. Do not be judgmental.

24. One of the rules of tactical safety that the paramedic must follow on all calls is:

a. wait to enter the scene with the police.
b. avoid danger by never entering the scene.
c. avoidance is always preferable to confrontation.
d. if you are not sure of a potential danger, call dispatch before entering the scene.

25. If you have to retreat from a dangerous scene, be sure to:

    a. document that you did not abandon the patient.
    b. make sure the dispatcher does not send any further EMS units directly into the scene.
    c. bring the patient with you.
    d. bring cover with you.

26. Which of the following is most correct about concealment for the paramedic?

    a. Concealment is positioning the paramedic or crew behind an object that hides them from the view of others.
    b. Concealment offers ballistic protection if the perpetrator begins to fire a weapon.
    c. An example of concealment is hiding behind a wooden picket fence.
    d. Concealment should be used when approaching a residence.

27. What can the paramedics do if an aggressor seems to be chasing them?

    a. Strike before the aggressor strikes you.
    b. Do not try to anticipate the moves of the aggressor.
    c. Use pepper spray or mace to slow the aggressor.
    d. Throw the equipment to slow or trip the aggressor.

28. All of the following statements about body armor are correct, *except*:

    a. Kevlar® has reduced protection when wet.
    b. body armor does not offer protection against high-velocity rifle bullets.
    c. body armor does protect against thin or dull-edged weapons.
    d. one should avoid having a false sense of security when wearing body armor.

29. In some cities, a limited number of EMS providers are trained in special tactics to accompany the police on high-risk operations. This program is called:

    a. CONTOMS.
    b. rescue EMS.
    c. tactical EMS.
    d. Superhero EMS.

30. The _____ program, started in 1989, was designed to meet the specialized medical training to support law enforcement operations and was funded by the Department of Defense.

    a. CONTOMS
    b. LEA/SWAT team
    c. SWAT–Medic
    d. TEMS

31. When removing clothing from a patient at a crime scene that is stained in blood or body fluids, the paramedic should avoid:

    a. cutting along the seam of the clothing.
    b. cutting through a knife or bullet hole.
    c. having law enforcement assist.
    d. placing items separately.

32. After removing the clothing from a patient at a crime scene, the paramedic should place the clothing in:

    a. a paper bag.
    b. a ziplock bag.
    c. a towel.
    d. the patient's bathtub.

33. If a person is found hanging and the paramedic is going to attempt a resuscitation, the paramedic should wear gloves and take the patient down by _____ the knot.

    a. untying
    b. cutting through
    c. getting the police to cut
    d. cutting to avoid

34. Wearing gloves while working at the scene of a crime may prevent the paramedic from leaving fingerprints, but it does not prevent:

    a. leaving the moisture from her skin at the scene.
    b. leaving the oil from her skin at the scene.
    c. destroying or "smudging" the perpetrator's prints.
    d. the spread of blood-borne disease.

35. The paramedic can minimize risks when working in a potentially dangerous situation by:

    a. not wearing a clip-on tie.
    b. keeping hands in his pockets to appear non-threatening.
    c. keeping a safe stance with feet apart, ready to react.
    d. keeping a stethoscope around the neck to look like a doctor.

Exam #50 Answer Form

	A	B	C	D		A	B	C	D
1.	❏	❏	❏	❏	19.	❏	❏	❏	❏
2.	❏	❏	❏	❏	20.	❏	❏	❏	❏
3.	❏	❏	❏	❏	21.	❏	❏	❏	❏
4.	❏	❏	❏	❏	22.	❏	❏	❏	❏
5.	❏	❏	❏	❏	23.	❏	❏	❏	❏
6.	❏	❏	❏	❏	24.	❏	❏	❏	❏
7.	❏	❏	❏	❏	25.	❏	❏	❏	❏
8.	❏	❏	❏	❏	26.	❏	❏	❏	❏
9.	❏	❏	❏	❏	27.	❏	❏	❏	❏
10.	❏	❏	❏	❏	28.	❏	❏	❏	❏
11.	❏	❏	❏	❏	29.	❏	❏	❏	❏
12.	❏	❏	❏	❏	30.	❏	❏	❏	❏
13.	❏	❏	❏	❏	31.	❏	❏	❏	❏
14.	❏	❏	❏	❏	32.	❏	❏	❏	❏
15.	❏	❏	❏	❏	33.	❏	❏	❏	❏
16.	❏	❏	❏	❏	34.	❏	❏	❏	❏
17.	❏	❏	❏	❏	35.	❏	❏	❏	❏
18.	❏	❏	❏	❏					

51

Basic Life Support (BLS) Resuscitation Issues

1. The care provided in the first few minutes of a life-threatening emergency is called:

   a. CPR.
   b. focused history and physical exam (FHPE).
   c. basic life support.
   d. ongoing assessment.

2. One of the major changes in the Guidelines 2005 was to improve the effectiveness of the delivery chest compressions by:

   a. emphasizing that all rescuers should push hard and fast.
   b. allowing more time between compressions for better chest recoil.
   c. increasing the compression rate and omitting ventilations for the lay rescuer.
   d. adding voice prompts in AEDs and defibrillators, which remind the rescuer to maintain the correct compression rate.

3. The general term now used to describe the spectrum of disease from acute angina to myocardial infarction is:

   a. heart attack.
   b. acute coronary syndrome (ACS).
   c. unstable angina.
   d. coronary illness.

4. In an effort to maintain the most effective delivery of chest compressions during a sudden cardiac arrest (SCA), it is recommend that the rescuers performing compressions switch positions every _____ minutes.

   a. two
   b. three
   c. four
   d. five

5. For the adult patient who is not breathing, each rescue breath should be provided:

   a. one second per breath.
   b. over two seconds.
   c. every six to eight seconds.
   d. every thirty seconds.

6. The new recommendation for one-rescuer CPR is for a compression ventilation ratio of:

   a. 30:2 for all rescuers.
   b. 30:2 for lay rescuers only.
   c. 15:2 for healthcare providers only.
   d. 30:2 for healthcare providers only.

7. The goal of the Guidelines 2005 was to develop widely accepted international resuscitation guidelines that were:

   a. based on a majority vote.
   b. based on the least cost to implement.
   c. based on scientific evidence.
   d. easy to read and explain.

8. Guidelines that are supported by very good evidence of effectiveness and safety in humans are class:

   a. I.
   b. IIa.
   c. IIb.
   d. III.

9. Guidelines supported by fair to good evidence of effectiveness and safety in humans with evidence of harm are class:

   a. I.
   b. IIa.
   c. IIb.
   d. III.

10. Actions or interventions with insufficient evidence to support a final recommendation for clinical use are placed into class:

   a. IIa.
   b. IIb.
   c. III.
   d. Indeterminate.

11. The Guidelines 2005 recommend that when attempting defibrillation:

    a. all rescuers deliver one shock followed by immediate CPR for two minutes.
    b. lay rescuers deliver one shock followed by immediate CPR for five minutes.
    c. using an AED, on children one to eight years old, the dose is the same as an adult.
    d. healthcare providers deliver three shocks followed by immediate CPR for one minute.

12. Terminating the code on a non-traumatic cardiac arrest victim, after an adequate trial of BLS and ALS has been done, to support the survivors would be an example of a Class _____ guideline.

    a. I
    b. IIa
    c. IIb
    d. III

13. All healthcare providers with a duty to perform CPR should be trained, equipped, and authorized to perform defibrillation is a class _____ guideline.

    a. I
    b. IIa
    c. IIb
    d. III

14. For the infant or child patient who is not breathing, each rescue breath should be provided:

    a. over two seconds.
    b. every one to two seconds.
    c. every three to five seconds.
    d. every six to eight seconds.

15. The recommendation for interruptions in CPR for pulse checks should:

    a. occur once every minute.
    b. take less than five seconds.
    c. take less than ten seconds.
    d. not occur more than once every five minutes.

16. When the rescuer performing the chest compressions allows the chest to recoil after each compression, this action:

    a. allows the heart to fill with blood.
    b. allows each ventilation to fill the lungs.
    c. reduces the amount of compressions delivered each minute.
    d. increases the amount of compressions delivered each minute.

17. When providing ventilations without an advanced airway in the patient experiencing cardiac arrest, the rescuer should avoid overventilation because:

    a. it impedes blood return to the heart.
    b. it increases the venous capacity of the heart.
    c. it reduces the threshold for cardioversion.
    d. it reduces the ventricular fibrillation threshold.

18. When an individual executes his right of self-determination and declares he does not want to be resuscitated if he becomes unresponsive, this is referred to as a/an:

    a. unrecognized determination.
    b. DNAR order.
    c. termination order.
    d. final rite.

19. The Guidelines 2005 are considered:

    a. the legal standard of care.
    b. national regulations.
    c. consensus standards.
    d. international law.

20. The initial dose for shocking ventricular fibrillation using a monophasic waveform for treatment is:

    a. 120 J.
    b. 200 J.
    c. 300 J.
    d. 360 J.

21. After the initial dose, subsequent shocks using monophasic waveform for treatment of ventricular fibrillation are:

    a. 150 J.
    b. 200 J.
    c. 300 J.
    d. 360 J.

22. If a patient received an adequate trial of ALS in the field, in which circumstance should you continue the arrest and transport to the local ED?

    a. a lengthy downtime
    b. the patient has a mortal injury
    c. a low body temperature
    d. rigor mortis is apparent

23. In the out-of-hospital setting, the five-year-old child who collapses from sudden cardiac arrest should first receive _____ .

    a. one minute of CPR
    b. two minutes of CPR
    c. ten cycles of CPR
    d. defibrillation with an AED

24. Of all the interventions available to the cardiac arrest patient, which has the most scientific evidence in its favor?

    a. CPR
    b. defibrillation
    c. compressions
    d. high-dose epinephrine

25. The use of the AED is encouraged for all patients over the age of:

    a. fifty.
    b. fifteen.
    c. eight.
    d. one.

26. Where is the best "bang for the buck" in saving cardiac arrest patients?

    a. adding more ALS units
    b. expanding the use of fibrinolytics
    c. removing barriers to implementing PAD
    d. training EMT-Bs to intubate

27. The Guidelines 2005 changes in healthcare provider "child" CPR now apply to:

    a. opening the airway.
    b. patients between one and eight years old.
    c. patients from one year old to the onset of puberty.
    d. two-rescuer, two-thumb-encircling-hands technique.

28. In what situation should you phone first instead of phone fast?

    a. a child with previous MI
    b. a child who may have drowned
    c. a child with a possible airway obstruction
    d. when you are not near a phone

29. In adults, when should the rescuer consider phoning fast instead of phoning first?

    a. cardiac arrest caused by electrical shock
    b. preexisting MI
    c. poisoning or drug overdose
    d. patients over sixty years old

30. When providing ventilations with a bag mask, the healthcare provider should provide smaller tidal volumes (400 to 600 ml) when:

    a. the patient is less than five feet tall.
    b. the patient weighs more than 100 kilograms.
    c. the patient weighs less than 100 kilograms.
    d. supplemental oxygen is attached.

31. When using a bag mask, the rescuer should:

    a. enlist a second rescuer to help squeeze the bag.
    b. use the "C"/"E" clamp hand position.
    c. provide breaths over one second.
    d. all of the above.

32. Where is the best position for the ventilator when using a bag mask on a supine patient?

    a. at the patient's side
    b. about 18" above the head of the patient
    c. straddling the patient
    d. lying flat on your stomach

33. Which statement is incorrect?

    a. Proper use of the bag mask requires practice.
    b. The jaw thrust can be used with one-rescuer technique on a trauma patient.
    c. Tidal volumes of 400 to 600 ml can be given over one second.
    d. The bag mask should be attached to 100% oxygen.

34. When smaller tidal volumes are used with the bag mask, the:

    a. patient should be hyperventilated.
    b. breaths need to be given faster.
    c. breaths need to be more forceful.
    d. chest should rise visibly.

35. If a rescuer is unable to cover both the mouth and nose of an infant with his own mouth, it is acceptable to:

    a. do mouth-to-nose breathing.
    b. skip the ventilations.
    c. defibrillate the patient.
    d. use a Combitube®.

36. When a victim suddenly collapses and has no signs of circulation, the rescuer should first provide _____ .

    a. two rescue breaths
    b. defibrillation with an AED
    c. one cycle of thirty compressions
    d. five cycles of thirty compressions followed by two rescue breaths

37. What evidence helped researchers recommend dropping the pulse check step for laypersons?

    a. No one checks it anyway.
    b. The patient often still has a faint pulse.
    c. It takes too much time to teach.
    d. They were frequently wrong in their assessment.

38. When biphasic waveform defibrillation is used on an adult in sudden cardiac arrest, the initial shock dose is:

    a. 150 J.
    b. 200 J.
    c. 300 J.
    d. 360 J.

39. If a foreign body airway obstruction is suspected in an adult patient, the healthcare provider should:

    a. call for the defibrillator.
    b. reposition the neck and reattempt to ventilate.
    c. simply give chest compressions.
    d. perform a blind finger sweep.

40. The initial shock dose for a child in ventricular fibrillation using a monophasic or biphasic manual defibrillator is:

    a. 1 J/kg.
    b. 2 J/kg.
    c. 3 J/kg.
    d. 4 J/kg.

41. If a person has a foreign body airway obstruction (FBAO) and is an adult:

    a. do not do chest compressions.
    b. chest compression may be helpful.
    c. reach down his throat to remove the object.
    d. ventilate twice as fast.

42. Where are the hands placed to do CPR compressions on an adult?

    a. on the bottom of the breastbone
    b. at the top of the breastbone
    c. on the seventh intercostal space
    d. in the center of the chest, between the nipples

43. At what rate should the chest be compressed for an adult patient in sudden cardiac arrest?

    a. 60 per minute
    b. 80 per minute
    c. 100 per minute
    d. 120 per minute

44. The compression-to-ventilation ratio for infants and children older than one year, when performed by two healthcare providers, is:

    a. 5:1.
    b. 15:2.
    c. 30:1.
    d. 30:2.

45. When providing chest compressions on a child in sudden cardiac arrest, the rescuer should use:

    a. the heel of only one hand to compress the lower half of the sternum.
    b. the heel of one or two hands to compress the lower half of the sternum.
    c. one hand to compress to a depth of one-quarter of the chest diameter.
    d. both hands to compress to a depth of one-quarter of the chest diameter.

46. The technique of using abdominal thrusts to relieve an FBAO is used:

    a. only on adults.
    b. on adults and children.
    c. on choking victims of any age.
    d. on adults and children older than eight years of age.

47. The first choice technique for chest compression in an infant when there are two rescuers is to do the:

    a. two-thumb-encircling-hands chest technique.
    b. two fingers at the center of the chest.
    c. one-handed technique.
    d. two-handed technique.

48. If the public is unwilling to do the ventilations of CPR, they should be taught:

    a. to not offer assistance.
    b. to keep reassessing the breathing.
    c. compression-only CPR.
    d. to call first with all patients.

49. Under certain clinical conditions, evidence shows that:

    a. the LMA is superior to an ET tube.
    b. the LMA and Combitube® are better than a bag mask.
    c. the Combitube® is a dangerous device.
    d. all EMT-Bs should be trained in the use of the Combitube®.

50. Who should decide if EMT-Basics are trained to use the LMA?

    a. the training officer
    b. the International Resuscitation Committee
    c. the AHA
    d. the agency's director

Exam #51 Answer Form

	A	B	C	D		A	B	C	D
1.	❑	❑	❑	❑	26.	❑	❑	❑	❑
2.	❑	❑	❑	❑	27.	❑	❑	❑	❑
3.	❑	❑	❑	❑	28.	❑	❑	❑	❑
4.	❑	❑	❑	❑	29.	❑	❑	❑	❑
5.	❑	❑	❑	❑	30.	❑	❑	❑	❑
6.	❑	❑	❑	❑	31.	❑	❑	❑	❑
7.	❑	❑	❑	❑	32.	❑	❑	❑	❑
8.	❑	❑	❑	❑	33.	❑	❑	❑	❑
9.	❑	❑	❑	❑	34.	❑	❑	❑	❑
10.	❑	❑	❑	❑	35.	❑	❑	❑	❑
11.	❑	❑	❑	❑	36.	❑	❑	❑	❑
12.	❑	❑	❑	❑	37.	❑	❑	❑	❑
13.	❑	❑	❑	❑	38.	❑	❑	❑	❑
14.	❑	❑	❑	❑	39.	❑	❑	❑	❑
15.	❑	❑	❑	❑	40.	❑	❑	❑	❑
16.	❑	❑	❑	❑	41.	❑	❑	❑	❑
17.	❑	❑	❑	❑	42.	❑	❑	❑	❑
18.	❑	❑	❑	❑	43.	❑	❑	❑	❑
19.	❑	❑	❑	❑	44.	❑	❑	❑	❑
20.	❑	❑	❑	❑	45.	❑	❑	❑	❑
21.	❑	❑	❑	❑	46.	❑	❑	❑	❑
22.	❑	❑	❑	❑	47.	❑	❑	❑	❑
23.	❑	❑	❑	❑	48.	❑	❑	❑	❑
24.	❑	❑	❑	❑	49.	❑	❑	❑	❑
25.	❑	❑	❑	❑	50.	❑	❑	❑	❑

52

Advanced Cardiac Life Support (ACLS)

1. The principles of _____ medicine classify interventions into one of five categories.

   a. diagnostic
   b. evidence-based
   c. homeopathic
   d. osteopathic

2. According to the Guidelines 2005, a Class _____ designation of a treatment is supported by excellent, definitive evidence of effectiveness in humans.

   a. I
   b. IIa
   c. IIb
   d. III

3. Class _____ interventions or actions are proposed guidelines with insufficient evidence to support a final recommendation for clinical use at this time.

   a. IIa
   b. IIb
   c. Indeterminate
   d. III

4. While performing CPR with an advanced airway in place, the rescuer delivering the ventilations should provide _____ ventilation(s) every _____ seconds.

   a. one; six to eight
   b. one; five to six
   c. two; fifteen
   d. two; thirty

5. The Guidelines 2005 require training in the use of a/an _____ by all healthcare providers.

   a. bag mask
   b. LMA
   c. Combitube®
   d. ET tube

6. The preferred method of medication administration during a cardiac arrest is through:

   a. an IV or IO.
   b. a synchronized IV drip.
   c. the endotracheal tube at normal dose.
   d. the endotracheal tube at double dose.

7. CPR is in progress on an adult when you arrive with a defibrillator. You quickly analyze the rhythm, detect pulseless ventricular tachycardia, and administer one shock. The next step is to:

   a. check the pulse, reanalyze the rhythm, and resume CPR for two minutes.
   b. reanalyze the rhythm, check the pulse, and resume CPR for two minutes.
   c. resume CPR for five cycles, then reanalyze the rhythm and check the pulse.
   d. reanalyze the rhythm, resume CPR for five cycles, and then check the pulse.

8. Which of the following devices provides a continuous visual display of the level of expired CO_2?

   a. capnometer
   b. capnography
   c. colorimetric device
   d. pulse oximetry

9. Which of the following is incorrect about the Combitube® airway device?

   a. The Combitube® is an advanced airway.
   b. This device is inserted blindly.
   c. It is placed orally and inserted past the hypopharyngeal space.
   d. This device requires extensive training to use.

10. One major change in the acute coronary syndrome (ACS) guidelines is that the:

    a. EMS dispatcher may instruct patients with symptoms of ACS to chew an aspirin.

    b. EMS dispatcher may instruct a family member on the use of a home AED on an unresponsive victim.

    c. patients with non-ST segment elevation myocardial infarction (STEMI) require rapid treatment with fibrinolytics.

    d. patients with unstable angina may require coronary artery bypass grafting (CABG).

11. During a cardiac arrest resuscitation emergency, cardiac drugs should be administered:

    a. after every shock.

    b. every two minutes during CPR.

    c. every three minutes during the rhythm check.

    d. during CPR, as soon as possible after rhythm checks.

12. _____ is a vasopressor that may be given to replace the first or second dose of epinephrine in cardiac arrest.

    a. Dopamine

    b. Vasopressin

    c. Dobutamine

    d. Isoproterenol

13. Pediatric post-resuscitation interventions that may improve the neurologic outcome include:

    a. avoiding hyperventilation.

    b. maintaining normal blood sugar levels.

    c. treating hyperthermia and allowing a mild hypothermia to exist.

    d. all of the above.

14. The use of high-dose epinephrine in pediatric cardiac arrest has been deemphasized for all of the following reasons, *except* that it:

    a. is very difficult to accurately dose to the patient's weight.

    b. can increase myocardial oxygen demand.

    c. can cause tachycardia and hypertension.

    d. can cause myocardial necrosis.

15. _____ is the preferred antiarrhythmic in the management of potentially fatal pediatric arrhythmias.

    a. Epinephrine

    b. Amiodarone

    c. Vasopressin

    d. Cardizem

16. One major change in neonatal resuscitation and the management of meconium staining is:

    a. routine suctioning is no longer recommended.

    b. endotracheal suctioning is a Class III treatment.

    c. aggressive suction must be started as soon as possible.

    d. endotracheal suctioning should be used first and exclusively.

17. You are treating a forty-five-year-old patient who is complaining of chest and left arm pain, nausea, and sweating. While you begin treatment and complete your assessment, you also consider whether or not the patient is a candidate for fibrinolytic therapy. For which of the following factors may this type of therapy be a contraindication in the patient you are treating?

    a. the patient's age

    b. the patient takes metoprolol

    c. the patient takes warfarin

    d. the patient's heart rate is fifty-six

18. An eighty-three-year-old female is complaining of palpitations. She denies chest pain but admits to being short of breath when walking. The patient is legally blind and, after talking to her, you find that she is questionable for compliance with the medications that control her heart rate. Her vital signs are: respirations 20/nonlabored, pulse 190, BP 140/90, and skin signs are pale, warm, and dry. The ECG shows an irregular rhythm with a narrow complex. Which of the following treatments is most appropriate for controlling the patient's heart rate?

    a. diltiazem

    b. adenosine

    c. amiodarone

    d. synchronized cardioversion

19. _____ has been shown to be effective for VF or pulseless VT, torsades de pointes, and dysrhythmias with known hypomagnesemia.

    a. Sodium bicarbonate

    b. Amiodarone

    c. Vasopressin

    d. Magnesium sulfate

20. _____ is an agent that appears to be as effective as epinephrine in cardiac arrest and lasts between ten and twenty minutes, so only one dose is recommended.

    a. Lidocaine

    b. Amiodarone

    c. Vasopressin

    d. Procainamide

21. You have responded to the home of a patient found in cardiac arrest. The patient's initial rhythm is asystole, and he was last seen alive thirty minutes ago. The patient is seventy years old and has a cardiac history. The patient's wife is asking you to do anything you can to save her husband, and more family members are arriving. What action is appropriate to take next?

    a. Ask the family if the patient has a healthcare proxy or any advanced directives.
    b. Offer the wife and family members the choice to observe the attempt at resuscitation.
    c. Begin resuscitation and assign a team member to remain with the family and answer questions.
    d. All of the actions listed above are appropriate and should be done.

22. For the patient who has tachycardia with pulses, the major change in the 2005 Guidelines is:

    a. beta-blockers are now a treatment option.
    b. the treatment is streamlined into one algorithm.
    c. synchronized cardioversion no longer requires sedation.
    d. there is no longer a need for expert consultation prior to providing treatment.

23. Acute MI and unstable angina are now recognized as part of a spectrum of disease known as:

    a. acute coronary syndromes (ACS).
    b. advanced coronary syndromes.
    c. ACLS disorders.
    d. acute cardiac disorders.

24. Cardiac patients who are not eligible for fibrinolytic therapy because of exclusionary criteria should be considered for transport or transfer to a hospital with _____ facilities.

    a. outpatient placement
    b. hyperbaric oxygen therapy
    c. primary angioplasty and intra-aortic balloon placement.
    d. primary beta-blocking central line

25. Intravenous fibrinolytics have been shown to improve neurologic outcome in stroke patients who meet the criteria, provided they are administered within:

    a. the first seventy-two hours after symptoms start to resolve.
    b. two hours after the symptoms start to resolve.
    c. three hours of the onset of stroke symptoms.
    d. three to six hours of the onset of stroke symptoms.

26. Overdose of tricyclic antidepressants has been shown to cause hypotension and/or:

    a. ventricular dysrhythmias.
    b. TIA or stroke.
    c. hypomagnesium.
    d. hypothermia.

27. The treatment of choice for an overdose of tricyclic antidepressants is the induction of:

    a. systemic alkalosis.
    b. an antiarrhythmic agent like lidocaine.
    c. procainamide.
    d. beta-blocker.

28. Cocaine overdose has been shown to be associated with serious:

    a. ventricular dysrhythmias.
    b. atrial dysrhythmias.
    c. hypomagnesium.
    d. hypothermia.

29. The Guidelines 2005 recommend all of the following for cocaine overdose, *except*:

    a. nitrates as a first-line therapy.
    b. benzodiazepines as a first-line therapy.
    c. alpha-adrenergic blocking agents as a second-line therapy when the first-line treatment fails.
    d. beta-blocking agents as a second-line therapy when the first-line treatment fails.

30. Recommended prehospital medications for all patients with ACS include _____ in the absence of contraindications.

    a. aspirin
    b. nitroglycerin
    c. beta-blockers
    d. none of the above

Exam #52 Answer Form

	A	B	C	D		A	B	C	D
1.	❏	❏	❏	❏	16.	❏	❏	❏	❏
2.	❏	❏	❏	❏	17.	❏	❏	❏	❏
3.	❏	❏	❏	❏	18.	❏	❏	❏	❏
4.	❏	❏	❏	❏	19.	❏	❏	❏	❏
5.	❏	❏	❏	❏	20.	❏	❏	❏	❏
6.	❏	❏	❏	❏	21.	❏	❏	❏	❏
7.	❏	❏	❏	❏	22.	❏	❏	❏	❏
8.	❏	❏	❏	❏	23.	❏	❏	❏	❏
9.	❏	❏	❏	❏	24.	❏	❏	❏	❏
10.	❏	❏	❏	❏	25.	❏	❏	❏	❏
11.	❏	❏	❏	❏	26.	❏	❏	❏	❏
12.	❏	❏	❏	❏	27.	❏	❏	❏	❏
13.	❏	❏	❏	❏	28.	❏	❏	❏	❏
14.	❏	❏	❏	❏	29.	❏	❏	❏	❏
15.	❏	❏	❏	❏	30.	❏	❏	❏	❏

Appendix A: Answers & Rationale for Questions

Chapter 1: The Well-Being of the EMS Provider

1. a. Health—Defined by the World Health Organization as not merely the absence of disease or infirmity; it is a state of complete physical, mental, and social well-being.

2. c. mental and emotional health.—The components of wellness include physical well-being and proper nutrition, as well as mental and emotional health.

3. d. weight control.—The principles of weight control (e.g., eating in moderation, limiting fat consumption, and exercise) must be understood and included in proper nutrition.

4. d. two-thirds—Eating too much animal food, fat, oil, and sugar, while eating too few complex carbohydrates, such as fresh vegetable and fruits, whole grains, and legumes, contributes to the development of degenerative diseases. These include the major killers like heart disease, diabetes, cancer, stroke, and obesity.

5. c. diabetes.—Poor diet and nutrition contribute to the development of degenerative diseases such as diabetes, hypertension, heart disease, and stroke.

6. a. limited access to choices of food types.—When you are only able to get meals on the run, and are limited to fast food choices, the choices are typically not the healthiest.

7. c. stopping for fast food when you are hungry and did not bring a meal.—Typical fast food is loaded with fat and calories. Stopping for good food fast is a better approach. Many fast food restaurants now have menus that include some items for those conscious of diet, nutrition, and their waistline.

8. b. making small changes with a slow transition—Extreme changes in diet tend to lead to failure in sticking to the diet. Look closely at the label for both fat and calorie content. Experts say it takes twenty minutes to feel full once you have started eating. Drink water before and during a meal to achieve that feeling to avoid overeating.

9. d. Snacks can fill the voids between meals and should be a part of your food plan.—Healthy snacks can help fill the void between meals, will decrease your appetite for the next meal, and can help to avoid overeating. High-fiber snacks are better for dental health, so include healthy snacks in your food plan.

10. a. attitude.—The elements of physical fitness include a positive attitude, strength, endurance, and aerobic conditioning. It is great to have a personal trainer and heart rate monitor, but not necessary. Running is not physically possible for many people. There are many other options for aerobic conditioning.

11. a. a physician will identify any specific limitations to consider.—This precaution is routinely given for those who are looking to begin a new exercise plan, or for other good reasons. The physician can make recommendations that will help to avoid injuries or excess stress on the body, based on age, past medical history, current weight, and general physical condition.

12. c. Lyme disease.—Hepatitis B, rubella, tetanus, and diphtheria are required immunizations. Paramedic students are required to have these prior to entering most colleges and clinical settings.

13. c. improved personal appearance and self-image.—Additional benefits include increased resistance to injury and illness; decreased blood pressure and resting heart rate; increased muscle mass and metabolism.

14. d. physical endurance.—Aerobic conditioning trains the heart to eject a larger volume with each stroke and does not need to pump as often. The oxygen-carrying capacity of red blood cells increases with improved physical endurance.

15. b. circadian rhythms—These biological cycles include hormonal and body temperature fluctuations, appetite and sleep cycles, and other bodily processes.

16. a. fatigued night-shift workers.—Three Mile island and the Chernobyl nuclear plant accidents can also be attributed in part to fatigued night-shift workers.

17. c. blood pressure.—Increased blood pressure may have serious long-term effects on the entire body. Additional considerations should include: cardiovascular endurance, total cholesterol, triglycerides, estrogen use, and stress.

18. c. high-level disinfection.—a product that is designed to kill all forms of microbial life, except high numbers of bacterial spores, is a high-level disinfection.

19. a. bending at the hips—The recommendation for safe lifting is to keep the back straight. Use the stronger muscles of the legs rather than the muscles of the back to lift. Bending at the waist when lifting can place the spine at risk for serious and permanent injury.

20. c. Leave yourself an exit and be prepared to retreat.—Safety should come first for you and your crew. This patient has an altered mental status (confused) with an obvious injury that needs medical care. Stay with her at a safe distance until further help arrives.

21. a. daytime, on clear, dry roads.—Ambulance accidents occur with high frequency in daytime hours on clear, dry roads, often in intersections.

22. b. there are limitations with these devices.—These emergency devices do not guarantee the right of way. The operator has the responsibility to drive with due regard while using these devices and is held to a higher standard than other drivers.

23. d. driving with due regard for the safety of other drivers—In most states, the emergency vehicle operator is held to a higher standard with regard to all others. Escorts increase the chance of a chain reaction collision, and are not recommended. Emergency lights and sirens should only be used on high-priority emergency calls.

24. c. Test all drivers on their knowledge of standard operating procedures (SOPs).—Other strategies to consider include: providing hands-on training; checking driver's license and qualifications; assuring familiarity with ambulance size, weight, use of mirrors, braking distances, steering and turning radius, and speed controls.

25. a. what to do when a collision occurs—Additional topics that should be included in SOPs include: how the agency qualifies drivers, who is not allowed to operate the ambulances, a policy on prudent speed, how to approach an intersection, and using a spotter when backing up the ambulance.

26. d. all of the above.—Depending on the type of collision, the safety equipment an EMS provider may use will range from eye protection and helmet to full turnout gear.

27. c. The blood pressure decreases.—Cigarette smoking causes the heart rate and blood pressure to increase. It also causes blood vessels to constrict, decreasing peripheral circulation.

28. c. one-half—According to the American Lung Association, many benefits of smoking cessation occur at different time intervals following your last cigarette.

29. b. For long-time smokers, stopping is not of any benefit.—Even heavy smokers show potentially significant improvement in both cardiac and pulmonary function after quitting.

30. a. nicotine has no effect on nerve cells—During the day, nerve cells become desensitized to nicotine.

31. b. addiction—A persistent, compulsive use of a substance, such as nicotine or heroin. A stimulant excites.

32. a. Stress is associated with positive events.—Stress is defined as a factor that induces bodily or mental tension. Stress is associated with both positive (eustress) and negative (distress) events.

33. c. alarm, resistance, and exhaustion.—The process and development of human stress is equated with the three stages: alarm reaction, stage of resistance, and stage of exhaustion.

34. a. level of resistance in the resistance phase.—During this stage, the body continues to adapt by actively using its homeostatic resources to maintain its physiologic integrity and resist the changes imposed on it.

35. d. susceptibility to physical and psychological ailments.—When one or more organ systems fail or become exhausted (stage of exhaustion) under the stress of adaptation, the organism can develop a disease of adaptation. Such diseases are also referred to as stress-related diseases (e.g., heart attack, gastric ulcer, stroke, or diabetes).

36. b. disorientation—Additional cognitive signs and symptoms of stress include: memory problems, poor concentration, and difficulty making decisions.

37. b. panic reaction.—Additional emotional signs and symptoms of stress include: fear, anger, denial, or feeling overwhelmed.

38. a. nausea and vomiting—Additional physical signs and symptoms of stress may include: difficulty breathing, chest pain, profuse sweating, flushed skin, sleep disturbances, or aching muscles and joints.

39. d. behavioral—Additional behavioral signs and symptoms of stress may include: crying spells, depression, changes in eating and sleep patterns, and increased alcohol consumption.

40. d. All of the above—Environmental stress is often caused by: siren noise, inclement weather, confined work spaces, rapid scene response, or life-and-death decision making.

41. a. a conflict with a supervisor or coworker.—Additional causes of psychosocial stress may include: stressed family relationships, a spouse or significant other who doesn't understand what EMS work or training involves, or abusive patients or their family members.

42. a. feelings of guilt.—Additional causes of personality and emotional stress in EMS may include: response to the death or injury of a child or coworker, personal expectations, feelings of anxiety or incompetence, or the need to be liked.

43. b. Coping—During this process, information is gathered and used to change or adjust to a new situation.

44. b. Controlled breathing—Examples of techniques used to manage stress include: reframing, controlled breathing, progressive relaxation, and guided imagery. Extensive information is available on each of these techniques in the "self-help" section in bookstores and libraries.

45. d. Critical incident stress management (CISM)—This process involves a network of peers and mental health professionals who support EMS providers who have been involved in a critical incident.

46. c. signs of gastrointestinal distress.—Signs of crisis-induced stress will vary for the individual and may include: headache, nausea, vomiting, anxiety, excessive humor or crying spells, or increased smoking, drinking, or drug use. The other answers listed are techniques used for reducing stress.

47. c. line-of-duty death or serious injury.—Crisis-induced stress reactions are also associated with disaster situations, emergency worker suicides, death of an infant or child, extreme threats to emergency workers, and death or injury of a civilian caused by the EMS provider.

48. c. increasing cigarette smoking.—Smoking increases heart rate and blood pressure, and impairs circulation.

49. a. allow them to express their feelings as best as you can.—Do not take this action personally or argue with the person. Avoid expressing any opinions or judgments.

50. b. six to nine years old—At this age, children are beginning to understand the finality of death. They will seek out detailed explanations for the death and want to understand the difference between a fatal illness and just being sick.

51. b. Tell the truth and be straightforward when talking about the death of a loved one.—This can be very difficult. Do not distort reality by saying that the person who has died has "gone to sleep" or "God took him." These phrases can lead to unnecessary fears.

52. b. shock.—There is no timetable on how long it generally takes for someone to go through the steps. The steps in order of occurrence are: shock, denial, anger, bargaining, depression, and acceptance.

53. d. sterilizing all ambulance equipment on a regular basis.—This is not practical or necessary. Sterilizing certain non-disposable items, such as laryngoscope blades, is appropriate.

54. a. exposure—An example of an exposure would be respiratory secretions sprayed into the face of the EMS provider.

55. c. completing the required medical follow-up.—Also included in the procedure for an exposure are properly reporting and documenting the situation in which the exposure occurred, and cooperating with the investigation.

56. c. actions taken to reduce chances of infection.—This may include: washing the affected area as soon as possible, seeking immediate medical attention when appropriate, and complying with recommended prophylaxis by your Medical Director or Infection Control expert.

57. b. Disinfection—There are three levels of disinfection: low, intermediate, and high.

58. d. prevent contact with body substances such as blood and urine.—BSI is a series of practices designed to prevent contact with body substances such as blood, urine, fecal material, vomitus, and so forth.

59. b. biofeedback.—A technique used for managing stress that uses mental control to manipulate the heartbeat or brain waves.

60. b. vaccination—Vaccinations are utilized for preventing diseases.

Chapter 2: Roles and Responsibilities of the EMS Provider

1. b. Cincinnati—A few years later, ambulance service was provided by the New York City Department of Health from Bellevue Hospital.

2. a. 1915—Air transport began in the military and was first employed during the retreat of the Serbian army from Albania.

3. b. mouth-to-mouth ventilation.—Doctor Peter Safar first demonstrated the effectiveness of mouth-to-mouth ventilation in humans.

4. d. CPR—Cardiopulmonary resuscitation was first demonstrated to be an effective treatment method for cardiac arrest patients in 1960.

5. b. Highway Safety Act—This act also required the secretary of the DOT, through their newly created EMS program, to develop a series of training programs to respond to the needs of patients injured on the highways.

6. d. National Highway Traffic Safety Administration—NHTSA was established in 1970 and, together with the DOT, serves to provide leadership to EMS, as well as to other federal and state agencies.

7. c. Ambulance Specifications.—This publication serves to standardize the design of ambulances. These "specs" continue to be revised every few years.

8. a. standard equipment to be carried on BLS ambulances.—The American College of Surgeons led the way in identifying and standardizing the equipment to be carried on BLS ambulances.

9. c. 1995—The last revision of the EMT-B curriculum included the application of the AED skills for EMT-Bs.

10. c. EMS system—The components of the emergency medical services system (EMSS) have evolved over the past thirty years from fifteen essential components (EMSS Act of 1973) to ten standard components (NHTSA Technical Assistance Program 1988).

11. b. licensure.—Examples of licenses include: a medical license or fishing license and, in some states, a paramedic license.

12. a. certification—This is usually used to refer to an action of a nongovernmental entity granting authority to an individual who has met predetermined qualifications to participate in an activity.

13. c. Critical Care Technician—The four levels of prehospital training recognized by the National Registry of Emergency Medical Technicians (NREMTs) are: First Responder, EMT-Basic, EMT-Intermediate, and EMT-Paramedic.

14. a. First Responder.—The role of the First Responder is initial and basic stabilization, and to interact with the EMS system. A First Responder could be a firefighter, police officer, or part of a responsive team at a work site.

15. d. all of the above—Each level of EMS responder has the role and responsibility of providing safety, initial assessment and treatment, and portraying a professional and positive appearance.

16. b. contributing to the development of professional standards.—The National Registry is also responsible for verifying competency, developing and administering practical and written examinations, simplifying the process of reciprocity or credentialing, and spreading the costs of exam development and validation across a larger user base than most states.

17. c. The current EMT-Paramedic curriculum does not contain recertification curricula.—This is true. NHTSA, however, issued a lengthy position paper emphasizing the need for states to move toward recertification by using continuing education and adhering to a form similar to that used by the National Registry.

18. c. Reciprocity—The process of issuing credentials based on prior training in another state.

19. d. refreshes knowledge and skills, and introduces new material.—Attending CE also increases the EMS providers' knowledge base and understanding of relevant EMS issues.

20. a. integrity—This means honesty in all of your actions and words. This important attribute is assumed by the public to be part of the responsibility of an EMS provider.

21. b. The expectations by society of healthcare professionals are high, both on and off duty.—EMS providers are very visible role models whose behaviors are closely observed. Image and behavior in public, both on and off duty, are extremely important.

22. b. Ethics—The principles of conduct governing an individual or group.

23. c. peer review.—A couple of examples are a coworker providing tips on how to lift a patient out of a tight spot or reviewing each other's paperwork for better ways to document what was done on the call.

24. a. integrity.—One of the most important attributes for the EMS professional is integrity. Examples of behavior demonstrating integrity are always telling the truth, never stealing, and providing complete and accurate documentation.

25. b. empathy.—Having empathy in emergency medicine means identifying with and understanding the feelings, situations, and motives of your patients.

26. a. Empathy—Examples of behavior demonstrating empathy include: showing caring and compassion, being supportive and reassuring, and demonstrating respect.

27. b. having a good understanding of your limitations.—Someone who is self-confident, but not overly confident, knows when to call for backup or consult with medical direction rather than getting in over one's head.

28. d. help to instill confidence in the patient and his or her family.—The manner in which you walk and carry yourself is important! Patients do not appreciate an EMS provider with bad breath, body odor, or too much aftershave or perfume.

29. d. is dressed appropriately and prepared to work when the shift begins.—Good patient care involves good time management skills. Examples include: prioritizing tasks during patient care; being punctual for meetings, appointments, and work shifts; and being prepared to work at the start of the shift.

30. c. works well as a team member.—The team includes: the emergency medical dispatcher, the public safety First Responder agency personnel, the BLS and ALS

personnel on the scene, medical direction, and the healthcare professionals at the receiving facility.

31. b. Diplomacy—Diplomacy is tact and skill in dealing with people and goes hand in hand with teamwork. Being a diplomat also involves saying and doing things that are considered "politically correct."

32. b. disagreeing with a coworker in public.—The patient's bedside is no place for interprofessional disagreements. Doing this in public, especially in front of a patient, is unprofessional and may negatively impact the image of you and your ambulance service.

33. d. be an advocate for your patient.—Part of your responsibility as the EMS provider is to advocate for your patient. Sometimes, this means not just delivering the patients to the busy ED, but staying with them for a few minutes to ensure that the ED staff fully understands the extent of the mechanism of injury (MOI) or nature of illness (NOI).

34. b. Telling a patient who smokes that he or she is really stupid for doing so.—Instead of scorning the patient, use this event as a teaching moment, and explain the risks associated with smoking and the benefits of cessation.

35. b. protecting the patient's confidentiality.—Protecting patient confidentiality is also a legal and ethical responsibility.

36. c. protecting the patient's furniture while moving your stretcher through the living room.—A good EMS provider pays attention to details. There may be times when the details are skipped due to the patient's severity, but most calls involve enough time for you to pay attention to things like wiping your feet before entering a patient's home.

37. a. ensure quality patient care.—The primary role of the Medical Director is to ensure quality patient care. The responsibilities include: authority over patient care and the authority to limit patient care activities of those who deviate from established standards; involvement with the ongoing design, operation, evaluation, and revision of the EMS system; and development and implementation of medical policies and procedures.

38. c. Protocols—Most protocols involve specific medical treatments and, as such, come under the domain of medical direction.

39. a. participating in the development of continuing education.—Additional typical roles include: participating in the personnel selection process, equipment selection, participating in quality improvement and problem resolution, interfacing between EMS systems and other healthcare agencies, and advocating within the medical community.

40. a. the ability to obtain real-time direction and orders.—Many patients have complicated problems that do not fit into specific protocols. Being able to obtain online direction can help the paramedic to provide better patient care with expanded treatment options.

41. b. protocols.—Off-line or indirect medical control utilizes guidelines (protocols) for the management of specific patient presenting problems. The protocols have appropriate "stop lines" to allow certain treatment options before having to establish online or direct medical control.

42. d. All of the above.—Confirm that the physician is a medical doctor who is willing to come with you and the patient to the hospital. Contact medical control to advise of the situation, and have the two physicians speak with each other.

43. d. by conforming to the standards of a healthcare professional providing quality patient care—Having a college degree, a lawyer on retainer, or knowing as many customers as possible in your area of response is fine, but not necessarily what one needs to be prepared to work as a paramedic.

44. a. clinical capabilities—Ideally, you would not bring a patient having a heart attack to a hospital that could not perform cardiac catherizations, or a serious burn patient to a non-trauma hospital.

45. d. replacing disposable items available from the hospital.—Restocking the ambulance with disposable items at the hospital in order to get the ambulance back in service as quickly as possible is a primary responsibility of the EMS provider.

46. a. It enhances visibility and a positive image of the paramedics and their agencies.—The primary benefits include: improving the health of the community regarding injury and illness prevention, ensuring appropriate utilization of resources by making sure the public knows when, where, and how to use EMS, improving the integration of EMS with other healthcare and public safety agencies, and enhancing visibility and a positive image of EMS providers and their agencies.

47. c. training to be a career paramedic/firefighter.—This is an example of a personal goal rather than an example of citizen involvement in EMS systems.

48. a. patient well-care visits.—One of the activities the *EMS Agenda for the Future* recognizes is the integration of health services. One example is to expand the EMS role in public health and involve EMS in community health monitoring activities.

49. b. the transportation alternatives are very costly.—When considering the system finance aspect, it is recommended that there be a collaborative effort with other healthcare providers and insurers to enhance patient care efficiency and develop proactive financial relations between EMS, other healthcare providers, and healthcare insurers.

50. c. integration of EMS with other healthcare providers to deliver quality care.—It also discusses expansion of the EMS role in public health in community health monitoring activities; being cognizant of the

special needs of the entire population; and incorporation of health systems within EMS that address special needs.

51. c. develop information systems that provide linkage between various healthcare services.—It also speaks to the development of academic institutional commitments to EMS-related research, and the allocation of federal and state funds for major EMS system research.

52. a. authorizing and funding a lead federal EMS agency.—It also discusses establishing and funding the position of state EMS Medical Director in each state, and implementing laws that provide protection from liability for EMS providers when dealing with unusual situations.

53. b. Collaboration with other healthcare providers.—It also addresses compensating EMS on the basis of a preparedness-based mode, reducing volume-related incentives, and realizing the cost of an emergency safety net.

54. a. conducting EMS occupation health research.—It also discusses developing a system of reciprocity for EMS-provider credentials, and developing collaborative relations between EMS and academic institutions.

55. a. require appropriate credentials for all those who provide online medical directions.—Other proposals include: appointing state EMS medical directors, and formalizing relations between all EMS systems and medical direction, with the appropriate resources to do so.

56. d. bridging and transitioning EMS programs with all health professions' education.—Since many courses in healthcare overlap, an example of this would be a course that would provide training to allow the student to graduate as a nurse and a paramedic, or a physician's assistant and a paramedic.

57. c. exploring and evaluating public education alternatives.—Other goals include collaborating with other community resources and agencies to determine public education needs, and engaging in continuous public education programs.

58. b. assess the effectiveness of resource attributes for EMS dispatching.—This includes assessing the effectiveness of personnel and requiring that personnel have the education, experience, and resources to optimally query the caller, make a determination of the most appropriate resources to be mobilized, and implement an effective course of action.

59. d. commit to a common definition of what constitutes baseline community EMS care.—Additional goals include establishing proactive relationships between EMS and other healthcare providers, and subjecting EMS clinical care to ongoing evaluations to determine its impact on patient outcomes.

60. c. develop a mechanism to generate and transmit data that are valid, reliable, and accurate.—Additional

goals include adopting uniform data elements and definitions, incorporating the elements into information systems, and developing systems that are able to describe an entire EMS event.

61. c. determine EMS effects for multiple outcome categories and cost-effectiveness.—Additional elements of the evaluation component include evaluating EMS effects for various medical conditions and developing valid models for EMS evaluations that incorporate consumer input.

62. b. uncover problems and provide solutions.—Specifically in the areas of medical direction, training, communication, dispatch, public information and education, mutual aide, and disaster planning.

63. d. research can be influenced by biases.—Quality EMS research is beneficial to the future of EMS, and biases can hinder and spoil research.

64. d. negatively affecting patient care.—The healthcare provider's philosophy is to "First do no harm."

65. a. what a randomized and controlled group is.—There are several basic research concepts that need to be understood, such as: the value of peer review and publishing research, types of research, how to randomize and select a control group, or how to select a sample using various methods. A statistics course can be very helpful in understanding the basics of research.

66. a. Collect the funding needs for the hypothesis development.—Funding is typically associated with working the hypothesis, rather than developing it.

67. c. providing results that lead to system improvements.—For example, research may reveal that repositioning emergency response units based on the location and frequency of calls can improve the average response time.

68. b. who developed the hypothesis?—The validity of research should be critically scrutinized by considering what type of data was collected and how, whether the data properly analyzed, and whether the research was peer reviewed.

69. b. Cardiac rescue technician—The three levels of EMS providers described in the DOT curriculum are: EMT-Basic, EMT-Intermediate, and EMT-Paramedic.

70. c. profession—Professions usually involve a specialized body of knowledge or expertise. They are often self-regulating through a licensure or certification process that requires competence validation.

71. a. Your image and behavior in the public's eye are not significant.—There are high expectations by society of healthcare professionals, both on and off duty.

72. d. patients and their families.—Certainly, empathy can be expressed in many ways to many people; however, the paramedic would typically express empathy to a patient, families of patients, or even other healthcare providers.

73. b. taking advantage of all learning opportunities—Self-motivation is the internal drive for excellence. Examples of this include taking the initiative to complete assignments, improve, and correct behavior, or taking advantage of as many learning opportunities as possible.

74. d. politically correct.—The paramedic job is very dynamic and, at times, includes playing the role of the diplomat, peacekeeper, negotiator, and tactician.

75. c. Most of what paramedics do involves communication skills.—Paramedics talk on radios, talk to coworkers and other emergency service providers, and, most importantly, establish a rapport with patients so a history and assessment can be obtained.

Chapter 3: Illness and Injury Prevention

1. d. Epidemiology—This is the branch of medicine that deals with the incidence, distribution, and control of disease in a population.

2. a. morbidity.—The state or incidence of a disease or injury.

3. a. heart disease—The CDC reports, for the year 2002, that disease of the heart remains the leading cause of death.

4. a. For ages one through forty-four, accidents were the leading cause of death.—This is why injury prevention is so important and why it is sensible for EMS providers to be involved in injury and illness prevention efforts in their communities.

5. b. There are more expectations for EMS services to provide care for patients being managed in the home setting.—As the hospitals have moved toward doing more procedures on an outpatient basis and are decreasing the number of hospital stay days for the treatment of injuries and illnesses, the reliance on EMS has increased.

6. a. accidents.—When death rates of Caucasians are compared to those of African Americans, the leading causes of death are the same except in two age groups. In the fifteen-to-twenty-four-year-olds, the leading cause was accidents in whites and homicide in blacks.

7. d. Injury risk—The definition of injury risk is a real or potentially hazardous situation that puts individuals at risk for sustaining an injury.

8. a. prevention and control efforts.—Injury surveillance is the ongoing systematic collection, analysis, and interpretation of injury data essential to the planning, implementation, and evaluation of public health practice. Timely dissemination of this data is needed for prevention and control efforts.

9. b. Secondary—This is where EMS has a great responsibility. For example, while extricating a victim with a possible cervical injury from a significant wreck, the EMS provider must assure adequate stabilization of the spine to prevent further (secondary) injury during the process.

10. b. tertiary injury prevention.—Examples of this would be preventing infection, or making modifications to a patient's home to accommodate a disability.

11. b. pick a cause that best suits your interest.—Select an interest you have always wanted to know something about and stretch a little to learn about the cause.

12. c. Over 95% of victims of bicycle-related head injuries were not wearing helmets when injured.—The solutions to the problem include education in injury prevention, legislation requiring the use of helmets, and distribution of helmets.

13. c. Requiring personal flotation devices (PFDs) to be worn whenever children or adults who cannot swim are on or near water.—The other recommendations listed are impractical or impossible.

14. d. getting everyone in the vehicle to wear seat belts.—The evidence from data clearly shows a direct correlation between wearing seat belts and lives saved.

15. d. use of child-resistant packaging of toxic substances for in-home use.—With more than 90% of poisoning exposures to children age five and under occurring in the home, the strategy behind this legislation was a push to educate the parents and older children to lock up the hazardous substances and label them appropriately.

16. c. homes.—This is why legislation was enacted in 1970 (Poison Prevention Act) to require the use of child-resistant packaging for toxic substances used in and around the home.

17. a. practice family fire escape plans every six months.—Additional strategies are to know what to do when your clothing catches fire, to change the batteries every six months, and to never smoke in bed.

18. a. educating riders to always wear a helmet and protective gear.—This is the most practical and proven strategy. Wearing a helmet reduces the chance of death and serious head injury as a result of a collision.

19. b. making sure that any surface that children may fall onto is soft and padded.—The best playgrounds have surfaces with at least six inches of mulch chips, pea gravel, fine sand, or shredded rubber to cushion a fall.

20. c. Injuries from falls affect the very young and the elderly more severely.—Childhood falls account for an estimated two million ED visits each year,

while one in every three adults age sixty-five or older falls each year.

21. b. Installing tiles in kitchens and baths.—Tiled surfaces can be very slippery, especially when wet.

22. c. drawstrings on curtains or blinds—Another common cause of strangulation is drawstrings on clothing (sweatshirts). They can become entangled in playground equipment, fences, and furniture, causing strangulation.

23. a. disassembling the National Rifle Association.—Some might argue that this is the best strategy for the prevention of firearm injuries and fatalities.

24. d. 50,000—Each year, approximately 82,000 pedestrians are injured in traffic crashes. This includes over 50,000 children, who often sustain a serious brain injury.

25. a. avoid drinking and walking.—Drinking and driving is known to be one of the biggest contributors to highway deaths and injuries. However, drinking and walking near traffic is unsafe too and contributes to highway death and injury.

26. b. set examples in all activities of the organization.—There are many ways EMS providers can make it acceptable and, within the mission of the organization, can be involved in prevention activities.

27. b. develop sensible policies and procedures promoting safety in all work activities.—The EMS leader also has the responsibility to provide EMS workers with appropriate personal protective equipment (PPE) and to provide all necessary safety training as required by OSHA.

28. c. extreme ambient temperatures.—The paramedic must able to recognize exposure to hazardous

materials, temperature extremes, vectors, communicable disease, assault, battery, and structural risks.

29. b. child protective services.—Additional resources to be cognizant of include: access to specialty equipment or devices, counseling services, alternative healthcare (e.g., free clinics), rehabilitation, grief support, and immunization programs.

30. b. recognizing the teachable moments.—Try to use concepts of effective communication such as: having a sense of time, being nonjudgmental, being objective, informing individuals about the use of protective devices, and informing the patient how he or she can prevent a recurrence.

31. d. all of the above—Some agencies use a special incident report to document hazards. Documentation of safety hazards should include: primary injury information, care provided, and any other specific information required by the EMS agency.

32. a. Scene conditions—Mechanism of injury (MOI), use of protective devices, absence of protective devices, and risks overcome are additional examples of primary injury data.

33. a. higher education attainment—Data have shown that higher education attainment is associated with a lower risk of death.

34. b. of their perspective offered in out-of-hospital care.—Paramedics come into the homes of the customers and have one of the best views or perspectives of any healthcare provider.

35. c. Primary injury prevention—An example would be not allowing diving in the shallow end of a swimming pool in an effort to prevent spinal injury or death.

Chapter 4: Medical/Legal Issues

1. c. legislative—Legislative law is made up of statutes that are voted on and passed by the legislature. An example of legislative law is a state's EMS Act.

2. a. legislative—Legislative law is made up of statutes that are voted on and passed by the legislature, be it the city council, county board, state legislature, or Congress.

3. c. "jury of your peers."—A jury may be selected by either the judge or the attorneys for each side.

4. b. EMS code.—The EMS code of rules and regulations that outline the specifics of the EMS law for each state will vary.

5. c. case—Case law is often used in a court to decide pending cases.

6. b. criminal—Criminal law deals with wrongs against members of society, such as homicide and rape. Federal, state, and local governments prosecute individuals for violating these laws.

7. c. civil—In a civil case the jury determines damages, such as money, for compensation, but the judge may modify the award. When there is no jury, the judge takes on both roles.

8. d. defendant.—The defendant is the person required to make answer in a legal action or suit.

9. b. hearing.—A hearing is a session in which testimony is taken from witnesses.

10. b. jury—In a court of law, a jury is comprised of persons legally sworn to give a verdict on some matter submitted to them according to the evidence.

11. b. may be appealed to a higher court.—An appellate court decision can uphold the decision of the trial court, overrule it, or send it back (remand) to the lower court for various reasons.

12. c. grand jury—An example of a case that may go to the grand jury is one involving allegations of wrongdoing during an ambulance collision. It is often the grand jury that decides if the DA will

charge the driver of the ambulance for actions that may have caused injury, death, or property damages.

13. b. negligence.—This is also called malpractice when speaking of a failure to exercise an acceptable degree of professional skill or competence.

14. c. civil court.—In civil court cases the jury determines damages, such as money, for compensation, but the judge may modify the award. When there is no jury, the judge takes on both roles.

15. b. breach of duty.—A breach of duty occurs if you have an established duty to act and do not comply with that duty (e.g., receiving an EMS call and refusing to respond).

16. a. nonfeasance.—Nonfeasance is the failure to perform a required duty or act.

17. a. proximate cause.—Proximate cause means that the damages to the patient were directly caused by the paramedic's act of omission or commission.

18. a. proximate cause.—Proximate cause means that the damages to the patient were directly caused by the paramedic's act of omission or commission.

19. b. gross negligence.—Gross negligence involves willful, wanton, intentional, or reckless actions, such as passing an endotracheal tube down the esophagus to see how long it takes for the pulse oximeter to drop below 80%.

20. d. abandonment.—An example of abandonment is delivering a patient to a busy ED, placing the patient onto a stretcher in the hall, and leaving without giving a report to the ED physician.

21. b. false imprisonment.—This is one of the major reasons why it is so important to get consent before taking the patient to the hospital.

22. c. slander.—Rumors or malicious spoken words about another person can hurt the reputation of that person.

23. a. libel.—Examples of libel might be written graffiti or anonymous notes.

24. b. delegation.—Delegation of authority is the granting of medical privileges by a physician, either online or off-line, to an EMS provider to perform skills or procedures within the EMS provider's scope of practice.

25. a. scope of practice.—The scope of practice is usually set by state law or regulation and by local medical authorities.

26. c. res ipsa loquitor—This term is used in reference to malpractice in which the cause of the damages does not require any special expertise to detect; the negligence is evident to a layperson.

27. c. negligence per se.—Negligence per se is the unexcused violation of a statute. An example of this would be an ambulance traveling through a red light at an excessive speed and injuring a pedestrian while doing so.

28. d. contributory negligence.—Contributory negligence arises when the actions of the plaintiff contribute to his own injury. As a result, the damages awarded the plaintiff may be reduced.

29. b. an investigation.—After an incident occurs, the plaintiff's representative investigates to see what facts can be uncovered. With the information discovered from the investigation, the plaintiff's representative will then decide whether to file a complaint and serve the defendant.

30. b. discovery.—Discovery may involve releasing documents such as dispatch tapes, patient records, and PCRs.

31. a. settlement.—At any time while the case is pending, an agreement may be made between the parties to settle the case.

32. a. interrogatories.—Obtaining interrogatories occurs during the discovery phase and allows the opposing sides to formulate their theories of the case and how they will present them, and to prevent surprise at trial.

33. c. liability.—Something for which someone is responsible.

34. b. statute of limitations.—The applicable time limits differ from state to state and are also dependent upon the cause of action.

35. c. seven—This is a good question to ask your service's attorney. Generally, seven years is a good period to save the records of interactions with adult patients.

36. a. expressed—Expressed consent is the when the patient directly agrees, either verbally or nonverbally, to receive care.

37. d. informed—Informed consent is given after full disclosure, or explanation, of information is provided to the patient.

38. b. emergency doctrine.—This type of consent applies to emergency intervention given to a patient who is physically or mentally unable to provide expressed consent.

39. a. no—This means that a parent or guardian must be contacted if the minor is involved in a medical emergency.

40. b. emancipation.—In most states, a child must be treated as an adult if he or she is emancipated.

41. d. full disclosure was provided to an alert patient.—A refusal of medical assistance (RMA) is considered legal if it is obtained in a proper manner with full disclosure to the patient of assessment findings, treatment recommendations, and the implications of refusal.

42. c. consult medical control.—It may be helpful in some instances to put the patient on the phone with the physician.

43. c. No, persons with an altered mental status are not usually able to make a competent decision.—As most EMS providers do not receive formal training to make the judgment about the level of intoxication and do not carry equipment to measure the

percentage of alcohol in the blood, the police should be utilized in these cases.

44. a. Not without additional training.—As most EMS providers do not receive formal training to make the judgment about the level of intoxication and do not carry equipment to measure the percentage of alcohol in the blood, the police should be utilized in these cases.

45. b. Yes, under the emergency doctrine.—Emergency doctrine or implied consent is the type of consent that applies to emergency intervention given for a patient who is physically or mentally unable to provide expressed consent.

46. b. A mental health officer.—Involuntary commitment requirements and procedures vary from state to state. Speak with your agency's attorney to learn what your state's laws are in this area.

47. b. protective custody.—The police can, in most jurisdictions, take a person into protective custody for a limited period of time if they feel the person may have a serious condition that could pose a life threat without the appropriate emergency care.

48. b. Involve the police for some assistance.—EMS providers are often put in a difficult position by family members who would like them to take the patient away against his will.

49. b. Civil Rights Act.—Services that employ EMS providers are responsible for complying with the Civil Rights Act (Title VII) of 1964, which is the federal law prohibiting discrimination based on race, color, religion, sex, or national origin.

50. d. all of the above.—A durable power of attorney or healthcare proxy allows a person to designate another person (agent) to act in cases where the person is unable to make decisions for him- or herself.

51. b. healthcare proxy—This is also referred to as a Healthcare Power of Attorney.

52. a. when a third party requires the information for billing—Release of patient information requires written permission from the patient or legal guardian, except when: a third party requires the information for billing, mandatory reporting by law (e.g., child abuse), in response to a subpoena, or to other healthcare providers who need to know how to provide care to the patient.

53. a. Humane restraints—The use of padded leather restraints or sheets are more acceptable to reduce the potential harm to the patient. Handcuffs are not considered humane restraints.

54. b. ethical—Typically there is no legal responsibility, but the paramedic does have an ethical responsibility to resuscitate all potential organ donors so that others may benefit from the organs.

55. c. the information has to be quickly available for billing.—The PCR is an important part of the patient's record, and a copy needs to go to the ED in the patient's chart. It should be completed while

information is fresh in the paramedic's mind. It also must be a record made "in the course of business" and not completed later.

56. a. his harmful actions.—Not all states allow plaintiffs to seek punitive damages. If awarded, these are usually not covered by malpractice insurance.

57. c. medical expenses—In a malpractice suit, a paramedic may be required to pay compensable damages such as medical expenses, lost earnings, and conscious pain and suffering.

58. b. plaintiff—The plaintiff brings the suit, so the burden of proof is on the plaintiff.

59. a. Scope of practice—Scope is the range of skills and knowledge in which the EMS provider is trained. The standard of care is based on national standards, national curricula, national testing standards, and the recognized treatment for patients in similar circumstances.

60. c. Freedom of Information Act—Sometimes called the Freedom of Information Law, or FOIL. The agency that is being requested to provide the information may charge a minimal fee for the duplication or preparation of the information, and must provide the information within a reasonable time of its request.

61. d. "borrowed servant"—If the paramedic is acting as a preceptor or in a supervisory capacity, he may be held liable for the actions of that intern.

62. c. false imprisonment.—The imprisonment of someone that is contrary to the law.

63. a. Was the signal that was given audible and/or visible to motorists and pedestrians?—Points that are considered include: was the signaling equipment actually used, was the signal that was given audible or visible to motorists and pedestrians, and was it reasonably necessary under all of the circumstances to use the signaling equipment?

64. d. does not warrant performance or quality, or authorize a person to perform any procedures on a patient.—The American Heart Association does not certify or attest to the skill level of the provider. A card verifying successful completion of a course is provided to graduates.

65. a. certificate—A certification is the act of certifying or the state of being certified.

66. b. The operator of the emergency vehicle assumes the extra burden of driving with due regard for others.—The operator has the added responsibility of ensuring that no one is injured and that no property becomes damaged because of his driving.

67. c. has hearing impairment—A qualified individual is one who has a disability that limits one or more major life activities. Temporary disabilities and illegal drug use are not covered under the ADA.

68. b. yes—There is usually no exemption to the provisions that mandate that the operator stop and exchange information immediately after an automobile

collision that results in property damage or personal injury.

69. b. FLSA—Fair Labor Standards Act is the federal law that regulates minimum wages and overtime in the workplace. In EMS, the law has an impact on issues such as on-call pay, compensatory time, long shifts, and overtime pay.

70. b. encourage the improvement of existing safety and health programs.—The purpose of OSHA is to develop standards and guidelines for employers and employees that reduce the incidence of deaths, injuries, and illnesses, and develop an enforcement procedure for safety and health standards. Those who are exempt from OSHA regulations are self-employed people, farms where only family members are employed, and those employed by federal agencies.

71. d. patients have a right to know who you are and your level of training.—The paramedic should always wear an ID tag or patch indicating level of training and name. It is a good practice to introduce yourself to your patient by name and level of training.

72. b. online and off-line supervision.—The Medical Director's liability for out-of-hospital care falls into two categories: online (direct) and off-line (indirect) supervision.

73. d. all of the above.—Even if you provide the correct care to your patient, you can still be sued.

74. c. protect himself and the crew.—Safety is always the first and foremost priority at any scene.

75. d. observations made of the patient's residence—This varies from state to state, but typically paramedics are required to make a report or personally notify a mandated reporter in the receiving facility of cases that may involve: child abuse or neglect, elder or spousal abuse, sexual assault, gunshot and stab wounds, animal bites, and communicable diseases.

Chapter 5: Ethical Issues for the EMS Provider

1. a. treatment protocols.—Also used are prospective and retrospective reviews of medical decisions.

2. a. a system of principles governing moral conduct.— Socrates defined ethics as how one should live. Actually, ethics comes from the Greek word "ethos," which means moral custom.

3. d. societal; personal—Morals relate to societal standards and ethics relate to personal standards. Acting in a lewd or crude manner might be considered immoral, whereas cheating on an examination is considered unethical.

4. d. "What is in the patient's best interest?"—Deciding what the patient wants should incorporate what the patient has said, what the patient has written, and family input.

5. c. Ethics can affect the extent to which you should persuade a patient to receive treatment.—The extent to which you attempt to persuade a patient to receive treatment or transport can be vague and may involve an ethical decision.

6. a. liability—This immunity from liability does not extend to a willful, wanton, or malicious disregard for the wishes of the patient.

7. b. use language/terms the patient can understand.— The best approach is to be honest and help the patient understand the ramifications of his decision in terms that are easily understood.

8. d. preplanned wills—A will is a legal instrument that attorneys deal with. The paramedic deals with "do not attempt resuscitation" orders (DNARs), living wills, and healthcare proxies.

9. d. make decisions on healthcare.—This is a fundamental element of the patient-physician relationship and is stated in the American Medical Association Code of Medical Ethics.

10. a. implied consent—When in doubt, always act in the patient's best interest.

11. a. capabilities of the hospital—The paramedic has a significant influence on the patient's decision about where to be transported. Consider this in all cases. "What would I do if this was my parent or child needing care for this presenting problem?"

12. c. Deciding whether or not to stop to render assistance when not on duty.—Deciding whether you should act as a Good Samaritan and stop to render assistance when not on duty can involve an ethical decision for some.

13. b. Ethics involve larger issues than a paramedic's practice.—Ethics have been described as "how one should live."

14. a. true parity—True parity is comparing what is fair for everyone. It is one of the criteria used in allocating scarce EMS resources.

15. a. True parity—True parity is comparing what is fair for everyone. It is one of the criteria used in allocating scarce EMS resources.

16. b. the patient's advanced directives.—The paramedic is accountable to the patient and the Medical Director, and to fulfilling the standard of care.

17. b. good faith—Avoid any emotional decisions, and use reason, morals, and good faith when considering your answer to an ethical question.

18. a. the patient's statements—For the alert patient who is unimpaired, the patient's wishes must be considered first and foremost. The best approach is to be honest and help the patient understand the

ramifications of his decision in terms that are easily understood.

19. d. When in doubt, resuscitate.—Sometimes it becomes an ethical decision whether or not to resuscitate when considering the patient's wishes and the presence or absence of an advance directive, and the family members do not agree. When in doubt, resuscitate.

20. b. Integrity—Integrity is derived from a combination of the words "integritas" and "integer." It refers to the putting on of armor; of building a completeness, a wholeness, a wholeness in character.

21. b. witnessing a coworker do something unethical and saying nothing.—This is a personal decision that you should think through before it occurs!

22. c. creating laws protecting patient's rights.—In addition, the use of preplans, such as wills and advanced directives, are used to make patient wishes known.

23. d. receiving a direct (online) order that is medically acceptable but morally wrong.—Occasionally, the paramedic is given a physician order that he believes is contraindicated, medically acceptable but not in the patient's best interest, or medically acceptable but morally wrong.

24. b. acting in the patient's best interest.—Be careful not to fall into the trap of making a value judgment; always act in the patient's best interest.

25. b. strengthen and validate our own inner value system.—It also serves to give direction to our moral compass and becomes the foundation upon which we can commit.

Chapter 6: General Principles of Pathophysiology

1. d. the study of how normal physiological processes are altered by disease.—The functional changes that accompany a particular disease or syndrome.

2. b. etiology.—The causes of disease or abnormal conditions.

3. c. exacerbation.—To cause a disease or its symptoms to become more severe.

4. d. the actions of a healthcare provider.—Iatrogenic disease requires a specific action or lack of action.

5. c. syndrome.—A commonly known syndrome is Down syndrome, a combination of a specific physical appearance and some degree of mental impairment.

6. a. atrophy.—The actual number of cells remains unchanged. An example is a leg that has been in a cast for six weeks or more. When the cast is removed, the muscle is typically atrophied.

7. c. cellular adaptation.—When cells are exposed to adverse conditions, they go through a process of adaptation. In some situations, the cells change permanently; in others, they change their structure and function temporarily.

8. d. hyperplasia.—This excess growth often causes tumors that may be malignant or benign.

9. a. dysplasia.—The growth may be normal or abnormal, as in a developing tumor.

10. a. neoplasia.—Neoplasia is a generic term for the growth of a new type of cell. These cells may be either benign or malignant.

11. d. virulence.—Virulence measures the disease-causing ability of a microorganism.

12. c. protect it from ingestion and destruction by phagocytes.—Not all bacteria are encapsulated, but they can still resist destruction.

13. b. septic shock.—Endotoxins are lipopolysaccharides that are part of the cell wall of gram-negative bacteria.

14. d. fever to develop.—Pyrogens act by affecting the hypothalamic thermoregulatory center.

15. b. viruses do not produce exotoxins or endotoxins.—Bacteria produce toxins, which are usually referred to as exotoxins or endotoxins.

16. a. inflammation.—White blood cells (WBCs) release endogenous pyrogens that cause a fever to develop.

17. c. Down syndrome.—In Down syndrome, the child is born with an extra chromosome, usually number 21.

18. b. It helps the cells in fighting off diseases.—Good nutrition is required to maintain good health and assist the cells in fighting off diseases.

19. b. changes in cell distribution with aging.—The cellular environment includes: the distribution of cells throughout the body; changes in cell distribution with aging and disease; the movement of water, sodium, and chloride in and out of cells; and acid-base balance in the cells and surrounding tissues.

20. c. 50–70%—The body consists primarily of water. About 50–70% of the total body weight is fluid.

21. b. intracellular fluids—Most (63%) of the body's fluid is in the cells and is called intracellular fluid (ICF).

22. b. 2,500 ml—The average adult takes in about 2,500 ml of water a day. Most is taken in by drinking, some comes from the water in foods, and the remaining is a byproduct of cellular metabolism.

23. a. sodium.—Sodium, the major extracellular cation, is often lost along with large amounts of fluid. The loss may affect nerve and muscle function, as well as extracellular fluid (ECF) volume.

24. c. extracellular—Extracellular fluid is broken down into the fluid that is between the cells (interstitial fluid), fluid inside the blood vessels (intravascular fluid), lymph, and transcellular fluid.

25. d. diffusion.—The movement of a substance from an area of higher concentration to an area of lower concentration.

26. c. endocytosis.—Endocytosis is one of several cell-specific ingestion processes.

27. d. phagocytosis.—Phagocytosis is one of several cell-specific ingestion processes.

28. b. osmotic—Water moves between intracellular fluid (ICF) and extracellular fluid (ECF) by osmosis. This is also referred to as osmotic pressure.

29. b. eighteen to forty—The distribution of body fluids changes with age and varies with gender. Women of this age group have approximately 51% body fluid weight, while the men have approximately 61%.

30. b. hypotonic—The solution with a lower solute concentration has a lower osmotic pressure and is referred to as hypotonic.

31. a. facilitated diffusion.—Facilitated diffusion is a form of passive transport and one of two general methods of water and dissolved particle movement.

32. a. albumin—Albumin is in blood plasma, muscle, egg whites, milk, and other substances, and in many plant tissues and fluids.

34. d. capillary colloidal osmotic pressure.—This is osmotic pressure generated by dissolved proteins in the plasma that are too large to penetrate the capillary membrane.

35. c. capillary hydrostatic pressure.—Because the pressure is higher on the arterial end than the venous end, more water is pushed out of the capillaries on the arterial end and more is reabsorbed on the venous end.

36. a. edema.—An abnormal excess accumulation of serous fluid in connective tissue or in a serous cavity.

36. a. ascites.—Accumulation of serous fluid in the spaces between tissues and organs in the abdominal cavity.

37. d. all of the above.—The clinical manifestations of edema may be local at an injury site or generalized.

38. b. decreased colloidal osmotic pressure.—Extensive burns cause an increased loss of plasma proteins, resulting in decreased colloidal osmotic pressure.

39. b. pitting edema.—Pitting edema can be significant in the patient with chronic heart failure.

40. c. to exchange three sodium ions for every two potassium ions.—If the pump is impaired due to insufficient potassium in the body, sodium accumulates and causes the cells to swell.

41. a. tonicity.—Changes in water content can cause a cell to shrink or swell. Tonicity refers to the tension exerted on cell size due to water movement across the cell membrane.

42. c. have the same osmolarity as intracellular fluid.—Solutions that body cells are exposed to are classified as isotonic, hypotonic, or hypertonic. When the cell neither shrinks nor swells, it is isotonic.

43. d. hypertonic; pulled out of—When the osmolarity of a solution is greater than the ICF, it is hypertonic.

44. b. lower; swell—When the osmolarity of a solution is less than the ICF, it is hypotonic.

45. c. sodium.—The average adult has 60 mEq of sodium for each kilogram of body weight. Most of the body's sodium is found in the ECF.

46. b. 500 mg.—Sodium is taken in with foods. As little as 500 mg/day meets the body's needs.

47. c. stimulating sodium reabsorption.—Angiotensin II is responsible for stimulating sodium reabsorption by the renal tubules. It also constricts the renal blood vessels, slowing kidney blood flow and decreasing the glomerular filtration rate.

48. a. renin.—Renin is a protein enzyme that is released by the kidney into the bloodstream in response to changes in blood pressure, blood flow, the amount of sodium in the tubular fluids, and the glomerular filtration rate.

49. b. aldosterone—Besides angiotensin II, three other factors stimulate aldosterone release: increased extracellular potassium levels, decreased extracellular sodium levels, and release of adrenocorticotropic hormone (ACTH).

50. b. hypernatremic.—Hypernatremia is defined as a serum sodium level that is above 148 mEq/L.

51. b. seizures and coma.—Any alteration of mental status is considered severe.

52. c. vomiting and diarrhea—Causes may include excess sweating from hot environments or exercise and GI losses through vomiting, diarrhea, or diuresis.

53. c. hyponatremia.—During prolonged or extreme periods of extreme exercise or hot environments, excessive sodium loss can cause symptoms associated with hyponatremia: weight gain, headache, confusion, weakness, abdominal cramps, nausea, vomiting, diarrhea, stupor, or coma.

54. b. potassium.—Potassium is necessary for neuromuscular control, regulation of the three types of muscles, acid-base balance, intracellular enzyme reactions, and maintenance of intracellular osmolality.

55. a. excessive vomiting or diarrhea.—Hypokalemia is defined as a decreased serum potassium level and can be caused by numerous conditions related to fluid imbalance.

56. c. low T wave and sagging ST segment.—Peaked T waves, depressed ST segments, depressed P wave, and widening QRS complex are associated with hyperkalemia.

57. c. renal failure.—A common cause of hyperkalemia is renal failure.

58. a. paresthesia and intestinal colic.—Potassium is necessary for neuromuscular control, regulation of the three types of muscles, acid-base balance, intracellular

enzyme reactions, and maintenance of intracellular osmolality.

59. c. widened QRS.—Peaked T waves, depressed ST segments, depressed P wave, and widening QRS complex are associated with hyperkalemia.

60. d. bones—The vast majority (99%) of the body's calcium is found in the bones.

61. a. strength and stability to bones.—The purpose of calcium is to provide strength and stability for the collagen and ground substance that forms the matrix of the skeletal system.

62. c. through the GI tract—Calcium enters the body through the GI tract and is absorbed from the intestine by vitamin D.

63. a. renal failure.—Some of the causes of hypocalcemia include: hypoparathyroidism, hypomagnesmia, vitamin D deficiency, impaired ability to activate vitamin D, renal failure, increased pH, increased fatty acids, and acute pancreatitis.

64. b. rapid transfusion of citrated blood.—Other causes include liver and kidney disease, hyperphosphatemia, and rapid transfusion of citrated blood.

65. a. skeletal muscle cramps.—The manifestations of hypocalcemia include: paresthesia, skeletal muscle cramps, abdominal spasms and cramps, hyperactive reflexes, carpopedal spasm, tetany, laryngeal spasms, hypotension, bone pain, deformities, and fractures.

66. b. calcium.—A decreased serum calcium level (hypocalcemia) may cause symptoms of skeletal muscle cramps, abdominal spasms, bone pain, deformities, and fractures.

67. d. hypocalcemia.—In addition to osteomalacia, the manifestations of hypocalcemia include: paresthesia, skeletal muscle cramps, abdominal spasms and cramps, hyperactive reflexes, carpopedal spasm, tetany, laryngeal spasms, hypotension, bone pain, deformities, and fractures.

68. b. excess calcium in the diet.—The causes of hypercalcemia include: excess vitamin D or excess calcium in the diet, excess milk or calcium containing antacids, increased levels of parathyroid hormone, malignant neoplasms, prolonged immobilization, thiazide diuretics, and lithium therapy.

69. c. hypercalcemia.—Additional manifestations of hypercalcemia include: increased thirst, nausea, vomiting, muscle weakness, atrophy, ataxia, loss of muscle tone, behavioral changes, stupor, coma, hypertension, shortening of the QT interval, and atrioventricular block.

70. a. hypercalcemia—Manifestations of hypercalcemia include: increased thirst, nausea, vomiting, muscle weakness, atrophy, ataxia, loss of muscle tone, behavioral changes, stupor, coma, hypertension, shortening of the QT interval, and atrioventricular block.

71. d. diabetic ketoacidosis.—Additional causes of hypophosphatemia include: antacids, severe diarrhea, lack of vitamin D, alkalosis, hyperparathyroidism, alcoholism, recovery from malnutrition, and renal tubular absorption defects.

72. c. hemolytic anemia.—Manifestations of hypophosphatemia include: ataxia, paresthesia, hyporeflexia, confusion, stupor, coma, seizures, muscle weakness, joint stiffness, bone pain, osteomalacia, anorexia, dysphagia, impaired WBC function, platelet dysfunction with bleeding disorders, and hemolytic anemia.

73. b. hyperphosphatemia.—Additional causes of hyperphosphatemia include: heat stroke, seizures, tumor lysis syndrome, potassium, deficiency, hypoparathyroidism, phosphate-containing laxatives, and enemas.

74. b. hypomagnesemia—The causes of hypomagnesemia include: alcoholism, malnutrition or starvation, malabsorption, small bowel bypass surgery, parenteral hyperalimentation with inadequate amounts of magnesium, and high dietary intake of calcium without concomitant amounts of magnesium.

75. a. hypomagnesemia.—Additional manifestations of hypomagnesemia include: personality change, athetoid or choreiform movements, nystagmus, tetany, tachycardia, hypertension, and cardiac dysrhythmias.

76. c. Trousseau's—Trousseau's sign is associated with hypomagnesemia.

77. c. 7.35–7.45—pH is the measurement of the hydrogen ion concentration. A blood pH greater than 7.45 is called alkalosis, and a blood pH of less than 7.35 is called acidosis.

78. b. greater; alkalosis—A blood pH greater than 7.45 is called alkalosis, and a blood pH of less than 7.35 is called acidosis.

79. b. metabolic acidosis.—Metabolic acidosis is an accumulation of abnormal acids in the blood for any of several reasons (e.g., sepsis, diabetic ketoacidosis, and salicylate poisoning).

80. a. respiratory acidosis.—Respiratory acidosis occurs when CO_2 retention leads to increased levels of pCO_2. It also occurs in situations of hypoventilation or intrinsic lung diseases.

81. c. respiratory acidosis.—Respiratory acidosis occurs when CO_2 retention leads to increased levels of pCO_2. It also occurs in situations of hypoventilation (e.g., depressed respiratory effort from a heroin overdose) or intrinsic lung diseases (e.g., asthma or COPD).

82. d. respiratory alkalosis.—Excessive "blowing off" of CO_2 with a resulting decrease in the pCO_2 causes respiratory alkalosis.

83. a. genetic histories of population.—Analyzing disease risk involves reviewing the rates of incidence,

prevalence, and mortality, as well as causal and noncausal risk factors.

84. b. Parkinson's disease.—Some diseases are more prevalent in men, such as lung cancer, gout, and Parkinson's disease. Women are more likely to get osteoporosis, rheumatoid arthritis, or breast cancer.

85. d. allergy.—Allergies are an acquired hypersensitivity. First, the person is exposed or sensitized to the antigen. Repeated exposures cause a reaction by the immune system to the allergen.

86. b. rheumatic fever—Rheumatic fever develops following a streptococcal infection (e.g., strep throat) and is characterized by myocarditis and arthritis.

87. a. recent weight gain—The American Cancer Society uses the acronym "CAUTION" to list the signs:
Change in bowel or bladder habits
A sore that does not heal
Unusual bleeding or discharge
Thickening or lung development
Indigestion or difficulty swallowing
Obvious change in a wart or mole
Nagging cough or hoarseness

88. c. asthma.—Asthma is exhibited by constriction of the bronchi, wheezing, and dyspnea.

89. d. asthma.—Acute asthma is a recurring condition of completely or partially reversible acute airflow obstruction in the lower airway. Asthma is the leading cause of chronic illness in children.

90. c. lung—Lung cancer is the leading cause of cancer deaths and the second leading cause of cancer cases in males and females.

91. c. Type I requires exogenous insulin.—Type I diabetic patients are absolutely dependent on exogenously administered insulin, while Type II diabetic patients typically are not.

92. b. Their digestive juices would destroy oral forms.—This is why insulin injections are necessary.

93. d. pancreas—Insulin is a hormone produced and released from the pancreas.

94. c. drug-induced anemia.—Drug-induced hemolytic anemia is a hemolytic anemia that is characterized by an increased destruction of red blood cells.

95. a. The cause is unknown.—The cause is unknown, but it has been associated with Marfan's syndrome, osteogenesis imperfecta, connective tissue disorders, cardiac, metabolic, neuroendocrine, metabolic, and psychologic disorders.

96. a. is inherited.—Hereditary prolongation of the QT interval may occur by itself or may be associated with other diseases.

97. b. hemophilia.—Hemophilia is a gender-linked hereditary bleeding disorder most commonly passed on from an asymptomatic mother to a male child.

98. b. cardiomyopathies.—There are a number of disease forms. The diseases cause the heart muscle to become thin, flabby, dilated, or enlarged.

99. d. cardiovascular disease—Almost half of all cardiovascular deaths result from coronary heart disease.

100. d. hypertension—Often referred to as the silent killer. Hypertension typically has no signs or symptoms.

101. c. gout.—The disease leads to inflammation of the joints due to a metabolic problem in the breakdown of proteins.

102. b. changing the size and shape of the heart.—The myocardial geometry (shape) changes that occur with chronic hypertension cause the hypertrophied heart to work harder to maintain a given output.

103. c. Nicotine causes vasoconstriction.—Arteries become damaged due to the excessive pressure of vasoconstriction and then become weakened. The weakened areas develop blood clots and thrombosis or they rupture and hemorrhage critically.

104. b. renal calculi.—Also called renal calculus.

105. c. males; thirty to fifty—Kidney stones are most prevalent in men between the ages of thirty and fifty.

106. c. ulcerative colitis.—A nonspecific inflammatory disease of the colon with no known cause.

107. b. lactose intolerance.—Lactose intolerance is likely the most common GI abnormality known to mankind. Some studies suggest that it affects more than half of the world's population.

108. a. peptic ulcers.—Peptic ulcer disease involves erosions of either the stomach or duodenum.

109. c. gallstones.—Cholelithiasis is the production of gallstones and the condition that results from it.

110. c. gallstones.—Gallstones can block the lumen, interfering with bile flow.

111. b. hypotension.—Hypertension is a health risk associated with obesity.

112. d. respiratory function impairment.—The formation of the adipose tissue around the neck, chest, and abdomen can impair normal respiratory function and cause sleep apnea.

113. b. Huntington's disease.—The disease produces localized death of brain cells and there is no cure. Symptoms do not usually develop until patients are over thirty years of age, and by then they may have already passed the gene to their own offspring.

114. a. multiple sclerosis.—MS is a demyelinating disease of the central nervous system. It is the major cause of neurological disability in young and middle-aged adults.

115. c. impaired cognition and abstract thinking.—In stage 2 of Alzheimer's disease, judgment and cognition become impaired and social behavior becomes inappropriate.

116. c. an extensive acute myocardial infarction.—Initially the signs and symptoms are the same as seen with ACS. As the body's compensating mechanism fails

and shock progresses, severe hypotension develops and organ tissues die.

117. c. Pericardial tamponade—Additional causes include: vena cava syndrome, dissecting aortic aneurysm, pulmonary embolism in the pulmonary circulation, and a ball valve thrombus in the cardiac chambers.

118. c. electrolyte loss from dehydration.—Additional causes of hypovolemic shock include: internal or external hemorrhage, plasma loss from burns or inflammation, trauma, anaphylaxis, and envenomation.

119. c. multiple organ dysfunction syndrome—MODS involves the progressive failure of two or more organ systems after severe illness or injury. The mortality rate is between 60 and 90%.

120. c. autoimmune—Autoimmunity occurs when a person's T cells or antibodies attacks the new red blood cells, causing tissue damage and organ dysfunction.

121. b. Vasodilation—The local effects of an inflammation response are vasodilation, increased capillary permeability, and the development of exudates.

122. a. fever.—The systemic responses to an acute inflammation include: fever, leukocytosis, and an increase in the circulating plasma proteins or acute phase reactants.

123. a. natural—Natural or native immunity is acquired either by getting the disease or receiving antibodies from your mother (also referred to as passive immunity).

124. c. complement.—The complement system plays a vital role in attracting WBCs to the site of the infection, as well as initially attacking bacteria. The activation of the complement system during a severe illness, though, may lead to "self-destruction" by activated components.

125. a. phagocytes—Phagocytes are one of the cellular components of inflammation, and their role is to engulf foreign matter and bacteria.

Chapter 7: Pharmacology

1. b. drug.—The two terms, drug and medication, are used interchangeably, yet there is a difference. A medication is a medicinal substance used as a treatment or remedy, whereas a drug is any chemical substance that, when taken into a living organism, produces a biological response.

2. a. pharmacokinetics.—Once a drug has been introduced into the body, it goes through five distinct stages: absorption, distribution, desired effect, metabolism, and elimination.

3. a. pharmacodynamics.—Specifically, it looks at the biochemical and physiological effects on, or interactions with, the target organ(s) or tissue(s).

4. d. biotransformation.—Biotransformation or metabolism is the chemical breakdown of the drug (stage 4) as it travels through the body.

5. d. research.—Medications are administered to achieve a therapeutic effect, a prophylactic effect, or a diagnostic effect.

6. a. drug action.—The interaction between a drug and a body organ or tissue is only a physiologic modification of the organ or tissue because drugs do not produce new functions. The drug-induced physiologic change to a body function or process is known as a drug action.

7. a. agonist.—A chemical substance capable of combining with a receptor on a cell and initiating a reaction.

8. b. target organs or tissues.—There are several ways by which a drug affects a body organ or tissue. This is called the drugs mechanism of action. The major mechanism by which a drug affects the body is by joining with receptors located on the target organs or tissues.

9. d. sympathomimetic.—This group of drugs is commonly used in the out-of-hospital setting, particularly within advanced cardiac life support (ACLS).

10. a. dopamine.—In addition to being a sympathomimetic drug, dopamine, an antecedent to the formation of epinephrine, can also act as a neurotransmitter in the sympathetic nervous system.

11. d. sympathomimetics.—This group of drugs is commonly used in prehospital emergency care, particularly within ACLS.

12. c. sympatholytics.—Beta-blockers (e.g., atenolol, metoprolol, and propranolol) are included in this group of drugs.

13. a. acetylcholine.—Drugs that perform similarly to acetylcholine and mimic the parasympathetic response are referred to as cholinergic or parasympathomimetic.

14. d. atropine.—Atropine primarily blocks parasympathetic stimulation of the heart, causing the rate to increase, but it also affects other body systems.

15. a. energy produced through a chemical reaction.—Active transport is the movement of chemical substance by the expenditure of energy through a cell membrane in concentration or electrical potential and opposite to the direction of normal diffusion.

16. d. cumulative effect.—The cumulative effect occurs when a dose is repeated before the prior dose has been metabolized.

17. a. idiosyncrasy.—Idiosyncrasy is an abnormal or unpredictable response to a drug that is peculiar to an individual rather than a general group.

18. b. blood-brain barrier.—The blood-brain barrier is a physiologic barrier that exists between circulating blood and the brain. This barrier protects brain tissue and cerebral spinal fluid from exposure to certain substances.

19. a. official—The official name is the same as the generic name and is followed by the initials USP (U.S. Pharmacopoeia) or NF (National Formulary), denoting its listing in one of these official publications.

20. b. angiotensin I from converting angiotensin II.—Angiotensin-converting enzyme (ACE) inhibitors work by affecting the renin-angiotensin-aldosterone system. This system supports the sodium and fluid balance of the body and maintains blood pressure.

21. a. ingredients.—A chemical assay is a test that determines the ingredients and their exact amounts.

22. d. label all dangerous ingredients in drug products.—In 1906, the U.S. government passed the first law to protect the public from impure or mislabeled drugs.

23. d. drug enforcement.—The Drug Enforcement Agency (DEA), in the Department of Justice, became the nation's sole drug enforcement agency in 1973.

24. b. the total body weight affects the distribution of the drug.—The total body weight and the amount of a drug given have a direct association to the distribution and concentration of a drug.

25. a. affinity.—The joining of a drug and a receptor site is called affinity, and is often compared to the connection of a lock and key. The drug is the key and the lock is the receptor.

26. d. antagonist.—When a drug inhibits a receptor, it is called an antagonist, which means "to block."

27. a. dopaminergic and adrenergic.—The two types of sympathetic receptors are adrenergic receptors and dopaminergic receptors. Adrenergic receptors are subdivided into the following four types: alpha 1 and 2, beta 1 and 2.

28. d. passive transport.—Passive transport of water and dissolved particle movement includes the following processes: diffusion, facilitated diffusion, osmosis, and filtration.

29. a. osmotic—Osmotic pressure is produced or associated with osmosis. It helps control the movement of water into or out of the cell.

30. c. drug interaction.—A drug interaction is the combined effect of drugs taken at the same time that alters the expected therapeutic effect.

31. b. potentiation—The combined effects of two drugs are better than either could have produced alone (e.g., 1 + 1 = 3 or more.)

32. a. additive—The additive synergistic effect of two agreeable drugs produces an effect that neither could alone.

33. d. antagonism.—The example described in the question is chemical antagonism. The charcoal binds with and absorbs the toxins present in the GI tract to inactivate them.

34. c. half-life—Half-life refers to the amount of time that a drug remains at a therapeutic level to produce a desired effect and the time it takes the body to metabolize or inactivate a drug's concentration by 50%.

35. a. controlled the sale of narcotics and drugs that cause dependence.—The Controlled Substance Act of 1970 superseded the Harrison Narcotic Act. This act sets forth the rules for the manufacture and distribution of drugs that have the potential for abuse.

36. d. V—Schedule V is the rating for the lowest abuse potential. Cough syrups and diarrhea medications fall into this schedule.

37. b. four—These phases include testing, approval, and marketing requirements before new drugs can reach the consumer.

38. b. The defect occurred before it left the manufacturer.—For the drug product liability to exist, the following three criteria must be met: the defect caused harm, the defect occurred before it left the manufacturer, and the product is defective or not fit for its intended reasonable uses.

39. b. therapeutic effect.—Because drugs are classified by their chemical class, mechanism of action, or therapeutic effect, looking at the medications a patient is taking can give you a lot of information about her medical history.

40. c. a quicker absorption rate than lower doses.—The dosage is a predominant factor for the absorption rate of a drug.

41. a. A loading dose is typically a single dose of a drug.—A loading dose is considered to be a single dose or the accumulation of several closely repeated single doses (boluses) used to obtain the therapeutic level to achieve a desired effect.

42. a. dehydration—Medications are often a cause of altered mental status, especially in the elderly. Improper diuretic use can lead to dehydration and electrolyte imbalances, especially with potassium. Colace is a stool softener.

43. b. decreased renal function—Impaired renal or liver function interferes with the body's ability to metabolize and eliminate drugs. This can lead to a cumulative effect and toxicity.

44. b. U.S. Pharmacopoeia.—A U.S. government publication and the only official book of drug standards in the United States since 1980.

45. d. drugs with weak acidity—Drugs that have a weak acidity, such as barbiturates, are absorbed better in the stomach than in the intestine. Drugs that have a weaker base, such as morphine sulfate, have a better reaction if given by a route other than orally so as to avoid the high acidity of the stomach.

46. b. it may elevate diagnostic enzyme levels.—The measurement of CK-MB (creatine kinase; M, muscle; B, brain) and troponin used in cardiac enzyme testing are a couple of examples.

47. b. Wear a face mask.—Wearing a face mask will reduce the chance of inhaling aerosolized particles, including medications and infectious particles.

Consider the use of a spacer with aerosolized medications to better direct the medication.

48. c. heart muscle—Most drugs are metabolized and eliminated by way of the liver, kidneys, GI tract, and lungs.

49. a. iatrogenic.—An adverse mental or physical condition inadvertently induced by a healthcare provider, medical treatment, or diagnostic procedure.

50. a. standardization.—Standardization is necessary because many drugs are made from plants. The strength from plant to plant may be different based on a number of variables, such as where it was grown and how it was processed.

Chapter 8: Medication Administration

1. b. indirect orders of medical control.—Indirect orders for medication administration are commonly used with specific circumstances such as an asthma attack or a cardiac arrest. These orders are written as standing orders and referred to as protocols.

2. a. avoid making medication administration errors.—This phrase refers to some of the universal principles of medication administration in an effort to avoid making an error when giving a patient a medication.

3. c. antiseptic.—Preventing or stopping the growth of microorganisms.

4. d. disinfectant.—A chemical agent that destroys microorganisms.

5. b. open ampule.—Sharps are any medical products that can cause a puncture or cut to anyone who handles them. An open ampule has an exposed glass edge.

6. a. local infection—The most common complication is that the patient develops a local infection at the site of injection. This is directly associated with poor (dirty) technique by the person who performed the skill.

7. c. twice a day—A Latin abbreviation (bis in die) used in writing prescriptions.

8. c. subcutaneous—An injection under the dermis into connective tissue or fat for slow absorption.

9. a. household—The household method is a system commonly used in the home, also called the United States system, and is based on the traditional English system.

10. c. gram.—In the metric system, the basic unit of mass (weight) is the gram; the basic unit of volume is the liter; and the basic unit of length is the meter.

11. c. either KVO or TKO.—Keep vein open or to keep open.

12. d. absorption effects are more predictable.—Drugs administered by IV have the fastest and most predictable absorption rates. Drugs administered by mouth will have many more factors that can affect the absorption rate, making this route slow and often unpredictable.

13. a. buccal—The space between the cheek and gum is the buccal area. Medications placed there dissolve through the buccal mucosa.

14. a. enteral—Because enteral routes are through the alimentary canal, which begins at the mouth and ends at the rectum, enteral drugs are taken orally (PO) or rectally (PR).

15. b. epidural.—This is a parenteral route.

16. b. 3.5 grams—$(3,500 \text{ mg}) \div (1,000) = 3.5 \text{ g}$

17. a. 0.0012 grams—First convert to milligrams $(1,200 \text{ mcg}) \div (1,000) = 1.2 \text{ mg}$. Next, convert milligrams to grams $(1.2 \text{ mg}) \div (1,000) = 0.0012 \text{ grams}$.

18. d. 2,500 ml—$(2.5 \text{ liters}) \times (1000) = 2,500 \text{ ml}$

19. c. 90 kg—kilograms = (lb) $\div$ (2.2). $(198 \text{ lb}) \div (2.2 \text{ kg}) = 90 \text{ kg}$.

20. c. 145 lb—pounds = (kg) $\times$ (2.2). $(66) \times (2.2) = 145.2$. Round down to 145 lb.

21. b. 120 mg—Convert pounds to kilograms = $(176 \text{ lb}) \div (2.2) = 80 \text{ kg}$. Next, multiply $(1.5) \times (80) = 120 \text{ mg}$.

22. b. 12 ml—The drug comes packaged as 100 mg in 10 ml. Two packages will be needed; all of one and 2 ml of the second, for a total of 12 ml.

23. b. 100 gtt/min—

$$\text{Administration Rate} = \frac{(\text{volume ordered}) (\text{drip set})}{\text{time}}$$

$$= \frac{(300 \text{ ml})(10 \text{ gtt})}{30 \text{ min}}$$

$$\frac{3000}{30} = 100 \text{ gtt/min}$$

24. b. 25—D-50 comes packaged in 50 ml, or 0.5 g/ml, or 25 grams.
25. c. Dilute the D-50 by one-half, then administer.—The pediatric dose is a lesser concentration (D-25), and the neonate dose is less (D-10).
26. c. 45 gtts— First mix the 200 mg lidocaine in the 50 ml bag for a concentration of 4:1 = 4mg/ml.

$$\text{Administration rate} = \text{gtt/min} = \frac{(\text{dose/min})(\text{drip set})}{\text{dose/ml}}$$

$$= \frac{(3 \text{ mg/min})(60 \text{ gtt/ml})}{4 \text{ mg/ml}} = 45 \text{ gtt/min}$$

27. c. 1.5 ml—Two vials with a total of 8 mg in 4 ml or 2 mg in 0.5 ml. You administer 5 mg in 2.5 ml, and what is left is 3 mg in 1.5 ml.
28. a. 37°—Temperature conversions:
Fahrenheit = F = (9/5C) + 32
Celsius = C = 5/9 (F − 32)

Fahrenheit temperature of 98.6°, and you desire to convert it into degrees on the Celsius scale. Using the above formula, you would first subtract 32 from the Fahrenheit temperature and get 66.6 as a result. Then you multiply 66.6 by five-ninths and get the converted value of 37° Celsius.
29. b. vial.—A small, closed container for fluids.
30. d. aspirin—Enteral drugs are taken orally (PO) or rectally (PR).
31. a. The absorption rate is fast.—Medications taken orally absorb much slower than medications administered by other routes.
32. c. PR allows for rapid absorption.—The rectum is vascular, allowing for rapid absorption that does not go through biotransformation in the liver before reaching its target organs.
33. b. use a single line to mark out the error, make the change, and initial it.—Erasing or deleting information gives the appearance of hiding information. Instead, mark a single line through the error, write your initials next to it, and then write the correction.
34. d. 70–80 mmHg—This range is tight enough to occlude venous return but not restrict arterial flow.
35. b. a reaction from the bee sting.—Hypotension is not typically a side effect of Benadryl®. The patient experiencing an allergic reaction has likely become hypotensive from vasodilation as a progression to anaphylactic shock.
36. a. kilo—(k) kilo = 1,000, (c) centi = 1/100 or 0.01, milli = 1/1,000 or 0.001, and (mcg or μg) micro = 1/1,000,000 or 0.000001.
37. c. 50 gtt/min—First mix 150 mg into 50 ml = 3:1 concentration or 3 mg/ml.

$$\text{Drip rate} = \frac{(X)(10 \text{ gtt})}{3 \text{ mg/ml}} = \frac{(15 \text{ mg/min})(10 \text{ gtt/ml})}{3 \text{ mg/ml}}$$

$$= 50 \text{ gtt/min}$$

Another method:
Order is to give 50 ml over 10 min.
1 ml = 10 gtt
10 ml = 100 gtts

$$50 \text{ ml} = 500 \text{ gtts} = \frac{500 \text{ gtt}}{10 \text{ min}} = \frac{50 \text{ gtt}}{\text{min}}$$

38. b. 25 gtt/min—First mix 2g (2000 mg) into 50 ml = 4:1 concentration or 40 mg/ml. You need to administer 2000 mg over 20 min = 2000 mg/20 min = 100 mg/min.

$$\text{Drip rate} = \frac{(X)(10 \text{ gtt/ml})}{40 \text{ mg/ml}} = \frac{(100 \text{ mg/min})(10 \text{ gtt/ml})}{40 \text{ mg/ml}}$$

$$= 25 \text{ gtt/min}$$

39. c. 25—Because D5W contains 5 grams of sugar per 100 ml of solvent, 500 ml contains five times as much, or 25 grams.
40. a. 19—1,600 mcg/ml in 250: (5 mcg)(100 kg) = 500 mcg/min

$$\text{Drip rate} = \frac{(500 \text{ mcg/min})(60 \text{ gtt/ml})}{1,600 \text{ mcg/ml}} = \frac{30,000}{1,600} = \frac{30}{1.6}$$

$$= 18.75 \text{ round up } 19 \text{ gtt/min}$$

41. a. 01. mg—First convert pounds to kilograms = 12 lb ÷ 2.2 = 5.45. Round down to 5 kg. Next (5 kg)(0.02 mg/kg) = 0.1 mg
42. d. 100—

$$\text{Drip rate} = \frac{(50 \text{ ml})(60 \text{ gtt/min})}{30 \text{ gtt/min}} = \frac{3,000}{30} = 100 \text{ minutes}$$

43. d. 120 ml—

$$\frac{(X \text{ ml/min})(60 \text{ gtt/min})}{60 \text{ gtt/min}} = \frac{(20 \text{ ml/min})(60 \text{ gtt/min})}{10 \text{ gtt/min}} \quad \frac{10}$$

$$= \frac{1200}{10} = 120 \text{ ml}$$

44. d. 23 mg—First convert pounds to kilograms = 200 lb ÷ 2.2 = 90.9. Round up to 91 kg.
Next (0.25 mg)(91 kg) = 22.75. Round up to 23 mg.
45. b. 5 cc—The package of medication has 25 mg in 5 ml, or 5 mg/ml. The dose is 23 mg, so the smallest syringe to use for one dose is a 5 cc syringe.
46. b. 15—You need to administer 150 mg over 10 min = 150 mg/10 min = 15 mg/min.
47. d. 30—One quart = 2 pints. If the total volume is 12 pints, 3.5 pints is 30%. (3.5) ÷ (12) = .29166, or approximately 30%.
48. d. 42 gtts/min—

$$\text{Drip rate} = \frac{(250 \text{ ml/hr})(10 \text{ gtt/ml})}{60 \text{ min}} = 42 \text{ gtt/min}$$

49. b. 29—350 liters at 12 lpm (350 L) ÷ (12 L/min) = 29 min
50. b. 23-ga and 0.5 inch needle—Subcutaneous injection is made using a small size needle (23–29 gauge) (1/2 to 5/8 inch) at a 45° angle.

Chapter 9: Life Span Development

1. b. 3.0–3.5 kg.—The average weight of a newborn is between 3.0 and 3.5 kilograms, or 6.5 and 7.5 pounds.

2. b. 5–10—There is a normal weight loss of 5–10% during the first week of life due to the excretion of extracellular fluid present at birth.

3. c. four to six months—During the first month, the infant grows by approximately 30 grams per day. As a result, the infant's weight should double by 4–6 months and triple by nine to twelve months.

4. d. The ductus arteriosus closes.—The circulatory changes lead to: closing of the ductus arteriosus, closing of the ductus venosus, and closing of the foramen ovale. When these changes are complete, the infant has made the shift from fetal circulation to normal infant circulation.

5. a. four weeks—Any occlusion of the nares during this time is the functional equivalent of an upper airway obstruction.

6. d. The ribs are positioned horizontally, causing diaphragmatic breathing.—The lung tissue on an infant is fragile and more prone to barotrauma. In the infant, there are fewer alveoli and the chest wall is less rigid. The accessory muscles are also immature and susceptible to early fatigue.

7. a. three months—The posterior fontanelle closes by three months of age, and the anterior fontanelle closes between nine and eighteen months of age.

8. c. nine to eighteen months—The posterior fontanelle closes by three months of age, and the anterior fontanelle closes between nine and eighteen months of age.

9. c. abnormal thyroid hormone levels—Abnormal levels of thyroid hormone and growth hormone can cause abnormally fast bone growth.

10. b. two—The rate of weight gain slows dramatically as the infant becomes a toddler. The average child gains only two kilograms per year during this period.

11. b. modeling—Modeling is imitation of another's behavior, dress, mannerisms, or attitudes.

12. c. school age—With each interaction, school-age children compare themselves with others. This leads to the development of self-esteem, either positive or negative.

13. b. secondary sexual development.—Secondary sexual characteristics are the external physical characteristics of sexual maturity resulting from the action of sex hormones. These include male and female patterns of body hair, fat distribution, development of external genitals, and deepening of the voice in males.

14. a. Gonadotropins released by the pituitary gland promote the production of testosterone.—These promote the production of testosterone by the testes, which contribute to further development of secondary sexual characteristics and to sexual maturity.

15. a. decrease in elasticity of the diaphragm.—In addition, a decreased muscle mass leads to relative chest wall weakness.

16. b. weakening of the chest wall.—This, combined with decreased elasticity of the diaphragm, leads to decreased respiratory function.

17. b. decrease in insulin production.—Insulin production decreases, leading to abnormalities in glucose metabolism and sometimes Type II diabetes.

18. d. changes in renal function.—Nearly 50% of functioning nephrons are lost during late adulthood. As a result, decreased excretion of fluid, salts, and waste products may occur.

19. c. their muscular sphincters become less effective with age.—Muscular sphincters (e.g., esophageal and rectal) become less effective, resulting in acid reflux and stool incontinence.

20. c. Growth spurts begin with enlargement of the feet and hands.—Most adolescents experience a rapid growth spurt lasting two to three years. It begins distally with an enlargement of the feet and hands.

21. a. infancy—During infancy, the kidneys are unable to concentrate the urine, resulting in a specific gravity usually no greater than that of distilled water.

22. a. moro—The reflex is elicited by striking the surface near the infant's head. This reflex is usually not obtainable after three months of age.

23. a. six months—Antibodies transferred from the mother maintain passive immunity throughout the first six months of life. By then, the infant's own immune system has begun to provide protection, at least to some extent.

24. d. 100—Rates below 80 bpm usually require CPR.

25. b. abnormal—At birth, the respiratory rate is normally between 40 and 60 breaths per minute. It drops rapidly after the first few minutes of life (30–40 breaths per minute), and slows to 20–30 breaths per minute by the time the infant reaches her first birthday.

26. b. triple—During the first month, the infant grows by approximately 30 grams per day. As a result, the infant's weight should double by four to six months and triple by nine to twelve months.

27. b. five to seven—The first baby teeth begin to erupt at five to seven months of age.

28. d. expectancy.—Life expectancy is the amount of time remaining before a person is expected to die. The average life expectancy depends on many factors.

29. b. accidents—Accidents are the leading cause of death in this age group.

30. c. middle adulthood—The cardiac output decreases throughout this period, and cholesterol levels tend to increase.

31. d. empty nest—The empty nest syndrome occurs when all of a parent's children become old enough to leave home. Often, this is very exciting for couples because they are able to spend previously unavailable time together.

32. d. Life span—Life span is a retrospective measurement. It measures how long a person actually lived.

33. b. orthostatic—Postural hypotension becomes more common because of inadequate compensatory mechanisms.

34. a. arteriosclerosis.—Vessel walls thicken, often due to arteriosclerosis. This results in an increase in peripheral vascular resistance with variable reductions in organ blood flow.

35. c. less elastic.—This leads to an increased workload on the aging heart.

36. b. Sick-sinus—Patients alternate from normal sinus rhythm to supraventricular tachycardias, to bradycardia and AV block, without apparent logic.

37. b. poor nutrition and malabsorption.—As a result, low-grade anemia is relatively common (though not normal) in late adulthood.

38. c. Anemia—This worsens oxygen delivery to tissues, including the myocardium.

39. d. They have a loss of normal mucous membrane linings.—As a result, inhaled air is less humidified.

40. a. pain perception—Virtually all sensory stems exhibit decreased responsiveness during late adulthood. The decrease in pain perception may result in the development of a serious disease with very few clinical signs or symptoms.

41. a. sleep-wake cycle.—Normal aging results in a loss of neurons and neurotransmitters. The clinical effects are variable. Generally, the sleep-wake cycle is disturbed.

42. c. osteoporosis of the spine—In late adulthood, no new growth takes place and height may decrease due to osteoporosis of the spine.

43. c. early adulthood—As a rule, all body systems are at optimal performance and a person reaches a peak in physical condition between nineteen and twenty-six years of age.

44. b. school-age—With each interaction, school-age children compare themselves with others. This leads to the development of self-esteem. Moral development varies considerably from child to child and depends on many facts. Individuals move through moral development throughout school age and young adulthood at very different paces.

45. b. three to four years—Hearing reaches peak (maturity) levels by three and four years of age.

46. c. permissive-indulgent—Parents who are low in authority and high in responsiveness are typified as engaging in an indulgent style of parenting. These parents are committed to their children and are tolerant, warm, and accepting, but they do not exercise much authority and make few demands for mature behavior on the part of the child.

47. c. understanding of body image.—This comes about in adolescence.

48. d. Presbycusis—A lessoning of hearing acuteness resulting from degenerative changes that occur in the ear, especially in the elderly.

49. c. a decrease in cortisol production.—Cortisol production by the adrenal glands is diminished by 25%. Because cortisol is produced during stress, the late adult is less equipped to handle bodily stresses (e.g., severe infection).

50. a. loss of normal cardiac pacemaker cells.—Degeneration of the cardiac conduction system may lead to a combination of brady- and tachydysrhythmias. This is often termed the "tach-brady" syndrome or "sick-sinus syndrome."

Chapter 10: Airway Management and Ventilation

1. a. alveoli—The alveoli are located within the lungs.
2. c. ring in the trachea.—The cricoid ring is the only complete ring in the trachea. In the pediatric patient, it is the narrowest portion of the trachea.
3. a. Infants and children have a more flexible trachea than adults.—The pediatric trachea is softer and more flexible than that of an adult. This is why airway positioning is critical in the unconscious pediatric patient.
4. d. They are proportionately larger and take up more space in the mouth.—Proportionately, the tongue and epiglottis are larger, softer, and more floppy than those of an adult.
5. d. ethmoid bone—The ethmoid bone is a structure in the nose.
6. a. warm, filter, and humidify the air we breathe.—It also includes the nose, which is the organ for the sense of smell.
7. c. exchange oxygen and carbon dioxide at the cellular level.—Normally, each alveolus is surrounded by a functional pulmonary capillary, where carbon dioxide passes from the blood and is eliminated by

breathing. Simultaneously, oxygen is absorbed from the alveolus into the capillary.

8. a. Ventilation; oxygenation—Ventilation refers to the movement of carbon dioxide out of the lungs during breathing. This process differs from oxygenation, the movement of oxygen into the lungs, though they are often interrelated.

9. c. 760; 100—At sea level the atmospheric pressure, measured in torr (mmHg and torr are interchangeable terms) should add up to 760 torr and should equal 100%.

10. b. 159.0—The partial pressure is the pressure exerted by a specific atmospheric gas. The normal concentration of oxygen in the atmosphere at sea level is 159.0 torr (20.84%).

11. a. There is less nitrogen and oxygen in the alveolar gas.—There is more carbon dioxide and water in the alveolar gas. Specifically, the concentrations are: nitrogen 569.0 torr (74.9%), oxygen 104.0 torr (13.7%), carbon dioxide 40.0 torr (5.2%) and water 47.0 torr (6.2%).

12. b. patient's metabolic status.—Especially the acid-base balance.

13. a. medulla—The rate of respiration is controlled by the medulla and pons in the brain. The medulla is the primary involuntary respiratory center. It connects to the respiratory muscles by the vagus nerve.

14. d. apneustic—The pons take over if the medulla fails to initiate breathing.

15. c. CSF.—The analysis sends messages to the brain to increase or decrease the respiratory rate.

16. a. aortic arch.—Chemoreceptors are most plentiful in the carotid sinus and the aortic arch.

17. b. high concentration of carbon dioxide—When chemoreceptors sense the level of carbon dioxide rising, they send a message to the brain to increase the respiratory rate to rid the body of the excess carbon dioxide.

18. c. trapped or retained CO_2.—The loss of normal alveolar structure leads to a decrease in the elastic recoil, which creates resistance to expiratory airflow. Air is trapped within the lungs, resulting in poor air exchange.

19. c. The risk of under-oxygenating this patient is greater than the risk of suppressing the stimulus to breathe.—The patient is in respiratory distress and appears to require higher oxygen concentrations. Observe the patient carefully for changes in the mental status and respiratory rate. If the patient begins to deteriorate, the oxygen concentration may be decreased. Bear in mind that problems other than excessive oxygen can cause these patients to deteriorate.

20. b. Smoking inhibits the normal movement of mucus out of the lung.—Cigarette smoking directly inhibits the normal movement of mucus via bronchial cilia out of the lung. As a result, the lung is unable to clear pathogens (e.g., bacteria and viruses) as effectively. Allowed to remain, these infectious agents multiply, resulting in pneumonia.

21. d. hypoxia.—A deficiency of oxygen reaching the tissues of the body.

22. c. Hypoxemia—Inadequate oxygenation of the blood.

23. b. hypoventilating and hypoxemic—Neurologic emergencies (e.g., stroke, seizure, brain injury, and tumor) cause abnormal respirations, altered mental status, paralysis, and vision, speech, and motor disturbances. Carefully assess the respiratory status for signs of hypoventilation and hypoxemia.

24. c. Cerebrovascular accident—Laryngeal spasm is often associated with cold-water drowning, post-extubation, and overly aggressive intubation attempts.

25. a. The patient is contagious.—Consider any patient with possible pneumonia to be contagious, and act accordingly.

26. a. severe allergic reaction—An FBAO (e.g., food or vomiting) can cause aspiration, which can result in exposure of pathogens into the lungs, infection, and destruction of lung tissue.

27. c. manual suction—The bulb syringe, V-Vac®, and foot pump style suction units are operated manually and require no oxygen or electric sources to operate.

28. d. deplete your oxygen source rapidly.—Unless you have an endless supply of oxygen, this can be a significant disadvantage.

29. c. suctioning the tracheobronchial region.—Sterile suctioning, also referred to as deep suctioning or closed suctioning, is the technique used to suction the tracheobronchial region through an endotracheal tube.

30. b. tickling the back of the throat.—The gag reflex, or vagal response, can be easily stimulated by suctioning the back of the mouth and throat.

31. a. prevent the tongue from obstructing the glottis.—OPAs are airway adjuncts designed to keep the tongue from becoming an obstruction.

32. b. they do not provide a secured airway.—Nasal airways can be suctioned through, can provide a patent but not secured airway, and can be tolerated by conscious patients. Nasal airways can be safely placed blindly and do not require the mouth to be opened during insertion.

33. b. The bevel is designed to face the nasal septum.—For this reason, nasal airways are usually designed to be inserted in the right nostril. That does not mean they cannot be used in the left if there is difficulty inserting one in the right.

34. c. collect in the lung tissue, causing a chemical aspiration pneumonia.—Water-soluble products are less irritating to the tissue if a small amount should get into the lungs.

35. a. systolic; inspiration—The cause is felt to be increased intrathoracic and pericardial pressures that decrease the venous return to the heart. A change in pulse quality may also be detected during inspiration.

36. b. during an asthma attack.—The cause is felt to be increased intrathoracic and pericardial pressures that decrease the venous return to the heart.

37. c. protective reflexes used by patients to modify their respirations.—Patients may modify their respiration with any of the following protective reflexes: cough, sneeze, gag reflex, sigh, or hiccup.

38. b. Sighing—Sighing increases the opening of alveoli to prevent localized collapsed areas of non-aerated lung.

39. c. Kussmaul's—Deep, gasping respirations representing hyperventilation to blow off excess CO_2 and compensate for an abnormal accumulation of metabolic acids in the blood or metabolic acidosis (e.g., kidney failure, sepsis, aspirin poisoning, alcoholic ketoacidosis, and diabetic ketoacidosis).

40. a. helps to make it easier to breathe.—Patients may modify their respirations by positioning themselves to make it easier to breathe. Often patients are not consciously aware that they took on a "special breathing position."

41. b. airway is not properly opened.—Gastric distension is an expansion of the stomach, usually due to an excess of trapped air. Excess air enters the esophagus and, ultimately, the stomach.

42. a. creating resistance to bag mask ventilation.—The enlarging stomach places pressure on the diaphragm and limits the lung expansion.

43. a. slowly applying pressure to the epigastric region.—Gastric distention can be relieved by being prepared to suction potentially large volumes, placing the patient in the left lateral position, and then slowly applying pressure to the epigastric region, suctioning as necessary to ensure that the patient does not aspirate.

44. b. It is tolerated by conscious patients.—The use of a gastric tube does not interfere with intubation, can be tolerated well by conscious patients, and mitigates recurrent gastric distention and nausea.

45. b. heart block.—Vagus nerve stimulation may lead to bradycardia, heart block, or asystole. The risk is greatest in persons with inferior wall myocardial infarction.

46. a. Terminate the procedure.—In most cases, patients respond promptly to termination of the procedure and atropine.

47. a. administering atropine.—In most cases, patients respond promptly to termination of the procedure and atropine. Be prepared to manage a cardiac arrest with high-quality compressions!

48. d. exposure to body fluids.—The risk of infection to the paramedic is serious due to the exposure to body fluids. Protect yourself from body fluids that could spread diseases such as hepatitis, tuberculosis, meningitis, or influenza.

49. b. valve stem—The regulator can be easily damaged, but if the valve stem breaks it could send the pressurized vessel flying like a missile, injuring everything and everyone in its path.

50. b. ten—OSHA has guidelines for the proper procedures for recording and documenting hydrostat dates.

51. a. react with the oxygen and cause a fire.—The oxygen could react with the adhesive and debris and cause a fire.

52. c. A therapy regulator is designed to be attached to the cylinder stem or wall of the ambulance.—It is generally set at 50 PSI, and the actual delivery to the patient is adjustable on the flow meter in liters per minute.

53. b. 30—The maximum pressure recommended for positive-pressure ventilation should not exceed 30 cm of water pressure.

54. d. exacerbated congestive heart failure patient—The patient has to be breathing to create negative pressure on the valve. The device then administers oxygen to the patient throughout inspiration.

55. b. When ventilating a *complete* laryngectomy patient, you do not need to cover the mouth.—If the patient has a partial laryngectomy, there may still be an open pathway through the mouth as well as a stoma. In this case, when ventilating through the stoma, you have to cover the mouth so the air does not exit there.

56. c. Ventilations can exit the pop-off valve without getting air into the patient.—There have been cases when a bag mask with a pop-off valve was used to ventilate a patient, and the EMS provider did not realize that all of the volume was exiting through the pop-off valve and no air was going to the patient.

57. a. two hands provide manual in-line immobilization.—Whenever the patient's head and neck is not taped down to the long board, there must always be two hands providing manual in-line stabilization until the neck is cleared in the ED.

58. b. when a patient has poor tidal volume—IPPB is not indicated in noncompliant patients (breathing patients that fight the device, patients with poor tidal volume, and small children).

59. b. it reduces the risk of overinflation.—IPPB can be self-administered, and it delivers a high volume and a high oxygen concentration. There is no oxygen wasted because it is delivered in response to the inspiratory effort.

60. a. biphasic positive airway pressure—Similar to a CPAP mask, the BiPAP device can help alleviate the need for intubation. This device can vary the degree of positive pressure during inspiration and

expiration separately. The ability to vary the pressure makes the system more comfortable and effective in most patients.

61. d. can eliminate the risk of aspiration.—An ATV does not eliminate the risk of aspiration. The patient must be observed constantly for possible aspiration.

62. d. Unconscious patients who are sedated.—ATVs are used in both intubated and unintubated patients who require extended ventilation. ATVs allow for control of the ventilation volume and rate.

63. c. Noninvasive ventilation—The first use of this technique originated in-hospital when continuous positive airway pressure (CPAP) was applied by mask to respiratory and cardiac patients.

64. a. intubation may be avoided where it may have previously been required.—The principle is that the patient constantly breathes against a small amount of positive pressure. The pressure causes previously collapsed airways to open, improving oxygenation.

65. b. atelectasis.—The term means to collapse due to inadequate aeration.

66. b. fractured ribs –Taking a large breath or sighing helps to open the small airway and prevents atelectasis. Taking a deep breath is very painful for patients with a fractured rib, and they avoid doing so. As a result, they decrease their tidal volume and their small airways collapse.

67. c. The right mainstem bronchus is straighter.—This anatomical difference in bronchial tubes is the reason for right mainstem intubation when the tube is inserted too far.

68. d. sniffing position—The sniffing position aligns the three axes of the airway, allowing for the best visualization of the vocal cords with a laryngoscope.

69. d. All of the above.—Just because the patient is improving doesn't necessarily mean he should be extubated right away. Removing an endotracheal tube often causes vomiting.

70. c. aspiration of vomitus—Removing an endotracheal tube often causes vomiting.

71. a. When pressure is applied improperly, airway obstruction results.—It is important that this pressure be on the lateral edge of the cartilage, rather than the middle; otherwise, visualization of the glottic opening may actually be more difficult, resulting in airway obstruction.

72. d. lateral edge; the cuff is inflated—It is important that this pressure be on the lateral edge of the cartilage, rather than the middle; otherwise, visualization of the glottic opening may actually be more difficult, and airway obstruction results.

73. b. has chest trauma.—The device cannot be used under high-pressure airway conditions (e.g., chest trauma, airway trauma, or restrictive COPD).

74. d. ETT—Of the three acceptable advanced airway devices, an endotracheal intubation is placed directly into the trachea. Properly inserted, it protects the airway from secretions and foreign objects.

75. a. there is a suspected cervical spine injury.—This technique is most helpful in an unconscious patient when either the larynx cannot be seen on direct laryngoscopy or there is a suspected cervical spine injury.

76. a. involves an invasive procedure beyond intubation.—Retrograde intubation involves placing a needle through the cricothyroid membrane. A guide-wire is then threaded upward toward the oropharynx. The ET tube is placed over the guide-wire into the trachea. The wire is removed when the tube is in place.

77. c. infrared—An infrared light beam measures the oxygen saturation of the blood.

78. c. Any condition that causes an altered hemoglobin molecule can cause a false reading.—The principle of pulse oximetry assumes normal capillary blood flow, normal hemoglobin concentration, and a normal hemoglobin molecule.

79. a. The hemoglobin concentration is low due to shock.—The pulse oximetry may not be reliable during shock and severe anemia. The infrared light beam measures the oxygen saturation of the hemoglobin in the blood. If the patient has a reduced hemoglobin count due to blood loss, and the few remaining are saturated, the reading will be high even though there is not enough to adequately perfuse the tissues. If the patient looks sick and the pulse oximetry reading is normal, the patient is still sick.

80. b. colorimetric—Colorimetric devices attach to the ET tube and detect exhaled CO_2 via color changes in the center of the device. This device is not used for continuous monitoring because the moisture in expired air ruins the paper filter in the device.

81. a. wash out any residual $EtCO_2$ that may be present in the esophagus.—This is especially necessary in non-perfusing patients to avoid false readings.

82. d. ingestion of fruits prior to obtaining a reading.—The ingestion of carbonated beverages prior to the use of capnography has been known to cause inaccurate readings in the first few ventilations.

83. b. esophageal intubation detector—A few studies have questioned the reliability of this device. Always combine your clinical intuition with other methods of verification to decide on proper ET tube placement.

84. a. Verify lung sounds.—The movement associated with transport can cause the tube to become displaced. Lung sounds should be reassessed frequently on any transport.

85. a. the technique does not require the use of a laryngoscope.—Nasotracheal intubation is performed without visualization of the vocal cords. When rapid sequence induction is not available or is contraindicated, nasotracheal intubation is an ideal option for the patient with clenched teeth.

86. a. is a blind technique.—Nasotracheal intubation is performed without visualization of the vocal cords. The patient must be breathing for this procedure.

87. b. nasotracheal intubation.—These devices are specially designed to facilitate nasotracheal intubation. The BAAM is a whistle placed on the end of the endotracheal tube, which provides a whistle sound when the patient exhales through the tube. The Endotrol® has a trigger that curves the tube to the airway anatomy.

88. c. Needle cricothyrotomy—A large bore angio is inserted through the cricothyroid membrane into the trachea to create an emergency airway.

89. a. through the cricothyroid membrane.—A means of providing ventilation through a large bore needle that is directly inserted through the cricothyroid membrane.

90. d. risk of hyperkalemia.—Succinylcholine is a safe and short-lasting neuromuscular blocking agent used in rapid sequence induction. It is contraindicated in patients with massive tissue damage (e.g., burns or severe crush injuries) due to the risk of hyperkalemia.

91. c. the cricoid cartilage narrows the trachea and serves as a functional cuff.—The smallest portion of the pediatric airway is the cricoid ring, which serves as a functional cuff. Passing a cuffed tube through this opening may be difficult and cause trauma to the area.

92. c. nasal airway—The nasopharyngeal airway is a very good airway adjunct for a patient with clenched teeth. It does not require visualization of the airway or the absence of a gag reflex.

93. b. use of a pediatric "pop-off" device that prevented adequate oxygenation of a patient—Ventilations can exit the pop-off valve without getting air into the patient. There have been cases when a bag mask with a pop-off valve was used to ventilate a patient, and the EMS provider did not realize that all of the volume was exiting through the pop-off valve and no air was going to the patient.

94. d. all of the above—Trauma to the neck from a rapid deceleration injury has the high probability of becoming a difficult airway to manage. The paramedic should suspect laryngeal edema and have smaller sized tubes ready, and be prepared to manage the airway with other backup adjuncts if the larynx is in spasm or is fractured.

95. a. Suction the airway and insert a nasal airway.—Manage the airway with the basic steps first and proceed to advanced techniques from there.

96. a. it has no face mask seal to maintain.—The mask fits into and shrouds the glottic opening, where it partially occludes the esophagus. The patient is ventilated with a bag mask device attached to the distal end of the tube.

97. d. Assist ventilations with bag mask device slowly and gently over two seconds.—It is important to allow sufficient time for exhalation when a patient is in bronchospasm. Slow and gentle ventilations can prevent barotrauma, especially in a patient with high airway pressures.

98. b. conscious, uncooperative patient in respiratory failure—An example of an ideal patient for RSI is a combative, head-injured patient. The sedative used can also reduce the anxiety level during the short period of neuromuscular paralysis.

99. d. neuromuscular blocking agents.—Succinylcholine is safe and short lasting (less than an hour), but can produce muscular tremors that are generally of no consequence in most patients. These tremors rarely lead to hyperkalemia.

100. a. LMA—The LMA cannot be used under high-pressure airway conditions (e.g., chest trauma, airway trauma, bronchospasm, or restrictive COPD). The device is designed for patients with normal airway pressures and will be ineffective or cause further complications under high-pressure airway conditions.

Chapter 11: Therapeutic Communications and History Taking

1. b. communication—The communication process used by the EMS provider is focused around a message.

2. a. speak with them.—Speaking with the patient is the best way to assess the mental status. Determine the AVPU (Alert, Verbal, Painful stimuli, Unresponsive) during the initial assessment and follow up using the Glasgow Coma Scale. During the patient interview, you should be able to determine whether the patient is conversing normally, is responding reasonably to questions, and is oriented.

3. a. receiver.—The message moves through various forms: written, verbal, nonverbal, encoding, message, decoding, receiver, and feedback.

4. a. complete health—This includes every surgery, hospital visit, illness, injury, immunization, and psychiatric problem. It also includes all medications, allergies, family history, activities, religious beliefs, daily routines, patient outlook, relationships, sleep patterns, and other personal stress factors.

5. b. present illness.—The acronym OPQRST is used in the out-of-hospital setting to remember the set of questions to be asked in order to obtain information about the present illness or injury.

6. c. Is this event similar to any previous events?—If the answer is yes, additional information to ask about should include: How many times has an event like this happened? When was the last event? and What treatment was received?

7. d. present illness or injury.—The acronym OPQRST is used in the out-of-hospital setting to remember the set of question to be asked in order to obtain information about the present illness or injury. It represents: Onset, Provocation, Quality, Relief (Radiation, Region, Recurrence), Severity, and Time of onset.

8. a. past medical history.—SAMPLE represents: Signs and symptoms, Allergies, Medications, Past medical history, Last oral intake or similar event, and Events leading up to this event.

9. d. tonsillectomy in childhood—The paramedic must quickly obtain information that is relevant to the present illness or injury.

10. b. Some patients may tell you what you want to hear rather than the truth.—Some patients may tell you what you want to hear rather than how they really feel.

11. a. Showing empathy helps to obtain more cooperation from the patient.—Showing empathy is a therapeutic communication technique to help the patient with his feelings and to obtain more information.

12. b. calling the patient "honey"—Using a patient's proper name, Mr., Mrs., or Ms. Jones, shows respect. If the patient gives permission to use another name, then it is okay to use that name. It is disrespectful to use terms of endearment (e.g., "honey" or "dear") or pet names (e.g., "chief" or "doll").

13. b. Why did you call us here today?—This question will, in many cases, get a nervous or confused patient talking and focusing on what the problem is.

14. d. embarrassed.—Take into consideration who else is present when you are interviewing a patient. The patient may not want family, coworkers, or bystanders to know certain information about herself.

15. d. open-ended—This type of question allows the patient to answer with more than a "yes" or "no."

16. b. when specific information is required—This can be especially important when the patient is unstable or critical (e.g., respiratory distress or chest pain). Attempt to get the answer to the most important questions before the patient is unable to answer any questions.

17. c. Native Americans—Other cultures take offense to where or how they are touched or spoken to. Consider obtaining more information about this topic.

18. d. The paramedic could lose the patient's trust.—It is better to explain what is happening and what is going to happen next. If the patient perceives that you are lying, you may not get the cooperation you need.

19. a. Do you have sharp chest pain?—If you asked, instead, "Are you having chest pain?" this would be a "yes or no" type question and not leading.

20. b. You don't smoke, do you?—Condescending or judgmental questions can make a patient uncomfortable, and this may cause him to lie about other information, or lead to information being withheld.

21. d. avoid the use of complicated medical terminology.—Stick to the use of lay terms as much as possible. If you are caring for a healthcare professional who understands medical jargon, it should become apparent quickly, and the use of medical terminology may be appropriate.

22. b. inattentiveness.—Inattentiveness can make a patient feel uncomfortable and lead to information being withheld.

23. c. Facilitation—Positive examples of facilitation include sitting close to the patient and making eye contact, while you nod or say, "I'm listening" or "Please tell me more."

24. d. reflection.—Reflection helps the patient feel that you are listening and can confirm information that is pertinent to the event.

25. a. Interpretation—An example would be to say, "It appears that when you exert yourself physically, you develop a shortness of breath."

26. a. the patient is blind—An overtalkative or symptomatic patient can be challenged when faced with limited time for interview and care, and, if the condition of the developmentally disabled patient is severe, information may be omitted.

27. c. Vial of life®.—This is an example of a commercial device available to provide medical and other emergency information about a patient to emergency medical providers.

28. a. Use positive body language while you begin care.—Ideally, the best solution is to find a translator. Otherwise, use positive body language, such as friendly facial expressions and slow movements to assess, take vital signs, and provide treatment.

29. d. ask permission to touch the patient before actually touching him or her.—This action is appropriate with most every patient, but especially with a blind person. You can avoid frightening the patient and reduce anxiety by first explaining prior to touching.

30. a. getting angry in return—Anger and hostility is often misdirected at the caregiver. Do not get angry in return; it is nonproductive and stressful.

31. c. depression.—Do not hesitate to ask a patient about her feelings. Depression is associated with some psychological illnesses.

32. d. Try using direct "yes or no" questions.—Attempt to get the patient to focus on one thing at a time by having him answer questions that require a "yes or no" answer. It may keep both of you from becoming frustrated.

33. c. Establishing a rapport with the patient—It begins from the time the call is dispatched and lasts until the patient is turned over to the ED.

34. a. direct.—With unstable and critical patients, ask questions that require a one- or two-word answer. With a patient in severe respiratory distress, ask questions that require nonverbal answers.

35. d. current vital signs—The current vital signs are part of your assessment. A history of irregular vital signs, such as hypertension or an irregular heartbeat, is considered part of the health history.

36. b. focused history.—A focused history is the chronological history of the present illness or injury.

37. b. Encoding—The communication process used by the EMS provider that is focused around a message. The message moves through various forms: written, verbal, nonverbal, encoding, message, decoding, receiver, and feedback.

38. c. MedicAlert® tags—There are a number of information sources found on patients in the field. Some wear necklaces or bracelets, while others use smart cards, computer chips, or wallet cards. The most common are the necklaces and bracelets available from the MedicAlert® Foundation, which maintains a twenty-four-hour Emergency Response Center.

39. a. ADA—The Americans with Disabilities Act includes a provision that requires the hospital to provide a sign interpreter within thirty minutes of the patient's arrival.

40. d. look to see if his hearing aid is on.—Many patients who have hearing aids do not wear them. Ask the patient if he has one, and help him to place it and turn it on.

Chapter 12: Techniques of Physical Examination

1. a. assessing vital signs—assessing mental status, obtaining a focused history, and making a treatment decision require little or no physical skill.

2. a. taking standard precautions.—Donning personal protective equipment (PPD) is part of taking standard precautions.

3. b. visual inspection—The physical assessment is typically performed by looking first, listening, and then feeling or palpating.

4. b. personal hygiene.—Sometimes the smell or odor is apparent before the visual inspection.

5. c. Percussion—A skill that is routinely used during a physical examination, but not as frequently by the prehospital provider.

6. a. warm hands before touching the patient.—It is attentive, considerate, and practical practice to warm hands or equipment prior to touching a patient.

7. b. the general appearance of the patient.—The general appearance of a patient is made from the first seconds to minutes of being with the patient.

8. a. fifth intercostal space at the midclavicular line on the left chest.—Apical heart sounds are best heard at the fifth intercostal space at the midclavicular line on the left chest.

9. b. inaccurately high reading—A blood pressure cuff that is too small can give an inaccurate reading that is higher than the actual pressure, while a cuff that is too large can give an inaccurate reading that is lower than the actual pressure.

10. d. Korotkoff sounds.—Korotkoff sounds are the sounds heard with a stethoscope while taking a BP that, when combined with readings on the gauge, indicate the systolic and diastolic readings.

11. b. systolic—Only the systolic reading may be obtained when taking a blood pressure by palpation.

12. a. ambient noise is too loud to hear pulse sounds.—Out of the hospital, noises are often too loud and interfere with the EMS provider's ability to hear with a stethoscope.

13. c. cause an inaccurate reading.—A blood pressure obtained on the arm on the same side as a mastectomy was performed can cause a patient discomfort and result in an inaccurate reading.

14. b. kidneys.—Diseases of the kidneys cause problems with fluid retention and contribute to the presence of edema peripherally or in the lungs.

15. d. connective tissue disease.—It is possible to have increased skin turgor due to increased tension or a connective tissue disease. Aging also affects skin turgor, and elderly people commonly have poor turgor due to loss of connective tissue.

16. a. tension pneumothorax.—The jugular veins are like a dipstick to the heart and give a measure of central venous pressure (CVP). Distention indicates

increased CVP, which can be caused by several conditions.

17. c. local vein blockage or restriction—Unilateral JVD is abnormal and may indicate a local vein blockage or restriction.

18. b. semi-fowlers with the head at the 30° angle—In this position the patient's jugular veins are observed to determine whether they are normal or distended. Then they are observed while simultaneously performing a deep palpation on the upper right quadrant of the abdomen for approximately thirty to sixty seconds. If an increase of more than 1 cm in JVD is noted, this finding may indicate right heart failure or fluid overload.

19. d. fluid overload.—If an increase of more than 1 cm in JVD is noted, this finding may indicate right heart failure or fluid overload.

20. a. otoscope.—The otoscope is placed into the nose or ear to inspect the inners structures, such as the eardrum, for redness, purulence, and foreign bodies.

21. b. ophthalmoscope.—The examiner looks through the ophthalmoscope at the patient's eye by focusing the scope with the lenses.

22. d. hemoglobin.—A pulse oximeter is used to assess the oxygen saturation of hemoglobin (SpO_2).

23. d. falsely high.—Pulse oximetry may give false high or low readings under certain conditions. Shock and hyperthermia can alter peripheral circulation and, therefore, affect the readings.

24. a. dull or flattened tone—Fluid in the body, when palpated, creates a dull or flattened tone.

25. b. one-half to two-thirds.—A carotid bruit can be heard when the lumen becomes occluded by one-half to two-thirds.

26. c. absence of sounds—This finding almost always indicates serious intra-abdominal pathology.

27. a. tenderness of the gallbladder—Murphy's sign is tenderness on deep palpation of the abdomen.

28. b. SpO_2 88% in a three-year-old having an asthma attack.—Any disease or condition that can alter the peripheral circulation can cause inaccurate pulse oximetry readings. A typical three-year-old should have very good circulation.

29. a. painful or injured.—Taking a blood pressure on an extremity that is injured or has pain can cause more discomfort for the patient and should be avoided if possible.

30. b. bruit—Bruits may be caused by the partial occlusion of an artery.

31. d. sacral area—Fluid or edema gravitates to the lowest point. For the non-ambulatory or bedridden patient, the sacral and presacral area tend to become edematous.

32. a. a baby with grunting respirations—Grunting on expiration is abnormal and indicates respiratory distress.

33. d. Subcutaneous emphysema—Air trapped under the skin, creating a "bubble wrap" feel when palpated.

34. b. eighteen-year-old male in a motorcycle accident—The head-to-toe examination is performed on trauma patient with a significant mechanism of injury (MOI).

35. a. watery discharge from the nose—Rhinorrhea is watery discharge from the nose.

36. a. disrupting plaque and possibly causing a stroke.—Ascultating for bruits in the carotid arteries in the out-of-hospital setting has been discouraged in recent years due to the possibility of disrupting plaque and possibly causing a stroke.

37. c. sitting up at 45°—This is the semi-Fowler's position, and it is important for assessing JVD because a patient who is sitting should have no JVD. When a person is supine, JVD is a normal finding.

38. c. fifth anterior axillary line and midaxillary line at the fifth rib level.—Always compare one side to the other before changing locations on the chest.

39. b. fluid.—Fluid in the sac around the heart will cause the heart sounds to be muffled or sound distant.

40. d. absence of bowel sounds—The most helpful finding is the complete absence of bowel sounds. This almost always indicates serious intra-abdominal pathology.

41. d. edema.—Edema can occur in a local area or be generalized throughout the body depending on the cause of the abnormal accumulation of fluids in body tissues.

42. a. the color or age.—You are looking at bruising to determine if it is new, old, or possibly a pattern indicative of abuse.

43. d. head.—HEENT is a commonly used acronym for head, eyes, ears, nose, and throat.

44. c. acute changes in hearing.—Acute changes are of concern and may indicate that a serious problem is occurring (e.g., stroke, tumor).

45. a. used to appreciate the size of the liver.—To assess the abdomen by deep palpation, the paramedic can use one or both hands to depress two to three inches in each abdominal quadrant. Often two hands are used with an obese or muscle tense abdomen. Deep palpation is used to appreciate the size of the liver and tenderness of the gallbladder, and to further evaluate any masses or enlarged organs.

46. d. extremities.—Range of motion may be used to assess the moving body parts (e.g., extremities, head, and neck).

47. c. carbon dioxide; exhalation—An end-tidal CO_2 monitor is a device that measures the amount of carbon dioxide during each breath at the end of exhalation.

48. c. Turgor—To assess the skin, gently pinch a small section such as the forearm or back of the hand. When the skin is released, it should return to its original shape quickly.

49. b. abnormal heart—To auscultate heart sounds, place the bell of the stethoscope at the fifth intercostal space at the midclavicular line. Listen to determine whether the heart sounds are normal or abnormal.

50. c. abdomen—Ascites is an abnormal accumulation of fluid in the spaces between the tissues and organ in the abdominal cavity.

Chapter 13: Overview: Patient Assessment

1. c. scene size-up.—Patient assessment begins with the scene size-up and ends when the patient is transferred to the ED.

2. d. general impression.—The general impression includes both the physical appearance and the psychological (emotional) presence.

3. b. circulatory status.—This includes the skin color temperature and condition, as well as the blood pressure.

4. a. location of the call—The uncontrolled environment makes EMS calls very dynamic and often unsafe.

5. c. omitted, deferred, or repeated.—The paramedic has to be flexible and quick to adjust to the unique dynamics of every call.

6. a. assessing the need for appropriate PPE—The paramedic determines the initial and appropriate PPE from the information gathered in the scene size-up.

7. c. an observation of the patient's environment.—The components of the general impression of the patient include observing and determining the patient's: age, gender, level of distress, and surrounding environment.

8. c. health history.—A partial or more thorough health history is obtained as part of the focused history.

9. d. transportation.—After completing the initial assessment, the paramedic should make a transport decision (high priority or low priority) for the patient.

10. c. focused on the patient's chief complaint.—After completing the initial assessment, the progressive direction of the exam is typically focused on the chief complaint.

11. b. head-to-toe exam.—The detailed physical exam (DPE) is the standard head-to-toe exam all prehospital care providers perform on patients where indicated (e.g., trauma patient with a significant MOI).

12. c. trauma patient with significant MOI—The detailed physical exam (DPE) is the standard head-to-toe exam all prehospital care providers perform on patients where indicated (e.g., trauma patient with a significant MOI).

13. c. asymptomatic after a fall of approximately three times the patient's height—This guideline is consistent for most trauma protocols.

14. d. minor damage to the front end of a car where the airbag deployed.—Unless the patient is complaining of cervical or back pain, this MOI is in most cases nonsignificant for spinal precautions.

15. a. Trending—Trending is an important tool in patient care. It is the process of obtaining a baseline assessment, repeating the assessment multiple times, and using the information to determine whether the patient is getting better, worse, or shows no change.

16. b. rapid trauma assessment—The rapid trauma exam is similar to the DPE, but not as thorough.

17. c. diagnostic—An ECG, SpO_2, or $EtCO_2$ reading and a blood glucose reading are examples of diagnostic information.

18. d. severity of the specific complaint.—The more severe and complex a patient's complaint is, the more often and detailed the ongoing assessment may become. For example, a patient with a possible stroke will need a neuro exam and vital signs repeated every five minutes, while a patient with an isolated extremity injury will need reassessment of distal pulse, motor, and sensation (PMS), and vital signs every fifteen minutes.

19. d. legal and ethical—Additional medicolegal and ethical components include: being accountable to the patient, respecting confidentiality and privacy, understanding advanced directives, and reporting accurate, factual, and nonjudgmental information.

20. a. positioning—As with the conscious patient, the ABCs are the highest priority. However, managing the ABCs in an unresponsive patient may take all available manpower, and positioning becomes critical.

21. a. focused trauma examination—After the initial assessment, the paramedic should be able to determine when an injury is truly isolated and begin to focus on that specific complaint.

22. b. determine the patient's mental status—The initial assessment is performed to determine a patient's mental status and find and manage any immediate threats to the ABCs.

23. b. cardiac and musculoskeletal—The cardiac and respiratory systems are often assessed simultaneously, as each is so closely affected by the other. The musculoskeletal system is assessed for possible defects that may contribute the respiratory distress (e.g., fractures ribs, strained muscles).

24. c. reflexes.—Babinski's reflex and other deep reflexes can provide valuable information when a patient is unable to answer questions.

25. a. legal—The paramedic has a legal obligation to document and report accurate, factual, and nonjudgmental information.

Chapter 14: Scene Size-Up and the Initial Assessment

1. b. initial assessment.—The scene size-up is the first component, which is followed by the initial assessment, focused history, and physical exam.
2. a. make use of door stops.—One of the best ways to keep a scene safe is to keep an exit open.
3. d. trip and fall from a standing position.—Near drowning, GSW, and a fall from a height of thirty feet are all significant MOIs.
4. a. Waddell's triad.—A triad injury pattern associated with pediatric patients struck by a motor vehicle.
5. a. the look test.—The general impression is your first impression of the patient as you approach. This has been referred to for years as the "look test," a "gut reaction," or your "assessment from the doorway."
6. a. determine the patient's mental status.—AVPU represents the patient's initial mental status as being: Alert, Verbal, Painful response, and Unresponsive.
7. c. recognizing hazards.—Safety first for the responders. Recognizing that hazards are present and then avoiding them is the first priority on any call. This is a dynamic process, and responders will continuously assess hazards throughout all phases of the call.
8. b. Three out of four family members are complaining of headache.—All of the scenarios described are potentially dangerous to the responder, but when three out of four members of the same household have a complaint of headache, the paramedic should first consider the possibility of high carbon monoxide levels and take the appropriate actions.
9. d. A potentially violent scene is safe for EMS.—Any potential hazard that can injure the responders, the bystanders, or further injure the patient makes a scene unsafe and unsecured (e.g., dangerous crowds, downed power lines, broken glass, or pets). When the actual or potential hazards are removed, the scene is considered secured.
10. a. a nighttime response to a house that has no lights on—For an EMS call in a residential area at night, you would typically see lights on and possibly someone outside waving to the ambulance. These instructions are provided by dispatches as part of the EMD protocol.
11. b. Continue to remove the patient and do not let anyone touch the gun.—Safety first, so do not allow anyone to touch the gun. Call a police officer over to secure the weapon. The patient is critical, so continue to rapidly extricate him from the vehicle. Once outside, a pat down should be completed for any additional weapons. This can be done while moving to the ambulance.
12. a. staging area—In many systems, dispatch will advise the ambulance to "stage in the area" or give a specific location on where to stage until police or fire notifies dispatch that the scene is secure or safe to proceed into.
13. b. a patient with a bad cough—A cough may seem relatively insignificant, but it can actually be a serious hazard. Many pathogens are spread through droplets by coughing and sneezing.
14. b. engage the emergency brake on a car that has been left in neutral—Setting the emergency brake, turning off the ignition and removing the key, and letting the air out of tires are all examples of simple and quick actions the paramedic can take to make the scene safer.
15. d. working in traffic at the scene of a collision—Working in traffic is one of the most common and dangerous aspects of the job for EMS responders, firefighters, police, and so forth.
16. c. twisting of the knee.—Falling or twisting of the knee is commonly associated with these sports. These MOIs often injure the supporting structures of the knee.
17. c. attempted hanging.—There is trauma associated with hanging (MOI), even though the nature of illness (NOI) that lead up to the attempt is a behavioral problem.
18. c. mechanism of injury—When the paramedic takes the time to learn about common MOIs, he can make some predictions or be better prepared to suspect specific injury patterns.
19. b. general impression—The general impression is your first impression of the patient as you approach. This has been referred to for years as the "look test," a "gut reaction," or your "assessment from the doorway."
20. c. Complete the assignment and search for the next patient.—Each responder is expected to report in, complete assignments as directed, and report back for additional assignments. Freelancing is one of the worst things to do in an incident command situation and can result in dangerous situations for others at the scene.
21. c. painful.—The patient is not aware of you by visual or verbal stimulation. He did respond to your touch and, therefore, is not unresponsive.
22. a. withdraw from pain—A purposeful withdraw from pain is an appropriate response and a good sign. No response, flexion, or extension are all inappropriate responses and indicate a serious problem.
23. d. asking the parent or caregiver to determine if the response is normal.—This is appropriate when the infant is not unconscious. The parent or caregiver can tell you if the infant is acting normal or not. If

the infant is not acting normal, they can tell you in what way the behavior is abnormal.

24. b. Level of consciousness—The level of consciousness is often used interchangeably with mental status, although they do have different meanings. The mental status is the appropriateness of the patient's thinking. The LOC is the degree of the patient's alertness, wakefulness, or arousability.

25. b. low-level—An unconscious patient who exhibits (decorticate or decerebrate) posturing is exhibiting neurological posturing. This may occur all the time or only when pain is applied. It is illustrative of low-level brain functioning.

26. b. metabolic causes.—Metabolic causes, such as severe diabetic ketoacidosis or sedative overdose, can cause neurological posturing.

27. a. broken jaw.—Fractures to the face can cause potentially serious airway problems. The paramedic must be alert to this and assess the need for airway management.

28. c. neck injury.—The MOI described has the potential to cause cervical spine injury and the paramedic must take the appropriate precautions.

29. a. Mental status—The level of consciousness is often used interchangeably with mental status, although they do have different meanings. The mental status is the appropriateness of the patient's thinking. The LOC is the degree of the patient's alertness, wakefulness, or arousability.

30. d. Minute—The minute volume is the amount of gas inspired or expired in a minute. An inadequate minute volume exists if the respirations are shallow and the rate is too slow.

31. b. close the airway.—When an infant's neck is hyperextended or hyperflexed, it can actually close off the airway. A neutral or slightly flexed position is best for an infant.

32. c. carotid artery—During the initial assessment, the pulse is assessed at the carotid artery for the "quick check" to determine whether the adult or child patient has a pulse. In infants, the pulse is assessed at the brachial artery.

33. a. radial; distal—When a patient has a distal (radial) pulse, this finding suggests the patient has an effective blood pressure.

34. b. color, temperature, and condition—The color, temperature, and condition (CTC) are the features that are assessed about the skin.

35. d. cyanosis—Blue, or cyanotic, skin is associated with a lack of oxygen resulting from inadequate breathing or heart function. A person with hepatic or renal failure is more likely to have skin that is jaundice (yellow) and pale. Red or flushed skin can be caused by heat exposure, hypertension, or emotional excitement in any patient.

36. d. palms or soles—The nail beds, lips, and eyes are additional areas of the skin to assess for skin color.

37. d. three-year-old asthmatic—The usefulness of capillary refill has been downplayed in adults because there are many unreliable factors that can interfere with the capillary refill time. However, in children, circulation is much better than in adults, and capillary refill is a useful assessment finding.

38. c. to determine the need for rapid transport and definitive care at the hospital.—The paramedic must make the determination of the need for rapid transport based on the patient's condition and location, and whether or not additional assistance is needed (e.g., helicopter or critical care transport unit).

39. d. in the OR—Severe trauma is not something that can be stabilized in the field. The basic rule is that the internal bleeding is stopped by the surgeon within the first hour (the golden hour) after the injury has occurred.

40. a. use of a short board immobilization device—When this step is skipped or expedited, it is called rapid extrication.

41. c. ongoing—The ongoing assessment includes reassessing vital signs and checking on interventions such as administered medications, IVs, or airway adjuncts.

42. b. focused—The focused physical exam is typically directed at the patient's chief complaint or life-threatening condition discovered in the initial assessment.

43. a. condition may be changing rapidly.—The initial assessment is repeated as needed throughout the call. It may frequently be repeated in critical patients and when the patient's condition is changing rapidly.

44. b. Trending—Trending is an important tool in patient care. It is the process of obtaining a baseline assessment, repeating the assessment multiple times, and using the information to determine whether the patient is getting better, worse, or shows no change.

45. b. conscious and unconscious.—The patient assessment algorithm for the medical patient subdivides patients into responsive and unresponsive.

46. a. significant and nonsignificant—The patient assessment algorithm for the trauma patient subdivides patients into two categories based on the MOI being significant or not.

47. c. any threat to life—Immediate threats to life are managed first in all patients.

48. d. Provide rapid transport to an OR.—The basic rule is that the internal bleeding is stopped by the surgeon; IVs can be started and maintained en route to the hospital, and should not delay transport.

49. b. sickle cell crisis—Sickle cell crisis is painful and potentially deadly. Symptoms include shortness of breath and severe abdominal pain.

50. a. patella dislocation—An isolated extremity fracture or dislocation is typically a stable condition, unless there is a loss of distal pulse, or motor or neuro function.

Chapter 15: Focused History and Physical Examination: Medical Patient

1. b. after the initial assessment has been completed.—The focused history often begins concurrently with the physical exam immediately after the initial assessment has been completed. When the patient is unresponsive, a rapid physical exam follows the initial assessment and management of the ABCs.

2. c. the patient's chief complaint.—With the conscious patient, the focused physical exam is typically directed toward the patient's chief complaint (e.g., for a patient with difficulty breathing, the paramedic will focus on the pulmonary, respiratory, and cardiac areas). When the patient is unresponsive, the initial assessment and management of the ABCs is started immediately. Because the patient is not able to provide a history, the rapid physical exam follows.

3. a. TIA.—The patient has described having neurologic symptoms (e.g., possible loss of consciousness, temporary loss of motor and neurologic function); therefore, the stroke/TIA should be considered first. Vitals signs, glucose reading, ECG, and a focused history and physical exam will help to rule out possible causes and narrow the differential diagnosis.

4. d. Determine if there is trauma associated with this event.—The dispatch information was for an unresponsive patient and you have found the patient lying on the floor. It is appropriate to determine if there actually was a loss of consciousness and if there are any injuries associated with a possible fall before proceeding with the other tasks.

5. c. the events that preceded this episode.—The acronym SAMPLE stands for Signs and symptoms, Allergies, Medications, Past medical history, Last meal–last similar event, and Events leading up to the current episode.

6. b. positive findings and pertinent negatives.—As part of the focused history, positive findings (such as a loss of consciousness prior to stroke symptoms) and pertinent negatives (such as the patient denying chest pain when she has difficulty breathing) are obtained by the paramedic.

7. d. difficulty breathing—The paramedic is asking about possible pertinent negative and positive findings associated with a respiratory complaint.

8. d. L—last meal—The last meal, last medication dose, last menses, or last similar event will help the paramedic to possibly determine why this event is occurring or how to proceed with treatment.

9. b. altered mental status.—AEIOU-TIPS stands for: Alcohol, Epilepsy, Infection, Overdose, Uremia, Trauma, Insulin, Psychoses, and Stroke (or shock).

It is used to remember the possible causes of altered mental status.

10. c. concurrent medical problems.—Many patients, especially the elderly, have a lengthy medication list for a number of concurrent medical problems. Always consider medications as a possible cause of new or worsened symptoms in any patient.

11. a. rapid physical examination.—When the patient is unresponsive, the initial assessment and management of the ABCs is started immediately and is followed by the rapid physical exam.

12. c. bronchodilator.—The patient's chief complaint is dyspnea. The chest pain changes with breathing, indicating a non-cardiac pain. The focused physical exam includes clear lung sounds and stable vital signs. Bronchodilator therapy is appropriate for this patient.

13. c. pertinent negative findings.—In a patient with respiratory distress, these are important pertinent negative findings, which help to differentiate the causes of the patient's distress.

14. b. good clinical judgment and experience.—The guideline for repeating the ongoing assessment is every five minutes for an unstable or critical patient and every fifteen minutes for a stable patient. However, there are many variables to each call, which can alter treatment and ongoing assessment. Good clinical judgment and experience should prevail.

15. c. associated signs and symptoms.—These are positive associated signs and symptoms for a respiratory distress patient.

16. c. neurologic—Dizziness and nausea may be signs of vertigo. A neurologic problem and the history of a recent cold could have caused an inner ear problem.

17. c. gain trust and cooperation from the patient.—Establishing a rapport with the patient is necessary to gain consent from most patients. Gaining a patient's trust and cooperation helps to move along the physical assessment and proceed with treatment.

18. a. responsiveness.—The patient assessment algorithm for the medical patient subdivides patients into responsive and unresponsive.

19. c. cardiac—Weakness, dizziness, and nausea are atypical cardiac symptoms, but in the elderly patient they may be the only signs of a cardiac problem.

20. d. chief complaint, initial assessment, and the focused PE findings.—The focused PE can be a dynamic process in the out-of-hospital setting. The way the focused PE is approached is based on the patient's chief complaint, the findings from the initial

assessment, the focused history, and other findings discovered along the way.

21. b. stabilize and transport.—Many of the presenting medical problems involve the same field management in the first thirty to sixty minutes, so it is not always necessary, or practical, to make a diagnosis in the field. Strive to assess emergent signs and symptoms, stabilize the patient to the best of your ability, and transport to the nearest appropriate facility.

22. a. cardiothoracic—Assess for the most serious potential problem first. Consider a cardiac problem first and intra-abdominal bleeding second.

23. d. obtain an ECG and pulse quality.—As the most serious possible problem may be cardiac in nature, an ECG, pulse rate, and quality should be assessed quickly.

24. a. OPQRST—The acronym OPQRST stands for: Onset, Provocation, Quality, Relief (Radiation, Region, Recurrence), Severity, and Time of onset.

25. b. neurologic—The new onset of problems affecting sensation, coordination, and bowel control are signs of a neurologic problem.

26. b. possible CO poisoning.—When two or more members of the same household have a complaint of headache, the paramedic should consider the possibility of high carbon monoxide levels first and take the appropriate actions.

27. a. skin.—The acronym DCAP-BTLS is used to remember what is assessed about the patient's skin. It stands for: Deformity, Contusion, Abrasion, Puncture/penetration, Burn, Tenderness, Laceration, and Swelling.

28. a. an unresponsive forty-year-old male—The rapid physical exam is performed on medical patients who are unresponsive or have a severely altered mental status.

29. b. findings from the initial assessment.—The components of the focused physical assessment are guided by the patient's chief complaint, the finding of the initial assessment.

30. b. neurologic—Assessment motor function and sensation are part of the neurologic exam.

31. c. Intracranial pressure can stimulate the vomiting reflex.—Nausea and vomiting are associated with many disorders. Frequently, but not always, vomiting is preceded by nausea. When brought on by injury, or accompanied by severe abdominal pain or headache, nausea and vomiting may indicate a serious condition. The vomiting reflex is located in the vomiting centers in the medulla.

32. a. vertigo is a vestibular disorder.—Vertigo is often used as a synonym for dizziness or lightheadedness. True vertigo is a vestibular disorder that includes motion sickness.

33. b. cardiac—Dysuria (difficulty urinating) and back pain are signs and symptoms of a urologic problem.

34. d. prevent complications from dehydration.—Some patients are medicated to prevent the complications from dehydration and GI distress. Cardiac patients are medicated to prevent the vagus stimulation that occurs with vomiting.

35. b. Vomiting is an active process in conscious patients, and regurgitation is not.—Regurgitation is a passive process in an unconscious patient.

36. d. stomach.—Sensory receptors in the stomach and intestine may stimulate the reflux due to infection, food irritation, or injury.

37. a. take c-spine precautions.—There is a lot of potential for traumatic injury in the bathroom (e.g., porcelain and tile showers, bowls, sinks, walls, and floors).

38. c. vasovagal—One of the common causes of syncope in the bathroom is a parasympathetic response from stimulation of the vagus (e.g., bearing down on the commode, shaving the neck and stimulating the carotids, or tying a tie, and pressing on the eye while manipulating contact lenses).

39. c. Vasovagal stimulation—Other non-cardiac causes of syncope include: dehydration, neurologic, hemorrhagic, pharmacologic, respiratory, and emotional.

40. a. beta-blockers.—Many drugs can cause syncope, and beta-blockers are one of the most common types of medications. Others include: diuretics, nitrate, digitalis, antihypertensives, antiarrhythmics, and narcotic analgesics.

41. d. blood pressure—Obtaining a baseline set of vital signs while getting a focused history is appropriate for this patient.

42. b. limbic system disorders.—Prolonged or frequent vomiting may produce GI bleeding as a result of the reflux of acid and bile. It may also cause Mallory-Weiss tears.

43. b. vagus stimulation.—In many cardiac conditions, the patient cannot tolerate the slow heart rate and its accompanying decrease in cardiac output, as well as the potential for myocardial irritability causing extra systoles.

44. a. bathroom.—One of the common causes of syncope in the bathroom is a parasympathetic response from stimulation of the vagus (e.g., bearing down on the commode, shaving the neck and stimulating the carotids, or tying a tie, and pressing on the eye while manipulating contact lenses).

45. c. heart block—A heart block can be an immediate, life-threatening condition, producing a heart rate too slow to provide adequate circulation.

46. b. post-syncope information, such as duration of LOC.—Additional information that should be obtained includes: what position the patient was in when the syncope occurred, whether there is a history of similar events, and, if so, when and how

many time it occurred, and what treatment was received.

47. a. cardiac dysrhythmias.—Cardiac dysrhythmias, such as SVT, Stokes-Adams syndrome, and sick sinus syndrome.

48. d. all of the above.—Orthostatic hypotension occurs due to sudden peripheral dilation with a compensatory increase in cardiac output. This is common in the elderly from prolonged bed rest, from certain medications, and from hypovolemia with a blood loss of greater than 1,000 cc.

49. b. positional symptoms.—There are wide variances in "normal ranges" for orthostatic vital signs. More significant are positional symptoms, especially if associated with significant pulse and blood pressure changes.

50. a. AMI.—Knowing the patient's baseline mental status is key to performing an accurate assessment.

Chapter 16: Focused History and Physical Examination: Trauma Patient

1. c. any injury that interferes with the ABCs—Life-threatening conditions include any injury that interferes with the airway, breathing, and circulation. The factor involved most often in traumatic injuries is shock.

2. b. one hour—Assessment-based patient care, not diagnostic-based care, provides the best chance for the survival of critical trauma patients. This is because it takes time to make a diagnosis. When you consider the golden hour, there is not enough time to diagnose injuries in the field, and often not even in the ED.

3. a. ten—For the best possible patient outcome, the EMS provider must consider the golden hour for critical trauma patients and take no longer than the "platinum ten minutes" to get the patient in the ambulance and on the way to the hospital.

4. d. rapid transport—Rapid transport is reserved for the critical trauma patient in most cases.

5. b. MOI—The most important aspect of trauma assessment is the MOI. Evaluating the MOI to understand the pathology of what happened is part of the foundation of excellent trauma patient care.

6. b. DCAP-BTLS—The acronym DCAP-BTLS is used to remember what is assessed about the patient's skin. It stands for: Deformity, Contusion, Abrasion, Puncture/penetration, Burn, Tenderness, Laceration, and Swelling.

7. a. Detailed—The detailed physical exam is a complete head-to-toe exam for injuries. The steps are similar to, but more thorough than, the rapid trauma exam.

8. d. transportation should not be delayed while waiting for ALS to arrive—For the best possible patient outcome, the EMS provider must consider the golden hour for critical trauma patients and take no longer than the platinum ten minutes to get the patient in the ambulance and on the way to the hospital. ALS can meet the ambulance en route to the hospital without delaying transport.

9. b. initial assessment—The information obtained at this point is enough to determine the patient's condition and to make the decision to "load and go" or "stay and play."

10. a. the MOI—The most important aspect of trauma assessment is the MOI. When the patient has sustained a significant MOI, the paramedic must consider the energy impact on the body and have a high index of suspicion for specific injury patterns.

11. b. every fifteen minutes—The ongoing assessment includes reassessing vital signs and checking on interventions such as administered medications, IVs, or airway adjuncts. It is repeated every five minutes for critical and unstable patients and every fifteen minutes for noncritical and stable patients.

12. d. IV—Level IV trauma centers are established for rural and remote communities. A Level IV may be a clinic rather than a hospital. The goal is to provide initial stabilization and then transfer the patient to a Level I, II, or III.

13. a. I—Most Level I trauma centers have a full range of resources, services, and programs.

14. d. traumatic cardiac arrest—The reason for this is that the survival rate of a traumatic cardiac arrest is so low that the closest facility that can provide stabilization may be the patient's best chance.

15. d. the loss of consciousness—The MOI, combined with the loss of consciousness and the confusion, are appropriate criteria for aeromedical transport.

16. b. Trauma Score—The trauma score was developed in 1980 as a scale to be used for triage and to predict patient outcome. Howard Champion, MD, is the physician responsible for the latest version of the trauma score referred to as the Revised Trauma Score.

17. a. fractures of the heels, ankles, and hips—When considering that the energy created by motion stays in motion from the point of impact (feet) through the entire body, the patient would also be likely to have spinal fractures.

18. a. full spinal immobilization—The long backboard serves as a splint for the entire body during the care of a critical trauma patient. Minor injuries should be attended to only after major and life-threatening injuries.

19. c. children—Trauma is the leading cause of death for people from one to forty-four years of age and, more specifically, is the number one killer of children in the United States.

20. b. decreased body fat minimizes the body's protection (padding) against traumatic injury.—Muscle and fat mass decrease with age.

21. b. Head injury—Trauma is the number one killer of children in the United States, and, more specifically, head trauma from falls is the most common cause.

22. a. falls.—Trauma is the number one killer of children in the United States, and, more specifically, head trauma from falls is the most common cause.

23. a. the presence of rib fractures is a critical finding.—Rib fractures are rare due to soft bones. When present, the risk of mortality in increased.

24. b. vomiting.—This increases the risk of aspiration as well. Always be prepared for nausea, vomiting, and airway management in the pregnant trauma patient.

25. c. 30%—During pregnancy, the mother's blood volume increases and reaches a nearly 50% increase.

26. a. thoracic aortic disruption.—The energy that can be absorbed by the body during an impact produces damage to the patient's body. The extent of the damage caused by this energy depends on the specific organs that have been affected. Fractured ribs, sternum, and trachea are injuries more consistent with a blow to the chest, such as a steering wheel impact.

27. c. spine, knee, and lower legs—When an unrestrained patient is found under the steering wheel, suspect knee, femur, hip, pelvis, and spine injuries.

28. c. broken steering wheel—Physical signs of the vehicle that lead you to suspect underlying injuries include: a starred or cracked windshield, a broken steering wheel, a broken dash, and intrusion into the side of the passenger compartment.

29. b. coup-contra coup—Coup injuries develop directly below the point of impact, and contra coup injuries develop on the opposite side of the point of impact. These are common when the back of the head is struck.

30. a. Waddell's triad—When struck by a vehicle, this is the injury pattern in children involving the legs, chest, and head: the legs from a direct blow, the chest from being thrown onto the car hood, and the head from being thrown clear of the vehicle when the vehicle comes to a stop.

31. d. cavitation.—Cavitation is the momentary acceleration of tissue laterally away from the projectile (bullet, knife, etc.) tract. This is like the ripple effect of a rock dropped into a pond. The tissue waves can cause damage and explain why a bullet near the spine can actually injure the spine. They also explain why the exit wound is usually larger than the entrance wound.

32. c. 1,300—It is estimated that the chances of a spinal injury increase up to 1,300 times when not wearing a seat belt and being thrown clear of the vehicle. Of course, this is assuming you are not run over by another vehicle.

33. d. epidural hematoma—Bleeding of an artery traveling along the inner surface of the cranium will result in a hematoma above the dura mater (epidural).

34. c. chest and abdomen.—Primary injuries are typically in the head, neck, and spine. Secondary injuries involve the chest and abdomen.

35. a. long backboard—The long backboard is a splint for the entire body, which can be utilized safety and quickly.

36. b. chest.—Paradoxical motion as seen in flail chest, crepitation associated with fractures, and asymmetry of the chest wall.

37. a. regional protocols.—Regional protocols typically provide specific information on when and where to transport trauma patients. State guidelines provide general information, as well as national guidelines, which are listed in many EMS texts.

38. d. Children compensate for shock better than adults in early shock.—Children in shock may appear better than they actually are because, initially, they compensate better than adults. When they begin to decompensate, it occurs quickly and is an ominous sign.

39. a. Rib fractures are rare in pediatric trauma.—Rib fractures are rare due to soft bones. When present, the risk of mortality in increased.

40. b. The use of MAOIs can interfere with the body's normal response to pain.—This statement is inaccurate.

41. c. intra-abdominal hemorrhage—Dizziness, diaphoresis, and pale skin color are signs and symptoms of shock. With the MOI, the paramedic should suspect intra-abdominal hemorrhage.

42. a. complicated airway—Airway, breathing, and circulation are the primary priorities of care in any patient.

43. d. wheezing is present with a hoarse voice—Airway, breathing, and circulation are the primary priorities of care in any patient.

44. b. Level I trauma center—Examples of criteria for transport to a Level I trauma center are severe burns or major trauma, especially when the patient is a pediatric, geriatric, or pregnant patient.

45. b. C3 and C4—Paralysis below the neck is associated with injury to C3 and C4 of the spine.

Chapter 17: Assessment-Based Management

1. b. assessment—An assessment is the foundation of care. It is difficult to report or manage a problem that you did not find.

2. c. history.—The history should be focused toward the organ systems that are associated with the complaint.

3. b. environment—A supermarket can be a loud and busy place, making a proper field assessment difficult. Consider moving the patient to the ambulance for privacy for the patient, and a more controlled environment for you and your crew.

4. c. rule out hypoglycemia—Any patient with an altered mental status should be considered for hypoxia and hypoglycemia early in the assessment.

5. a. frequent flyer—Labeling patients is unfair, because they may not be afforded the full attention that all patients deserve.

6. a. organ systems associated with the complaint.— The history should be focused toward the organ systems that are associated with the complaint. One's knowledge of a disease and its assessment findings, as well as maintaining a degree of suspicion about a particular problem, affects the quality of a history taken from the patient.

7. b. Recognition of various injury patterns can help the paramedic be better prepared to provide the proper emergency care.—With this understanding, the paramedic can potentially make a significant difference in the patient's outcome.

8. c. equipment to conduct the initial assessment of the patient's ABCs—The "first-in" equipment should contain the following items: airway, breathing, and circulation control equipment, scissors and blanket to expose the patient, ECG monitor or AED, and pad and pen for notes.

9. b. guidelines for care.—There are both benefits and disadvantages to protocols, standing orders, and patient-care flow charts. One benefit is that they provide some structure for the EMS provider, and a major disadvantage is that they do not fit every patient.

10. a. The paramedic has a bias against people who do not have a similar background to her.—Having a biased or prejudicial "attitude," or attempting to classify patients by a social status, can cause the EMS provider to miss vital pieces of information, often short-circuiting the information-gathering process.

11. c. a biases or prejudicial "attitude"—Having a bias against people who do not have a similar background or attempting to classify patients by a social status can cause the EMS provider to miss vital pieces of information, often short-circuiting the information-gathering process. Tunnel vision or myopia can be very dangerous!

12. d. accompany the patient through definitive care.— The team leader is usually the EMS provider who will accompany the patient through definitive care. The team leader takes on many responsibilities, including: establishing a dialogue and rapport with the patient, obtaining a history, performing the physical exam, presenting the patient, completing documentation, coordinating transport, and designating tasks.

13. c. acting as the initial EMS command in an MCI.— Typically, this is the role of the team leader.

14. a. equipment needed to conduct the initial assessment of the patient's priorities.—This also includes the equipment to manage the ABCs in the first few minutes of a call. Many agencies carry this equipment in a "first-in" bag, together with an AED or cardiac monitor.

15. a. a poor assessment and care were made.—A good oral presentation suggests effective patient assessment and care; a poor presentation suggest poor assessment and care.

16. d. dispatch information.—As part of the job, the paramedic will communicate patient information face to face, over the telephone or radio, and on the prehospital care report (PCR).

17. b. people skills and customer service.—EMS is a business, and the patients are the customers.

18. a. have and practice a preplan.—You should have a preplan to avoid the appearance of confusion. Practice the preplan before you need it.

19. a. Choreography—The paramedic must learn to be proficient at choreographing the scene of a call. This includes maintaining overall patient perspective and designating tasks at all types of calls, ranging from a two-person crew to EMS command at a multiple casualty incident (MCI).

20. b. seeing a local drug abuser and immediately blaming his disorientation on the drugs rather than looking for a medical problem.—Labeling patients can be very destructive to the assessment process. Even the frequently intoxicated patient or people whom you feel abuse your services get sick and injured once in a while.

21. d. make the appropriate management decisions.— Decisions are only as good as the information they are based on.

22. d. An unorganized approach can lead to important information being overlooked.—An organized approach allows for a complete and smooth assessment.

23. c. it allows for a complete and smooth assessment.— With one EMS provider, there is sequential information gathering and treatment. With two, there can be simultaneous information gathering and treatment, which is more efficient. When multiple responders are present, the team leader should designate to avoid confusing the patient or missing answers to questions asked by different responders.

24. b. existing treatment protocols.—Treatment decisions involve a combination of information obtained from the history, the physical exam, recognition of injury patterns and disease processes, the field impression, and existing BLS or ALS treatment protocols.

25. b. The paramedic's knowledge of a disease and its assessment findings.—The history should be focused toward the organ systems that are associated with the complaint. One's knowledge of a disease and its assessment findings, as well as maintaining a degree of suspicion about a particular problem, affects the quality of a history taken from the patient.

26. b. Important information can be missed by performing a cursory physical exam.—For most EMS responders, there are time constraints. However, you cannot benefit from the information obtained from the physical exam if you overlook some part or just do a cursory physical exam.

27. c. there is a "thinking cook."—It is important to understand that protocols are "guidelines for care" and dictate when and how the EMS provider may deviate from a protocol if the patient's condition warrants.

28. a. more efficient.—With two, there can be simultaneous information gathering and treatment, which is more efficient than one. When multiple responders are present, the team leader should designate to avoid confusing the patient or missing answers to questions asked by different responders.

29. d. preplanning and practicing with her crew.—Some agencies assign critical roles or positions based on the equipment an EMS provider carries into the call. For example, the person who carries the drug box and defibrillator may be the team leader, and the person carrying the oxygen and advanced airway kit may go right to the patient's head for airway control.

30. c. watching everyone's back to make sure no one gets hurt.—The patient care provider is also responsible for gathering scene information, obtaining vital signs, performing skills as requested by the team leader, and performing triage at an MCI.

Chapter 18: Ongoing Assessment and Clinical Decision Making

1. c. scene size-up—The key aspects of ongoing assessment are: trending, adapting, time constraints, manpower limitations, anticipating changes, and altering or modifying care.

2. b. improved muscular strength—The natural hormonal responses include: improved reflexes and muscular strength, enhanced visual and auditory acuity, diminished concentration and assessment abilities, and impaired critical-thinking skills.

3. b. stimulants of the "fight or flight" response for paramedics.—There are many stimulants and variants for the individual. The most common stimulants are: alarms, pagers, dispatch information, cell phones, emergency lights, sirens, traffic, and other hazards.

4. a. short transport time—With an unstable patient, managing the ABC's may take all available resources; if the transport time is short, it may alter how the ongoing assessment is completed.

5. d. The time interval for repeating the ongoing assessment for the critical trauma patient is the same for the critical medical patient.—The ongoing assessment of the critical patient, either trauma or medical, is repeated every five minutes. For the noncritical patient, it can be repeated every fifteen minutes.

6. a. Trending—Trending is an important tool in patient care. Treatment is continued as is, or modified, using the information obtained from trending.

7. b. subtle changes in the patient's mental status.—An example is the head-injured patient whose condition may deteriorate quickly. The earliest indications are often subtle changes in the patient's mental status.

8. a. Isolated measurements are generally less helpful than changes over time.—This is why trending is such an important tool.

9. d. think and work under pressure.—The out-of-hospital environment is uncontrolled and dynamic. Gathering information, evaluating, and processing information while developing and implementing appropriate patient management is different for every call.

10. b. evaluating and processing information.—The essential concepts of clinical decision making include: gathering, evaluating, and processing information, while implementing appropriate patient management.

11. d. all of the above.—Based on the ongoing assessment and evaluation, a new plan may be formulated and additional interventions may be required.

12. b. The hospital is a relatively controlled environment.—The out-of-hospital environment is uncontrolled and dynamic.

13. c. isolated extremity injury without neurologic compromise—This is an example of a non-life- or limb-threatening injury. The patient's distal pulse, motor, and sensory (PMS) functions are reassessed as part of the ongoing assessment.

14. c. the patient's level of discomfort—For the patient presenting with cardiac chest pain, your goal is to reduce and eliminate the pain while quickly transporting the patient to the most appropriate facility.

15. d. achieving and maintaining an adequate body of medical knowledge.—As with any healthcare provider, this is an ongoing process, because the medical field is dynamic and continually improving.

16. a. Criticizing the actions of the first responders.—This action is non-productive and make the next call with the first responders more difficult.

17. c. Look up the correct dose in your protocol book.—Never guess, especially with medications. Take a few seconds to look up the information you need, like all other medical professionals do.

18. d. Identifying and managing medical ambiguity—Other fundamental elements of critical thinking include: gathering and organizing data, forming concepts, analyzing and comparing similar situations, differentiating between relevant and nonrelevant data, articulating and documenting decision-making reasoning, and constructing valid arguments.

19. a. clearly define performance parameters.—In addition, they provide a standard approach to patient care and speed the application of critical-care interventions, while providing structure for the EMS provider.

20. c. They can speed the application of critical interventions.—Additional benefits of using protocols and standing orders include promoting a standard approach to patient care, defining performance parameters, and providing some structure to patient care.

21. d. Rephrase—The "six Rs" of putting it all together are: read the patient, read the scene, react, reevaluate, revise, and review.

22. a. Collect information and formulate concepts, interpret and process information, apply treatment, reevaluate, and reflect.—The flow of the critical-thinking process should follow a logical plan that resembles this format.

23. a. location of the patient—Reading the scene includes considering: the mechanism of injury, environmental conditions, and immediate surroundings.

24. a. identifying the chief complaint—Reading the patient also includes assessing the ABCs and skin condition, ruling out life threats, obtaining baseline vital signs, and triage.

25. a. Stop and think before acting.—Mental preparation tricks to use when critical thinking becomes clouded include: staying calm, anticipating and planning for the worst, reassessing frequently, and pausing to take a deep breath.

26. a. planning for the worst scenario.—Mental preparation tricks to use when critical thinking becomes clouded include: staying calm and stopping to think before acting, anticipating and planning for the worst, reassessing frequently, and pausing to take a deep breath.

27. c. critically life-threatening.—Other examples of critically life-threatening patient situations include: end-stage chronic disease process, major multisystem trauma, or major single-system trauma.

28. b. potentially life-threatening.—Minor multisystem injuries and concurrent disease presentations are examples of potentially life-threatening patient situations.

29. c. ask the patient for a signature on a billing form.—This action is required by most EMS agencies; however, in many cases it is done near the end of a call or at the hospital.

30. a. An unrestrained victim of a MVC sustained facial lacerations on the windshield.—It would be appropriate to use a teaching moment with a patient who is an alert and stable patient after experiencing injuries that could have been prevented.

31. a. CUPS—In some areas, the acronym CUPS—Critical, Unstable, Potentially unstable, and Stable—is used to describe a patient's priority after completing the initial assessment.

32. a. manage similar experiences.—For most, the more an individual is exposed to an experience, the better she is able to avoid panicking, manage similar experiences, and generally be able to overcome having a bad day.

33. b. trending mental status and vital signs.—These are repeated every five minutes for a critical patient and every fifteen minutes for a noncritical patient.

34. d. treat as he goes, correcting life threats first.—"React" means to treat life-threatening injuries as you find them (e.g., suction the airway before you control bleeding).

35. a. Take a deep breath, and revert back to assessing the ABCs.—Reassess the airway, breathing, and circulation. This will help you to refocus and will give you information to proceed.

Chapter 19: Communications

1. d. the code summary on a monitor-defibrillator unit.—Pulse oximeters, capnography, electronic BP, and temperature devices are other examples of electronic communication used by paramedics.

2. c. detection.—Occurrence is the first phase of communication necessary to complete a typical EMS call, and detection is the second phase.

3. b. treatment.—In the treatment phase of communication necessary to complete a typical EMS call, the paramedic may choose to contact medical control to discuss treatment options for the patient.

4. b. Receiver gives feedback.—The basic model of communication has six steps: sender has a message; sender encodes the message; sender sends the message; receiver receives the message; receiver decodes the message; receiver gives feedback to the sender.

5. c. the patient's family physician.—Although this is not required, there are times when calling the patient's physician can be helpful. For example, when the patient initially refuses transport for evaluation for a serious condition (e.g., chest pain), the physician can help persuade the patient to go to the hospital.

6. c. add an unnecessary level of complexity.—Many services that previously used special radio codes have changed to plain English to prevent confusion or the possibility of multiple interpretations.

7. c. global positioning device—Many cell phones already have a global position system, and, in the near future, all cell phones will have this technology.

8. b. semantics.—Semantics and technical terminology are two factors that tend to impede verbal communication.

9. a. avoid technical terms.—To help avoid confusion, select your words and phrases with the audience in mind.

10. b. it helps avoid cutting off the first few words.—This is called "keying the microphone."

11. b. The operator may be unfamiliar with your community.—In most cases, dialing "0" will delay the appropriate response to an emergency.

12. a. close proximity to computers—Sometimes, 60-cycle interference can occur when the radio is too close to a computer, fluorescent light fixture, or electronic motor.

13. b. prearrival instructions.—The emergency medical dispatcher (EMD) is trained to give prearrival instructions to the caller. These instructions may include helping the caller deliver a baby, providing bleeding control, or the compression of CPR.

14. a. Is the patient conscious?—The other three key questions are: Is the patient breathing? What is the patient's approximate age? What is the patient's chief complaint or the type of incident?

15. d. queue—During this time, the dispatcher determines the type of call, the most appropriate units to dispatch, and their response mode.

16. b. the scene time may be inaccurately lengthened.—On calls where it takes a while to find the patient, the scene time can be extended. This extra scene time should be explained on the PCR.

17. b. a lengthy extrication.—An extrication can take minutes or hours, depending on the type of entrapment.

18. a. in enhanced 9-1-1, a computer displays the caller's phone number.—The caller's phone number appears on the dispatcher's terminal just before the ring comes in.

19. b. second-party caller.—The first party is the patient calling for herself.

20. d. all of the above.—The FCC is responsible for regulating all aspects of the communication industry.

21. d. Jeff Clawson, MD—Dr. Clawson developed the Medical Priority Dispatch® system.

22. b. pre-arrival instructions—The emergency medical dispatchers trained using Jeff Clawson's system provide prearrival instructions that effectively create a "zero-minute" response time.

23. b. CAD.—Computer-aided dispatch.

24. c. give them time to prepare for the patient.—A verbal report over the radio or telephone helps prepare the ED for the arrival of the patient.

25. a. patient's name—The airways are public and open for all to hear. Never say anything over the radio, including divulging the patient's name, that you would be uncomfortable saying on public television.

26. a. drugs administered on standing orders.—The other choices listed are information that would normally be provided in the standard radio report.

27. d. APCO.—Association of Public Safety Communications Officials.

28. c. say each digit for clarity when transmitting a number.—This technique is a basic principle of proper radio system usage.

29. b. digital transmitters do not require voice transmission time over the radio.—Some EMS systems have mobile data terminals that can receive a call from a dispatcher and print it out.

30. b. frequency.—Depending on the range, radio frequency may be very high (VHF) or ultra high (UHF).

31. a. call simplex.—On this system, it is not possible to transmit and receive at the same time.

32. d. repeater.—Repeaters can be used on radio towers or ambulances.
33. d. UHF.—The 460 MHz range is most commonly used for EMS communications.

34. b. FM; AM—Frequency modulation is more reliable than amplitude modulation.
35. b. analog transmission.—Analog is a voice transmission.

Chapter 20: Documentation

1. b. an indication of poor assessment.—Some say the paperwork is almost as important as the care itself. Whether or not your assessment and care were optimal, poor documentation is a difficult hurdle to overcome.
2. a. Documentation serves as a legal record of the incident.—The documentation that is completed for out-of-hospital care provides a professional link between the field assessment and in-hospital management.
3. a. NHTSA—The National Highway Traffic Safety Administration has defined the minimum data set in order to standardize and compare data from different agencies and systems.
4. c. disposition of the call—The patient data includes patient name, address, date of birth, gender, age, nature of the call, mechanism of injury, nature of illness, location of the patient, SAMPLE history, signs and symptoms, assessment findings, treatment, changes in patient condition, and disposition of the call.
5. d. level of training of the crew members—The run data includes: the date, times, service name, unit identifier, and the names and level of training of the crew members.
6. d. DNAR.—The do not attempt resuscitation order (DNAR) or DNR is prepared by the patient and his physician.
7. b. the patient's address—Patient demographic information includes the patient's name, address, age, date of birth, phone number, Social Security number, and so on.
8. c. Remove patient's name from documentation.—The patient's name must be removed or completely covered if the forms will be used for discussion with providers other than those who were present on the specific call.
9. a. Vital signs should be documented before and after a medication administration.—Vital signs are documented before and after interventions to determine the effect.
10. b. being objective, specific, and concrete.—When documenting, use objective language. Be precise by writing exactly what you see, hear, feel, or smell, and avoid making judgments.
11. b. both sides.—Circum –around; Ambl/y –dim, dull, or lazy; Ant –against or opposed to.
12. b. development, formation.—dynia –a painful condition; -plasty –a surgical repair; -plegia –paralysis.

13. d. "speaks for itself."—A PCR should, by itself, provide a complete and accurate portrait of the patient's needs and the care given.
14. c. averting further legal action during the "discovery phase" of a lawsuit.—The proper documentation of patient care is one more step toward keeping clear of legal entanglements.
15. d. "The patient stated she vomited four times last night."—Remain objective and be precise by writing exactly what you see, hear, feel, or smell, and avoid making judgments.
16. d. the length and design of stylet used to facilitate the intubation—Unless there is something very unique about this piece of equipment, this information is irrelevant.
17. a. A patient struck his head in MVC and denies a loss of consciousness.—A pertinent negative is a negative response, such as the answer to a question that adds to the assessment. Pertinent negatives are valuable data that are routinely documented on PCRs.
18. a. Subjective—This information consists of symptoms or answers to questions.
19. c. Objective—This information is exactly what you read, see, hear, feel, or smell.
20. d. held in confidence.—HIPAA laws help to ensure this.
21. c. pale, diaphoretic skin—Objective findings are things you can see or measure, such as vital signs or the patient's skin CTC.
22. b. to show trends in the patient's condition.—Take vital signs every five minutes for critical or unstable patients and every fifteen minutes for stable patients.
23. c. had something to hide.—The proper documentation of patient care is one more step toward keeping clear of legal entanglements.
24. b. dorsiflexion—bending backward; protraction—pushing forward; lateral rotation—rotating outward away from the body's midline; cephalad extension—stretching or moving in a straight line toward the head.
25. c. who adjusted the drip rate.—Unless there is an extenuating circumstance, this is extraneous information. The paramedic has oversight of this and is responsible for any amount of fluid infused.
26. b. the patient's medical insurance information—In most agencies, this information is recorded on a separate billing form or included with the PCR. Narcotic use is documented on the PCR and often requires special documentation on another

form, both of which are separate from the billing form.

27. b. triage tags—This a form of documentation used in special situations (multiple casualty incident [MCI]).

28. b. follow your state and local guidelines.—Each state has its own guidelines for mandatory reporting of suspected child abuse or neglect.

29. d. Erase the entry.—Erasing an entry may appear as if the record is being altered.

30. c. Radio failure delayed contact with medical control and subsequent medical orders.—Any unusual occurrence during the call that affects the patient should be documented on the PCR. In addition, a special incident report may be needed depending on the service's standard operating procedures.

31. a. Adequacy of the neurovascular supply before and after immobilization.—Excellent documentation of pre- and post-splinting (or immobilization) findings may be vital when defending your care.

32. b. document the statement in "quotes."—Examples of statements to quote include a dying statement, admission of guilt to a crime, or a threat of suicide.

33. c. standardized and professional.—Many agencies and regions have approved lists of terms or abbreviations to use or avoid in documentation.

34. b. q.i.d.—This information may be found on prescription drug bottles or in a patient's medical records. When discovered by the paramedic, this information must be passed on to the next healthcare provider.

35. c. patient's marital status.—The information may be included in the narrative by the paramedic in a statement such as "The patient's wife reported. . . ."

36. c. compare data from different agencies.—The National Highway Traffic Safety Administration has defined the minimum data set in order to standardize and compare data from different agencies and systems.

37. a. The record contains everything it should in a clear, legible, and concise fashion.—When the PCR "stands on its own," you or anyone else should be able to refer to it in the future and be perfectly clear about what happened.

38. a. SOAP and CHART.—CUPS and AVPU are used for level of consciousness and to assess mental status. SAMPLE, OPQRST, and PMHX are used to obtain a focused history, and APGAR is used for assessing the newly born.

39. c. professional responsibilities—Often, decisions about the patient's care are made based on PCR documentation. The PCR must accurately reflect what the paramedic found and what was done for the patient.

40. c. a police officer who is a friend of the patient—Patient's have a legal right to have their medical information held in confidence, and breaching that right may cause harm or embarrassment to the patient and her family.

41. d. all of the above—Documenting special situations may require additional forms or may need to be cleared through the supervisor or another superior. There are correct and incorrect methods of correcting documentation errors.

42. a. The specific recommendation for care and transport, and consequences of refusing care.—Document the competency of the patient and avoid nonprofessional statements.

43. c. at the ED, after transfer of the patient to a bed.—Ideally, the PCR should be completed while the information is fresh in your mind. Then a copy of the record should be left at the hospital as part of the patient's permanent record.

44. a. narrative.—The administrative and demographics sections are usually in a format that requires filling in or checking boxes.

45. d. all findings should be recorded—Each finding is important and should be documented. Often, decisions about the patient's care are made based on PRC documentation. The PCR must accurately reflect what the paramedic found and what was done for the patient.

46. d. Libel—Slander is false or malicious statements in the form of spoken words.

47. a. All personnel and resources involved in the call should be recorded.—This is called covering yourself. Be sure to include duty supervisors also.

48. d. superficial—The other terms have different relationships to the body.

49. a. —stasis—stomy –a surgical opening; scopy –to see; plasty –surgical repair.

50. a. Nephr/o—Hepat/o –relates to the liver; Ganglio –a knot; Dacry/o –a tear.

Chapter 21: Pulmonary and Respiratory

1. d. perfusion.—The flowing of fluid through organs.
2. a. Ventilation; oxygenation—PO_2 measures oxygenation, and pCO_2 measures ventilation.
3. c. rightward; leftward—Shifts to the right or to the left affect the affinity of hemoglobin for oxygen.
4. b. does their oxygen need.—With increased body temperature, the body automatically tries to provide more oxygen to the tissues.
5. a. decreased body temperature—Decreased body temperature and alkalosis are the most common causes of a leftward shift of the curve.

6. c. 35–40—Levels over 40 mmHg can cause an increase in the blood acid level, and decreased levels result in a decreased blood acid level.

7. d. acid.—Levels over 40 mmHg can cause an increase in the blood acid level, and decreased levels result in a decreased blood acid level.

8. a. 0.1—Blood gases are very straightforward, and there is a direct relationship between pH and pCO_2. They always move in opposite directions by a 10:0.1 ratio.

9. d. 80—Lower levels lead to hypoxia.

10. b. The only predictable and reproducible relation in blood gases is between the pH and pCO_2.—Blood gases are very straightforward, and there is a direct relationship between pH and pCO_2. They always move in opposite directions by a 10:0.1 ratio.

11. c. pCO_2.—This can also occur in situations of hypoventilation or intrinsic lung diseases (e.g., asthma or COPD).

12. a. respiratory acidosis—Respiratory acidosis occurs when CO_2 retention leads to increased levels of pCO_2.

13. a. tonsillitis—The other answers are associated with the lower airways.

14. b. epiglottis—Epiglottis can cause upper airway obstruction.

15. b. anemia—Other perfusion-related factors that may impair gas exchange include: hypovolemia, impaired circulatory blood flow, and chest wall pathology.

16. c. impairment of chest wall movement.—Neuromuscular diseases can impair movement of the chest wall by causing phrenic or spinal nerve dysfunction.

17. a. asthma.—Stridor is an abnormal sound caused by blockage or constriction of the upper airway. Asthma is in the lower airways.

18. c. out against a partially closed epiglottis.—In infants and toddlers, grunting is a sign of respiratory distress.

19. b. pallor and diaphoresis—The other findings are clearly identifiable signs of respiratory distress.

20. b. mentation—Confusion suggests hypoxemia or hypercarbia, while lethargy or coma is a sign of severe hypoxia or hypercarbia.

21. a. an indicator of severe pulmonary disease.—More information about the previous intubation should be obtained quickly, if possible. This information can help the paramedic decide how aggressively or not to treat the patient.

22. b. beta-blockers—In addition, allergic reactions to any medication may lead to wheezing and exacerbate underlying respiratory conditions.

23. d. spontaneous pneumothorax—The sharp chest pain is often localized to the side of the lung involved. Decreased breath sounds are present on the affected side, and the respiratory rate is increased.

24. c. a congenital bleb.—A congenital bleb is an air-filled sac on the surface of the lung that has been present since birth.

25. d. bradycardia—Tachycardia is a sign of hypoxemia and fear. A slowing respiratory rate in the face of an unimproved condition suggests patient exhaustion and impending respiratory failure.

26. d. Cheyne-Stokes.—Can occur with emergent conditions such as brain injury (cerebral) or drug overdose.

27. b. ataxic.—This breathing pattern often precedes agonal gasps and apnea.

28. c. Kussmaul's.—A pattern of very deep, gasping respirations. This breathing pattern is associated with coma and metabolic acidosis.

29. a. right heart failure.—As a result, blood backs up into the venous system, especially the neck veins, peripheral edema, and sometimes ascites.

30. c. right-sided heart failure—Distended neck veins, peripheral edema, and ascites are the most common manifestations of right-sided congestive heart failure, whatever the underlying cause. The liver and spleen are also engorged with blood backed up through the portal circulation.

31. a. barrel chest; increased—Trapped air leads to hyperinflation of the lungs, resulting in a widening of the anterior-posterior diameter of a person's chest.

32. a. both.—Crackles or rales usually result from fluid in the airways, in the interstitial tissue, or in both.

33. c. Carpopedal—The change in pH from respiratory alkalosis increases the binding of calcium to albumin. This leads to a decreased level of unbound calcium in the blood. Because calcium participates in nerve transmission and muscle contraction, both are affected, leading to spasm.

34. a. sleep apnea.—CPAP may be helpful in some cases of acute pulmonary edema.

35. a. end-tidal CO_2.—pO_2 and pCO_2 are blood levels, and peak flow is the measured effectiveness of exhalation.

36. b. COPD.—COPD is sometimes subdivided into emphysema and chronic bronchitis, though many patients have clinical features of both.

37. a. Administer Versed 0.05 mg/kg.—An asthma patient who required intubation will need to stay intubated for evaluation at the ED. Post-intubation sedation is appropriate with either Versed or etomidate.

38. b. wheezing.—The transmitted sound becomes high pitched and somewhat squeaky.

39. a. irritation—People with asthma have extra-sensitive bronchial airways that are easily irritated.

40. c. Respiratory infections—This includes cold, the flu, and sinus infections. These illnesses trigger asthma attacks because they temporarily inflame and damage the lining of the air tubes, causing bronchospasm, increased mucus production, and swelling.

Barnes & Noble Bookseller
1200 Airport Boulevard
Pensacola, FL 32504
(850) 969-9554
03-07-08 S02926 R007

CUSTOMER RECEIPT COPY

EMS Field Guide ALS Vers	21.95
9781890495329	
Rnotes: Nurse's Clinical	23.95
9780803613355	
Paramedic Exam Review	35.95
9781418038182	

SUB TOTAL	81.85
SALES TAX	6.14

TOTAL 87.99

AMOUNT TENDERED

AMEX 87.99

CARD #:	***********1011
AMOUNT	87.99
AUTH CODE	584490

TOTAL PAYMENT 87.99

A MEMBER WOULD HAVE SAVED 8.20

Thank you for Shopping at
Barnes & Noble Booksellers
#373536 03-07-08 06:44P MarshG

Valid photo ID required for all returns, (except for credit card purchases) exchanges and to receive and redeem store credit. With a receipt, a full refund in the original form of payment will be issued for new and unread books and unopened music within 30 days from any Barnes & Noble store. For merchandise purchased with a check, a store credit will be issued within the first seven days. Without an original receipt, a store credit will be issued at the lowest selling price. With a receipt, returns of new and unread books and unopened music from bn.com can be made for store credit. Textbooks after 14 days or without a receipt are not returnable. Used books are not returnable.

Valid photo ID required for all returns, (except for credit card purchases) exchanges and to receive and redeem store credit. With a receipt, a full refund in the original form of payment will be issued for new and unread books and unopened music within 30 days from any Barnes & Noble store. For merchandise purchased with a check, a store credit will be issued within the first seven days. Without an original receipt, a store credit will be issued at the lowest selling price. With a receipt, returns of new and unread books and unopened music from bn.com can be made for store credit. Textbooks after 14 days or without a receipt are not returnable. Used books are not returnable.

Valid photo ID required for all returns, (except for credit card purchases) exchanges and to receive and redeem store credit. With a receipt, a full refund in the original form of payment will be issued for new and unread books and unopened music within 30 days from any Barnes & Noble store.

41. b. cold—Cold weather irritates the bronchial airways.
42. b. respiratory alkalosis—The change in pH from respiratory alkalosis increases the binding of calcium to albumin. This leads to a decreased level of unbound calcium in the blood. Because calcium participates in nerve transmission and muscle contraction, both are affected, leading to spasm.
43. c. Adult respiratory distress syndrome—Administering 100% oxygen often requires a ventilator in a hospital setting, and arterial blood gas measurements are needed to confirm a diagnosis of ARDS.
44. b. Status asthmaticus—Its onset may be sudden or insidious, and is frequently caused by a viral respiratory infection.
45. a. inadequate use of anti-inflammatory medication.—These medications include steroids and leukotriene blockers.
46. b. Chronic bronchitis—These patients have a productive cough for at least three months per year for two or more consecutive years.
47. c. Emphysema—The decrease in elastic recoil creates resistance to expiratory airflow. Air is trapped within the lungs, resulting in poor air exchange.
48. b. cigarette smoking—Industrial inhalants, air pollution, and tuberculosis also contribute to the condition.
49. d. come on relatively quickly—The patient with an acute COPD episode complains of a shortness of breath with symptoms gradually increasing over a period of days.
50. a. FBAO—Small children explore and learn by putting things in their mouths. Suspect a foreign body airway obstruction first in a child with a sudden onset of respiratory distress, with isolated wheezing or stridor.
51. b. bronchodilating—Nebulized bronchodilators, such a albuterol and epinephrine are commonly used in the out-of-hospital setting.
52. d. anti-inflammatory—Steroids are beneficial in the chronic treatment of nearly all asthmatic patients and many COPD patients.
53. b. fewer—The inhaled forms of steroids are not free of side effects. Additional oral or IV steroids underlie the successful treatment of acute obstructive airway disease.
54. a. take at least one or two hours to work.—Initiating therapy in the field can help the patient to a quicker discharge a few hours later.
55. c. Leukotrienes—Specific medications that directly attack leukotriene production or action have emerged in the past few years.
56. a. smooth muscle relaxing—It is not known exactly how magnesium sulfate helps some patients with severe bronchoconstriction. However, magnesium sulfate is a smooth muscle relaxer and this may be the action that helps.

57. c. us to breathe.—The carbon dioxide drive stimulates breathing centers in the brain when the CO_2 levels rise.
58. a. movement of mucus via bronchial cilia out of the lungs.—As a result, the lung is unable to clear pathogens as effectively. Allowed to remain, these infectious agents multiply, resulting in respiratory infection and pneumonia.
59. b. weakened immune system caused by ethanol.—In addition, drinkers are especially likely to get aspiration pneumonia during passing-out spells.
60. d. all of the above—Additional risk factors include: cigarette smoking, alcoholism, abnormal immune system, extremes of age, and prolonged acute or chronic hypothermia.
61. b. The clinical approach to viral or bacterial pneumonia is the same.—In the out-of-hospital setting, it is impossible to tell whether a person has bacterial versus viral pneumonia.
62. b. hypoxic drive.—If the level of oxygen in the blood goes very low, brain breathing centers are stimulated, leading to the reflex response of breathing.
63. c. nonproductive cough—A cough productive of purulent (rust colored or green) sputum is a typical finding with pneumonia.
64. d. syncope.—Other atypical symptoms associated with viral pneumonia include: nonproductive cough, fatigue, nausea, vomiting, diarrhea, and continuous fever and chills, versus the acute onset that occurs in typical pneumonia.
65. c. exposure to a contagious patient—Consider any patient with possible pneumonia to be contagious, and act accordingly.
66. a. Ventolin—A sympathomimetic that stimulates beta-2 receptors of the bronchi, leading to bronchodilation.
67. a. viral—Influenza is an acute and highly contagious viral disease.
68. b. cultures.—In the out-of-hospital setting, it is impossible to tell whether a person has bacterial versus viral respiratory infection.
69. c. with or without antibiotics.—URI is an acute, usually self-limited infection of any part of the upper respiratory tract. Most commonly, the mouth, throat, and ears are affected. Most people have a spontaneous resolution of symptoms within seven days. People who have underlying disease may develop more severe infections, such as pneumonia or sepsis.
70. a. Some URIs cause bronchoconstriction.—URI is used interchangeably with the "common cold," and serious complications can develop in patients with underlying diseases, such as COPD or cancer.
71. c. spleen—Patients who have had their spleen removed lose resistance to common organisms that often cause a bacterial URI. For these patients, this can become a life-threatening illness.

72. c. cigarette smoking.—Other diseases, such as coal miner's lung and asbestosis, also predispose people to lung cancer, but cigarettes often still play a role.

73. a. cardiac arrest—Altered mental status, severe cyanosis, or profound hypotension also suggest the presence of a life-threatening embolus in a proximal location.

74. a. nausea, vomiting, and weakness—The most common side effects from chemotherapy are nausea, vomiting, diarrhea, and hair loss. Some patients become significantly dehydrated following therapy.

75. d. dry cough or shortness of breath—More commonly, patients are asymptomatic but may experience dry cough. Scar tissue from radiation treatment may restrict lung expansion, leading to shortness of breath.

76. b. raising; calcium—The patient may complain of weakness, depression, and abdominal pain.

77. d. cardiac ischemia—Sometimes people with severe CHF develop pulmonary edema. Typically, they do not.

78. c. CHF is a spectrum of conditions associated with decreases in cardiac function.—Pulmonary edema is a general term for fluid in the lung, for any of several reasons.

79. a. the recumbent position increased venous return to the heart.—The result is an increase in the preload or amount of blood that the heart must pump out.

80. c. vasodilation of both veins and arteries.—Nitroglycerin causes non-selective vasodilation of blood vessels. This may result in a drop in blood pressure.

81. d. increased cardiac preload.—Lasix vasodilates, causing a decrease in the cardiac preload (venous return).

82. a. Reduces cardiac preload and afterload.—This may result in a drop in blood pressure.

83. b. the conversion of angiotensin I to angiotensin II in the lungs.—Angiotensin II is a powerful vasoconstrictor. By blocking it, vasodilation occurs, leading to a decrease in cardiac work.

84. b. increase intrathoracic pressure.—Increased airway pressure causes the expansion of previously atelectic (collapsed) portions of the lung and improves overall ventilation. It may also increase intrathoracic pressure and counteract increased pulmonary capillary hydrostatic pressure.

85. c. spontaneous pneumothorax—The sharp chest pain is often localized to the side of the lung involved. Decreased breath sounds are present on the affected side, and the respiratory rate is increased. The reasons for the association of smoking and bleb rupture are not clear.

86. d. IUD contraceptive use—Birth controls pills and patches are associated with increased risk of pulmonary embolism.

87. a. pulmonary arterial circulation.—Usually, the obstruction is due to a piece of blood clot that has broken away from a pelvic or deep leg vein.

88. a. bronchospasm—The release of histamine from white blood cells causes bronchoconstriction and may be responsible for localized wheezing sometimes heard during the physical exam.

89. b. AMI—The patient may experience classic symptoms of an acute myocardial infarction or spontaneous pneumothorax (e.g., dyspnea, tachypnea, and chest pain).

90. a. The presence of absence of pleuritic chest pain.—Pain that is clearly worsened by breathing is more likely due to a lung or chest wall problem than myocardial ischemia.

91. d. tachycardia.—Breath sounds are usually normal, though localized wheezing is heard occasionally. SpO_2 may be normal, and, after several hours, a pleural friction rub (grating sound) may be heard.

92. c. young, tall, male smoker—These patients are the most likely to develop pneumothorax from the rupture of a congenital bleb, the most common cause of spontaneous pneumothorax.

93. a. low; increases—The change in pH results in respiratory alkalosis.

94. c. Assuming that the patient is experiencing a simple anxiety attack.—Many disease states and serious conditions cause hyperventilation (e.g., asthma attack, COPD, MI, pulmonary embolus, spontaneous pneumothorax, CHF, increased metabolism, central nervous system lesions, hypoxia, drugs, increased metabolic acids in the body, and psychogenic factors). A conservative approach demands that you assume the patient is seriously ill until proven otherwise.

95. b. Offer the patient a nasal cannula.—Putting a mask over the patient's face may make him feel like he is suffocating, which worsens the patient's anxiety and overall condition.

96. a. pulmonary embolism—Fat released from the bone marrow of a fractured long bone can cause pulmonary embolism.

97. a. fat embolus from bone marrow—Fat released from the bone marrow of a fractured long bone can cause pulmonary embolism.

98. c. spontaneous pneumothorax—These patients are the most likely to develop pneumothorax from the rupture of a congenital bleb, the most common cause of spontaneous pneumothorax. The reasons for the association of smoking and bleb rupture are not clear.

99. d. carpopedal spasm—Stress and anxiety may cause the patient to hyperventilate.

100. a. providing high flow oxygen and watching for changes in mental status.—Many disease states and serious conditions cause hyperventilation. A conservative approach demands that you assume the patient is seriously ill until proven otherwise.

Chapter 22: Cardiology

1. a. pulmonic and aortic—The tricuspid and mitral valves are known as the atrioventricular valves.
2. a. stenotic.—Stenosis can occur in any or all valves and may produce a murmur.
3. b. right atrium.—The coronary sinus empties into the right atrium.
4. c. deficit.—Pulse deficit is associated with atrial fibrillation.
5. a. paradoxus.—This is a symptom of various conditions (e.g., pericarditis).
6. c. mitral and tricuspid—This sound is the louder of the two normal heart sounds.
7. d. heart failure.—S3 is a soft, low-pitched sound heard about one-third of the way through diastole.
8. b. pericardial friction rub.—A pericardial friction rub sounds like a grating or scraping noise and is sometimes mistaken for a cardiac-related sound. The sound stops when the patient holds his breath.
9. c. endocardium.—Endocarditis is a potentially fatal bacterial infection of the endocardial layer of the heart, most commonly the heart valves.
10. b. 50—The abnormal collection of pericardial fluid is called pericardial effusion. The rapid accumulation of as little as 50 ml can result in pericardial tamponade and death.
11. c. endocarditis.—Endocarditis is a potentially fatal bacterial infection of the endocardial layer of the heart, most commonly the heart valves.
12. b. diastole—The passive expansion of the chambers of the heart during which they fill with blood.
13. d. Starling's law of the heart.—This refers to the preload of the heart. It is based on the fact that the greater the initial length or stretch of the cardiac muscle, the greater the degree of shortening that will occur.
14. b. decrease heart rate—Chronotropism relates to influencing the rate of the heart beat.
15. c. increase force of muscular contractility—Inotropic is influencing the force of muscular contractility. Positive inotrophy is an increase in the force.
16. a. somatic—Somatic pain is often characterized as sharp, constant, and aggravated by movement or coughing.
17. c. visceral—Visceral pain impulses are carried by nerve fibers that return to the spinal cord at several levels from both sides of the body; the pain is typically perceived by the patient as being poorly localized and ill-defined.
18. b. neuropathy.—The loss of pain sensation is why patients who develop ulcers wait until they are quite advanced before seeking treatment.
19. b. diabetes—A diabetic patient may suffer atypical symptoms from myocardial ischemia due to neuropathy.
20. a. ischemia—Ischemia means lack of oxygen. Prolonged ischemia will progress to infarction (cell death).
21. b. pulmonary embolism.—They are also used to treat deep vein thrombosis, arterial thrombosis, arterial embolism, and arteriovenous cannula occlusion.
22. a. referred pain.—A patient with chest pain may also feel pain in the neck and arm because, during embryonic life, the heart, neck, and arms originate together.
23. c. history.—In a significant number of cases, it is difficult to diagnose ACS based on any one component of an examination or test. The history is a significant aspect to the diagnosis of an acute myocardial infarction (AMI).
24. d. Prinzmetal's—Chest pain may be severe and can occur at rest, similar to unstable angina. Oxygen, nitroglycerin, aspirin, and drugs that influence calcium metabolism by the myocardium are of benefit.
25. a. coronary thrombosis.—Blood clot occurs about 90% of the time.
26. b. weakness.—Weakness is not a classic symptom associated with ischemic chest pain in the young adult, but in the elderly may be the only initial indication of cardiac ischemia.
27. b. QRS complex.—The QRS is usually composed of a group (three separate waves) of wave forms.
28. c. Sedate the patient and begin transcutaneous pacing.—The patient has symptomatic bradycardia with a third-degree heart block. The heart rate needs to be corrected. Sedation and pacing is the recommended treatment, and a dose of atropine and a fluid bolus should be considered while awaiting pacing or if pacing is ineffective. Another consideration is that the blood pressure may be too low for sedative medications.
29. c. acute pericarditis and Prinzmetal's angina.—Many things can cause ST segment elevation or depression. This is an abnormal finding, and, in most cases, you must assume that these represent ACS until proven otherwise.
30. a. nitroglycerine.—This is because, with reduced right ventricular function, the patient needs a high preload to maintain forward flow through the lungs. These patients often respond to fluid administration.
31. c. II, III, and a VF—These leads provide a view of the inferior wall and normal conduction pathway of the heart.
32. b. V_3 and V_4—These leads provide a view of the left anterior ventricle.
33. a. V_1 and V_2—These leads provide a view of the septal wall of the heart.

34. b. cardiac dysrhythmias—A wide range of abnormal ECGs and dysrhythmias may result from these conditions.

35. d. Adams-Stokes syndrome—Also called Stokes-Adams Attack, this is a disorder found more commonly in the elderly.

36. a. reduces the chance of post-shock dysrhythmias.—Synchronization is used to avoid shocking the heart in the relative refractory phase of the conduction cycle.

37. c. external pacing.—The use of this device is a temporary measure until an invasive pacemaker can be placed in the patient.

38. d. Wolff-Parkinson-White syndrome.—This condition is also referred to as pre-excitation syndrome. These changes may be asymptomatic or may be associated with paroxysmal supraventricular tachycardia or atrial fibrillation.

39. b. kidney disease—These risk factors carry potential dangers from excessive bleeding.

40. b. automaticity.—These tissues automatically fire at a given rate under certain conditions, without external nerve stimulation.

41. a. self-excitation.—The ability of cardiac muscle to conduct impulses rapidly throughout the heart.

42. a. hypokalemia—A deficiency of potassium in the blood.

43. c. slow heart rate.—Too much potassium (hyperkalemia) or too little (hypokalemia) slows the heart rate.

44. d. calcium.—Calcium is important for initiating muscle contractions.

45. a. use of supplemental salt tablets—Too much salt (hypernatremia) slow the heart.

46. a. SA node—The sinoatrial node is the normal pacemaker for the heart.

47. c. escape foci—The heart has multiple backup pacemakers.

48. b. lowers stroke volume—Acetylcholine also slows the heart rate.

49. b. norepinephrine—Both epinephrine and norepinephrine are released during sympathetic activation.

50. d. SA and AV nodes.—These nerves affect the heart rate and the contractility of the heart by the use of the natural chemicals acetylcholine, epinephrine, and norepinephrine.

51. c. accessory pathway.—Reentry, aberration, and accessory pathways are related to the conduction pathway of the heart.

52. a. reentry.—Reentry, aberration, and accessory pathways are related to the conduction pathway of the heart.

53. c. the preload and afterload are directly affected.—As a result, the circulation of blood does not effectively reach all areas of the body, and a backup of fluid develops in other areas.

54. d. hypertrophy.—Enlargement of the heart muscle, typically the left ventricle.

55. d. renal failure.—The kidneys become damaged and shut down.

56. b. permanent organ damage.—The organs most likely to be at risk are the brain, heart, and kidneys.

57. d. hypertension.—If cerebral autoregulation is lost, such as during a stroke or after head injury, the only way for the brain to maintain adequate perfusion is to elevate the arterial BP.

58. a. cerebral autoregulation.—This occurs with the opening and closing of sphincter muscles in the small arterioles of the brain.

59. a. phlebitis.—It can develop from intimal damage to the vein from catheters, injection of irritating substances, and the use of oral contraceptives.

60. d. spontaneous rupture of the aorta—These patients develop aneurysms that typically involve the aortic arch.

61. c. claudication—Similar to angina, it typically occurs with exertion and subsides with rest. The calf is most commonly affected.

62. c. preload.—Starling's law of the heart is based on the fact that the greater the initial stretch of the cardiac muscle, the greater the degree of shortening that will occur.

63. a. venous congestion—When the heart fails to pump effectively, blood backs up in the venous system.

64. b. sympathetic nervous system.—The system circulation is stimulated to increase the tone in the blood vessels to provide better venous blood flow to the heart.

65. d. chronic hypertension.—Often this is a cumulative problem as a result of multiple heart attacks.

66. b. shock.—Cardiogenic shock is the most severe form of pump failure resulting in inadequate cardiac output due to left ventricular malfunction. Out-of-hospital treatment begins with treating for shock.

67. a. ascites.—This occurs when blood is not pumped adequately from the system circulation into the lungs.

68. a. the use of fibrynolytics.—Clot busters may be a treatment option for some patients.

69. c. hypothermia—The hypothermic heart may be resistant to defibrillation and first-line cardiac drugs.

70. b. decreasing preload.—Positioning the patient is a primary treatment step. When possible, the patient sitting upright with legs dangling assists in venous pooling and helps to decrease the preload.

71. c. ventilatory support—Assisted ventilations with bag mask, CPAP, or intubation may be necessary.

72. a. cardiogenic shock.—Cardiogenic shock greatly diminishes blood flow throughout the body; tissues deteriorate rapidly, and death ensues. The most common cause is as a result of an extensive MI.

73. d. past medical history of heart disease.—Sometimes it is really impossible to tell a difference, but past history may be helpful. Look for a history of heart disease because this tends to be consistent with APE, while a history of COPD is consistent with CHF. However, the patient may have both.

74. b. cardiac tamponade—This life-threatening condition quickly progresses from decreased cardiac output to cardiac failure and cardiogenic shock.

75. a. CHF versus APE.—Many providers, when in doubt, give both furosemide and an inhaled bronchodilator. This generally covers both conditions, as long as careful attention is paid to the basics of the ABCs.

76. b. ACS.—The most common cause is as a result of an extensive MI. As the body's compensating mechanism fails, shock progresses, severe hypotension develops, and organ tissues die.

77. a. chronic CHF—Peripheral edema and neck vein distension are far more common in chronic CHF than in acute pulmonary edema. Do not make the error of excluding the possibility of acute pulmonary edema simply because no peripheral edema is present.

78. b. Positioning the patient upright.—Positioning the patient is the primary treatment step. When possible, the patient sitting upright with legs dangling assists in venous pooling and helps to decrease the preload.

79. d. paroxysmal nocturnal dyspnea.—Most people sleep in a prone or near-prone position. Blood pools in the lungs, leading to pulmonary congestion and difficulty breathing. Typically, the patient wakes suddenly from sleep and is extremely diaphoretic and short of breath.

80. d. blood glucose—Two conditions that must be ruled out quickly with any patient who has an altered mental status are hypoxia and hypoglycemia. Administer oxygen and obtain a blood glucose reading quickly.

81. d. hypertensive emergency.—Hypertension is a devastating disease that affects the cardiovascular system. A hypertensive emergency is a life-threatening, sudden, and severe increase in BP that can lead to serious, irreversible end-organ damage within hours if left untreated.

82. b. heart failure.—Heart failure occurs when the heart has been injured and cardiac pumping is insufficient to meet the circulation demand of the body.

83. a. preload—The afterload is the force against which the ventricles contract. Refractory period and action potentials are used in reference to the depolarization and repolarization of the heart.

84. a. pain.—As the bulging of the sac continues to grow, the pressure it exerts on other structures often causes symptoms such as abdominal or back pain.

85. d. sudden death.—It may leak, causing pain, or grow and burst like a balloon. The significant and rapid blood loss from the rupture results in sudden death.

86. a. rapid transport.—Rapid, gentle transport and early notification to the ED is the best approach.

87. b. headache, vision disturbance, and confusion.—Backache, chest pain, and dyspnea are not typical symptoms, but may be present with concurrent emergency conditions.

88. d. primary problem.—Treat the primary problem first. The hypertension may be a compensatory mechanism for another emergency, such as intracranial hemorrhage, pulmonary edema, MI, toxemia, or aortic dissection.

89. a. bradycardia—Too much potassium (hyperkalemia) or too little (hypokalemia) slows the heart rate.

90. d. dissecting abdominal aortic aneurysm.—As the aneurysm grows, the pressure it exerts on other structures often causes symptoms such as abdominal or back pain. As it leaks or ruptures, the blood loss causes other symptoms, such as syncope, dyspnea, and pain or numbness in the lower extremities.

91. b. restore perfusion.—Aspirin is used to decrease the risk of vascular mortality with suspected acute MI. Aspirin produces inhibition of platelet aggregation, helping to restore perfusion.

92. b. Kussmaul's—Kussmaul's signs may be observed during the physical exam.

93. d. location of the damage.—This rather simple device has saved many people whose hearts cannot beat effectively alone.

94. c. left chest area—The site of implantation is usually the left chest area, although it may be placed in other areas.

95. d. dysrhythmias.—Cardiac irritability from hypoxia or other causes typically produces dysrhythmias.

96. a. Beck's triad—Beck's triad is a combination of three symptoms (hypotension, JVD, and quiet heart sounds) characteristic of cardiac compression (tamponade).

97. b. relieve cardiac compression.—This is accomplished by placing a needle directly into the pericardial sac (pericardiocentesis) to remove the fluid.

98. d. accessory.—Reentry and aberration are also related to the conduction pathway of the heart, and intrinsic means from within the heart.

99. b. junctional escape—The intrinsic rate of the junctional pacemaker is 40–60. The QRS is narrower than NRS, and the P wave may be before the QRS with a short P-R interval, during, or after the QRS.

100. b. Administer nitroglycerine and aspirin.—The patient's blood pressure is more than adequate for nitroglycerin. Due to the patient's cancer, you should ask the patient if he can tolerate aspirin.

Chapter 23: Neurology

1. a. monitor internal changes of the body.—The nervous system is the most complex of the body systems. It acts as the control center of the body.

2. b. cerebrum.—Also called telencephalon, this is the location of higher cognitive abilities such as learning, analysis, memory, and language.

3. b. telencephalon—Also called cerebrum; this is the location of higher cognitive abilities such as learning, analysis, memory, and language.

4. c. basilar artery.—Brain gets its blood supply from the two internal carotid arteries and the basilar artery, which connect into a cerebral arterial circle (circle of Willis).

5. c. circle of Willis.—If for any reason blood flow gets disrupted, the circle of Willis may provide for collateral cerebral circulation, reducing the chances for serious complications.

6. b. midbrain, pons, and medulla oblongata.—These structures are critical to the maintenance of vital functions.

7. a. pineal body—It functions primarily as an endocrine organ.

8. c. cerebellum.—It is located in the back of the skull beneath the cerebrum and surrounding the brain stem.

9. d. subarachnoid space.—SCF is produced in the ventricles of the brain and is completely replaced several times a day.

10. d. help the brain to recognize changes in CO_2 levels.—The brain monitors changes in the CSF CO_2 level and activates responses in the respiratory centers to regulate the CO_2 and pH of the body.

11. b. Hydrocephalus—Sometimes this condition results in increased pressure within the skull (increased intracranial pressure).

12. b. pia mater—The pia mater is the innermost layer of meninges.

13. c. CSF—Meningitis may be life-threatening, especially when caused by bacteria.

14. a. not covered with myelinated fibers.—White matter is the white fibers of the brain and spinal cord that are covered with myelin (myelinated). Myelin is a layer or coating that protects the axon process and increases the conduction of nerve impulses.

15. b. neuron.—Also called nerve cells, these are dependent on aerobic metabolism, meaning they require oxygen to function.

16. d. myelin.—A soft, white, fatty material that forms a thick sheath around some axons.

17. c. glucose.—The brain cannot create or store either of these, so it relies heavily on the supporting cells as a source of energy.

18. a. multiple sclerosis.—Some disease processes, such as multiple sclerosis, interfere with the myelin sheath.

19. d. synapses.—The synapse (junction) is the place where impulses are transmitted to the axons and dendrites of other neurons.

20. a. reticular activating system—The RAS controls the degree of activity of the central nervous system, as in maintaining sleep and wakefulness.

21. b. peripheral—The peripheral nervous system (PNS) consists of twelve pairs of cranial nerves and thirty-one pairs of peripheral nerves exiting the spinal cord between each vertebra.

22. b. ALS—Amyotrophic lateral sclerosis is a rapidly progressive disorder leading to atrophy of all body muscles and death.

23. c. multiple sclerosis—A demyelinating disease marked by patches of hardened tissue in the brain or the spinal cord.

24. d. hydrocephalus—This condition is caused by either a blockage or decreased reabsorption of CSF, and sometimes results in increased pressure within the skull.

25. c. ruptured aneurysm—Cerebral aneurysm is a congenital defect on the wall of a cerebral artery. This is the fourth leading cause of cerebrovascular disorder in the United States.

26. b. atherosclerosis—Vascular dementia is caused by atrophy and death of brain cells due to decreased blood flow.

27. b. secondary—Medical research has demonstrated that all brain damage does not occur at the moment of impact. Rather, it occurs over the next few hours and days.

28. c. concussion.—Symptoms most commonly include headache, memory loss, and irritability, which usually resolve in two hours but may persist for months.

29. c. Rapidly transport the patient to a trauma center.—The greatest reduction in mortality and morbidity of the head-injured patient includes: prompt resuscitation, rapid transport to a trauma center, CT scanning, prompt evacuation of significant intracranial hematomas, ICP monitoring, and treatment.

30. c. This is a chronic disorder that does not require emergency care.—The condition described is Parkinson's disease. These symptoms are associated with the chronic and slowly progressive disorder. There is no information that suggests that this patient requires emergency care.

31. c. the TIA has no lasting effect.—A TIA or ministroke is a temporary occlusion of an artery to the brain caused by a blood clot. It is believed to be a warning sign of future CVA.

32. b. a major stroke.—TIAs are strong predictors of stroke risk and may occur days, weeks, or months before a stroke.

33. c. seizure.—Seizures occur in patients of all ages, though the causes of seizures vary slightly in each age group.

34. b. atonic—Lack of physical tone.

35. b. complex partial—The aura with this type of seizure may include hallucinations of sounds, visuals, smells, and tastes.

36. a. brain damage can occur.—Prolonged seizures tend to present with very little or no body movement (fixed gaze only). This does not mean the patient has stopped seizing. The patient's neurons are burning out, so treat and stop the seizures.

37. c. medication.—There are many common home medications that may be the culprit of a syncopal event.

38. a. by speaking with the patient—Subtle changes in the patient's mental status are usually the earliest indicator of nervous system dysfunction. Talking to the patient and performing serial assessments is the best way to pick up on the subtle changes.

39. a. performing serial assessments—Subtle changes in the patient's mental status are usually the earliest indicator of nervous system dysfunction. Talking to the patient and performing serial assessments is the best way to pick up on the subtle changes.

40. a. GCS—The Glasgow Coma Scale is a numerical tool used to assess and score a patient's best response to eye opening, verbal, and motor response.

41. d. apneusis.—An abnormal respiratory pattern associated with neurological emergencies.

42. c. Cheyne-Stokes respirations.—This abnormal breathing pattern occurs when the brain stem has been injured.

43. b. autisms.—When autisms are present together with an altered mental status, this may indicate the presence of a lesion in the lower brain stem.

44. c. Ataxic—This abnormal breathing pattern is also associated with lesions in the lower brain stem.

45. b. binocular vision.—Binocular vision is controlled by the forebrain. If this reflex fails, double vision occurs.

46. a. accommodation—A normal function of the eyes that allows the normal eye to focus on objects closer than 20 feet.

47. c. nystagmus.—Nystagmus may be induced by alcohol intoxication, irritation of the inner ear, blindness, and neurologic diseases.

48. d. miosis.—Miosis is seen in the early stages of meningitis, as well as in some types of drug overdose, brain lesions, and sunstroke.

49. a. anisocoria.—Always ask the patient if this finding is normal for her before assuming that it is an abnormal finding.

50. a. chorea.—This involuntary movement may be blended with voluntary movements that can hide the involuntary motions.

51. b. athetosis.—Chorea often occurs simultaneously with athetosis.

52. c. Tourette's syndrome.—This disorder begins in childhood and is three times more prevalent in boys than girls.

53. c. Assess the six cardinal positions of gaze.—As assessment of the six cardinal positions of gaze is used to evaluate cranial nerves III, IV, and VI, in order to detect midbrain and pontine dysfunction.

54. d. V—Assessment of the cranial nerves can help clue you in to the location of a brain injury or insult. Cranial nerve V is linked to speech, swallowing, chewing, and the blinking reflex.

55. b. Ataxia—The inability to coordinate voluntary muscular movements.

56. a. spinal cord injury.—When this finding is present during the exam of a patient with a suspected spinal cord injury, the paramedic should mark the level on the chest for comparison with serial assessments to follow.

57. b. heat stroke—These signs include: altered mental status, neurological dysfunction, elevated temperature, and hot and dry skin.

58. d. behavioral changes.—This occurs because the cerebral hemispheres are the most susceptible to injury.

59. a. pons.—Arm and leg extension is also referred to as decerebrate posturing.

60. c. Decorticate—Characteristics include muscle rigidity with arms flexed and held tightly to the chest, clenched fists, and legs extended and internally rotated.

61. b. late—The three signs of rising ICP are: rising BP, changing respiratory patterns, and a decreasing pulse rate.

62. a. pyramidal—Babinski's reflex or sign is a reflex movement in which, when the sole of the foot is tickled, the great toe turns upward instead of downward.

63. a. the corpus callosum—The cerebrum is the largest part of the brain and is connected by nerve tissue called the corpus callosum.

64. b. parietal—It also controls speech and memory.

65. d. hypothalamus—It is responsible for many important functions for survival and pleasure, such as: eating, drinking, temperature regulation, and sex.

66. c. ventricles of the brain—CSF is present in the subarachnoid space, cavities, and canals of the brain and spinal cord.

67. d. tentorium.—The tentorium process of dura mater separates the cerebrum and cerebellum and supports the occipital lobes.

68. a. venous—Arterial bleeding is associated with epidural hematoma.

69. d. interneurons—Interneurons connect afferent and efferent neurons in the brain and spinal cord.

70. b. Dendrites—Axons carry impulses away from the cell.

71. a. myelin.—A soft, white, fatty material that forms a thick sheath.

72. b. epidural and subdural.—The two most common hematomas that may develop within the brain are epidural and subdural hematomas, named by the location in relation to the meninges.

73. c. spina bifida.—A malformation of the spinal column with an opening in the membrane that covers the vertebra.

74. a. Poliomyelitis—Also called polio.

75. b. contusion—Concussion, amnesia, and aphasia cannot be seen on a CT scan of the brain.

76. d. Retrograde—This type of amnesia presents with a loss of memory of events that occurred before an adverse event.

77. d. subarachnoid hemorrhage—Hypertension with a headache is more likely to be associated with subarachnoid hemorrhage.

78. a. Ischemic—The out-of-hospital treatment for stroke is the same for all causes of stroke. The definitive (in-hospital) therapy, however, varies.

79. c. uncontrolled hypertension—The blood pressure inclusion factor for the use of thrombolytics is a systolic BP between 90 and 200.

80. a. atropine—Some opthalmic drops will also cause dilation or constriction of the pupils.

81. b. dolls-eye maneuver—With the patient's eyes opened, the head is turned quickly from side to side or up and down. The normal response is for both eyes to move in conjugate gaze to the opposite side of the head turning, similar to the doll with counterweighted eyes.

82. a. one—Another abnormal finding is a dilated pupil greater than 4 mm.

83. b. Aphasia—Aphasia is categorized as expressive or receptive.

84. b. irregular breathing pattern—Additional neurological deficits to look for in the unconscious patient include: abnormal eye movement, (including pupil reaction), Babinski's reflex, muscle tone, and signs of rising ICP (early versus late.)

85. b. mean different things to different people.—These are nonspecific antiquated terms that have different meanings to different people.

86. b. irregular breathing pattern—Additional neurological deficits to look for in the unconscious patient include: abnormal eye movement, (including pupil reaction), Babinski's reflex, muscle tone, and signs of rising ICP (early versus late).

87. b. rising ICP.—Loss of extraocular movement on the affected side due to increased pressure on the cranial nerves.

88. a. herniated disc—Pressure on the spinal nerves (pinched nerve) may cause pain in the extremities.

89. c. Bell's palsy.—Paralysis of the facial nerve causing distortion on one side of the face.

90. d. during sleep—The patient awakens with symptoms of a stroke or is difficult to awaken.

91. a. epilepsy.—This is the patient's first seizure, which precludes epilepsy. Epilepsy is more common in children than in infants or toddlers.

92. c. tonic.—This phase typically lasts fifteen to twenty seconds and alternates with muscle spasms (clonic) lasting up to five minutes.

93. c. syncopal—Fainting.

94. c. neoplasm—A new growth of tissue serving no physiological function.

95. c. hypertension—The other choices are neurologic disorders.

96. b. V—Also called trigeminal neuralgia.

97. a. heredity.—Glaucoma is a disease in which elevated pressure in the eye, due to an obstruction of the outflow of aqueous humor, damages the optic nerve and causes visual defects.

98. b. glaucoma—Symptoms may occur suddenly and are sometimes accompanied by nausea and vomiting. If untreated, glaucoma may result in permanent blindness within a few days.

99. d. sensory function—There are at least six types of tactile receptors located in the skin and tissues below the skin.

100. a. frontal lobe—The cerebrum is also responsible for higher cognitive abilities such as learning, analysis, memory, and language.

Chapter 24: Endocrinology

1. c. diabetic problems—Diabetes and related complications affect approximately 6% of the U.S. population.

2. a. hyperlipidemia—This is a risk factor associated with heart disease.

3. a. Diabetes—The most common of the endocrinologic emergencies is diabetic problems, which occur more frequently than all of the rest put together.

4. a. chemical—The normal secretion of hormones is tightly regulated by a feedback mechanism involving the: hypothalamus, pituitary gland, target gland, and end-organ.

5. d. nervous—The nervous system acts as the control center of the body; together with the endocrine system, the body's internal physiological balance is monitored and controlled.

6. b. Hormones—Hormones move through the body and produce specific effects on target cells and organs.

7. d. blood.—In the blood, they move through the body and produce specific effects on target cells.

8. b. a pancreas transplant.—At the current time, Type I diabetes is without a cure, except for a pancreas transplant.

9. c. pituitary—The pituitary gland is associated with hormones that directly and indirectly affect most basic bodily functions.

10. a. parathyroid—Four small endocrines glands that are adjacent to the thyroid gland and secrete a hormone that regulates the metabolism of calcium and phosphorus in the body.

11. c. pancreas—The pancreas secretes the hormones insulin and glucagon as well as hormones that aid in digestion.

12. d. adrenal—Either of a pair of organs that are located on top of the kidney. The adrenal glands secrete the hormones epinephrine and norepinephrine.

13. b. Excessive hormone production—Endocrine emergencies also occur when normal hormone production fails and with failure of feedback inhibition systems.

14. b. glucagon.—The pancreas secretes the hormones insulin and glucagon.

15. a. stored.—In addition, insulin prevents the breakdown of fat tissue in the body.

16. a. Type I diabetes—Type I diabetes is an autoimmune type of disease.

17. c. many diabetics have some form of neuropathy.—Many diabetic patients (both Type I and II) have an acquired dysfunction of the peripheral nervous system (neuropathy).

18. d. permanent neuronal damage.—A period of hypoglycemia is far more dangerous to the patient than an equivalent period of hyperglycemia.

19. c. dehydrated; fluids—The most important immediate problem in hyperglycemia is dehydration. Identify and correct it as soon as possible following local protocols. Always look for other sources of symptoms, especially if the patient has an altered mental status.

20. a. amino acids—Free fatty acids, amino acids, and sugar fail to enter the cells properly, resulting in hungry cells.

21. a. ketones and ketoacids—As the patient's blood sugar rises significantly and the fatty tissue breaks down, the body forms compounds called ketones and ketoacids from the fat tissue. These substances change the acid-base balance in the body, harming the patient.

22. d. total body potassium.—The elevated blood sugar level makes the patient urinate more frequently than usual, leading to dehydration and a loss of body chemicals, particularly potassium.

23. b. infection.—The stress of the infection results in an increased insulin requirement in the body. Unless the diabetic patient recognizes the need to increase the daily dose of insulin when sick, metabolism and the regulation of blood sugar level become abnormal.

24. b. Not every patient with hyperglycemia will have DKA.—Whether symptomatic or not, patients who develop hyperglycemia may not have DKA or hyperosmolar hyperglycemia nonketotic coma (HHNC).

25. c. stored fats—Free fatty acids from stored triglycerides are released and metabolized in the liver to ketones. When ketones dissolve in the blood, they form ketoacids.

26. a. blood; high—When ketones dissolve in the blood, they form ketoacids. If the level of ketones is high enough, the patient is not only ketotic but develops an acidosis. The combination is called ketoacidosis.

27. b. hyperosmolar hyperglycemic nonketotic coma.—Not all people with elevated blood sugar levels have DKA or HHNC. Many people have glucose intolerance and hyperglycemia with absolutely no symptoms.

28. a. early warning signs from the counter-regulatory hormones fail.—The production of glucagon and epinephrine in response to low blood sugar normally causes symptoms of tachycardia and diaphoresis. This early warning system may fail, and the patient remains asymptomatic until the sugar level drops low enough to result in loss of consciousness.

29. d. caffeine—Caffeine increases a person's sensitivity to hypoglycemia.

30. d. glycogenolysis.—Glycogenolysis, together with gluconeogensis (enzymes that cause the liver to manufacture more glucose), tends to raise the blood sugar.

31. c. thyrotoxicosis—Acute thyrotoxicosis, also known as thyroid storm, is a potentially life-threatening acute exacerbation of ongoing hyperthyroidism.

32. a. atrial fibrillation and fever.—Additional signs and symptoms include: flushing, sweating, tachycardia, CHF, agitation, restlessness, delirium, seizures, coma, nausea, vomiting, diarrhea, and fever out of proportion to other clinical findings.

33. b. hypothyroidism—Hypothyroidism is a clinical syndrome due to a deficiency of thyroid hormones. The group of hypothyroid symptoms is often referred to as myxedema.

34. d. hyperglycemia.—Hypoglycemia is more common as the condition goes untreated and progresses to coma.

35. c. sinus bradycardia—Myxedema is characterized by hypothermia, extreme weakness, altered mental status, hypoventilation, and hypoglycemia. Sinus bradycardia is the most common dysrhythmia.

36. a. Cushing's syndrome—The production of excess corticosteroids by the adrenal or pituitary glands produces an abnormal condition resulting in excess body weight and muscular weakness.

37. d. Cushing's syndrome—Rounding of the face (moon face) and dorsocervical fat pad (buffalo hump) are recognizable characteristics of this disorder.

38. a. Cushing's syndrome—Because most people's acute complaint is not related to Cushing's syndrome, symptom-based assessment and management is the key to patient management.

39. c. Addison's disease—The condition is characterized by weight loss, extreme weakness, low blood pressure, GI disturbances, and brown pigmentation of the skin and mucous membranes.

40. b. cortisol and aldosterone—Steroid use is the most common cause of exogenous adrenal suppression.

41. a. the use of oral or inhaled steroids.—Steroid use is the most common cause of exogenous adrenal suppression.

42. d. decreased pigmentation.—An increased pigmentation (brown) on the exterior surfaces, creases of the palms, and oral mucosa are signs of adrenal insufficiency.

43. a. hypovolemia.—The acute life threats in adrenal insufficiency are hypotension and hypoglycemia.

44. a. hyperthyroidism.—If this finding is present during thyroid storm, it is helpful. However, less than 50% of patients with acute thyrotoxicosis have visible eye changes.

45. a. Novolin—Regular insulin is exogenous unmodified insulin.

46. c. human—Many insulin preparations are available. Made from various sources, some are faster acting than others, while some are longer lasting than others.

47. b. malnourished.—Thiamine may benefit any hypoglycemia patient who is also undernourished (e.g., due to cancer, AIDS, or other chronic diseases).

48. c. administer $D_{50}W$—IV administration of dextrose must be given first, as the patient is hypoglycemic. IV fluid hydration is appropriate next because of the hypotension. The patient may be experiencing acute adrenal insufficiency due to the steroid use.

49. a. acute adrenal insufficiency—The patient may be experiencing acute adrenal insufficiency due to the steroid use. The acute life threats in adrenal insufficiency are hypotension and hypoglycemia.

50. a. adrenal—The resultant excess affects carbohydrate, protein, and lipid metabolism.

51. b. hyperglycemia—Until a blood glucose reading is obtained, hypoglycemia should be suspected. However, the history and the physical findings (e.g., Kussmaul's respirations, warm and dry skin, and dehydration) suggest possible hyperglycemia.

52. c. Deep respirations are a response to increased acid levels from excess ketones.—Kussmaul's respirations are the body's response to attempts to blow off excess acid in the body.

53. b. High-flow oxygen, IV fluid boluses, and transport.—The most immediate problem in hyperglycemia is dehydration.

54. d. administer another 25 grams of dextrose—Manage the airway and breathing with BLS techniques until the patient receives additional dextrose.

55. b. diabetic emergency—For any patient with an altered mental status, the paramedic must rule out hypoxia and hypoglycemia first.

56. b. glucose reading—For any patient with an altered mental status, the paramedic must rule out hypoxia and hypoglycemia first.

57. a. Beta-blockers will conceal compensatory signs of shock.—Decreased blood sugar levels result in the production of glucagon and epinephrine in the body's attempt to raise the sugar. This causes a sympathetic response (tachycardia and diaphoresis). Beta-blockers inhibit this response and mask the signs.

58. b. the amount of glycogen reserves in the liver—Glucagon increases the sugar level in the blood by breaking down glycogen in the liver.

59. b. glucagon—Insulin and glucagon are both produced in the pancreas. Glucagon increases the sugar level in the blood by breaking down glycogen in the liver.

60. d. all of the above—Abdominal pain may be the first indication of a diabetic or endocrine disorder, especially in infants and the elderly.

61. a. moon face—The other findings are associated with other endocrine disorders or emergencies.

62. a. typical findings—Excess growth of body hair is another classic finding.

63. b. DKA—When ketones dissolve in the blood, they form ketoacids. If the level of ketones is high enough, the patient is not only ketotic but develops an acidosis. The combination is called ketoacidosis.

64. c. pancreas—The pancreas produces the hormones insulin and glucagons, as well as hormones that aid in digestion.

65. d. pituitary—Also called vasopressin, it increases blood pressure and exerts an antidiuretic effect.

Chapter 25: Allergies and Anaphylaxis

1. c. immune response.—An immune response is a bodily response occurring when a foreign substance tries to invade the body.

2. c. allergic reaction—Damage to the tissue includes swelling and cell wall breakdown.

3. a. basophils and mast cells.—The reaction causes the release of histamines, leukotrienes, and other mediators.

4. b. angioneurotic edema.—This may occur as a result of anaphylaxis or other types of reactions (e.g., cold or drugs).

5. d. blood products.—The other examples are common allergens.

6. c. bradycardia.—A person experiencing symptoms of a severe allergic reaction would show signs of compensating shock.

7. a. GI tract—Signs and symptoms include: cramping, nausea, vomiting, and diarrhea.
8. d. 0.3; 0.15—The epinephrine auto-injector is prescribed to patients with known allergic reactions for emergency use and may be used by trained EMS providers with permission from medical direction.
9. b. antihistamine—Benadryl® is routinely administered to counteract the effects of histamine release.
10. c. latex sap is chemically related to these fruits and vegetables.—This results in a "cross-reactivity" of antigens to IgE.
11. d. When peripheral circulation is so poor SQ injections will be ineffective.—The peripheral circulation shuts down as shock progresses. SQ injections will not be effective in this condition, and obtaining IV access becomes more difficult as well.
12. c. markings of the animal—Distinguishing the type of bite may be difficult at best. A good history describing the markings of the animal is most helpful.
13. b. Latex—It has been shown that multiple skin contacts or inhalation exposures to the proteins found in natural rubber latex can cause a latex allergy.
14. a. slow histamine release.—Solumedrol or hydrocortisone may be helpful over the first few hours following a reaction.
15. b. increased arterial pressure.—Histamine release causes vascular permeability, bronchoconstriction, nausea, and vomiting.
16. a. transferred from breast milk.—This is one of many reasons why experts favor breast-feeding.
17. c. competes with histamine at the receptor sites, blocking the effects of histamine.—Benadryl® is routinely administered to counteract the effects of histamine release.
18. d. skin, respiratory, and GI tracts.—This is why the most common findings in anaphylaxis are urticaria, wheezing, and abdominal pain.
19. b. bronchospasm—Epinephrine is the main treatment as a bronchodilator.

20. b. increase dilation of the capillaries.—Histamine release also causes contraction of smooth muscle and stimulation of gastric acid secretion.
21. a. the airway.—Not all of the following signs and symptoms are present in every case; however, the patient may develop hoarseness, stridor, pharyngeal edema or pharyngeal spasm in the upper airway and hypoventilation, labored accessory muscle use, abnormal retractions, prolonged expirations, wheezes, and diminished lung sounds in the lower airways.
22. c. SC epinephrine 0.01 mg/kg (1:1,000).—The pediatric dose of epinephrine for an allergic reaction is 0.01 mg/kg of 1:1,000.
23. c. epinephrine—Epinephrine is the primary treatment as a bronchodilator.
24. a. degree of sensitivity.—The severity of the reaction varies significantly form patient to patient and exposure to exposure.
25. b. Adjust the pump to stop the flow of antibiotic.—Stop the infusion of the suspected cause of the allergic reaction first! Follow local protocol.
26. b. repeat epi and give fluid boluses—All patients with any type of acute anaphylactic reaction need to be treated with epinephrine. Fluids are needed to treat for shock.
27. b. Start administration of a vasopressor.—Vasopressors may be helpful for hypotension not responsive to fluids alone.
28. a. blood vessels dilate and become permeable.—As a result of the vascular dilation, plasma escapes into the tissues, causing urticaria and angioedema.
29. d. Antihistamines block H_1 receptors in blood vessels.—Antihistamines do not block all of the released mediators, only histamine. Therefore, treating an anaphylactic reaction with antihistamines alone is potentially fatal.
30. c. renal and mesentery artery vasodilation—Low dosages cause renal and mesenteric vasodilation and should be avoided.

Chapter 26: Gastroenterology and Urology

1. c. referred.—Referred pain is pain that originates in one area but is sensed in another area.
2. b. Somatic—An example of somatic pain is the sharply localized lower-right quadrant pain of the later phase of appendicitis.
3. a. Visceral—This type of pain is typically described as crampy, gaseous, and often intermittent.
4. b. gallbladder—There are several characteristic patterns of referred pain. Biliary pain commonly radiates around the right side to the back and angle of the scapula.

5. a. PID, diverticulitis, and ovarian cyst.—These conditions are associated with pain in both the right and left lower quadrants.
6. c. ruptured aneurysm.—Some patients will experience numbness in the lower extremities or a syncopal event with the rupture of an abdominal aortic aneurysm.
7. d. swallowed blood from epistaxis—The most common "false alarm" in GI bleeding calls is swallowed blood from a nosebleed that is subsequently vomited back up.

8. d. esophageal varices—The other conditions are causes of lower GI bleeding.

9. b. diverticulosis—The other conditions are causes of upper GI bleeding.

10. b. renal colic.—The pain from kidney stones is excruciating even for those with a high pain threshold.

11. a. It appeared tarry and black.—Melena is tarry, sticky black stool and may indicate upper GI bleeding or the ingestion of iron or bismuth preparations, such as antacids.

12. b. treatment for shock.—Administer fluids per your local protocol.

13. b. Cholecystitis—An inflammation of the gallbladder.

14. d. acute hepatitis—Acute hepatitis refers to an inflammation of the liver for any reason. Often jaundice and upper-right quadrant tenderness are present.

15. b. 15–20—The patient may complain of dizziness and experience changing vital signs (e.g., increased heart rate, decreased BP) when moved to an upright or erect position.

16. d. reflux esophagitis—This condition may range from asymptomatic to severe chest pain, or any degree of symptoms in between. Even if a patient has a history of heartburn, assume that chest pain is due to myocardial ischemia until proven otherwise.

17. b. history—Sudden, abrupt pain suggests an acute perforation, strangulation, torsion, or vascular accident. Inflammatory lesions and obstructive phenomena are slower in their development.

18. a. appendicitis—Typically, the pain gradually increases with appendicitis, whereas the other conditions present with acute pain.

19. a. cholecystitis—Ingestion of fatty foods may precipitate an attack of acute cholecystitis.

20. c. peritoneal inflammation—Somatic pain is caused by a stimulation of nerve fibers in the parietal peritoneum due to chemical or bacterial infection. The patient usually lies quietly with the thighs flexed to relax the peritoneum.

21. c. absence of sounds—Realistically, in the out-of-hospital setting, it is difficult to differentiate specific conditions by the presence of bowel sounds. More helpful is the total absence of bowel sounds in all four quadrants.

22. d. peritoneal irritation.—Any maneuver that jars the inflamed peritoneal cavity should result in rebound tenderness. This includes: the direct release of palpation pressure, moving the stretcher quickly, and percussion of the soles of the feet.

23. a. <thirteen—The tilt test (orthostatic) is more reliable in adults than in children.

24. c. lactose intolerance.—Lactose intolerance is probably the most common GI abnormality worldwide. Some studies suggest that it affects more than half of the world's population.

25. d. irritable bowel syndrome.—Also called "spastic colon," IBS is often associated with emotional stress.

26. b. ascites.—An accumulation of serious fluid in the spaces between the tissues and organs in the abdominal cavity.

27. b. the release of digestive enzymes often worsens the condition.—Food causes the release of digestive enzymes that often worsen most abdominal conditions.

28. d. Dialysis—The most common emergency from peritoneal dialysis is an acute infection of the peritoneum.

29. c. oxygen as tolerated, IV fluids, IV Phenergan, and morphine—Until the patient's nausea passes, oxygen by cannula is appropriate. The patient needs fluids, pain relief, and an antiemetic.

30. a. appendicitis—The "classic" presentation of appendicitis is periumbilical crampy pain that then localizes in the lower-right quadrant. Nearly all persons with acute appendicitis have anorexia.

31. a. avoiding taking a BP in any extremity with a fistula.—Another special consideration for the dialysis patient is to avoid the dialysis vascular access site for drawing blood or giving IV fluids.

32. b. UTI—Clinically, a UTI is diagnosed on the symptoms described. Next to respiratory infections, uncomplicated UTIs are the most common problem encountered in EDs.

33. b. ectopic pregnancy—Acute urinary retention may be the initial presenting symptom of ectopic pregnancy.

34. a. torsion of the testicle—Testicular torsion is an acute urological emergency that threatens the male's future reproductive capabilities. The condition is usually unilateral, although cases of bilateral torsion have been reported.

35. a. ice—Ice and elevation may be helpful for men with scrotal discomfort. Use pain medications as per your local protocol.

36. a. maintaining proper balance between water and salts in the blood.—The renin-angiotensin-aldosterone mechanism is responsible for the kidneys' regulation of sodium, potassium, and water in the body.

37. c. oxygen and morphine—The administration of nitrates within twenty-four hours of a patient taking Viagra® may result in patient death. Morphine is far safer in treating acute pulmonary edema or suspected myocardial ischemia under these circumstances.

38. b. chlamydia.—Women are commonly asymptomatic, while men often have urethral burning, especially during urination, and a discharge.

39. b. pain management.—The pain from kidney stones is excruciating even for those with a high pain threshold.

40. d. Crohn's disease.—Crohn's is a chronic condition resulting in bowel inflammation, usually of the small intestine.
41. d. Bright red blood can occur with bleeding in the lower or upper GI tract.—Bright red discoloration of stool may be due to vegetables in the diet. The most immediate concern is GI bleeding.
42. a. Referred—There are several characteristic patterns of referred pain. For example, blood or pus under the diaphragm presents as aching pain in the top of the shoulder.
43. a. upper—A lower GI bleed involves bleeding located more distally to the duodenojejunal junction.
44. b. bright red blood in the stool—Hematochezia may be seen with upper GI bleeding and acute transit, or left colon, or sigmoid colon bleeding.

45. d. unreliable.—It takes only drops of blood to turn the entire bowl red.
46. b. small piece of stool.—As the obstructed appendix distends, its blood supply is cut off.
47. b. bile flow.—Blockages are typically caused by gallstones. These are particles of variable size that block the lumen, interfering with bile flow.
48. c. Colitis—The most common causes of colitis are: infections, inflammatory disease, and sexually transmitted disease.
49. d. varices.—Alcoholic varices are secondary to cirrhosis caused by alcohol ingestion. Nonalcoholic cirrhosis and varices are four times as likely to bleed from varices as from peptic ulcer.
50. b. hemorrhoids.—Hemorrhoids are a common cause of lower GI bleeding and are rarely hemodynamically significant.

Chapter 27: Toxicology

1. a. the patient's home.—Over 80% of exposures occur in the home.
2. c. twenty to forty-nine—Over 50% of poisoning fatalities occurred in twenty- to forty-nine-year-old individuals.
3. b. unattended children—Failure to supervise children properly and childproof the home are major reasons that children are at high risk for toxic exposures, especially ingestion.
4. c. the development of pulmonary edema.—Inhaled irritant gases cause pulmonary edema and severe hypoxia.
5. a. insect stinger—Needles and insect stingers may inject toxic poisons.
6. b. absorption.—Pesticides and agricultural chemicals are often absorbed this way.
7. a. the type of poison.—Some poisons affect the central nervous system while others affect the peripheral and autonomic nervous systems.
8. d. sea urchin—Other sea creatures that can sting include: Portuguese man-of-war, lionfish, and jellyfish.
9. a. salivation and nausea—Nerve agents produce SLUDGE: salivation, lacrimation, urination, defecation, GI upset, and emesis.
10. a. Toxidromes—They are useful for remembering the assessment and management of toxicological emergencies.
11. d. aspirin—Normally an antipyretic, toxic doses cause metabolic acidosis.
12. b. bradycardia.—Other drugs that cause bradycardia include: beta-blockers, pesticides, clonidine, calcium channel blockers, local anesthetics, and cholinergic agents.

13. c. Anticholinergics—Mydriasis is also caused by sympathomimetics, mushrooms, and substance withdrawal.
14. d. constricted.—Narcotics and opiates cause miosis.
15. b. Botulism—Symptoms include: headache, blurred vision, and respiratory paralysis.
16. c. tricyclic antidepressants and mushrooms.—Antihistamines, anti-diarrheals, over-the-counter cold remedies, and antipsychotics are all anticholinergics.
17. b. narcotics—Opiates also cause these assessment findings.
18. a. sympathomimetics—These include: amphetamines, over-the-counter diet pills, caffeine, and cocaine.
19. c. ingestion—Deliberate ingestions often consist of more than one substance. This results in a potentially bewildering variety of signs and symptoms.
20. c. ensure your own safety first.—Take care of number one first.
21. a. poisoning involves exposure to a substance that is generally harmful and has no beneficial effects.—Overdose suggests excessive exposure to a substance that has normal treatment uses, but taken in excess results in harm.
22. c. aspirin.—Gastric dialysis and the induction of vomiting is appropriate treatment for many substances in the ED. Follow your local protocols.
23. c. has a decreased mental status.—An altered mental status may cause aspiration.
24. a. strychnine—Other substances to avoid inducing vomiting include ingested: corrosives, petroleum products, and drugs that may cause a sudden altered mental status.

25. a. activated charcoal.—Gastric dialysis is effective for many common household substances and drugs, such as phenobarbital, theophylline, tricyclic antidepressants, salicylates, and iron.

26. c. consider administering activated charcoal—Activated charcoal has been shown to absorb many different ingested toxins from the stomach.

27. a. hypoxia.—Systemic toxins such as carbon monoxide often result in severe hypoxia, shock, and death.

28. d. carbon monoxide exposure.—There are many poisonous gases to consider exposure to, following a fire (e.g., cyanide, chlorine).

29. a. seizures—Additional assessment findings associated with theophylline toxicity include: nausea, vomiting, altered mental status, and cardiac dysrhythmias.

30. c. dissolves easily—These substances are the most likely to cause poisoning by absorption.

31. a. paralysis.—Signs and symptoms will vary depending on the particular substance involved. General symptoms include: burning and tearing of the eyes, respiratory distress, GI distress, excessive sweating and salivation, headache, dizziness, seizures, and altered mental status.

32. b. CNS toxicity.—This is a part of a toxidrome that includes insecticides and pesticides.

33. c. Monitor her ABCs and administer oxygen.—Manage the airway, breathing, and circulation. Specific antidotes are available only for a few agents.

34. b. The substance is absorbed at the alveolar level, leading to systemic toxicity.—This is the case with carbon monoxide poisoning where the gas competes for receptor sites on the hemoglobin molecules at a rate 200 times greater than oxygen.

35. c. reversal of the respiratory depression—Narcan is administered to reverse the effects of narcotics (e.g., respiratory depression).

36. c. wax—People suffering from a poison that has been absorbed through the skin may not be immediately aware of their exposure. Always wear gloves when touching a patient and take a careful history.

37. b. atropine—Most herbicides and pesticides are nerve agents.

38. c. He had an excessive exposure to insecticides.—Most herbicides and pesticides are nerve agents.

39. b. tolerance.—When a person develops a tolerance to a substance, more and more of the substance is required to achieve the same effect. That person may accidentally take too much and develop toxicity.

40. c. dependence.—Drug dependence is a psychological problem, not a physical one.

41. a. smuggling from Colombia—Many illegal drugs are smuggled into the United States from Central and South American countries such as Colombia.

42. c. cocaine.—Cocaine is also referred to as coke, nose candy, flake, and snow.

43. b. tricyclic antidepressants.—These drugs block the reuptake of serotonin and norepinephrine.

44. b. alcohol.—Alcohol (ethanol) overdose decreases inhibitions, causes visual impairment, muscular incoordination, slowed reaction time, slurred speech, ataxia, hypothermia, hypoventilation, and hypotension.

45. d. tricyclic antidepressants—Beware of delayed toxicity.

46. a. huffing.—Found in solvents and manufacturing hydrocarbons, these are highly volatile.

47. a. iron—An overdose of iron is serious and results in an initial critical state, followed by an apparent recovery phase, a relapse into metabolic acidosis, and organ failure.

48. c. a hyperbaric chamber.—Hyperbaric therapy helps to rid hemoglobin of carbon dioxide so that oxygen can bind normally.

49. c. rebound hypertension—Withdrawal syndromes can result from the sudden stoppage of several prescription medications that are not considered addictive by most criteria.

50. b. lead poisoning—The toxidrome of symptoms describe lead poisoning.

Chapter 28: Environmental Conditions

1. d. atmospheric pressure.—The other choices are predisposing risk factors.

2. c. small children and geriatrics—People at the extremes of age are at greater risk for environmental emergencies. Older patients lose their ability to internally regulate their temperature, and small children have large body surface area and a very limited ability to compensate for acute major changes in temperature.

3. c. cancer—Anyone who has a serious underlying medical condition, especially if he is undernourished, is more susceptible to environmental influences.

4. b. diabetes—Many diabetics have a decreased sensation in the extremities.

5. a. tricyclic antidepressants—Many common medications have anticholinergic side effects. The result is an impaired ability to sweat and dissipate heat.

6. b. diving—Diving illness and high-altitude illness are examples of pressurization illnesses.

7. d. cold diuresis—Hypothermia can cause peripheral vasoconstriction, which results in cold diuresis and hypovolemia in many patients. The principal types of environmental illnesses include: heat, cold,

pressurization, and local injuries (e.g., burns or frostbite).

8. c. central blood vessels—The peripheral blood vessels are components of the body's thermoregulatory mechanism.

9. c. metabolic—This includes the breakdown of glucose, proteins, and fats to energy.

10. a. Thermoregulation—As the body temperature increases, changes occur in each organ system. If an individual gradually exposes himself to a hot environment, the body acclimates or becomes used to the heat.

11. a. convection—Heat is gained or dissipated from the body by four mechanisms: radiation, conduction, convection, and evaporation.

12. b. conduction.—The transmission of heat from warmer to cooler objects in direct contact.

13. d. evaporation—High humidity seriously impairs heat dissipation because evaporation occurs slowly.

14. a. dehydration.—The patient loses significant fluid and electrolytes, especially sodium. The result is increased concentrations of sodium (sometimes potassium) in the serum, with resultant symptoms.

15. b. diaphoresis and flushing.—Increased skin temperature and flushing may be present.

16. b. disrupt sodium concentrations.—People who are acclimatized to warm temperatures are less likely to suffer heat illness. Proper acclimatization requires at least a week of gradually increasing heat exposure.

17. a. urban—Cold stress among the elderly, intoxication, or debilitation can cause fatal hypothermia (urban hypothermia).

18. b. exhaustion—A more severe loss of fluid and salt than occurs in heat cramps. Some patients simply develop dehydration without further signs or symptoms of heat exhaustion.

19. a. treat for dehydration.—There is a high incidence of heat exhaustion in young children, individuals on water pills, and the debilitated (who are unable to maintain an adequate oral water intake), or those having prolonged bouts of diarrhea.

20. c. hypothermia—This finding is common in people who are relatively immobile, such as in a nursing facility.

21. c. antihistamines—The anticholinergic side effects impair the ability to sweat and dissipate heat.

22. a. take diuretics.—There is a high incidence of heat exhaustion in young children, individuals on water pills, and the debilitated (who are unable to maintain an adequate oral water intake), or those having prolonged bouts of diarrhea. Some patients simply develop dehydration without further signs or symptoms of heat exhaustion.

23. a. pyrogens—Fever usually results from an infection, though other illnesses (e.g., hyperthyroidism) may also increase the body temperature.

24. b. Fever; heat stroke—Fever is a normal response based on an intact thermoregulatory system. Heat stroke develops when that system fails and the body is no longer able to keep the temperature from rising.

25. a. wool—A natural fiber wool is an excellent clothing material for cold and wet conditions.

26. d. hyperglycemia—The other conditions may directly cause or contribute to the development of hypothermia.

27. d. AMI—There are many common predisposing factors for hypothermia, including: extreme ages (young/old), medications, accidents, limited mobility, chronic disease, and low income. Acute MI is not a common predisposing factor.

28. b. signs and symptoms.—The severity of hypothermia is determined by the CBT and the presence of signs and symptoms. There is no reliable correlation between signs or symptoms and a specific CBT. Always obtain a reliable CBT reading.

29. c. 85°F—The presence of signs and symptoms, together with a CBT of less than 85°F, indicates severe hypothermia.

30. b. subacute—Comes on over minutes to hours. The prognosis may be better than the acute onset form unless the patient is not rescued or treated for a long period of time.

31. d. urban—This occurs to individuals who may be inside but lack appropriate thermoregulation.

32. a. stroke.—Endocrine disorders (hypothyroidism, malnutrition, and hypoglycemia) may cause hypothermia as well.

33. b. ventricular fibrillation—It may occur as the CBT drops, but it is more common in the rewarming phase.

34. a. Cold may affect the potency of first-line cardiac drugs.—Avoid lidocaine and procainamide in hypothermia because they paradoxically lower the VF threshold, increasing resistance to defibrillation. Follow your local protocols.

35. b. V-fib and asystole.—The risks of V-fib are related both to the depth and duration of hypothermia. Severe hypothermia mimics clinical death. It may be impossible to distinguish a patient who is still alive, but profoundly hypothermic, from the victim of a cardiac arrest.

36. d. the patient is handled roughly during care and transport.—There is no increased risk of inducing V-fib from orotracheal or nasotracheal intubation as long as the patient is adequately preoxygenated.

37. b. hypothermic—Many immersion victims are hypothermic.

38. d. stop ongoing heat loss.—Remove the patient from the cold environment.

39. c. ice crystals—These crystals damage the blood vessels and other tissues.

40. a. deep frostbite skin has a white, waxy appearance.—Generally there is also a complete loss of sensation that does not recover within a short period.

41. b. lack of oxygen.—The patient may say that the affected area feels "like a stump." This feeling is due to a lack of oxygen in the affected area.

42. a. the use of alcohol and mind-altering drugs.—Studies have shown that anywhere from 35–75% of drowning victims have elevated blood alcohol levels.

43. a. they may appear normal and unaffected.—Secondary drowning may occur within a few minutes or up to four days later, and present in the form of pulmonary edema or aspiration pneumonia after a successful recovery from the initial incident.

44. b. hypoxia.—The mechanisms of lung damage from seawater and freshwater submersion are very different, but the endpoints are the same: decreased pulmonary compliance results in pulmonary edema and hypoxia.

45. a. metabolic acidosis.—No matter the type of water involved, the endpoints in submersion are metabolic acidosis, pulmonary edema, and aspiration injuries. Cerebral hypoxia often precipitates neurogenic pulmonary edema, worsening an already bad situation.

46. b. secondary.—Secondary drowning is the recurrence of respiratory distress after a successful recovery from the initial incident. It can occur within a few minutes or up to four days later.

47. a. persistent laryngeal spasms.—The other choices are examples of complications that can occur following a submersion incident.

48. b. time to the first spontaneous gasp following removal from the water.—The shorter this period, the better the neurological prognosis.

49. c. Secondary—The patient develops pulmonary edema or aspiration pneumonia after a successful recovery from the initial incident.

50. c. self-contained underwater breathing apparatus.—SCUBA.

51. c. Dalton's law—Room air, for example, is a mixture of nitrogen and oxygen. The total pressure in a diving tank equals the sum of each individual partial pressure.

52. a. Boyle's—In other words, as the pressure increases, the gas volume decreases.

53. a. decrease; expand.—This relates to Boyle's law of gases.

54. c. pneumothorax—Failure to exhale upon ascent from a dive causes the lungs to expand and pop.

55. b. nitrogen bubbles—Also called "the bends." This releases previously absorbed excess nitrogen from the tissues into the bloodstream in the form of bubbles.

56. a. bends.—Pain in the legs or joints is present in 90% of the cases. The most commonly involved joint is the shoulder, though multiple joints may be involved in serious cases. Recurrent pains are common.

57. b. Henry's—Henry's law states that, at a constant temperature, the solubility of any gas in a liquid is directly proportional to the pressure of the liquid. The deeper one dives, the greater the pressure and threat the soluble gas that becomes dissolved in the blood and tissue.

58. b. Asthma—Mucous plugs can trap air that cannot be exhaled properly during ascent.

59. a. air embolism—This is the most serious diving-related emergency. Because divers most commonly ascend in a vertical position, bubbles of air in the bloodstream often travel to the brain.

60. c. Consider decompression therapy.—Hyperbaric 0_2 is beneficial for both air embolism and decompression sickness.

61. d. Did the patient fly in an airplane more than twenty-four hours ago?—More important is flying within a minimum of twenty-four hours after diving, as this can increase the risk of developing decompression sickness.

62. d. air embolism—Even late recompression of decompression sickness problems can be accomplished with relief of symptoms and morbidity.

63. a. lack of recognition of symptoms.—Often there is wishful thinking that symptoms will just go away.

64. a. air embolism.—While waiting to begin the dive, many people experience motion sickness from rough waves, hyperventilation from anxiety, physical injury while leaving the boat or encountering marine animals, or submersion.

65. b. descent—Gas-associated problems (hypoxia due to equipment failure or carbon monoxide poisoning) commonly occur at this point also.

66. d. high-altitude pulmonary edema (HAPE)—HAPE occurs when increased pulmonary artery pressures develop from hypoxia. This leads to the release of various vasoactive substances that increase alveolar permeability. Fluids leak into the alveoli, and pulmonary edema occurs.

67. b. hypoxia.—The most common altitude syndromes are acute mountain sickness (AMS), high-altitude pulmonary edema (HAPE), and high-altitude cerebral edema (HACE).

68. a. skydiving—High-altitude illness occurs as a result of decreased atmospheric pressure that causes hypoxia. Typical skydiving does not allow enough time in the conditions that would cause these syndromes.

69. a. AMS—This condition occurs after rapid ascent by an unacclimatized person to altitudes in excess of 8,000 feet.

70. a. administer high-flow oxygen.—The most important treatments are rapid descent and oxygen.

71. d. all of the above—At room temperature, 75% of heat dissipation occurs by radiation and convection. Evaporation accounts for about 25% of heat loss.

72. a. diabetes and smoker—Neuropathy can mask the typical decreased sensation over the affected area, allowing a progression to deep frostbite before the patient recognizes what is happening. Smoking constricts the blood vessels and aggravates hypoxemia to the involved area.

73. c. ears and sinuses—Squeeze syndromes are caused by excess pressure involving the ears and sinuses.

74. c. His glucose stores are depleted.—As the energy stores (liver and muscle glycogen) are exhausted, shivering will cease and the CBT will drop.

75. a. impaired thinking—Nitrogen narcosis, often referred to as "rapture of the depths," is the development of an apathetic, slight euphoric mental state due to the narcotic effect of dissolved nitrogen. This effect is analogous to excessive ethanol levels.

76. c. 55—High humidity seriously impairs heat dissipation because evaporation occurs slowly.

77. b. drink warm fluids.—Warm fluids will help warm the patient and restore energy.

78. c. providing high-quality CPR—Continue CPR and stabilize the spine due to the MOI.

79. a. gastric distention—The stomach may contain water from the drowning and aggressive ventilations, and overfill as a result. Consider abdominal decompression.

80. a. decompress the stomach.—The stomach may contain water from the drowning and aggressive ventilations, and overfill as a result. Consider abdominal decompression.

Chapter 29: Infectious and Communicable Diseases

1. b. pathogen.—Bacteria that cause disease are called pathogens.

2. a. normal flora.—Normal flora is found over the entire body and on the protective coverings of the respiratory, GI, and genitourinary systems.

3. b. protozoa.—Protozoa can be found in almost every kind of habitat.

4. d. virus.—Viruses are known to cause infectious diseases.

5. c. mucous membranes.—The mouth, nares, or rectum.

6. d. latency period.—The duration of this stage varies by specific disease.

7. c. skin—The external barriers on the body are skin and normal flora.

8. b. latency—Once a host is infected, the first stage is the latency period. The duration of this stage varies by specific disease.

9. b. incubation—This is the third stage, and its duration varies by specific disease.

10. d. disease—The duration of a disease period varies by specific disease.

11. b. hospital—Healthcare facilities are also responsible for reporting communicable diseases seen by healthcare providers.

12. c. forty-eight—Notification is made by a designated officer who acts as a liaison between the hospital and exposed EMS provider.

13. a. Federal—Other federal agencies involved in disease outbreaks include the U.S. Department of Health and Human Services, Centers for Disease Control (CDC), National Institute for Occupational Safety and Health (NIOSH), and the U.S. Department of Defense.

14. a. HCV.—No vaccine or prophylactic post-exposure treatment for HCV is available currently.

15. a. HBV, HCV, and HIV—Pneumonia and URI are not caused by needle sticks.

16. d. hand washing.—This is still the best protection against the spread of disease.

17. c. No further titers are necessary, even after an exposure.—The whole point of the postvaccination titer is to make sure the series of shots had its desired effect of protection against HBV. If there is no response to the first series, a second series is administered. If there is no response to the second series, no further series are recommended.

18. c. hypothermic geriatric—Severe infection (sepsis) may actually result in hypothermia when the body's fever-producing centers are overwhelmed. This finding is common in people who are relatively immobile, such as in a nursing facility.

19. c. hepatitis—More than 700,000 new infections occur annually, making this the most serious infectious disease in the United States.

20. c. seven—This infectious disease causes inflammation of the liver, which interferes with liver functions. Seven types exist (A–G), but only the first four are common in the United States.

21. c. complete only the third dose—This is the current recommendation.

22. a. sexual contact.—HCV may also be contracted through blood transfusions.

23. b. HCV—No vaccine or prophylactic post-exposure treatment for HCV is available currently.

24. b. oral-fecal—It is spread by direct contact with feces, usually through food or water contact by an infected person who has not washed after using the toilet.

25. a. productive cough—TB spreads through droplets from coughing and sneezing. The bacteria are inhaled and settle in the lungs. From the lungs, it is transported in the blood to other organs in the body.
26. b. rabies—An acute viral infection of the CNS.
27. d. bacteria—Helicobacter pylori, or H. pylori, is the cause of most gastric ulcers.
28. b. rabies.—Without intervention, the disease progresses rapidly and death results.
29. a. Salmonella—Salmonella are gram-negative bacteria that live in the intestinal tracts of humans and other animals. Food may also become contaminated by an infected person who has not washed his hands after using the toilet.
30. a. salmonella—There are over 1,400 species of salmonella that can cause mild gastroenteritis or severe and often fatal food poisoning.
31. d. thirty-six to forty-eight—Signs and symptoms begin with an expanding rash around the area of the bite. Flu-like symptoms and muscle joint aches follow, with or without a rash.
32. c. Lyme disease—Further progression of the infection leads to altered mental status, paralysis, paresthesia, stiff neck, sensitivity to light, dysrhythmias, and chest pain.
33. b. meningitis—A history of recent respiratory illness or sore throat often precedes symptoms of fever, headache, vomiting, and the classic stiff neck. Changes in mental status follow, and dehydration may lead to shock. The finding of a stiff neck was not given in the case, due to the altered mental status.
34. b. an inflammatory response.—Internal barriers work through the inflammatory and immune responses.
35. b. designated officer.—The Ryan White Act of 1990 requires that all EMS providers be notified by the hospital or healthcare facility if they have been exposed to infectious diseases. Notification is made by a designated officer who acts as a liaison between the hospital and exposed EMS provider.
36. c. U.S. Fire Protection Administration—The other national agency involved in disease outbreak is the National Fire Protection Agency (NFPA).

37. b. Varicella—Chicken pox vaccination.
38. a. BSI—Body substance isolation. The concept is to wear gloves for all patient contact.
39. d. staph—This is why hand washing is still the best preventative measure for spreading disease.
40. c. red—The exact guidelines for decontamination and disposal of contaminated equipment should be posted or easily available for reference in every EMS agency.
41. b. puncture-proof containers—The exact guidelines for decontamination and disposal of contaminated equipment should be posted or easily available for reference in every EMS agency.
42. b. shingles—Herpes zoster, or shingles, is caused by a varicella-zoster virus, the same virus that causes chicken pox. Pain and inflammation occur on unilateral nerve tracts and may follow the path of one or more adjacent dermatomes.
43. b. titer—Titers are used to determine if adequate immunity has been achieved through immunization.
44. c. employer—The exact guidelines to follow for an exposure should be posted or easily available for reference in every EMS agency.
45. d. tuberculosis—One reason why TB is making a comeback is that more resistant strains are developing. Estimates are that nearly eight million new cases occur each year, with only one in five getting treatment.
46. c. Gastroenteritis—This condition usually is not serious in healthy individuals. Children, the elderly, and patients with chronic illness can develop complications, such a dehydration.
47. b. arbovirus—Arbovirus is a group of viruses that is transmitted to humans by mosquitoes and ticks.
48. c. Lyme disease—Signs and symptoms begin with an expanding rash around the area of the bite. Flu-like symptoms and muscle joint aches follow, with or without a rash.
49. a. pneumonic.—Plague is an acute febrile, infectious, and highly fatal disease caused by gram-positive bacteria.
50. b. Colorado.—Bubonic plague is the most prevalent type and is a primary disease found on rats and rodents.

Chapter 30: Behavioral and Psychiatric Diseases

1. b. emotion—A psychic and physical reaction subjectively experienced as strong feelings and physiological changes.
2. b. mental disorder.—Also called emotional disorder.
3. a. In the United States, behavioral and psychiatric disorders incapacitate more people than all other health problems combined.—Some researchers indicate that one in seven people will require treatment for an emotional illness at some time in his or her life.
4. c. Having a mental disorder is cause for embarrassment and shame.—Though some people still feel this way, it is a result of inappropriate pressure from society rather than any scientific evidence.

5. d. lose control and become aggressive.—Impulse-control disorders involve an abnormal inability to resist a sudden and often irrational urge or action.

6. a. cognitive—Cognitive disorders affect a person's thinking and judgment.

7. b. Schizophrenia—These individuals suffer from delusions and hallucinations. They are often withdrawn from interaction with society and display disorganized thought.

8. d. bipolar.—Mood disorders include depression and mania. When these moods alternate, it is called a bipolar disorder.

9. c. anxiety—The common theme with anxiety disorders is that apprehension, fears, and worries dominate a person's life.

10. a. psychologic—Dependence is a psychological problem, not a physical one.

11. b. Somatoform—The major types of somatoform disorders are somatization syndrome and conversion disorders.

12. a. dissociative—Also called multiple personality or schizophrenia. The result is an altered state of consciousness or confusion in the patient's identity.

13. c. Personality—This large group of disorders is often broken down into three clusters: Cluster A (paranoid, schizoid, schizotypal), Cluster B (antisocial, borderline, histrionic, narcissistic), and Cluster C (avoidant, dependent, obsessive-compulsive).

14. d. Some type of psychological aspect accompanies every illness and injury.—The degree to which it affects a particular patient varies widely. Healthcare providers must always consider a patient's emotional, as well as physical, needs.

15. c. crisis intervention.—Each state, and sometimes locality, has specific regulations governing the handling of mentally ill individuals, including patients who exhibit self-destructive behavior.

16. b. state laws—Each state, and sometimes locality, has specific regulations governing the handling of mentally ill individuals, including patients who exhibit self-destructive behavior.

17. c. neurotransmitters.—Sometimes the cause of the disorder is an organic illness. Either an excess or, more commonly, a deficit of certain neurotransmitters results in some types of behavioral and psychiatric disorders.

18. d. migraine headaches.—One example is the use of antidepressants for treating migraine headaches.

19. a. pain.—Be alert for other possible causes of apparent emotional or psychiatric illnesses, especially in older patients. The most common "offenders" are medications and severe infections.

20. a. poor hygiene.—Some people with behavioral problems exhibit an abnormal lack of regard for their own personal hygiene.

21. d. Phobias—These fears can interfere with normal daily activities, affecting both personal and societal relationships.

22. b. when the patient exhibits a danger to others—The patient must be transported in any situation where the patient is a danger to himself or to others.

23. a. phobias—These fears are out of proportion to reality and compel the patient to avoid the feared object or situation.

24. b. delirium.—Delirium tremens is a violent delirium with tremors that is induced by excessive and prolonged use of alcohol.

25. d. Assuming the patient's actions were not an actual suicide attempt.—A common clinical myth is that people who engage in suicide gestures never really attempt suicide. This is a naïve and potentially deadly assumption.

26. d. suicide gesture—The person performs the act in a potentially reversible way, such as taking a small amount of pills.

27. c. unable to cope.—People manage stress in a variety of ways by adapting to new situations from past experience. When a person's coping mechanism fails and the person feels overwhelmed, a behavioral emergency can develop.

28. a. Psychosis—The person truly believes his situation or condition is real. Often the psychotic person hears voices.

29. b. the "talk-down" technique.—This is done by gently and calmly talking to the person and reassuring him that everything is OK.

30. a. paranoia—The other signs and symptoms are associated with depression.

31. c. medications.—Be alert for other possible causes of apparent emotional or psychiatric illnesses, especially in older patients. The most common "offenders" are medications and severe infections.

32. d. mood—Mood disorders include depression, mania, and bipolar.

33. c. Addiction—A true addiction is a psychological and physical craving for the drug, as well as for the effect.

34. b. Intoxication—An abnormal state that is essentially a poisoning.

35. c. addiction—Addiction is a condition characterized by an overwhelming desire to continue taking a drug to which one has become "hooked."

36. b. worsens.—There is often an interrelationship between people with psychiatric disorders and substance abuse. In some cases, there is a direct cause-effect relationship. In other cases, the link is more anecdotal or based on stories of prior incidents.

37. d. posture.—For example, a paranoid individual may posture by keeping the face hidden and the extremities crossed close to the body.

38. c. confusion—Confusion results in bewilderment and the inability to act decisively.

39. c. affect—For example, a flat affect means a lack of any apparent verbal or body language expression of emotion.
40. d. engage in active listening—Other positive interview techniques include: engaging in active listening, being supportive and empathetic, limiting interruptions, allowing the patient to express anger and frustration verbally, forming an alliance with the patient, and avoiding continuous eye contact.
41. b. attempt to build a good rapport with the patient.—Attempt to do this by using positive therapeutic interviewing techniques that calm the patient and encourage him to cooperate with you.
42. c. keep talking to the patient—Continue to attempt to calm and reassure the patient and encourage him to cooperate with you.
43. a. no prior history of suicide attempts.—The other factors increase the risk that a person is suicidal.
44. b. women have better support systems.—Support systems (family, friends) are an integral part of a person's coping mechanism.
45. c. psychosomatic illness—The physical ailments are very real, despite the patient's emotional origin.
46. c. may develop violent behavior.—The aspects of domestic violence, pacing back and forth, and bragging about how tough she is are clues that a patient may develop violent behavior.
47. b. People with neurosis are not crazy.—Neurosis is a mental and emotional disorder that affects only part of the person's personality.
48. a. severely depressed.—Depression may present as another disease.
49. d. Phobias can interfere with daily living activities.—These fears are out of proportion to reality and compel the patient to avoid the feared object or situation.
50. a. They are used to encourage better patient responses.—These types of questions are used to allow the patient to express herself.

Chapter 31: Hematology

1. c. hematopoietic—The formation of blood or blood cells in the living body.
2. b. bone marrow.—The liver, spleen, and bone marrow make up the components of the hematopoietic system.
3. d. bone marrow.—The majority of blood cells are formed in the bone marrow.
4. c. 7.40—The average pH is slightly lower in venous than in arterial blood.
5. b. 70—In an adult man, this amount equals approximately five or six liters of blood. Women have slightly less, 65 cc per kg.
6. d. spleen.—The liver and the spleen produce red blood cells (RBCs) during fetal life. After birth, the majority of normal blood cell production occurs in the bone marrow in the long and flat bones.
7. b. stem cell.—All blood cells are derived from one common stem cell. This cell is capable of reproducing itself, but is also capable of differentiating into any of the marrow elements.
8. c. 120—After that, they are absorbed by tissues of the spleen.
9. a. bilirubin.—Cellular components are recycled and hemoglobin byproducts are excreted as bilirubin.
10. c. hematocrit.—Normal hematocrit (Hct) levels indicate a normal number of RBCs; a high Hct meant too many RBCs (polycythemia), and a low Hct level means too few (anemia).
11. d. anemia.—A high Hct meant too many RBCs (polycythemia), and a low Hct level means too few (anemia).
12. a. thirty-six to forty-six.—The normal range for men is slightly higher: forty-one to fifty-three.
13. c. forty-one to fifty-three.—The normal range for women is slightly lower: thirty-six to forty-six.
14. b. granulocytes.—Granulocytes are one of two types of white blood cells (WBCs).
15. b. monocytes.—Monocytes are one of two types of WBCs.
16. c. maintain host defenses against infection.—Leukocytes defend against infections, particularly bacterial infection.
17. c. kidneys and liver; bone marrow—Body feedback systems continuously monitor intravascular volume, as well as the numbers of circulating platelets and red and white blood cells. If more are needed, the kidneys and liver produce compounds that stimulate the bone marrow to manufacture additional cells.
18. a. humoral immunity.—Humoral immunity primarily involves antibodies that are produced by a specialized WBC, the B lymphocyte.
19. a. leukopenia.—This condition may result from congenital problems, acquired anemia, leukemia, viral infection, drug reaction, immunosuppression, destruction of WBCs in the peripheral blood, and pooling of WBCs.
20. b. seven to ten—Platelets are formed from stem cells in the bone marrow and they are removed by the spleen.
21. c. anti-inflammatory drugs.—Many anti-inflammatory drugs and some herbals decrease the aggregation of platelets. Though this may have a beneficial effect

(e.g., stoke and MI), these drugs may also result in a bleeding tendency.

22. c. Blood vessels dilate and develop increased permeability.—This response increases blood flow, producing the signs of heat and redness.

23. c. fibrin.—Intrinsic and extrinsic clotting systems are the chemical reactions that lead to the formation of fibrin. This substance completes the blood clot, which now consists of injured vascular epithelium, a platelet plug, and intertwined strands of clot formation.

24. b. red blood—Blood groups are classified into four types: type A, B, AB, and O.

25. c. AB—They may receive blood from people with any ABO blood type.

26. d. O—Their blood may be given safely to people with any ABO blood type.

27. b. sickle cell crisis—All conditions may produce dyspnea. The severe abdominal pain is more specific to sickle cell crisis.

28. c. hemophilia.—A hereditary deficiency of clotting factors VIII resulting in excessive bleeding after minor wounds, insignificant trauma, and spontaneous bleeding into joints, abdomen, or central nervous system.

29. d. Leukemia—This type of cancer results in the rapid and uncontrolled proliferation of abnormal numbers and forms of leukocytes.

30. a. thyme—Aspirin, ibuprofen, and ginseng are blood thinners.

31. a. Fobrinolysis—Small injuries often lead to the activation of the clotting cascade. To prevent these small clots from developing into clinically significant thrombi, plasminogen is activated to form plasmin. Plasmin lyses the clots, returning things to a hemostatic baseline.

32. b. leukocytosis—A condition that results in too many WBCs.

33. c. eosinophils and basophils—These are two types of granulocytes (WBCs) that are important in allergic reactions.

34. b. hemoglobin.—The Hct and hemoglobin (Hb) are direct reflections of the number of RBCs. Each normal RBC contains the same amount of Hb. Thus, if we have a normal number of RBCs, the Hb concentration is normal.

35. a. anemia—The other conditions listed can produce a state of anemia, thus creating the same symptoms.

Chapter 32: Gynecology and Obstetrics

1. b. urethra—The urethra is part of the genitourinary tract.
2. a. ovaries—The ovaries produce sexual hormones and oocytes, the precursors to mature eggs.
3. c. Fertilization of the ovum usually occurs in one of the fallopian tubes.—Then the fertilized egg proceeds through the fallopian tube to the uterus for implantation.
4. a. fundus.—The main portion of the uterus is called the fundus.
5. b. embryo.—During the embryonic period, all the major organ systems begin to develop.
6. d. returning oxygenated blood from the placenta to the fetus.—The two arteries return deoxygenated blood from the fetus to the placenta.
7. c. endometriosis.—The relocated cells respond to the same hormonal stimuli as the normal cells. Symptoms include abdominal pain, pelvic pain, lower back pain, dysuria, irregular menses, and infertility.
8. a. the secretory phase.—This phase begins at the time of ovulation and lasts until the corpus luteum breaks down (about twelve days after ovulation).
9. d. Premenstrual dysphoric disorder—Formerly called premenstrual tension syndrome or PMS. The cause is not clear at this time.
10. d. aimed at relieving the symptoms.—The cause of premenstrual dysphoric disorder is not clear, so the treatment is aimed at relieving the symptoms.

Analgesia, mild diuretics, and mood-lifting medications may be taken to relieve the symptoms.

11. a. estrogen—Estrogen also induces the development of female sexual characteristics.
12. b. progesterone.—Progesterone also helps to prevent rejection of the developing embryo or fetus.
13. a. zygote.—After fertilization, the zygote begins cell division and forms a hollow ball called a blastocyst as it moves into the uterine cavity, where it implants on the uterine wall.
14. a. pregnancy—Amenorrhea, or the suppression of menstruation, is normal during pregnancy and abnormal in other circumstances.
15. d. PID—Pelvic inflammatory disease is an infection in the female reproductive and surrounding organs that can lead to complications such as sepsis and infertility.
16. d. chlamydia—Chlamydia infections remain the most common of all bacterial STDs occurring in both men and women.
17. c. urinary tract infection—UTIs may produce blood in the urine (hematuria).
18. b. bladder—The symptoms are urinary frequency and pain with urinations. The condition can be acute or chronic.
19. b. abruptio placenta.—Abruptio is characterized by severe constant pain with or without bleeding and occurs after twenty weeks' gestation.

20. b. Treat for shock and begin transport.—The premature separation causes blood loss that is not always apparent because it may be trapped behind the placenta. If the separation is complete, most often the fetus will die.

21. b. destroy fetal cells.—After the termination of any pregnancy, either by birth or abortion, the mother is given an injection of immune globulin to suppress her immune response.

22. c. pulmonary embolism—This condition occurs frequently and has a high mortality rate. It results from a blood clot in the pelvic circulation. This can occur during pregnancy, labor, or postpartum.

23. d. rapid transport for a life-threatening condition.—Appropriate treatment includes high-concentration oxygen and vascular access with gentle but rapid transport to an appropriate facility.

24. a. hypertension—Pregnancy-associated hypertension (≥140/90) is an indication of possible toxemia. Preexisting hypertension requires close monitoring.

25. b. slowed peristalsis.—The slower digestion results in the stomach remaining fuller for a longer period of time.

26. a. size of the baby's head.—During active labor, the baby's head should be down in the cervix as opposed to the top of the uterus (fundus).

27. a. spine—Rubbing the patient's lower back during labor can help to ease the discomfort.

28. c. oxytocin—Stretch receptors in the uterine walls sense the increased stretch produced by the movement of the uterus, and this triggers the pituitary gland to secrete the hormone oxytocin.

29. b. Labor is two weeks early, but the mother is mentally competent and refuses.—Any adult patient who is alert and competent has the right to refuse any or all care offered.

30. d. holding one hand on the baby's head while the mother is pushing.—This may help to reduce tearing of the perineum.

31. b. inspect for a nuchal cord.—Nuchal cord is common and must be recognized and corrected quickly to prevent strangulation and hypoxia.

32. a. laterally.—The baby's head will turn to the left or right, then the shoulders will appear.

33. a. reflex and color.—Each sign is rated 0, 1, or 2, depending on the findings at one and five minutes after birth.

34. c. the baby will be easier to manage and assess.—Typically there is no hurry to cut the cord, unless the baby or mother is in distress. If the cord is not cut immediately, the infant should be kept at a level lower than the placenta to prevent placental transfusion.

35. b. at a lower level than the placenta—This is a gravity thing. If the baby is raised above the level of the placenta, the baby's blood will drain out.

36. c. umbilical vein cannulation—Umbilical vein cannulation is preferred in neonatal resuscitation because the vein is so easy to identify and cannulate. The skill does take practice, and a special umbilical catheter is used.

37. c. the right side of the board elevated slightly.—This position helps to keeps the fetus off the mother's vena cava in an effort to allow adequate blood return to the heart.

38. a. aggressive fluid replacement.—Appropriate management of this patient includes aggressive management of the ABCs and rapid transport to a trauma center.

39. d. in the clinical setting and not in the field.—Assessing the fetal heart rate is the standard of care in the clinical setting to determine if the fetus is in any distress.

40. a. They can be relieved by drinking milk.—Each of the other facts has a substantial basis.

41. d. shunting of blood from the fetus.—The mother's body will begin to decrease circulation to non-vital organs (skin and GI) when it goes into shock. In a state of shock, the mother's body treats the fetus as a foreign object and shunts blood from the placenta to its own heart, brain, and lungs.

42. b. STDs—The other injuries are considered primary injuries from a sexual assault.

43. a. Place any items removed from the patient into separate bags.—Handle the clothing as little as possible, and bag each item separately. Avoid using plastic bags for blood-stained articles because they degrade the evidence with moisture.

44. b. providing emotional support.—The paramedic must treat the whole patient and respond to her physical and emotional needs.

45. a. one in three—It is also estimated that only 10–30% of these crimes are reported.

46. b. Menopause—In most women, menopause occurs in the late forties.

47. d. ruptured ovarian cyst—The other examples involve different body systems.

48. d. Mittelschmerz—The pain is self-limiting and benign. The complication that arises is making a differential diagnosis from other causes of abdominal pain.

49. b. Endomeritis—The infection can originate from an STD, trauma, use of an intrauterine device (IUD), or an abortion.

50. c. shock and death.—Uncontrolled bleeding can lead to hypovolemia, shock, and death.

51. b. Prepare for imminent delivery.—A multiparous woman will know when she is about to deliver. Listen to her, and prepare to assist with the delivery. This can be done in the ambulance, and transport may be started.

52. c. Observe the birth canal for crowing.—Crowning is a clear indication that birth is about to happen.

53. a. Start an IV and prepare an OB delivery kit.—A breech delivery may turn into a complicated delivery. The IV is appropriate, as is contacting medical control.

54. c. Allow the cord to deliver and support the body.—The head may require extra attention in passing through the vaginal opening. Support the body to prevent tearing of the neck muscles and blood vessels.

55. b. Treat for shock and begin transport.—Significant blood loss can occur with postpartum hemorrhage, and this must be managed aggressively. If possible, bring the placenta to the hospital for inspection. An incomplete placenta could be the cause of the bleeding, and inspection can help rule out a cause.

56. d. the presence of an undelivered fetus.—If the patient has a midwife, most likely she has had prenatal care and would be aware of multiple fetuses.

57. b. begin a Pitocin® drip.—Not all EMS agencies carry Pitocin®. This means continued care remains an aggressive treatment for shock.

58. b. Nearly 40% of twin deliveries are preemies.—One baby is larger than the other and is typically born first.

59. d. cephalopelvic disproportion.—A condition in which the size of the mother's pelvis is small in relation to the size of the child's head. Emergency caesarian section is required in many cases.

60. b. cover the protruding tissue with moist, sterile dressings.—This is a true emergency that requires aggressive treatment and rapid transport.

Chapter 33: Trauma Systems and Mechanism of Injury

1. c. transportation incidents.—In 2004, the leading cause of work-related deaths was transportation incidents (43%).

2. a. MVCs, poisonings, and falls.—The top five causes of trauma deaths in all ages are: MVCs, poisonings, falls, suicides, and homicides.

3. b. many MOIs have predictable patterns for specific injuries.—EMS providers are trained to consider the forces that were applied to the body and to look for specific injury patterns, even when the injuries are not visibly apparent.

4. a. >1%—Despite the fact that few injuries are life-threatening, inappropriate identification and treatment may result in high mortality rates per injury.

5. b. anatomic structures that are involved.—The extent of damage caused by the energy absorbed by the body depends on the specific organs that have been affected.

6. b. incident.—EMS providers can help to minimize further injury or death by responding and working safely on every call.

7. a. MOI—Early recognition of the MOI and the possible injuries associated with those forces can help save the patient's life.

8. d. filling out an organ donor card.—This action may be helpful, but it is not a prevention strategy.

9. c. minimizing scene time when appropriate.—The golden hour is the first hour after the injury occurs. In serious trauma, the best chances of survival for the patient are a result of reaching the hospital's operating suite and having the bleeding controlled within that hour. EMS providers can do their part in helping achieve this goal (surgical intervention in <sixty minutes) by limiting scene time to a "platinum ten" minutes. That's ten minutes for assessment and management at the scene of a critical trauma patient.

10. d. White Paper.—Released in 1966, the White Paper depicted a very poor emergency care system and was credited as the "match that sparked" the future development of modern EMS systems.

11. b. hospice care.—The other components of a trauma system include: out-of-hospital care, ED care with interfacility transport as necessary, rehabilitation, and data collection.

12. a. registry—Two software programs produced by the American College of Surgeons (ACS) are National Tracs® and the National Trauma Data Bank™.

13. c. A delineated criterion for a trauma center includes use of air-medical transport.—Not all hospitals meet the criteria involving appropriately trained and experienced in-house surgical staff, specialty equipment, and services, as well as an administrative commitment. Trauma centers do not have to operate their own helicopter.

14. c. traumatic cardiac arrest—These patients have extremely small chances of survival even with brief periods of ROSC. This is why they are transported to the nearest hospital.

15. a. access to a remote area—The other choices listed are contraindications or relative contraindications for air-medical transport.

16. a. traumatic cardiac arrest—These patients have little or no chance of survival from a possible reversal. This is why they are transported to the nearest hospital by ambulance.

17. d. Conservation of energy—This is one of the physical laws of energy. This is an important concept

when you consider the MOI and the potential for injuries.

18. c. Newton's first law of motion.—One of the physical laws of energy. This is an important concept when you consider the MOI and the potential for injuries.

19. a. Kinetic energy—One of the physical laws of energy. This is an important concept when you consider the MOI and the potential for injuries.

20. c. Cavitation—Cavitation can be caused by both blunt and penetration trauma.

21. b. velocity—The value of speed (the velocity) is squared in the kinetic energy formula; the value of the mass is merely divided by two. The more speed involved, the greater the potential KE.

22. a. foot-pounds—Total kinetic energy is expressed in foot/pounds. Example: the impact of a person weighing (mass) 150 pounds moving at a speed (velocity) of 30 mph will strike with a force of 67,000 foot-pounds (total KE).

23. c. immediately after the injury is sustained—The golden hour is the first hour after the injury occurs.

24. a. The third collision occurs when the internal organs strike against the inside of the body.—The first collision is the car striking the concrete barrier; the second collision is the driver striking the steering wheel or dashboard. Any of the three collisions may result in severe damage.

25. d. Tumbling creates greater tissue damage.—The leading edge of the bullet does not enter the patient; rather, the bullet is tumbling through space and the entire side surface of the bullet can enter the body.

26. d. rapid acceleration and deceleration—The rear-end collision is where the rapid acceleration occurs (whiplash), and the stopping of the vehicle in the ditch is where the rapid deceleration should be suspected.

27. d. GSWs—Don't assume that a projectile, such as a bullet, always follows a straight path between the entrance and exit sites. Projectiles may ricochet inside the body, especially off bones, and travel many different pathways.

28. c. tertiary—In this phase, injuries can result from the patient becoming a flying object and striking other objects.

29. b. flying articles.—Injuries can be blunt from compression, or penetrating from lacerations.

30. a. high-power rifle—The more speed there is involved, the more energy there is to exchange with the body, and the higher the possibility for tissue damage.

31. d. 60 kg patient traveling at 60 mph—The more speed there is, the more energy there is. The value of speed (the velocity) is squared in the kinetic energy formula; the value of the mass is merely divided by two.

32. b. compression—In the primary phase of a blast, there is a pressure wave that causes major effects on the lungs and GI tract.

33. d. tertiary—In this phase, injuries can result from the patient becoming a flying object and striking other objects.

34. a. frontal—This is a common MOI. The rider is ejected up and forward with both legs striking the handle bars, resulting in bilateral femur factures.

35. b. rear-end—This is due to the whiplash effect of flexion and then extension. Head restraints, if properly positioned, can be helpful in reducing this type of injury.

36. c. smoke condition in the room in which the patient was found—With this common MOI, the paramedic should have a high index of suspicion that the patient has suffered smoke inhalation resulting in injury to the airways and difficulty breathing.

37. c. CO_2 inhalation—The inhalation of poisonous gases is very likely the cause of the patient's present state of unconsciousness.

38. d. the combination of forces involved—Getting a complete and accurate account of the incident is one of the best ways to suspect and look for injuries that may not be visibly apparent.

39. a. contusion, fracture, or rupture.—When a bullet is fired into the body, the energy forces from the bullet are transferred to the tissues. This causes momentary acceleration of tissue laterally away from the tract of the projectile, creating a cavity (cavitation).

40. d. type of empty shell casings—Shell casings may help providers understand the type of wound created (e.g., gunshot, buckshot, hand gun, or high-power rifle).

41. b. crush injuries—The initial impact with the leg, arm, shoulder, and hip against the car causes crush injuries. The fall and skid after the initial impact cause fractures and abrasions.

42. a. brain contusion—In the third collision, internal organs strike the body. This causes contusions, hematomas, and shearing of organs suspended by ligaments.

43. a. ten—The "platinum ten" minutes. In serious trauma, the best chances of survival for the patient are a result of reaching the hospital's operating suite within the golden hour. EMS providers can help patients reach that goal by working within the first ten "platinum" minutes to get the patient off-scene and en route to the trauma center.

44. c. cavitation.—When a bullet is fired into the body, the energy forces from the bullet are transferred to the tissues. This causes momentary acceleration of tissue laterally away from the tract of the projectile, creating a cavity (cavitation).

45. b. lungs and GI tract—This type of MOI may cause injuries such as pneumothorax, ruptured organs, and an air embolism.

46. b. rupture of an organ or air embolism.—The lungs and the GI tract are the organs primarily affected.

47. d. being run over by the vehicle.—The other choices describe injuries that occur in the first and second phases of an auto-pedestrian collision.

48. c. 300—One of the key strategies for teaching motorcycle safety is educating the riders about wearing a helmet and protective gear when riding.

49. b. Airbags may produce minor facial and forearm abrasions.—These injuries are insignificant compared to the potential injuries that can result without the use of airbags.

50. a. They prevent hyperflexion of the upper torso.—The other choices are incorrect.

Chapter 34: Hemorrhage and Shock

1. c. internal and external.—External bleeding is usually due to trauma, whereas internal bleeding can be from either trauma or a medical cause.

2. b. occult GI bleeding.—The most common site of nontraumatic bleeding is in the GI tract (e.g., peptic ulcer, diverticulosis, and esophageal varies).

3. b. artery.—Arterial bleeding is characterized as spurting or pulsing with each heartbeat.

4. c. three—Also referred to as decompensated shock, this stage of shock involves between 25 and 35% intravascular loss.

5. c. 25 to 35%—The patient will have the classic signs of hypovolemic shock.

6. b. two large bore IVs en route—Consider the need for IV fluid replacement en route to the hospital. If a patient is continuing to bleed, he can easily lose more blood in the time it takes to start the IV than the IV fluids will actually replace.

7. b. decompensated—When the body's compensatory mechanisms can no longer sustain the patient, decompensated shock will ensue (e.g., tachycardia, tachypnea, decreasing blood pressure, altered mental status, loss of distal pulses, and decreased urine output).

8. c. 70 cc—The stroke volume is the amount of blood ejected from the left ventricle with each contraction of the heart. This is usually approximately 70 cc of blood per beat, or approximately 4,900 cc per minute.

9. b. increasing the heart rate.—The heart rate can increase to improve the cardiac output (CO), or the systemic vascular resistance (SVR) can be increased through the constriction of the peripheral vessels.

10. b. increase in diastolic pressure—An early sign of hypovolemic shock is a narrowing pulse pressure. The systolic pressure drops slightly (due to volume loss) and the systolic pressure increases (representing vasoconstriction as a compensatory mechanism).

11. c. aerobic exercise on a regular basis—The body cannot increase the stroke volume on a moment's notice by a large amount. In order to increase the SV, you need to do aerobic exercise for more than twenty minutes, three or more times a week, for months. The effect of this type of exercise is the thickening of the left ventricle to increase the SV, making the muscle a more efficient pump.

12. b. vasoconstriction.—The alpha-1 effects of epinephrine cause vasoconstriction, an increase in peripheral vascular resistance, and an increase in afterload from arteriolar constriction.

13. c. positive dromotropic effects—The dromotropic response affects conductivity of the myocardium.

14. c. arginine vasopressin.—AVP, also known as antidiuretic hormone, is released from the anterior pituitary gland and increases free water absorption. It also decreases urine output and visceral vascular constriction.

15. d. angiotensin II.—It is also a positive inotrope (force of contraction) and chronotrope (rate of contraction).

16. b. hyperglycemic.—Insulin secretion is diminished by circulating epinephrine. Poor perfusion impairs the effect of insulin on peripheral tissue, leading to the failure of cells to take up glucose. This contributes to the hypoglycemic states seen following injury and volume loss.

17. c. myocardial blood supply increases.—In addition, there are capillary and cellular changes that ultimately lead to irreversible shock.

18. b. washout—The third of three phases the cells go through during decreased perfusion states. Here the post-capillary sphincter relaxes, causing hydrogen, potassium carbon dioxide, and thrombosed erythrocytes to wash out into the circulation. Metabolic acidosis results, and the CO drops even further.

19. b. vasomotor center failure.—This occurs in the stagnation (second) phase.

20. c. Irreversible—Even aggressive treatment at this stage does not result in a recovery. It is not possible in the out-of-hospital setting to differentiate decompensated shock from irreversible shock, so all patients should be managed aggressively.

21. a. chief complaint of chest pain—Cardiogenic shock is differentiated from hypovolemic shock by one or

more of the following: complaint of dyspnea, chest pain, tachycardia, bradycardia, signs of CHF, and dysrhythmias.

22. d. flushed skin—Distributive shock is differentiated from hypovolemic shock by the presence of one or more of the following: warm, flushed skin, absence of tachycardia, and an MOI suggestive of vasodilation such as spinal cord injury, drug overdose, sepsis, or anaphylaxis.

23. b. presence of JVD—Obstructive shock can be differentiated from hypovolemic shock by the presence of distended neck veins and a narrowing pulse pressure, as seen with cardiac tamponade or tension pneumothorax.

24. a. isotonic—Normal saline or Ringer's lactate have the same tonicity (osmolarity) as plasma.

25. b. one-third—Consider the need for IV fluid replacement en route to the hospital. If a patient is continuing to bleed, she can easily lose more blood in the time it takes to start the IV than the IV fluids will actually replace.

26. a. interstitial space—Only about one-third of the infused fluid stays in the intravascular space, and it does not carry hemoglobin like a transfusion of whole blood does.

27. d. They do not carry hemoglobin.—Only about one-third of the infused fluid stays in the intravascular space, and it does not carry hemoglobin like a transfusion of whole blood does.

28. a. compensated—The compensated stage of shock involves 15–25% intravascular loss. The cardiac output is maintained by arteriolar constriction and a reflex tachycardia.

29. b. internal bleeding.—The potential for blood loss from femur fracture is approximately a liter, and intraabdominal bleeding can produce much more.

30. b. aortic arch—They sense a decreased flow and activate the vasomotor center, which, in turn, causes vasoconstriction of the peripheral vessels.

31. c. vasoconstriction of the peripheral vessels.—In addition, the sympathetic nervous system is stimulated.

32. c. adrenal glands.—The sympathetic nervous system sends the message from the brain down the spinal cord to the adrenal glands, which are located on top of the kidneys.

33. a. narrowing pulse pressure—The other events described are not signs that can be measured in the out-of-hospital setting.

34. a. endocrine responses.—These include the release of hormones: growth hormone, renin-angiotensin, glucagon, ACTH, and antidiuretic hormone.

35. b. 2–3—The fluid controversy is ongoing. Since only about one-third of the infused fluid stays in the intravascular space and does not carry hemoglobin, after two or three liters of a volume expander, the patient needs to receive fluid that carries hemoglobin (e.g., blood, blood products, or blood substitutes).

36. c. stabilization of pelvic fractures—Many EMS systems have relegated use of MAST/PASG to the stabilization of pelvic and femur fractures.

37. b. ACEP—The American College of Emergency Physicians still recommends that the MAST/PASG be available for immediate use in hospital EDs.

38. d. loss of vasomotor tone.—Distributive shock can occur with spinal injury, sepsis, and anaphylaxis.

39. c. Aldosterone—Secreted by the cells in the adrenal cortex, aldosterone protects the fluid volume.

40. a. arterioles in the kidney.—It is also a positive inotrope (force of contraction) and chronotrope (rate of contraction).

Chapter 35: Soft Tissue Trauma

1. a. crushing injury.—When treating a patient with a crush injury, one of the most important points is observing for the presence of ECG changes or dysrhythmias.

2. a. secondary infections.—Soft tissue injuries can be fatal, even without deep injuries.

3. b. physical forces—Activities such as contact sports and those involving high speed increase the risk of soft tissue trauma. MVCs, falls, assaults, and violence all contribute significantly to the risk of soft tissue injury.

4. c. superficial lesion—A lesion is an abnormal growth involving one or more layers of skin.

5. b. epidermis—The outer layer of skin.

6. a. dermis.—The layer of skin covered by the epidermis.

7. d. deep fascia—Binds together muscles and other internal structures.

8. a. tension lines.—There are two types of tension lines: static and dynamic. Static tension is the constant force due to the taut nature of skin. Underlying muscle contraction causes dynamic tension.

9. a. Hemostasis—In the first phase, there is reflex vasoconstriction for ten minutes, and then clotting begins.

10. b. collagen synthesis.—One of the phases of normal wound healing.

11. a. Epithelialization—One of the phases of normal wound healing.

12. c. body region—Other factors that can affect wound healing include: static skin tension, dynamic skin tension, and pigmented and oily skin.

13. c. corticosteroids—Normal healing may be slowed if the patient is taking any of the following medications: corticosteroids, nonsteroidal anti-inflammatory drugs, penicillin, colchicines, anticoagulants, and antineoplastic agents.

14. c. acne—There are a number of medical conditions and diseases that can affect normal wound healings.

15. c. human bites—Other wounds that have a high risk for infections include: bites from animals or humans, foreign bodies, wounds contaminated with organic matter, injected wounds, wounds with significant devitalized tissue, and crush wounds.

16. a. keloid scar.—These are more common in dark pigmented people and often occur on the ears, upper extremities, lower abdomen, and sternum.

17. b. cosmetically acceptable healing.—Plastic surgery is often requested for wounds to cosmetic regions such as the face, lip, and eyebrow.

18. a. degloving—Large, gaping wounds require closure (e.g., wounds over tension areas, degloving injuries, ring injuries, and skin tears).

19. b. hepatitis.—Hepatitis is easily transmitted by persons with no signs or symptoms of the disease. Healthcare providers are at risk of exposure when PPE is not used with every single patient.

20. a. contusion—With a contusion, the epidermis remains intact. Blood accumulates, causing pain and ecchymosis.

21. c. incision—These injuries are similar to lacerations except the wound ends are smooth and even. They tend to heal better than lacerations due to the constriction of the vessels.

22. d. avulsion.—This type of injury can involve a small or large area of skin.

23. a. laceration.—The jagged wound is caused by forceful impact with a sharp object, and the ends usually bleed freely.

24. b. ring injury—The other injuries are all types of amputations.

25. c. secondary and tertiary—The secondary injuries are due to flying debris striking the patient, and the tertiary injuries are caused when the patient is thrown from the blast and strikes a hard object.

26. b. crush—The patient may develop "crush syndrome," also called traumatic rhabdomyolysis.

27. d. sodium bicarbonate to neutralize the buildup of acids.—When the cause of the crush injury is moved or lifted off, the patient may suddenly go into cardiac arrest due to the massive release of toxins from the ruptured muscles into the blood stream.

28. d. crush injury—Crush injuries occur as a result of compressive force sufficient to interfere with the normal metabolic function of the involved tissue. Prolonged compression can result from an improperly applied cast.

29. b. anaerobic metabolism—As a result of anaerobic metabolism, various compounds accumulate and cause local inflammation.

30. d. six to eight hours—With compartment syndrome, a prolonged period of ischemia, greater than six to eight hours leads to tissue hypoxia and anoxia, and ultimately cell death.

31. d. capillary hydrostatic—This causes ischemia in the affected muscle tissue.

32. c. weakness and pain—A patient experiencing a compartment syndrome may complain of pain, paresthesia, paresis, and pressure passive stretch pain. Pulselessness may be an assessment finding, but is not something the patient complains of.

33. a. palpation.—The "Ps" of compartment syndrome are the signs and symptoms a patient may experience: pain, paresthesia (the sensation of pins and needles), paresis (weakness), pressure, passive stretch pain, and pulselessness.

34. c. in a confined space.—The full effect of the blast is experienced within confined spaces. The patient also has an extremely high potential for inhalation injuries.

35. c. considering that both internal and external injuries are possible.—When you consider the MOI, remember the three phases of blasts and the injuries associated with each.

36. d. indirect pressure—The methods of hemorrhage control include: direct pressure, elevation, pressure dressing, pressure points, and tourniquet application.

37. a. Direct pressure—Applying direct pressure on a bleeding wound is the first and most efficient method of bleeding control.

38. b. promote localized clotting.—Once the bleeding has been stopped, normal wound healing begins with reflex vasoconstriction (hemostasis), and clotting begins.

39. b. elevation—Do not elevate the extremity if there is a possible musculoskeletal injury to the involved extremity or a large impaled object in the extremity.

40. d. The bandage should not occlude or impede arterial blood flow.—After applying a pressure bandage, check for a distal pulse. If there is no pulse, loosen the bandage enough for the return of the pulse.

41. c. pregnant trauma patient with an abdominal evisceration—A pressure dressing is indicated for hemorrhage control when direct pressure and elevation have not controlled the bleeding.

42. a. artery runs over a bone and close to the skin.—When pressure is applied correctly over a pressure point, the artery is compressed against the bone, distal bleeding will minimize or stop, and clotting will be promoted.

43. a. direct pressure.—Direct pressure, elevation, and a pressure bandage should be employed prior to applying pressure to a pressure point.

44. c. there is too much bone—A tourniquet placed in this area will not adequately control the bleeding. The most common pressure points used are femoral and brachial arteries.

45. b. lose the limb to save the life.—Use of a tourniquet is considered a last resort of bleeding control. It is considered only after all other methods of bleeding control have failed.

46. a. the process to eliminate bacteria from the dressing material.—This type of dressing is used when infection is a concern.

47. a. passage of air—This type of dressing is useful for wounds involving the thorax and major vessels. It may prevent pneumothorax and air embolism.

48. d. non-adherent—This type of dressing is often used after wound closure.

49. b. adhesive—This type of dressing can also assist in controlling acute bleeding.

50. d. decreased risk of wound infection—The other choices are likely to occur with an improperly applied dressing.

51. b. Explain that a tetanus shot and sutures are necessary.—Transportation considerations for this type of wound include: the need for proper wound cleansing and dressing, the need for a tetanus booster, and the need for sutures due to the depth and location of the injury.

52. c. Do not allow the dressing to get wet.—A wet dressing will act as a wick and draw bacteria into the wound.

53. c. every ten years—Currently, the recommendation for a booster is every ten years.

54. a. covering the wound with a dry, sterile dressing.—Nonsterile dressings are used when something clean is acceptable and infection is not a concern.

55. b. be wrapped in sterile, moist gauze pad.—The amputated part should be wrapped in a sterile, moist gauze pad and placed in a plastic bag. Then, place the bag on ice. Be careful to ensure that the tissue does not freeze.

56. c. gangrene—Some experts recommend hyperbaric therapy to prevent gangrene and improve healing in crush injuries.

57. a. the observation of the presence of ECG changes or dysrhythmias.—Calcium chloride (1 to 3 cc IV in an adult) is indicated in this case. Of course, follow your local protocols.

58. b. subcutaneous layer—The other choices listed are the other layers of the skin (e.g., epidermis, dermis).

59. b. inflammation—These mediators include granulocytes, lymphocytes, and macrophages.

60. a. Hypertrophic scar—These are more common in areas of high tissue stress, such as flexion creases across joints.

Chapter 36: Burns

1. a. house—Each year, an estimated 1.25 million people are burned severely enough to seek treatment. Those who are at the highest risk are the elderly and children.

2. b. toddler and preschool—Smoke inhalation, scalds, contact, and electrical burns are especially likely to occur in children younger than four years old.

3. d. impairment of mobility or sensation.—Those who are at the highest risk for burns are the elderly (from impairment of mobility or sensation) and children (from child abuse).

4. c. turning down the thermostat on the hot water heater to 120°F.—Setting the thermostat to 100°F is the recommendation for preventing accidental burns.

5. a. decreased catecholamine release—An increase in catecholamine and dysrhythmias is a system complication of burn injuries.

6. c. full thickness—A full thickness burn involved all layers of the skin and may include charring of tissue.

7. b. deep fascia—This is a layer of connective tissue covering or binding body structures together.

8. b. second—Also referred to as a partial thickness burn.

9. c. eschar.—Eschar is the scab or immediate scar that forms on the skin following a burn injury.

10. a. body surface area burned.—The rule of nines is one method of estimating the amount of body surface area affected by a burn injury. There are two versions, one for adults and one for pediatrics.

11. b. requires transport to the nearest hospital.—Additional examples include: burns greater than 30% of BSA in adults, 15% of BSA in children, burns of the head or perineum, and burns associated with multiple trauma or serious medical problems.

12. b. the patient's gender—The other factors have a significant impact on the management and prognosis of the burn-injured patient.

13. c. the kidneys—Preexisting problems with the kidneys, lungs, or heart may make it difficult for the patient to handle the tremendous movement of body fluids that occurs with a burn injury.

14. d. 24%—The front and back of each lower leg is 6% (6 × 4). This equals 24% for both lower legs.

15. b. compensation—The phases of burn shock include the emergent, fluid shift, resolution, and hypermetabolic phases.

16. b. release of catecholamines—The patient will have tachycardia, tachypnea, mild hypertension, and anxiety.

17. c. fluid shift—During this phase, there is a massive shift of fluids from the intravascular to the extravascular space.

18. c. resolution—In this phase, the extravasation of fluid diminishes and equilibrium is reached between intravascular space and interstitial space.

19. a. carbon monoxide poisoning.—MOIs associated with inhalation injury include: toxic inhalations, smoke inhalation, carbon monoxide poisoning, thiocyanate intoxication, and thermal and chemical burns.

20. d. Eschar—The scar formation is thick and nonelastic. If large enough, it may impair circulation or respiration.

21. a. circulatory compromise—When this condition develops, the patient will require an escharotomy, a life- or limb-saving procedure in which physical cuts are made into the eschar formed on the skin with a scalpel.

22. b. fluid replacement amounts—This is a consideration in the management of the burn patient.

23. a. Maintain body heat.—Moving the patient to safety and stopping the burning process are the initial steps of care. Maintaining body heat, so the patient does not become hypothermic, is a priority over pain management.

24. b. determine fluid replacement—The formula is to administer four times the BSA, times the patient's weight in kilograms. The first half is given in the first eight hours. For example, a 100 kg patient with 40% BSA full thick burns (4 × 40 × 100 = 16,000) should receive 8,000 cc in the first eight hours.

25. c. crawling on the floor in a room with flames—The coolest area of a burning room is always the floor.

26. a. hoarseness—Other clues to look for include: singed nasal hairs, black soot in the sputum, stridor, and inspiratory wheezing.

27. c. hyperbaric oxygen—Though once reserved for only the very ill, some data suggest that treatment of patients with fairly low levels of carbon monoxide is also beneficial.

28. b. hot tar—Tar sticks to the skin, creating a longer exposure time. The temperature of hot tar ranges from 400°–500°F.

29. b. brushing it off and calling the poison control center for decon procedures.—Figure out what the chemical is before just washing it off. Some chemicals react with water and produce heat or develop a substance that is toxic to inhale.

30. a. continuous irrigation—Remove contacts and provide continuous irrigation. Take care with the runoff so as not to burn other areas of the body.

31. a. one; two—The burning effects of both of these substances can be minimized when the patient is instructed to avoid rubbing his eyes or face.

32. a. get the patient to blow his nose and spit out any residue.—The patient should also be instructed to avoid rubbing his eyes or face.

33. b. remove the lenses with a gloved hand or assist the patient in doing so.—The contact lens must be removed promptly to stop the burning process and allow for proper irrigation.

34. d. The path of electricity through the body may cause serious complications.—Always try to define the entry and exit points of the current because anything in the pathway is fair game for injury.

35. b. 1,000—The cause of death is usually attributed to the electrical effect on the heart, massive muscle destruction occurring from the current traveling through the body, or thermal burns from contact with the electrical source.

36. c. identify the source of the electricity prior to approaching the patient.—Personal safety first! Prior to approaching the patient, be sure you know what the source of the electricity injury was, and if it is still a live source.

37. b. less dangerous than AC.—The effects of AC on the body depend on the frequency. Low frequency currents of 50 to 60 Hz, which are commonly used, are more dangerous than high frequency currents, and are three to five times more dangerous than DC currents of the same voltage and amperage.

38. c. 60—Prolonged exposure causes more severe burns.

39. b. Escharotomy—A lifesaving or limb-saving procedure in which the physician cuts into the eschar formed on the skin with a scalpel.

40. d. moist mucous membrane (mouth)—Body resistance is highest with dry, intact skin with thickly calloused areas (e.g., palm of the hand or sole of the foot).

41. a. anything in the path is "fair game" for injury.—The body is a great conductor of electricity. Assume that any tissue anywhere in the path of the current was damaged.

42. c. malocclusion—The other signs and symptoms are frequently associated with electrical injuries.

43. a. There is nothing you can do.—There is no treatment for preventing airway swelling with this MOI. The paramedic should assess the need for assisting ventilation and intubating, and provide what is necessary for the patient before the swelling becomes a complete airway obstruction. When the patient is conscious, sedation is often necessary. Call for the additional resources needed and follow local protocol.

44. a. lightning strike—Lightning rarely produces entrance and exit wounds. Typically, lightning flashes over the patient as opposed to achieving a direct hit.

45. c. The potential for internal injury is less than a thermal injury.—The potential for internal injury is often much greater. Thermal burns are typically associated with injury to the body's surface.

46. c. hands.—The hands, followed by the head, are the most common entry point. The most common exit point is the foot.

47. b. singed nasal hairs—This finding is more common with blast and inhalation injuries.

48. d. feet—The hands, followed by the head, are the most common entry point. The most common exit point is the foot.

49. a. ionization—Ionization can result from X-rays, gamma rays, and particle bombardment.

50. a. when the history is inconsistent with injuries—When a child's injuries or pattern of injuries do not appear to be consistent with the patient's, parent's or caregiver's history of the MOI, the paramedic should consider the possibility of abuse.

51. b. Neutrons—The other types of radiation are non-ionizing.

52. b. Beta particles—They cause less local damage than the alpha particles, yet can be dangerous if inhaled or ingested.

53. d. neutrons—Neutrons have ten times more penetration than gamma rays.

54. a. Alpha particles—They are generally a minor hazard unless taken internally by ingestion or inhalation.

55. d. roentgen equivalent in man (REM).—For practical purposes, RAD and REM are equivalent in their clinical value to the EMS provider.

56. c. ionizing—This can occur acutely (from a single large exposure) or chronically (from exposure to dangerous levels over a period of time).

57. a. by the severity of symptoms—Obtaining a Geiger counter reading is the best indicator for determining the severity of an exposure. However, most paramedics do not have immediate access to a Geiger counter.

58. b. White blood cells—WBCs are very sensitive to radiation.

59. d. nausea and vomiting—This is a very common side effect following radiation therapy.

60. c. In a dirty accident, the patient continues to be a hazard of exposure to responders.—These patients need to be monitored with a Geiger counter and decontaminated by the appropriately trained personnel.

Chapter 37: Head and Facial Trauma

1. c. airway compromise.—Consider the ABCs. With this type of injury, there is a high risk of potential for complications of the patient's airway.

2. d. gunshot wounds (GSW).—The other choices are not examples of penetrating MOIs; they are blunt trauma.

3. d. cervical spine injury—The paramedic must take C-spine precautions with any patient who has an MOI with a blunt force above the shoulders.

4. d. there is an associated injury to the major blood vessels.—Throat injuries may be fatal, usually due to associated injury to the airway or the main blood vessels (e.g., carotid and jugular). Vocal cord injury may lead to hoarseness or respiratory compromise.

5. d. hyphema—A collection of blood in the front of the eye.

6. c. blowout fracture.—A blowout fracture occurs because blunt trauma is applied to the eye socket.

7. a. punch—More severe injuries to the mouth are rare and often involve penetrating trauma.

8. a. complicated airway.—LeFort fractures are based on X-ray or CT scan findings. These injuries involve the mouth, nose, eyes, and cheeks.

9. c. X-ray or CT scan findings.—Some experts now contend that the differentiation is artificial and not helpful.

10. d. cranial nerves 1–5.—The vagus nerve (tenth) is the only cranial nerve that extends out of the skull into the thorax.

11. c. external—The key assessment point is to note if CSF is draining from the ear.

12. b. eardrum.—The key assessment point is to determine if there is acute gross hearing loss.

13. d. cones.—Conical-shaped photoreceptive cells in the retina are called the cones.

14. d. cornea—The cornea can be easily injured from exposure to chemicals and other substances, or from blunt force trauma.

15. b. Eyelids—Also called palpebra.

16. b. rods—Rod-shaped photoreceptive cells in the retina.

17. a. hypoglossal—The pair of twelfth cranial nerves, which are the motor nerves that supply the muscles of the tongue and hyoid.

18. a. hyoid.—The only unarticulated bone in the body.

19. b. malocclusion.—Determine if the malocclusion is normal for the patient or new as a result of traumatic injury.

20. c. movement from conjugate gaze of the uninjured eye.—Conjugate gaze refers to the use of both eyes to look steadily in one direction.

21. c. million—Most head injuries are minor. Major head injury is the most common cause of death from

trauma in trauma centers. Statistics show that over 50% of all trauma deaths involve a head injury.

22. b. males; fifteen to twenty-four—Also at high risk are infants, school-age children, and the elderly.

23. a. MVC.—Other common MOIs for head injury include: sports, falls, and penetrating trauma from GSWs.

24. d. galea—It is comprised of the hair and subcutaneous tissue, which contains the major scalp veins that, when injured, can bleed profusely.

25. c. be strong yet light in weight.—The head also has sinuses (hollow cavities) that help to lighten the weight.

26. b. cerebrum—This area of the brain contains the cortex controls that are responsible for voluntary skeletal movement and the level of awareness component of consciousness.

27. c. occipital—This area of the brain is the origin of the optic nerves.

28. c. III; X—The third cranial nerve controls pupil size. The tenth cranial nerve is the vagus, which innervates the sinoatrial (SA) and atrioventricular (AV) nodes, as well as the stomach and GI tract. Stimulation of this nerve causes bradycardia.

29. d. reticular activating system—The RAS is responsible for the level of arousal and must be intact for cortical function to maintain wakefulness.

30. a. venous blood vessels that reabsorb CSF.—The arachnoid member is the middle layer of the meninges and loosely covers the central nervous center.

31. c. 20—The brain also requires many nutrients, (e.g., glucose and thiamine), but does not have the ability to store nutrients.

32. c. autoregulation—Perfusion of the brain can be affected by conditions that interfere with cerebral perfusion pressure (CPP), such as edema, bleeding, or hypotension.

33. a. coup—Coup injuries develop directly below the point of impact.

34. b. concussion—A concussion results in a transient episode of neuronal dysfunction with a rapid return to normal neurological activity. The injuries are most commonly the result of blunt trauma to the head.

35. b. focal—Focal injuries are specific, grossly observable brain lesions (e.g., cerebral contusion, intracranial hemorrhage, and epidural hematoma).

36. d. Diffuse axonal injury—It is often a mild or classic concussion, but it can be moderate or severe.

37. b. concussion—The injuries are most commonly the result of blunt trauma to the head. The patient is often initially confused and disoriented and may not remember the event.

38. c. Battle's sign—This is a finding (bruising behind the ear) associated with a basilar skull fracture.

39. a. linear—Leaking of SCF may not occur for twenty-four hours. If there are no other associated injuries, there is typically no danger.

40. a. Acute subdural—This type of hemorrhage results from the rupture of bridging veins between the cortex and dura and may be acute, chronic, or delayed.

41. b. tachycardia.—Bradycardia would be a more typical finding due to pressure on the vagus nerve.

42. a. four to six—This response is a late and ominous finding associated with brain herniation.

43. d. elevated blood pressure—The usual response within the brain is elevated BP due to the loss of cerebral autoregulation. This is the only way that the body can continue perfusion to the injured tissue.

44. d. cerebral cortex and upper brain stem—The effects of an expanding hematoma on the cerebral cortex and upper brain stem may include Cushing's reflex and reactive pupils, and Cheyne-Stokes respirations may be present. Initially, the patient will have a purposeful response to pain. As the mental status deteriorates, this sensation is lost and the patient withdraws from pain. Flexion or decorticate posturing will occur in response to a painful stimuli.

45. a. Vegetative functions are temporarily impaired because of the pressure.—At this late point in brain herniation, the patient's injury is not considered survivable.

46. b. 8 to 12.—A severe head injury is less than 8.

47. c. subarachnoid—The arachnoid membrane is composed of venous blood vessels that reabsorb CSF.

48. a. pads of the fingers—When the depression is visually obvious, there is no reason to palpate the site. When performing a focused exam of the skull for a possible injury, use the pads of the fingertips, which are dexterous and sensitive enough to assess a potential skull depression without causing further injury.

49. c. tachycardia and tachypnea—Bradycardia and abnormal respirations are associated with enlarging intracranial hematomas.

50. a. frontal lobe—Trauma to this area of the brain may result in personality changes, placid reactions, or seizures.

51. b. aggressive hyperventilation.—It is now believed that hyperventilation produces a marked reduction in cerebral blood flow. Decreased cerebral blood flow may lead to or exacerbate ischemia, enhancing rather than reducing injury. It also decreases coronary perfusion pressure in cardiac arrest.

52. a. another organ or injuries besides the brain.—Typically, bleeding from the head is not significant enough to produce hypotension.

53. d. paralysis prior to intubation—Pharmacological-induced paralysis keeps the patient from becoming anxious and combative, both of which can worsen head injury.

54. b. only when hypoglycemia is confirmed.—Exogenous glucose can increase brain swelling and should

only be administered when hypoglycemia can be confirmed.

55. b. assure adequate tidal volume.—Ensure a patent airway, adequate ventilation, and oxygenation.

56. a. systolic; 70—Ensure adequate circulation, but do not administer too much fluid. Manage hypotension with fluid boluses, not to exceed a systolic of 90–100 mmHg in the adult male patient.

57. c. nasal intubation—Ensure an adequate airway, but avoid nasal intubation because it may increase the ICP.

58. a. the history of the MOI—Getting a good story of the MOI may be the only way to recognize the presence of brain injury.

59. c. 5—Eye response = 1, verbal response = 1, motor response = 3, for a total of 5.

60. a. linear—This is the most common type of skull fracture and can only be determined by X-ray. If there are no associated injuries, the fracture may be missed. Getting a good story of the MOI may be the only way to recognize the presence of brain injury.

Chapter 38: Spinal Trauma

1. b. men, sixteen to thirty—This occurs primarily due to sports, as well as inexperienced and immature drivers.

2. c. 25—This includes bystanders pulling patients out of cars and swimming pools without proper spinal immobilization.

3. d. all of the above.—Nerves and blood vessels are also interconnected with the spine. Injury to any of these components may result in neck or back pain.

4. b. posterior longitudinal.—The four key ligaments that support the spine are the anterior and posterior longitudinal ligaments, and the cruciform and accessory atlantoaxial ligaments.

5. c. cruciform.—Cruciate means shaped like a cross. This very complete ligament supports the atlas vertebra.

6. c. axis.—The atlas is the first cervical vertebra and the axis is the second.

7. d. transverse.—The atlantoaxial ligament attaches the axis and atlas, as well as the transverse ligament that serves to hold the odontoid process close to the anterior arch.

8. a. dens—A fracture of the odontoid process results in death in most cases.

9. b. thoracic.—The spine is thickest in this area and has the additional protection of the ribs.

10. c. thirty-one—Also called peripheral nerves, they exit the spinal cord between each of the vertebra.

11. a. coccyx—The coccyx joins with the sacrum from above and is the terminus of the spine.

12. b. transverse process.—These processes can fracture and break off as a result of blunt force trauma.

13. b. spinous process.—These processes can fracture and break off as a result of blunt force trauma.

14. d. nucleus pulposus.—Trauma, degenerative disk disease, and improper lifting may cause herniation (a tear in the capsule enclosing the nucleus pulposus) of the intervertebral disk.

15. c. L-2—The spinal cord ends at the level of second lumbar vertebra.

16. b. It is manufactured in the ventricles of the brain.—CSF protects and supports the brain and spinal cord. CSF is completely replaced several times a day.

17. a. white matter.—The white matter is located in the anatomical spinal tracts, which are longitudinal bundles of myelinated nerve tracts. Myelin is a soft, white, fatty substance that forms a thick sheath around certain nerves. The gray matter is located in the core of the cord.

18. b. ascending nerve tracts.—There are two groups of ascending nerve tracts: spinothalmic tracts and the fascicular gracilis and corneatus tracts.

19. c. descending nerve tracts.—The descending nerve tracts carry motor impulses from the brain to the body. There are three groups: corticospinal, reticulospinal, and rubrospinal tracts.

20. a. a group of nerve fibers with a similar function—The funiculi function like a coaxial cable. They conduct sensory impulses from the skin, muscle tendons, and joints to the brain for interpretation as sensations of touch, pressure, and body movement.

21. c. conduct impulses of pain and temperature to the brain.—The lateral and anterior spinothalmic tracts are located in the lateral and anterior funiculi, and the impulses cross over at the spinal cord.

22. b. dermatome.—Dermatomes can be mapped out by the level of the spinal nerve. They are a useful tool to determine the specific level of spinal cord injury (SCI).

23. d. T-4—The motor and sensory dermatomes at the nipple line are located at the fourth thoracic vertebra.

24. a. C-3—The nerve roots C-3, 4, and 5 have a relationship to the motor function of the diaphragm.

25. b. resistance to movement.—Two exceptions for not moving a patient into a normal anatomical position for immobilization are extreme pain or resistance from the bones in gently moving the neck.

26. d. Have the patient sign a refusal for the collar and immobilize her without it.—Any competent adult patient has the right to refuse any or all care offered.

27. b. The patient experienced hyperflexion.—The classic "lipstick" sign results from hyperflexion of the head as it is forced down to the chest with rapid acceleration.

28. b. thoracic—Paraplegia can occur with transection of the lumbar level, as well. When a patient has a complete spinal cord transection, all cord-mediated functions below the transection are permanently lost.

29. c. The spinal cord may be injured without accompanying bone or soft tissue injury.—The other statements are inaccurate.

30. d. it should not be used at all—If the decision is made to immobilize a patient in the field, the patient should get both a collar and spine board.

31. b. full spinal immobilization with the parent providing support—The patient has more than one indication for providing full spinal immobilization (e.g., fall from twice his height and loss of consciousness).

32. c. mental status—A patient who is alert, calm, cooperative, sober and oriented, and has had no loss of consciousness is considered reliable and able to refuse any or all care.

33. c. fully immobilize the spine.—New neck pain or tenderness after any MOI is an indication for the application of full spinal immobilization.

34. b. Tender areas may not hurt unless palpated.—Always palpate over the spinous processes before concluding that a patient has no neck pain. Some providers simply ask the patient and never perform a physical exam.

35. b. paresthesia in the left leg after, not before, immobilization—A change in the patient's condition that is more severe is significant. Recognizing the change is good assessment; correcting the problem is good care.

36. a. vertical compression of the spine—Also referred to as axial loading, usually to the top of the head from a sudden deceleration (e.g., a brick falling onto someone's head). It may cause a compression fracture without an SCI or a crushed vertebral body with an SCI.

37. d. distraction of the neck—This type of force may cause a stretching of the spinal cord and supporting ligaments (e.g., hanging that did not break the odontoid).

38. a. rotational neck injury—T-bone collisions are associated with excessive rotation of the neck beyond the normal range of motion. A rupture of the supporting ligaments may also occur.

39. a. concussion.—The spinal cord can be injured in a number of ways. A cord concussion is a temporary disruption of cord-mediated functions.

40. b. spinal shock.—Spinal shock refers to a temporary loss of all types of spinal cord functions distal to the injury. The patient will be flaccid and paralyzed distal to the injury site. It is important to manage the patient carefully to avoid a secondary injury.

41. d. Brown-Sequard syndrome—This syndrome is caused by a penetrating injury that produces a partial transection of the spinal cord. It is referred to as a hemisection of the cord and involves only one side of the cord.

42. c. variable segment instability.—The degeneration of a disc may cause the vertebrae to come in closer contact with one another.

43. c. 60–90—The usual cause is a lumbar nerve root problem. This syndrome affects men and women equally up to the age of sixty, when it increases in women.

44. b. The head moves around inside the helmet.—The helmet is not the right size when the head moves around and should be removed in order to properly immobilize the cervical spine.

45. b. spondylolysis—A structural defect of the spine involving the lamina or vertebral arch. It usually occurs between the superior and inferior articulating facets.

46. a. palliative care—The goal is to make the patient comfortable by decreasing any pain or discomfort from movement.

47. c. metastasis—Tumors are often accidentally discovered with an X-ray following a traumatic event.

48. b. 10; 15—This is a major reason for placing a patient with a suspected SCI on a backboard. This neutral position allows the most space for the cord, helping to reduce excess pressure and cord hypoxia.

49. c. They totally eliminate neck movement.—Cervical collars alone do not totally eliminate neck movement. They are used together with an immobilization device to prevent neck movement.

50. b. airway management—When the airway cannot be adequately managed with the helmet in place, it must be removed promptly without causing further injury.

51. a. compensating shock—Rapid extrication should only be used with the critical patient or when hazardous conditions will further harm the patient or rescuers.

52. c. Passenger involved in a high-speed MVC complaining of a headache after the collision.—The MOI is one of the most significant factors in the assessment and treatment of any trauma patient.

53. c. when it is necessary for the patient to be supine—In most cases, a toddler can be immobilized in a child seat. If it becomes necessary for the child to be placed in the supine position, the child should be rapidly extricated out of the car seat onto a backboard.

54. b. position is the most comfortable for the patient.—This position is uncomfortable for most patients. Many patients complain of increased pain after being immobilized.

55. a. The goal is to prevent further injury.—Preventing secondary injury following the primary injury is paramount. The first step is to recognize the actual or potential primary injury and manage it appropriately.
56. d. lumbar and cervical—These areas of the spine are most susceptible to injury.
57. a. Palpate over each of the spinal processes.—Each process is palpated for deformity, step-offs, and free-moving bones.
58. b. foot dorsiflexion.—The patient is asked to pull up and push down against the resistance of the examiner's hands.
59. a. directions of force.—These forces include: acceleration, deceleration, flexion, hyperflexion, extension, hyperextension, vertical compression, distraction, and deformation.
60. b. neurogenic shock—A temporary loss of the autonomic function of the cord at the level of injury that controls the cardiovascular function.

Chapter 39: Thoracic Trauma

1. b. second—Head injuries are number one.
2. d. disruption of the bellows action.—The other conditions interrupt gas exchange rather than impair ventilations.
3. a. tearing of a great vessel.—Tearing occurs with rapid deceleration and penetrating MOIs.
4. b. tear—Tearing occurs with penetrating MOIs.
5. c. massive lung contusion to develop.—There is also a potential for respiratory burn injuries from the inhalation of superheated gases. Contusion or bruising reduces the area available to exchange oxygen and carbon dioxide (CO_2).
6. c. perforated lung tissue—The accumulation of air under the skin may also be caused by a tracheobronchial injury.
7. b. mesotendons—This is found in joints containing synovial fluid.
8. a. Sternocleidomastoid—A muscle used in breathing, as well as in flexion and extension of the head.
9. b. trapezius.—This muscle lies over the scapula.
10. d. mainstem bronchi.—It bifurcates (splits) into the right and left mainstem bronchi.
11. a. Parenchyma—The essential and distinctive tissue of a specific organ.
12. d. inferior vena cava.—The largest vein in the body.
13. a. aorta—The largest artery in the body.
14. b. trachea—The mediastinum contains the great vessels (e.g., aorta, vena cava, heart, esophagus, and trachea).
15. c. positive intrathoracic pressure pushes air out of the lungs.—The other choices are accurate regarding ventilation.
16. b. accessory muscles of breathing—These injuries can occur from deceleration, compression, or penetrating trauma.
17. a. serous pleural fluid.—Two other key components of gas exchange with respiration are cardiac circulation and red blood cell interface.
18. b. carotid sinus—These constantly measure the CO_2 levels in the blood. Respiratory centers in the brain adjust the rate and depth of breathing to maintain normal CO_2 concentrations.
19. a. contusions on the lung tissue—Other mechanisms that can impair gas exchange as a result of chest trauma include collapsed alveoli (atelectasis) and blood accumulation, and disruption of the respiratory tract from a cut to the trachea or major respiratory anatomy.
20. d. all of the above.—Observe the patient for ECG changes, ST segment or T wave elevations or depressions, and conduction or rhythm disturbances.
21. a. splenic rupture.—The spleen lies beneath the lower ribs and is highly susceptible to laceration and rupture from blunt trauma. Because it is highly vascular, it can produce life-threatening hemorrhage.
22. a. expand all the air sacs.—This will help prevent atelectasis and pneumonia from developing.
23. b. 4 to 9—The most common locations of rib fractures are in the axillary line and around the sternum.
24. c. severe trauma—This ribs are protected by the clavicle. The force required to fracture these ribs is significant.
25. c. 20 to 40—Mortality is increased with advanced age, seven or more ribs fractured, three or more associated injuries, shock, or a head injury.
26. d. The arterial blood flow is impaired, resulting in a ventilation-perfusion mismatch.—This type of injury impairs venous return.
27. a. pulmonary contusion—The contusion causes a decrease in the lung compliance and hemorrhage in the intra-alveolar capillaries and alveolus, making it even more difficult to ventilate and exchange gases at the cellular level.
28. d. deceleration compression—This occurs when the chest strikes the steering wheel or dashboard. This is a very serious injury that involves a 25–45% mortality rate.
29. c. because of the associated injuries.—If the thorax receives enough force to fracture the sternum, then

we must assume that the same force was transmitted to the heart, great vessels, lungs, and diaphragm.

30. b. shoulder or arm on the affected side.—An abnormal accumulation of air in the apexes of the chest can cause pain in the shoulder or arm on the affected side.

31. c. hypoventilation.—Ventilation perfusion mismatch occurs as a result of shunting, hypoventilation, hypoxia, and the development of a large, functional dead space.

32. b. respiratory effort is ineffective.—If the size of the hole is greater than the glottic opening, little to no air comes in through the glottis.

33. d. a serious reduction in cardiac output caused by deformation of the vena cava reducing preload.—The mediastinum shifts to the contralateral side, and this leads to right-to-left intrapulmonary shunting and hypoxia.

34. b. hyporesonance and mediastinal shift to the ipsilateral side—These findings should be detected on the affected side.

35. d. 50—Hemothorax can occur from penetrating or blunt trauma to the lung, chest wall vessels, the intercostal vessels, or the myocardium itself.

36. a. 2,000 to 3,000—A large volume of blood can bleed into the pleural space and chest cavity.

37. c. parenchyma.—The pulmonary parenchyma is a low-pressure vascular system. When a massive hemothorax is present, consider another cause for the bleeding (e.g., great vessel or heart).

38. b. respiratory distress.—The major problem following a massive hemothorax is the development of shock and respiratory compromise.

39. b. positive pressure ventilation.—Airway and ventilatory management are first and foremost. Positive pressure ventilation may be helpful to re-expand the injured lung, which in turn may help reduce the bleeding.

40. c. the high incidence of other associated injuries.—The mortality is between 14% and 20%.

41. d. cyanosis to the face and neck—The other findings are typical with pulmonary contusion.

42. d. abdominal—Patients with pulmonary contusions also tend to have other severe thoracic and abdominal injuries. Always assume multiple potential injuries are present.

43. a. prevent the kinking of the great vessels.—It attaches the great vessels at the base of the heart.

44. b. ventricular diastolic filling—The accumulation of fluid in the pericardial sac impairs diastolic filling of the heart, with a subsequent decrease in cardiac output.

45. c. JVD and narrow pulse pressure.—Other signs and symptoms may include: respiratory distress and cyanosis of the head, neck, and upper extremities, pulsus paradoxus, ECG changes, and Beck's triad.

46. b. myocardial contusion—If the thorax receives enough force to fracture the sternum, then we must assume that the same force was transmitted to the heart, great vessels, lungs, and diaphragm. The fractured ribs are more local over the heart. Myocardial and pulmonary contusions are very likely.

47. a. sinus tachycardia without obvious hypovolemia.—Other ECG changes to be alert for as a clue to this problem include: persistent tachycardia, ST segment elevation, T wave inversion, right bundle branch block (RBBB), atrial flutter or fibrillation, and PVCs or PACs.

48. d. all of the above—Evaluate the need for advance airway insertion and contact medical control, while transporting to the nearest appropriate facility.

49. c. CHF or pulmonary edema—The history of a recent trauma and a new onset of CHF or pulmonary edema are clues to a possible myocardial rupture.

50. b. falls.—This is a very critical injury, where 85–95% of the patients die instantaneously.

51. d. 85 to 95—Aortic dissections are present in 15% of all blunt trauma deaths.

52. c. pleuritic pain in the neck.—Pleuritic pain occurs in the chest.

53. c. Trendelenburg position—This position may make the respiratory distress worse. Gravity will push the abdominal contents and diaphragm further up into the chest cavity, impeding expansion of the lungs.

54. a. cardiac event.—Other signs and symptoms may include: chest pain, fever, hoarseness, dysphagia, respiratory distress, shock, subcutaneous emphysema, and ECG changes.

55. c. the skin below the crushed area is cyanotic.—Cyanosis may be present in the face and upper neck.

56. a. IV fluids for hypotension.—Airway and ventilatory management are primary, as with any patient. After the compression is released, typically the patient will experience hypotension, which should be managed with IV fluids.

57. c. both blunt and penetrating chest trauma.—This type of injury occurs in less than 3% of chest injuries, but has a mortality rate of greater than 30%.

58. d. tachy-brady dysrhythmias—The tear from this injury can occur anywhere along the tracheal-bronchial tree. There is a rapid movement of air into the pleural space, often making the tension pneumothorax refractory to a needle decompression.

59. c. penetrating trauma.—Penetrating trauma from a bullet or a knife can cause an esophageal injury.

60. a. diaphragmatic injury.—When the MOI causes a high-pressure compression to the abdomen, the result can be a diaphragmatic rupture with extravasation of abdominal contents into the chest.

Chapter 40: Abdominal Trauma

1. a. second—Major hemorrhage can occur rapidly and go unrecognized. This is why abdominal trauma is a major cause of trauma death and the second leading cause of preventable trauma death.
2. b. 1.5—The adult abdominal cavity can hide a significant blood loss easily before showing any signs of distention.
3. d. associated chest injuries.—Based on the MOI, certain syndromes are common. People with abdominal injuries often have a chest injury, as well.
4. c. MOI—When the MOI is penetrating, the obvious wound is the clue to potential injury to underlying organs. When the MOI is blunt, the potential for injury is often underappreciated or not recognized at all.
5. c. rapid deceleration—MVCs often produce the rapid deceleration that can cause these types of injuries.
6. b. jejunum—The jejunum has larger, thicker walls, and is more vascular than other sections of the small intestine.
7. c. ileum—This section lies between the jejunum and the large intestine.
8. b. hernia repair—Surgical repair of a hernia.
9. a. liver—The liver is very vascular, and the blood loss from an injury can be fatal.
10. a. Visceral—The visceral peritoneum receives input from both sides of the spinal cord. This causes pain to present as diffuse rather than localized.
11. a. somatic—Somatic pain is caused by direct irritation of the parietal peritoneum. As such, it is more localized. Visceral pain is more diffuse.
12. d. liver and gallbladder—These organs are located in the upper left quadrant of the abdomen.
13. b. intraperitoneal bleeding and/or irritation.—The location of pain often does not correspond to the actual source. However, there are referral patterns and pain associated with many conditions.
14. a. Cullen's sign.—This sign may be identified twelve to twenty-four hours after the initial injury.
15. c. testicular torsion—This condition is usually unilateral. Frequently, the patient complains of a sudden onset of extreme pain in his testicle, occurring during or after physical exertion.
16. c. Move the patient into his position of comfort, then administer analgesia and an antiemetic.—

Management is primarily palliative to decrease any pain or discomfort and ease the nausea.

17. c. Manage his pain and transport gently.—Testicular torsion is an acute urological emergency that threatens the male's future reproductive capability. Manage the patient's pain and nausea while transporting to the hospital.
18. a. prompt surgery.—Even with prompt treatment, some studies report a semen analysis to be abnormal after unilateral torsion.
19. a. perforations and hemorrhage.—Perforations are common in both males and females. They are caused by foreign objects inserted into the vagina or rectum. Signs and symptoms include acute abdominal pain, tachycardia, tachypnea, fever, and a rigid abdomen.
20. b. contamination from fecal matter—All of the signs and symptoms described above are due to contamination from fecal matter.
21. a. Keep the patient in a position of comfort.—Monitor the patient for signs of shock, and treat for shock if present.
22. d. nausea and vomiting.—Treat nausea with an antiemetic.
23. c. intra-abdominal bleed.—Isolated head injury rarely causes hypotension. Intra-abdominal bleeding must be suspected when signs of shock are present but no other apparent cause for bleeding can be immediately discovered.
24. c. IV fluid replacement.—This should be done en route to the hospital.
25. d. peritonitis.—This can result at a later point, as a result of the infection from perforation.
26. c. 35%—Maternal circulation increases by nearly 50% by full term. She can lose a significant amount of blood before signs and symptoms begin to appear.
27. a. uterine inversion.—A condition where the uterus turns inside out after delivery.
28. b. shoulder—This is an established referral pattern of pain associated with diaphragmatic irritation.
29. c. pancreas—The other organs are located in the abdominal cavity.
30. d. Ileus—A bowel obstruction that is painful and impairs peristalsis.

Chapter 41: Musculoskeletal Trauma

1. b. become more porous.—This causes the bones to become brittle.
2. a. bony thorax.—The thorax protects the vital organs in the chest (e.g., heart, lungs, aorta, and vena cava).
3. d. clavicle and scapula.—This structure supports the upper extremity.
4. a. tendons—The tendon allows for power of movement across the joints.

5. b. fibrous, cartilaginous, and synovial.—These are the structural classifications of joints.

6. d. producing red blood cells.—Bones also store salts (e.g., calcium) and metabolic materials.

7. a. parts of a long bone.—The ends, shaft, and covering of long bones.

8. a. Metaphysis—The area of the bone that transitions between the epiphysis and the diaphysis.

9. c. the olecranon—The process on the ulna that articulates with the humerus and forms the elbow.

10. d. ulna shaft—The radius is the bone on the thumb side of the lower arm.

11. a. acromioclavicular joint.—The joint connecting the acromion and the clavicle.

12. b. pelvis—If the fracture is complicated, such as one that severs the femoral artery, the patient can easily bleed to death.

13. d. femur—The femur is the bone of the upper leg.

14. b. condyle—The distal ends of the femur and humerus have condyles.

15. a. anterior; medial malleolus—The shin bone.

16. d. all of the above.—The range of motion of a specific bone depends on its location.

17. d. posterior; lateral—The smaller of the two lower leg bones.

18. c. axial—The three muscle types are cardiac, skeletal, and smooth.

19. a. Smooth—Smooth muscle can relax or contract to alter the inner lumen diameter of vessels.

20. b. cartilage.—A cartilaginous joint is one in which there is cartilage connecting the bones.

21. c. Ligaments—A sprain is an injury to the ligaments around a joint.

22. b. Smooth muscle—Found in the lower airways, blood vessels, and intestines. It is under the control of the autonomic nervous system.

23. c. padded by cartilage.—Ligaments hold the joints together.

24. a. automaticity.—Only cardiac muscle has this capability.

25. b. Skeletal muscle—Smooth muscle includes the major muscle mass of the body and allows for mobility.

26. c. elbow and knee.—The hip and shoulder are ball and sockets joints, and the digits are pivot joints.

27. a. symphysis—The articulation of bones may be formed of cartilage.

28. b. gomphoses.—An example of gomphoses is teeth in the jaw bone.

29. c. Syndesmoses—Bone ends that are connected by ligaments.

30. d. synovial—Examples of synovial joints include: hinge, pivot, saddle, and ball and socket joints.

31. c. greenstick—The fracture appears similar to how a live green tree splits.

32. d. synovial—The knee, hip, fingers, and shoulder are examples of synovial joints.

33. b. transverse—These types of fractures are obvious and gross, and may be open or closed.

34. a. 500—A complicated fracture involving a laceration to an artery can produce life-threatening hemorrhage.

35. a. subluxation.—A subluxation usually produces a great amount of damage and instability.

36. b. dislocation.—When the bone is moved from its normal position within a joint, it becomes dislocated.

37. d. occupational repetitive motions.—Carpal tunnel syndrome is associated with occupational repetitive motions, such as typing (keyboarding).

38. b. tibia; posterior—Dislocation of the knee and elbow is serious because they have a high probability of blood vessel and nerve damage.

39. c. brachial artery and blood supply to the arm.—Dislocation of the knee and elbow is serious because they have a high probability of blood vessel and nerve damage.

40. b. painful, swollen deformity.—These are typical findings associated with many uncomplicated fractures.

41. b. bursitis and gouty arthritis.—Tendonitis is another common cause.

42. d. relieve the muscle spasms that can worsen the injury.—Controlling the spasm of the strong muscles surrounding the femur helps to minimize overriding by the broken bone ends.

43. d. transportation is long or delayed.—Delayed or prolonged transport may require a different approach. Follow your local protocol.

44. a. a knee dislocation involves the tibia popping out of the knee joint.—A patella dislocation is the movement of the knee cap from its normal position.

45. a. pelvic—Many EMS systems have relegated use of MAST/PASG to the stabilization of the pelvic or bilateral femur fractures.

46. b. Loosen the sling, then swathe and reassess.—If this does not work, consider repositioning the extremity and reassessing.

47. a. initial swelling has gone down.—Heat is not used in the emergency care of a sprain, fracture, or dislocation.

48. d. forearm.—Commonly occurs from falls, skating, snowboarding, and skiing. Wrist guards significantly reduce the risk of Colles' fractures.

49. c. allowing the bone to protrude through the skin.—Open fractures become complicated because of the significant risk of infection.

50. c. diaphoresis—Diaphoresis may occur as a result of the pain produced by a fracture or dislocation, but not at the site of injury.

Chapter 42: Neonatology

1. d. foramen arteriosus.—The other vessels are part of the fetal circulation.
2. c. ductus venosus—In utero, the ductus venosus empties into the inferior vena cava.
3. a. foramen ovale—The opening in the septal wall between the right and left atria in the fetus.
4. a. persistent fetal circulation—Hypoxia or acidosis can trigger the pulmonary vascular bed to constrict and reopen the ductus arteriosus, creating fetal circulation as in utero. The danger here is that the majority of the circulation is then shunted from the right heart to the left heart, bypassing the lungs.
5. c. stimulating the newborn to breathe.—In addition, the baby must be kept warm and assisted with oxygenation and ventilation as required.
6. d. apnea of infancy.—This condition usually resolves itself, but does need to be monitored until such time.
7. b. mixed.—A combination of central and obstructive apnea that may occur when the baby is awake or asleep.
8. b. three—The extra genetic material disrupts their physical and cognitive development.
9. d. flat facial profile with a small nose and depressed nasal bridge—The tongue is very large, the eyes have an upward slant and a small fold on the inner corners, and the ears are small with an abnormal shape (dysplastic ears).
10. d. an excessive space between the large and second toe.—Other distinguishing features include: a single deep crease across the palm of the hand, overall weak body muscle tone, and excessive ability to extend the joints.
11. b. exposed spinal structures.—There are three common types of spina bifida: occulta, meningocele, and myelomeningocele.
12. b. no prenatal care—Inadequate or no prenatal care is an avoidable factor that can affect childbirth.
13. b. prolonged labor—Other factors include: preterm labor, prolapsed cord, abnormal limb or fetal presentation, meconium staining or aspiration syndrome, and a mother's use of narcotics just before delivery.
14. a. Birth defects—Approximately 3–5% of the four million infants born annually in the United States are born with birth defects.
15. b. prolonged labor.—This is a significant antepartum factor that classifies a newborn as high risk.
16. a. 500–2,500—Low birth weights run between 500 and 2,500 grams.
17. c. placenta previa—Prenatal drug use increases the risk of miscarriage, premature labor, fetal stroke, death, abruptio placenta, low birth weight, birth defects, feeding problems, sleep disorders, SIDS, and the slowed development of motor skills.
18. d. respiratory effort, pulse rate, and skin color.—The initial assessment is the same as with any other patient: airway, breathing, and circulation.
19. c. appearance, pulse, grimace, activity, and reflex.—APGAR is assessed and given a score of 0, 1, or 2 at one and five minutes after birth.
20. d. metabolic—Specific tests vary from state to state.
21. b. poor growth and mental retardation.—This is an example of a condition that may be screened for at birth.
22. a. low birth weight, small head, and small eye openings—Fetal alcohol syndrome (FAS) results from maternal alcohol consumption. Even the consumption of very small amounts of alcohol during pregnancy can have serous effects on a developing fetus.
23. a. FAS does not occur with consumption of very small amounts of alcohol during pregnancy.—Even the consumption of very small amounts of alcohol during pregnancy can have serous effects on a developing fetus.
24. c. decreased mental status of the newborn—Maternal narcotic use within four hours of delivery can depress the fetus and is associated with respiratory depression at birth.
25. c. Administer oxygen, assist ventilations, and administer Narcan®.—Treatment is similar to adult narcotic overdose.
26. a. barotrauma.—Barotrauma is associated with positive pressure ventilation.
27. b. fractured clavicle—This occurs when the shoulders are too large to fit through the birth canal.
28. b. Assist with ventilations by bag mask.—The next step in resuscitation is to assist with ventilations by bag mask. If this fails to stimulate the child to breathe and increase the heart rate, compressions are started.
29. d. Start CPR.—If assisted ventilations fail to stimulate the child to breathe and increase the heart rate, compressions are started.
30. a. keeping the baby warm and continuing oxygen delivery.—Follow local protocols and medical direction for additional interventions.
31. a. hypoxia.—Poorly developed lungs and respiratory muscles and drive increase the need to provide assisted ventilations.
32. b. surfactant—Surfactant is not present in adequate quantities until after thirty-four weeks' gestation.
33. a. excessive heat loss through breathing.—Neonates can lose heat rapidly due to all of the other choices listed.
34. a. hypoglycemia.—Additional causes include alcohol or drug withdrawal and, less commonly, genetic or metabolic disorders.

35. b. immature thermoregulatory system.—An infection from a virus or bacteria is the most common cause of fever in neonates. Due to the immature thermoregulatory system, any fever is serious and requires evaluation.

36. d. before, during, and after.—This is a fact.

37. c. bilirubin.—This condition usually disappears within five to seven days after birth. The most common treatment is exposing the infant to ultraviolet lights to help break down the extra bilirubin so the baby's liver can process it.

38. c. two to three days—Jaundice occurs when a baby's immature liver cannot dispose of excess bilirubin.

39. a. drug withdrawal.—Complications can result from the aspiration of vomitus, electrolyte imbalance, or dehydration due to the loss of fluids.

40. d. electrolyte imbalance.—A congenital abnormality of the pyloric valve (pyloric stenosis) leads to vomiting within a few days after birth.

41. b. all stools are loose.—A general guideline is to consider more than six stools a day to be excessive.

42. b. hernias.—Intestinal obstruction and congenital abnormalities are other causes of abdominal distention in the neonate.

43. b. to watch the baby's airway.—Full stomachs and vomiting go hand in hand with babies.

44. a. ETT—IV and IO are safer and more reliable, accepted routes for medication administration. IO is a rapid way to obtain vascular access.

45. b. diaphragmatic herniation—This is a congenital disorder.

46. c. umbilical—An opening or weakened muscles around the bellybutton permit a bulge when the infant cries, coughs, or strains.

47. b. oxygenation—Basic treatments are applied before advanced interventions.

48. c. fluid imbalance—Airway and fluid imbalance problems are the most common potentially life-threatening disorders that affect neonates.

49. c. concentrated lemon juice—Teratogens are drugs or other substances that can cause fetal malformations.

50. b. always have their own placenta.—This is an accurate statement.

Chapter 43: Pediatrics

1. c. toddler—Generally speaking, toddlers do not like to be touched by strangers or separated from their parents. They do not like their clothing removed, they frighten easily, and they often overreact. They do not want to be "suffocated" by an oxygen mask.

2. c. preschool—Children in this age group may believe that their illness is a punishment for being bad. They fear pain, blood, and permanent injury.

3. d. adolescent—They want to be treated as adults. They may feel they are indestructible, but may also have fears of permanent injury and disfigurement.

4. d. The largest diameter of the airway in an infant is at the cricoid ring.—The smallest diameter of the infant's airway is at the cricoid ring.

5. b. six—A stuffy nose or mucus in the nose can be a complete, serious airway obstruction.

6. a. head injury.—In a healthy infant, the fontanels are normally soft and flat. They may sink when dehydrated or in shock, and bulge when crying or when there is increased pressure in the head (ICP).

7. b. Abdominal or "belly breathing" is normal in this age group.—The infant's respiratory muscles are not well developed, and they use their abdominal muscles to help them breathe. The infant becomes fatigued easily, and, in cases of severe respiratory distress, as the child attempts to compensate, sternal retractions occur.

8. a. They do not have the ability to shiver to create body heat.—Infants have immature and underdeveloped thermoregulatory systems, making it difficult for them to maintain their body temperature.

9. d. Trauma—The leading cause of trauma death in pediatrics is MVCs.

10. a. respiratory depression—Many of the ingested products cause life-threatening symptoms in the respiratory, CNS, and circulatory systems.

11. b. Injuries to the head, face, and neck occur with more frequency in children than in adults.—Due to the relatively larger size of the child's head, face, and neck, these areas are injured more frequently than in adults.

12. a. during the winter months.—Other risk factors that have been identified include: male, premature, and low-birth weight infants are at high risk; infants with respiratory infection are at high risk; and maternal smoking, placing the infant on the stomach, and a family history of SIDS are also high risks.

13. a. access to drugs and alcohol.—Even children have a choice about drinking and taking drugs.

14. b. viral infections.—Cold or flu are the most common triggers. Other common triggers include: exposure to smoke, irritants, or strong odors, exercise, allergies, respiratory infections, and stress or emotions.

15. a. headache and muscle ache.—Stomachache and lack of energy are also common physical complaints.

16. a. emotional—Child abuse and neglect occur when a child is injured or allowed to be injured by someone who was entrusted with their care.

17. b. the location and color of each bruise.—Be objective and report exactly what you see.

18. b. signs of malnourishment—The others are signs of physical abuse.

19. a. severe head trauma.—Because infants have weak neck muscles and heads that are proportionately larger than their bodies, small rips and tears occur in the brain. This can result in a subdural hematoma from the bleeding, swelling of the brain (edema), and/or retinal hemorrhages.

20. b. under one year old when trauma is inflicted.—Other predisposing risk factors include: male child (60%), young parents, families below the poverty level, and a baseline with a preexisting medical or physical disability.

21. a. the same—The risk factors vary in each age group.

22. c. meningitis—To date, there is no vaccination for meningitis.

23. a. rash and feces.—The disease is spread by direct contact with rashes and fecal matter. Frequent hand washing helps to prevent the spread of this disease.

24. c. saliva or blood.—This disease is spread by direct contact with blood and saliva.

25. c. meningococcemia meningitis—This type of bacterial meningitis requires special isolation procedures, since it is highly contagious.

26. a. Febrile seizures have no lasting neurological effects.—These seizures are associated with a rapid rise in body temperatures. The post-ictal period is usually brief, but the child remains tired from the event.

27. d. Asthma—Asthma can occur at any age but is prominent in the three-to-twelve-year-old age group.

28. b. presenting with Reye's syndrome.—This disease process affects multiple body systems and is characterized by severe edema of the brain, increased ICP, hypoglycemia, and liver dysfunction. The cause is unknown, but it is usually associated with a previous viral infection. There is also an association between the administration of aspirin for fever, particularly with flu and chicken pox.

29. b. IV fluids and seizure precautions.—Out-of-hospital treatment is supportive of the ABCs, with IV fluids and seizure precautions.

30. c. inflammation, excess mucus production, and bronchoconstriction—To date, it is still unknown what causes asthma. However, there are various triggers that are well known.

31. c. Bronchiolitis—Bronchiolitis is produced by a viral infection. Symptoms are often indistinguishable from asthma.

32. d. asthma attack—Air trapping and difficulty exhaling are major characteristics of asthma.

33. c. nebulized Ventolin.—Keep the child calm and provide continuous nebulized bronchodilators (e.g., albuterol, ipratropium, epinephrine, or levalbuterol).

34. d. Pneumonia—Ask about a recent history of upper respiratory infection.

35. a. under; above—Croup is caused by viral or other infections, including ear infections that may cause the tissue of the upper airway to swell.

36. d. As airways enlarge, some children outgrow the condition.—There is a tendency for some children to outgrow the condition.

37. c. decreased level of consciousness.—When the child can no longer compensate and becomes physically exhausted, ventilatory failure and respiratory arrest quickly follow.

38. a. prolonged infection.—Sepsis, metabolic disorders, or brain disorders affecting thermoregulatory centers can be the cause of hypothermia in pediatrics.

39. c. hyperglycemic.—High blood sugar, excess thirst (polydipsia), and urination (polyuria) are the signs of new onset diabetes mellitus.

40. d. while the fetus is developing in utero.—These defects occur while the child is developing and are present at birth.

41. a. disrupt normal blood flow.—There are more than thirty-five different types of heart defects.

42. a. stenosis.—Many conditions can be corrected surgically due to significant advances in surgery.

43. d. asystole.—Irregular rhythms, murmurs, and bundle-branch blocks are generally not as common in children as adults.

44. c. hypoxia—Hypoxia leads to acidosis and suppression of the SA node, causing bradycardia. Correction of the hypoxia with oxygen usually corrects the bradycardia.

45. b. conjunctivitis.—Also called pink eye.

46. d. dehydration.—A common childhood condition caused by one or a combination of the following: fever, nausea, vomiting, diarrhea, burns, loss of appetite, and poor feeding.

47. d. gentle cooling measures—Febrile seizures, in most cases, do not require aggressive or invasive treatment modalities. Gentle cooling and fever reducers (acetaminophen) work in most cases. If seizures persist, Valium is indicated.

48. c. epiglottitis.—A relatively rare, potentially life-threatening infection that causes a severely inflamed and swollen epiglottis. Infection can occur at any age, but three to six years of age is the most common.

49. b. Visualize the airway for an obstruction.—Allow the child to take the most comfortable, but safe, position. Keep the child calm, and avoid alarming the child by looking in the airway, slamming ambulance doors, using excessive speed, or using the siren.

50. a. Consider the use of blow-by oxygen.—It is paramount to keep the child calm and avoid agitating

him, as this can worsen the condition. The swollen epiglottis has the potential to completely obstruct the airway.

51. a. immediate but calm transport.—The safest means of transport is to use the child's own car seat. The child is familiar with its own seat and tends to stay calm there. Keep a parent next to the child, within the patient's eyesight.

52. b. the patient's mental status.—Respiratory depression and depressed mental status are the concerns with methadone overdose.

53. c. 0.1 mg/kg naloxone.—If respiratory depression needs to be reversed, administer naloxone slowly to bring the patient to a more alert status. Be prepared to manage an agitated and possible physical patient!

54. b. head, chest, and lower extremities—By the MOI, head injury is probably the reason for unconsciousness. The size of the patient places the child at risk for specific injury patterns that involve the head, chest, and lower extremities.

55. b. Waddel's triad.—The child is tall enough that the bumper strikes the femurs (1); the child is thrown up onto the hood, striking the chest (2); and the child is thrown to the ground, where he strikes his head (3); creating a predictable triad of injuries.

Chapter 44: Geriatrics

1. d. Gerontology—The comprehensive study of aging and the problems associated with aging.

2. b. loss of elastic fiber.—The loss of sebaceous glands and vascularity in the skin affects thermoregulation.

3. b. decreased muscle and bone mass.—Consistent weight-bearing exercise can slow this process.

4. a. decreased gag reflex responses increase the risk of aspiration.—This can occur with some disease processes but is not related to aging.

5. b. catecholamine—Cardiac output decreases with age, and coronary artery disease predominates in the elderly.

6. d. increased depression—The other choices are sociological rather than psychological.

7. a. decrease in thyroid function.—These changes bring about a long list of symptoms: fatigue, weakness, cold intolerance, muscle and joint aches, hypertension, and many more.

8. b. the drop in sexual hormone levels.—The ovaries begin to produce less of the three sex hormones: estrogen, androgen, and progesterone.

9. c. menopausal syndrome.—Some of the symptoms include: fatigue, depression, headaches, irritability, nervousness, insomnia, stress, incontinence, decreased sexual drive, and vaginal dryness.

10. b. five—Most of the baby boomer generation will be age sixty-five or older by this year.

11. d. all of the above—Women are still living longer than men, as well as the groups described.

12. c. quadruple—Depressive symptoms are an important indicator of the general well-being and mental health of older Americans.

13. a. heart disease—Risk factors for heart disease include obesity, hypertension, diabetes, smoking, elevated cholesterol, poor diet, and lack of exercise.

14. d. brain and vessels tear on the sharp, bony edges inside the skull.—The brain atrophies (shrinks) with age. The subdural space enlarges, and veins become stretched. When the patient experiences rapid acceleration or deceleration forces, the brain and vessels tear on the sharp, bony edges inside the skull.

15. b. Younger adults tend to die from ACS rather than heart failure.—Heart failure is more common in those over sixty-five. The underlying cause of heart failure may be from an acute MI, dysrhythmia, aneurysm, anemia, fever, or hypertension.

16. a. diminished pain perception.—A decreased catecholamine response affects the ability to increase the heart rate in response to stress and exercise. This may mask the typical pain a younger person might experience. Certain medications (beta-blockers) have the same effect.

17. c. hypertension—One of the main problems associated with hypertension is that it is often asymptomatic until severe complications (e.g., stroke) occur.

18. d. pulmonary embolism—The history suggests pulmonary embolism: a patient that presents with difficulty breathing that progressively worsens, pleuritic chest pain, anxiety, leg pain, and typically no cough or fever. Often the patient is overweight with a history of heart failure, recent surgery or immobilization, and estrogen use.

19. a. IV access only.—The patient has a cardiac history with respiratory distress. She also has a history that suggests the possibility of a pulmonary embolus. Contact medical control for early notification and any other orders.

20. d. neurologic—Behavioral emergencies include: anxiety, paranoia, hostility, wandering, and uncooperativeness; psychiatric—depression; and metabolic—dehydration, infection, and drug toxicity.

21. b. injuries from falling.—Emergencies in Parkinson's patients usually result from falls, dementia, and dysphagia.

22. b. Alzheimer's—A major, leading cause of death in the elderly. It can run its course in just a few years or last as long as twenty years; the average is nine years.

23. c. Depressive symptoms—Higher rates of depressive symptoms are associated with higher rates of physical illness, functional disability, and higher healthcare resource usage.

24. a. hypothermia.—Symptoms associated with hypothyroidism include: fatigue, weakness, cold intolerance, muscle and joint aches, hypertension, and many more.

25. b. the elderly have decreased susceptibility to certain infections.—Diabetes increases the risk of developing infections and complications associated with them.

26. c. hemorrhoids and colorectal cancer.—Other common causes include: peptic ulcer, diverticular disease, and angiodysplasia.

27. a. bowel obstruction—Signs and symptoms of a bowel obstruction are acute onset of pain, cramps, vomiting, distention, and constipation.

28. b. stable with a bowel obstruction—The patient states that she is in a lot of pain. The acute onset of pain with cramps suggests a bowel obstruction. Her vital signs are stable.

29. d. hydrocodone—Pain medications (e.g., codeine) often cause constipation.

30. b. Paget's disease—For bone diseases, Paget's is second only to osteoporosis in frequency.

31. c. ibuprofen—This is one of the most common nonsteroidal anti-inflammatories (NSAIDs). The most serious side effect of NSAIDs is GI bleeding.

32. d. drug toxicity.—Geriatric patients have a higher risk of an adverse reaction. If a patient is taking a medication, assume that it could be contributing to just about any health problem.

33. d. senior retirement facilities—The other choices are types of nursing homes, to which federal regulations apply.

34. a. intermediate care facility—This is one type of nursing facility.

35. c. Fractures from falls cost an estimated one billion dollars annually in the United States.—The cost is considerably more just for medical care costs each year.

36. b. the tasks of daily living.—Affective disorders, such as forgetfulness, distractibility, or difficulty following directions, interfere with the tasks of daily living. Injuries commonly occur with driving, falling, wandering, and cooking.

37. a. digitalis—With aging, there is a decrease in circulation as well as renal and liver functions, which in turn causes a decrease in the metabolic rate and results in more drugs in the system. The increased amount of drugs in the system can reach lethal levels, commonly referred to as drug toxicity. Some of the most common drugs that produce drug toxicity are digitalis, lidocaine, and various beta-blockers.

38. c. Pressure sores—The greatest incidence occurs in those of sixty-five years of age. Prevention is the best medicine.

39. c. severe infection.—Because of a decrease in the function of the thermoregulatory system and the body's impaired ability to maintain homeostasis, even a modest elevation or subnormal temperature is an indication for concern. This is especially true when it is associated with confusion, loss of appetite, or other behavioral changes. Consider that hypothermia in the elderly is due to a severe infection (e.g., pneumonia, urinary tract infections, and sepsis) until proven otherwise.

40. d. family members.—Abusers can be anyone that an older person comes in contact with.

41. c. resistance abuse—The other choices are forms of elder abuse.

42. b. obtaining infectious pulmonary diseases.—The cilia in the airway act as a filter. When the filter and cough reflex become less effective, the risk of developing a respiratory illness increases. A diminished gag reflex increases the risk of aspiration.

43. a. cause any additional injury.—The older patient can be very fragile. Bones can be easily fractured during a move.

44. a. severe infection—Because of the decreased function of the thermoregulatory system and the body's impaired ability to maintain homeostasis, even a modest elevation or subnormal temperature are indications for concern, especially when is associated with confusion, loss of appetite, or other behavioral changes.

45. b. vertebral fractures.—Hip fractures in older people increase their mortality significantly during the following year. This is true even if the patient is in good health prior to suffering the fracture.

46. a. developing dementia—Dementia is not a normal part of aging. In fact, only 30% of patients over eighty-five years of age show a significant progressive decline in cognitive function.

47. c. hypoglycemia—Hypoxia and hypoglycemia must be ruled out first in any patient with altered mental status, not just the elderly.

48. d. all of the above.—When confusion is not acute, get a good history from the family or caretakers and do a thorough physical exam to begin to rule out each of the conditions listed.

49. b. Diabetes—Complications of diabetes lead to many other diseases.

50. c. Hospice programs—Hospice care emphasizes comfort measures and counseling to meet physical, spiritual, social, and economic needs. This care is under medical supervision.

Chapter 45: The Challenged Patient

1. c. sensorineural—One of two types of hearing impairments. The nervous system is unable to perceive or transmit sound impulses due to damage to nerve or brain tissue.

2. d. unless you are making direct eye contact.—Many people with borderline hearing impairment are unaware that they have a problem. If a patient frequently asks you to repeat what you said, suspect a hearing impairment.

3. b. Speaking slowly with exaggerated lip movement.—Many deaf and hearing-impaired people are able to read lips. Speak slowly, but do no exaggerate your lip movements. Lip readers are trained to read normal lip movement, not exaggerated ones.

4. c. strokes and CNS infections.—The two most common etiologies of visual impairment are injury and disease.

5. a. acute head injury—Sometimes acute head injury may cause transient blindness.

6. a. fluency—Stuttering may also be associated with psychiatric or developmental disorders.

7. a. aphasia.—Common causes include: stroke, head injury, brain tumor, delayed development, hearing loss, lack of stimulation, or emotional disturbance.

8. b. dysarthria.—An articulation disorder; patients often have slurred, indistinct, slow, or nasal-sounding speech.

9. d. voice production—Though the neuromuscular pathways are intact, voice production disorders result from factors that impair the proper functioning of the vocal cords.

10. a. hearing loss with an acute onset—An acute loss is often associated with an emergent event (e.g., trauma or stroke).

11. a. a low metabolic rate.—Other etiologies include excess insulin production and the use of steroids.

12. c. psychoses—The person with psychoses truly believes his situation or condition is real.

13. b. talk—In a drug-induced psychosis, hallucinogens or stimulant agents cause the patient to lose touch with reality. Often, the patient develops hyperactive and sometimes dangerous behavior.

14. b. the brain.—Developmental disabilities result in an inability to learn at the usual rate.

15. d. they have abnormal intestines.—The other choices are special consideration for Down syndrome patients.

16. d. deficiency of neurotransmitters.—Psychosis is when the patient has no concept of reality. This condition may also be induced by drugs.

17. a. maladaptive behavior.—This means that a person is unable to properly adapt to various challenging circumstances for a variety of different reasons.

18. a. Decreased range of motion may limit the physical exam.—More time than usual may be necessary to complete a physical exam and to move the patient.

19. a. transdermal medication patches.—Be alert for these, as they are not always obvious. Too much pain medication can cause altered mental status, respiratory depression, and other problems necessitating the call for EMS.

20. c. understands everything you say and do.—Cerebral palsy is a nonprogressive disorder of movement and posture. Most patients are highly intelligent.

21. b. is prone to mood disorders.—This is a common problem associated with multiple sclerosis patients.

22. a. many common medications may worsen an exacerbation.—Always contact medical control prior to administering any drugs other than oxygen.

23. a. catheters—If present, catheters may need attention. Problems with shunts may also be the purpose of an EMS call, but care of these problems is managed in the hospital.

24. a. six to twelve months—The phrase "terminally ill" is subject to widespread interpretation. For EMS providers, it usually means the patient has a condition that, regardless of any current available treatment, will result in death within the next six to twelve months.

25. a. DNAR status.—The most important consideration for the paramedic is a clear understanding of the patient's "end of life" decisions. Follow your local protocol for "no code," "living will," and other related determinations. Whenever possible, follow the patient's wishes.

26. c. try to convince him that his health should be the first priority.—Competent patients do have the right to refuse any or all care offered. When a patient has a financial concern, knowledge about your local resources may make the difference.

27. b. Acknowledge that the competent patient has a right to refuse care.—Competent patients do have the right to refuse any or all care offered.

28. a. injury or earwax.—Conductive deafness is caused by an obstruction, usually in the external ear canal.

29. b. high-pitched—This is why you should avoid shouting and use low-pitched sounds directly in the ear canal.

30. b. multiple sclerosis—There are many disease processes that cause both temporary and permanent vision loss.

31. c. Pad the contractures and use extra care during the move.—Gentle handling may take extra time, but it is necessary. Make the patient as comfortable as possible and never force an extremity, as it may cause an injury.

32. a. respiratory support—This may include oxygenation, assisted ventilation, CPAP, or suctioning.

33. b. pointing to an area of the body before touching it.—A calm and professional manner goes far. Facial expressions are universal.

34. d. culturally based preferences may conflict with a paramedic's learned medical practice.—Be aware of cultural differences, but not to the point of limiting your thinking about the other person.

35. a. All people share common problems or situations.—Making this presumption may be a mistake. A patient's culturally based preferences may conflict with the learned medical practice of the EMS provider.

36. d. appropriately sized diagnostic devices.—One example is the need for an extra-large blood pressure cuff.

37. b. Speak in English first to determine if she can understand even a little of the language.—Attempt to obtain a reliable interpreter as soon as possible, and notify the ED in advance so they can do the same.

38. a. describe everything she is going to do before actually doing it.—Don't hesitate to ask patients about the best way you can help them navigate.

39. a. expressive aphasia—Patients often know what they want to say but are unable to speak their thoughts. This often leads to frustration, anger, and depression for the patient.

40. a. The patient is most likely very alert and frustrated by this deficit.—Allow the patient time to respond to questions and provide any aids (e.g., writing tablet, pictures) necessary, if available.

41. c. trauma.—The most common cause of para- or quadriplegia is spinal cord injury.

42. a. involving the alert and oriented patient in any decisions regarding movement and transport.—Chances are good that the patient has gone through the move before. The patient often knows more about his own particular needs than you do.

43. a. psychotic person—When psychosis is drug induced (e.g., hallucinogens or stimulants), it is common for the patient to develop hyperactive and sometimes dangerous behavior.

44. c. 20–30%—There are numerous underlying and often related causes.

45. b. three—Moving and transporting a very large person may present special challenges.

46. b. minor symptoms.—An example is a minor cough in an otherwise healthy older person. This person can unknowingly infect every healthcare person with whom she comes into contact with an infectious disease such as tuberculosis.

47. d. Not wearing prescribed corrective lenses—When possible, allow the patient to wear or bring glasses to the hospital.

48. b. drooping eyelids and difficulty swallowing.—Patients may have vision problems, difficulty speaking, chewing, or swallowing.

49. b. supportive care and transport.—Other accommodations will vary depending on the presentation.

50. c. There has been a recent change in the patient's behavior.—There is no typical appearance or presentation for previously head-injured patients. Ask about the patient's baseline mental status and behavior, and if there have been any recent changes. This is of concern and most likely the reason EMS has been called.

Chapter 46: Acute Interventions in the Home Care Patient

1. a. offer supportive healthcare of the patient living at home.—The other choices are more specific to one or the other, not both.

2. b. can provide emergency advanced cardiac life support.—Paramedics are trained in ACLS.

3. b. post MI.—Unless there are specific complications, the other patient examples do not require home health services.

4. a. complications from infections.—Other examples include airway conditions, circulatory pathologies, and wound care.

5. b. Palliative care—The goals of palliative or comfort care are to alleviate pain and other distressing symptoms for patients with potentially life-threatening illnesses and their families and friends.

6. a. shopping service—The other choices are skilled services.

7. b. dental care.—This is an example of a skilled service rather than a support service.

8. a. hospice programs.—Hospitals also provides services for the patient's family.

9. c. obstructed shunts.—This is an example of a typical complication associated with shunts. Often the patient requires transport to the ED to have the shunt cleaned or replaced.

10. a. These services help to reduce expensive inpatient stays.—These services also help to shorten inpatient stays. For most patients and their families, the preference is to receive services in their own homes and communities, rather than in institutional settings.

11. d. economic—Hospice programs and services provide significant support for the dying person and the family members as the death experience come to a culmination.

12. b. Home—There are a number of community services available that can provide care at home.

13. c. Hospice—Hospice offers services to put advanced directives in place and to help carry out the final wishes of the patient.

14. c. requires high maintenance—Neglect and abuse are high risks for this group of patients.

15. d. infections—Other complications include: sepsis, respiratory and cardiac failure, and emergencies with defective or inoperative equipment and access devices (plugged tubes, dislocated or accidentally removed tubes).

16. a. Palliative—Also called comfort care.

17. b. obstructed tubing—Problems arise with airway devices when they are improperly placed or become obstructed, and when oxygen tubing becomes blocked or the oxygen runs out.

18. c. pulmonary function meter—This device is a pulmonary exerciser commonly used at home.

19. c. PPEK—Each of the other devices is often effectively used to increase the patient's oxygenation. BiPAP (biphasic continuous positive airway pressure), CPAP (continuous positive airway pressure), and PEEP (positive end-expiratory pressure) are the modifications of traditional positive pressure ventilation.

20. c. BiPAP—Both BiPAP and CPAP may be administered by nasal cannula or face mask without endotracheal intubation.

21. a. apnea monitor.—These devices are used at home to monitor babies who have infantile apnea and with adults who have sleep apnea.

22. b. discomfort—Easing the discomfort associated with a new vascular access device (VAD) can be managed at home by a skilled healthcare provider.

23. d. Extracath®—The other devices are well known VADs used both in the hospital and at home.

24. a. embolism—Problems that arise with VADs are due to infection, clotting, dislodgement, extravasation, hemorrhage, embolism, or an infusion given too rapidly.

25. a. ventilatory support as needed and rapid transport.—Oxygenation and ventilatory support are the primary concerns with embolism.

26. a. Canadian catheter®.—The other devices are well-known urinary catheters used both in the hospital and at home.

27. d. P-tubes—The other devices are well known GI tract devices used both in the hospital and at home.

28. b. UTI and urinary retention.—These devices may be short or long term.

29. c. leaking catheter—The other choices may be discovered during an assessment but are not problems associated with failure of the device.

30. b. choose the place to die and time of death.—The patient also has the right to: know the truth, confidentially and privacy, consent to treatment, and determine the disposition of his body.

31. b. five—When a person first learns he is dying, he typically experiences shock and disbelief. Then acceptance comes after moments or months, and the person enters the second state, "anger." Bargaining is followed by depression. Finally, acceptance is achieved in the final stage of detachment.

32. b. anger.—Many dying patients experience anger as well as the other stages: shock, bargaining, depression, and acceptance.

33. d. detachment.—Acceptance comes in the last stage.

34. a. squamous.—The other choices are wound-closure devices that patients may be sent home with.

35. c. urostomy—The other devices are gastric emptying devices.

36. b. ostomy.—Ostomys are common in the home care setting.

37. a. VAD—VADs and medication ports are common in home care settings. They are used to administer medication, maintain long-term vascular access, and provide nutritional support.

38. c. systemic infection—The signs and symptoms suggest a systemic infection.

39. d. all of the above—All of the questions are necessary to ask when a patient has a complaint of abdominal pain.

40. c. obstruction—No bowel movement in two days is abnormal for most people. Obstruction should be suspected, but keep an open mind about other potential problems.

41. c. position of comfort and supportive care.—There is no indication to provide any other specific treatment.

42. d. any of the above—A urinary tract infection (UTI) is common and very likely with patients with urinary catheters.

43. b. supportive care and routine transport.—Fever and altered mental status (confusion) are commonly associated with UTIs.

44. a. they often know more about the patient's special needs than anyone else.—Do not hesitate to ask for their expertise, if needed.

45. a. Wait for hospice to arrive and then leave.—Sometimes the family gets nervous and calls EMS. Hospice serves an important role, and EMS providers should cooperate fully with the family and hospice representatives to comply with the patient's wishes.

Chapter 47: Ambulance Operations and Medical Incident Command

1. b. State—Minimum standards for ambulance operations specify the worst they could let things get and still be allowed to operate.

2. d. ambulance design and manufacturing requirements.—These specifications are an attempt to influence safety standards, as well as standardize the look of ambulances.

3. d. as a risk-management tool.—Completing the ambulance equipment and supply checklist helps make the work environment safer for the EMS provider.

4. c. Restock items to be obtained from the hospital.—The list is dynamic and changes from call to call.

5. a. routinely checking expiration dates.—Many expiration dates fall at the beginning or end of the month.

6. c. after the transport of any patient with a potentially communicable disease.—OSHA is charged with setting and enforcing standards for worker safety.

7. b. cleaning requirements.—This plan must also state how personnel should clean up a blood spill in the ambulance.

8. b. ambulance deployment.—Deployment is often based on the location of existing facilities to station the ambulance, location of hospitals, geographic considerations, and the anticipated call volume in each area of the community.

9. d. Reserve capacity—Some services ask off-duty personnel to carry pagers or sign up for backup coverage.

10. b. system status management.—This is one method of deployment that has become popular in recent years.

11. a. its resources.—The standards of reliability of a response agency take into consideration the percentage of the time that high-priority calls are responded to within an agreed-upon system response time.

12. d. patient.—This clearly relates to the ambulance operator, as well as to the EMS providers.

13. d. all of the above.—The effect on your agency's reputation in the community is another cost to consider.

14. c. due regard.—Due regard is a responsibility that the operator of an emergency vehicle takes on when operating an emergency vehicle.

15. b. higher—Nowhere in the motor vehicle laws does it say any other driver is responsible for the safety of all other motorists.

16. c. the posted parking regulations.—Some allow exemptions from posted speed limits, the posted direction of travel, and the requirement to stop and wait at a red light.

17. c. 50 to 100—Do not rely solely on the lights and siren to alert the other motorists. Be sure to leave plenty of room around your vehicle and get a face-to-face commitment from other drivers that they understand where your vehicle is going.

18. c. use the siren at all times while the lights are on.—Some states have specific laws, or services have SOPs, that address the actual use of the siren. Some states have very old laws that do not even use the word "siren" (e.g., audible device). Always assume that another driver is going to behave erratically when she suddenly notices the siren or red lights. Expect the unexpected!

19. a. increase its visibility.—Alternating headlamps should only be used on nighttime calls if they are installed in a secondary lamp.

20. a. 50 feet in front of—Park at least 50 feet in front of the wreckage if your ambulance is the first emergency vehicle on the scene, so your warning lights can warn approaching motorist before flares can be set up.

21. d. Maryland—The Maryland state police medevac program continues to set the gold standards, which other programs try to emulate.

22. b. multiple casualty incident—Sometimes the term MCI is used for a mass casualty incident. This is misleading because it gives providers the impression that the MCI plan should be saved for the "big one."

23. a. specific location of the incident.—The report should also include the extent of the incident and the approximate number of patients.

24. d. closed—An example of a closed incident is an overturned bus where there is limited access to the passengers inside.

25. b. equipment and facilities.—ICS also consists of procedures for controlling personnel and communications.

26. c. the requirement for management and operations no longer exists.—Though originally developed for the fire service, ICS has been adapted to serve all emergency response disciplines.

27. b. Planning—Planning is also responsible for the collection, evaluation, dissemination, and use of information about the development of the incident and the status of the resources.

28. b. span of control—It can be very easy to lose track of your workers at an incident if they are not assigned to small units.

29. d. developing the incident action plan.—The IC is also responsible for assessing incident priorities and determining the strategic goals.

30. a. making it easy to identify the command officers.— These can be easily donned over the uniform and outer coat.

31. c. triage—It is not a good idea to take a physician or nurse who is not familiar with the workings of your EMS system and put her in a sector officer position.

32. b. they do not take any training to use.—Triage tags can be very useful tools. The hardest part is getting the crews to pull them out and start using them.

33. d. commanders can critique without the fear of offending anyone.—There is something to be learned from each incident so we can do a better job the next time. In a nonthreatening manner, the commanders of each emergency service should schedule a critique to discuss the incident.

34. d. the function they serve.—During an MCI is not the time to begin figuring out another agency's "code system."

35. c. to work cooperatively with other emergency commanders—Responsibilities also include managing the EMS response, designating the EMS division or sector officers, and establishing a command post and remaining there.

36. a. open—An open incident is one where the patients are accessible and the EMS providers will have safe access to the patients.

37. c. logistics—The size of the incident will help determine when and how much logistics are required.

38. d. unified command.—A unified command structure is the more common and key component of an ICS.

39. b. unified command post.—This means that all involved agencies contribute to the command process by determining the overall goals and objectives, joint planning for tactical activities, and maximizing the use of all assigned resources at the incident.

40. d. simple triage and rapid transport.—The START process permits a few rescuers to triage large numbers of patients very rapidly.

41. a. the most serious patients are treated and transported first.—In situations where there are many serious patients and limited ambulances, the very critical patients who have a small chance of survival are given the lowest priority.

42. a. to never let the driver, keys, or stretcher get separated from their ambulance.—This mistake has resulted in unnecessary fatalities and delays in patient care.

43. b. identify the location and size of the ambulance.— The vehicle must be clearly visible from 360° to all other motorists.

44. c. open rear doors—Always assume that oncoming traffic does not see you, and that, even if they do, they often won't pull over or slow down.

45. a. remote regions, such as parts of Alaska.—In addition, these aircraft are often used to bring critical patients who sustain serious medical emergencies or injuries while traveling from faraway places back to a hospital closer to their home.

46. b. limited treatment area in the aircraft.—Depending on the specific aircraft used, the cabin size can place limitations on the crew members, equipment carried, and configuration of the stretcher in the aircraft.

47. c. 100×100—All EMS providers should be capable of selecting a landing zone (LZ) and describing the terrain, major landmarks, estimated distance to the nearest town, and other pertinent information to the pilot of the helicopter on a designated frequency.

48. a. Convert IV bags over to pressure infuser bags.— Problems arise during ascent and descent when pressures change with altitude.

49. d. strengthen the safety of the aviation transport environment.—CAAMS also serves to promote the highest quality of patient care.

50. a. cabin size.—Depending on the specific aircraft used, the cabin size can place limitations on the crew members, equipment carried, and configuration of the stretcher in the aircraft.

Chapter 48: Rescue Awareness and Operations

1. c. awareness—Awareness-level training implies enough knowledge to comprehend the hazards and realize that additional expertise is needed to effect the rescue.

2. c. the patient's medical condition—Because there is no rescue if there is no patient, all rescues should be driven by patient need. Just as in patient care, the first concern is rescuer safety.

3. a. comprehend the hazards.—Failing to train EMS providers in rescue awareness eventually ends in injury to the EMS personnel or patient.

4. c. a combination of a and b.—Rescue involves a combination of medical and mechanical skills, with correct amounts of each applied at the appropriate time.

5. d. all of the above.—The paramedic's role may be more involved depending on how much training he has.

6. b. when it is or is not safe to gain access.—One of the major benefits of rescue awareness training is to avoid a provider attempting a rescue for which he is not trained.

7. a. helmets and eye protection—Personal safety must be the paramount issue in any rescue situation. For most rescues, the minimum PPE should include eye protection, a helmet, and the appropriate gloves.

8. b. They do not withstand severe impact.—The best rescue helmets have a four-point, nonelastic suspension system, in contrast to the two-point system found in construction hard hats.

9. d. climbing helmets—Climbing helmets are often used for confined space and technical rescue situations.

10. a. ANSI.—The eye protection should include both goggles, vented to prevent fogging, and industrial safety glasses held by an elastic band. These should be ANSI (American National Standards Institute) approved.

11. d. industrial safety glasses.—The face shield on most fire helmets is inadequate protection for your eyes.

12. c. leather work gloves.—In addition to disposable rubber or latex gloves for BSI purposes, leather work gloves, such as those used for gardening, are usually best for protection against cuts and punctures.

13. a. provide limited flash protection.—These materials provide limited flash protection and should be strongly considered as part of the EMS provider's personal protection.

14. b. aluminized rescue blankets—A variety of protective blankets should be available to shield patients from debris, fire, or weather. Aluminum rescue blankets protect from fire, heat, or glass dust.

15. c. backboards—Short and long backboards and other commonly found equipment can be used as shields to protect patients.

16. c. surgical mask—Surgical masks or commercial dust masks are adequate for most occasions. These should be routinely supplied to all EMS units.

17. d. Go—The water rescue model is Reach-Throw-Go.

18. d. hypothermia.—Compared to the normal human body temperature of 98.6°F, almost any body of water is colder and causes heat loss.

19. c. SOPs.—Standard operating procedures should include sections on all types of anticipated rescue and specify the required safety equipment, particular actions required or prohibited, and any rescue-specific modifications in assignments. SOPs should include a statement requiring a safety officer and describing his relationship to command.

20. d. arrival and size-up, hazard control, and gaining access to the patient.—The last four phases are medical treatment, disentanglement, patient packaging, and transportation.

21. d. safety officer.—The safety officer should be someone with the knowledge and authority to intervene in unsafe situations.

22. b. provide immense psychological support.—This is especially true in situations where the patient is entrapped and disentanglement will take a significant amount of time.

23. b. Improvement of personnel safety and operational success.—Preplan also generates ideas on the efficient use of existing personnel and equipment, and anticipates the need for additional equipment, rescuers, or expertise.

24. d. all of the above.—This is the purpose of logistics as a functional component of an IMS.

25. c. coffee.—Caffeine is actually a diuretic, which should be avoided when hydration is needed.

26. a. conduct a scene size-up.—The first arriving crew must immediately establish medical command and conduct a scene size-up to determine the number of patients and appoint a triage officer and other personnel as necessary.

27. b. to determine if it is a body recovery—The decision about whether the incident is a search, a rescue, or a body recovery must be made quickly.

28. c. creating a safe perimeter.—The EMS provider's approach should be limited to creating a safe perimeter, attempting to identify the substance involved from a safe position, and keeping bystanders and EMS personnel away from the hot zone.

29. c. Wearing the appropriate PPE—Additional precautions include making sure all EMS personnel are clearly visible and always alert to traffic.

30. a. A confined space—A potentially hazardous confined space may be a cave or a mine.

31. c. an on-scene SAR specialist.—If possible, ask dispatch to send an on-scene specialist (search and rescue team member) to meet the crew. Search dogs, electronic detection devices, or an experienced search manager may be required to find the patients.

32. a. after gaining access—After gaining access, medical personnel can begin to make patient contact. No EMS provider should enter an area to provide patient care unless she is protected from hazards with PPE and has the technical skills to reach, manage, and remove patients safely.

33. c. protected from hazards with PPE.—All EMS personnel must have on the PPE appropriate for the specific type of rescue.

34. c. disentanglement.—Disentanglement literally means removing the wreckage from the victim, not the other way around.

35. c. just removed from a pool.—In many situations, the best overall patient care requires the rapid basic stabilization and immediate removal of the patient rather than ALS interventions done at the site of an incident. This example is not typically one of those situations.

36. b. risk of injury to the rescuers.—Final positive patient outcome may depend on the initial sacrifice of definitive patient care so the patient and rescuers can be removed from imminent danger.

37. c. disentanglement—The methods used to disentangle the patient must each be analyzed for their risk versus benefit to the patient's medical needs and the estimated time they take to perform.

38. b. means of egress.—Some patient packaging can be more complex than others, considering the specialized rescue techniques required to get them out of the situation they were found in.

39. b. SKED.—The SKED can be a useful substitute for a Stokes® in tight places. If the patient has a possible spine injury, place him on the long backboard first, then put him into the SKED.

40. c. Wear a PFD around water or ice.—Also consider learning to swim if you don't already know, and take a basic water rescue course.

41. d. Hypothermia can set in rapidly.—Compared to the normal human body temperature of 98.6°F, almost any body of water is colder and causes heat loss.

42. d. 92—The colder the water, the faster the loss of heat. Compared to the air, water causes heat loss at a rate twenty-five times faster.

43. b. loss; 25—Compared to the air, water causes a heat loss at a rate twenty-five times faster. Immersion for more than fifteen to twenty minutes in 35°F water is likely to be fatal.

44. b. They may be dehydrated from cold diuresis.—A horizontal position can help to avoid orthostatic stressed.

45. b. HELP—The heat-escape lessoning position (HELP) involves floating with the head out of the water and the body in a fetal tuck. Researchers estimate that someone who has practiced with HELP can reduce his heat loss by almost 60% as compared to treading water.

46. b. past history of submersion—Other factors to consider include: temperature and speed of the water, number of patients, and the environmental conditions present and expected.

47. d. Recirculating water is difficult to get out of.—The low head dam produces a "drowning machine" as the water recirculates, making it nearly impossible to swim clear of the dam.

48. a. Float downstream, feet first.—Steer with your feet and point your head toward the nearest shore at a 45° angle, or continue to float downstream until you come to an area where the water is slow enough for you to swim to the river's edge.

49. a. a large boulder in the water.—The current can force a patient up against a strainer, making if difficult to be removed due to the power of the water flow.

50. d. outside; faster than the inside—If you are being carried rapidly downstream, steer to the inside of the next curve in the river.

51. c. 50—Many states have enacted tough laws to restrict the operation of a boat while intoxicated.

52. d. each boater wearing a PFD—Wearing a PFD around water can reduce drownings considerably.

53. b. mammalian diving reflex.—The mammalian diving reflex, which can increase the chances of a cold-water submersion patient's survival. Because of the reflex, saved lives have been documented from cold immersions of up to sixty-six minutes.

54. a. the precise location where the patient went under.—Try to establish a location of the submerged patient based on quick interviews with witnesses.

55. c. three—Backboarding and extrication from the water requires at least three EMS providers in the water and additional rescuers at the water's edge.

56. d. 60—The major problem with confined spaces is that they often are oxygen deficient. Consequently, as a rescue category, confined-space rescues have the highest fatality rate among potential rescuers.

57. a. They are oxygen deficient.—Most confined spaces appear, at first glance, to be relatively safe. As a result, rescue procedures may appear far less difficult, time consuming, or dangerous than they actually are.

58. d. Most employers are required to develop a confined-space rescue program.—These programs provide training for their employees who work in and around confined spaces. These employees may be called upon to perform on-site rescues.

59. c. It can create an explosive hazard.—The patient can get buried in fine solid materials that can flow like sand, such as grain, coal, or dust. Dust also creates an explosive hazard.

60. c. a trench cave-in.—Most trench collapses occur in trenches less than 12 feet deep and 6 feet wide. Patients are suddenly covered with heavy soil, resulting in hypoxia.

61. b. establishing a perimeter.—If the collapse caused burial, a secondary collapse is likely to occur. Call for the team specializing in trench rescue and do not allow entry into the trench or cave-in area. Specially trained personnel should make safe access only after shoring in place.

62. a. shoring is in place.—Specially trained personnel should make safe access only after shoring in place.

63. d. traffic—The greatest concern is the traffic itself. Studies have shown that drivers who are drugged, intoxicated, or tired actually drive right into the emergency lights.

64. a. the risk of fire or explosion.—There may be a natural gas or high-pressure tank at risk of fire or explosion. Electrical-powered vehicles have storage cells that may be very dangerous.

65. b. not be directly exposed to traffic.—Ambulance lights to warn traffic are often obstructed when the doors are open for loading.

66. b. turn on only a minimum of warning lights.—When too many lights are used, it is very confusing and blinding to the oncoming traffic.

67. a. direct the flow of traffic away from emergency workers.—As soon as the first unit arrives on the

scene, flares or cones should be placed to direct traffic away from the collision.

68. a. The potential for a fire hazard is increased.—Under each vehicle is a catalytic converter (which has a temperature around 1,200°F), which is a good source of ignition for a fire.

69. b. If loaded, they may release when unexpected.—The bumpers on many vehicles have pistons in them and are designed to withstand a slow-speed collision to limit the damage to the front or rear of the vehicle. Sometimes these bumpers become loaded in the crushed position and do not immediately bounce back out.

70. d. it can inflate when not expected.—Airbags that have not deployed during a collision, have been known to deploy in the middle of extrication.

71. b. stabilize the vehicle.—Remember to turn off the ignition and set the vehicle in park. If trained to do so, temporarily stabilize the vehicle ropes, chocks, or a come-a-long until the vehicle rescue team has arrived at the scene.

72. c. Stabilize the vehicle with cribbing.—Setting cribbing and chocking the wheels are simple measures the paramedic can take to stabilize a vehicle.

73. b. firewall.—The firewall can collapse on a patient's legs when involved in a high-speed, head-on collision. Sometimes the patient's feet may go through the firewall.

74. c. Nader pin.—The Nader pin must be disengaged to make it possible to pry the door open unless hydraulic jaws are used.

75. b. safety—The safety glass that is used in the windshield is designed to crack when struck with an object such as a flying stone. When shattered or broken, safety glass stays intact.

76. c. safety—It does produce glass dust and shards of glass that can easily cause cuts or get into the eyes, nose, mouth, or wounds, so it is essential to cover the patient whenever removing this type of glass.

77. a. tempered; sharp—Tempered glass is used in the side and rear windows of a vehicle, and is designed to withstand blows with a blunt object without breaking.

78. d. Nader pin—The Nader pin must be disengaged to make it possible to pry the door open unless hydraulic jaws are used.

79. d. try to open all four doors first.—Always try to open a door that may be unlocked prior to breaking any glass.

80. c. gain access through the window farthest away from the patient.—This reduces the risk of furthering injury to those inside.

81. b. inner circle.—The inner circle is where the rescue takes place. The outer circle is where equipment staging and additional personnel should wait until they are assigned a duty.

82. b. low angle.—The types of hazardous terrain are divided into low angle, high angle, or flat with obstructions.

83. b. Stokes®—The Stokes® stretcher is the standard for rough terrain evacuation. It provides a rigid frame for patient protection and is easy to carry with an adequate number of personnel.

84. a. wire and tubular metal.—The wire-mesh Stokes® baskets are the strongest of the types and provide better air and water flow through the basket.

85. d. The patient should be restrained in a body bag.—The other choices are precautions that should be taken when packaging the patient into a basket stretcher.

86. c. 6—There should be a minimum of six personnel on the Stokes®, and extra teams of six should be rotated in situations where there is a long way to carry the basket.

87. a. haul on the lines as instructed.—Any rescue requiring hauling needs plenty of helpers to assist with the hauling.

88. a. belay the basket with a rope.—When a basket is being slid down a ladder, the litter must always be belayed to prevent it from falling off.

89. d. short haul.—Many rescue helicopters use short hauls or sling loads of equipment or personnel as opposed to rappel-based rescues, which can be very dangerous.

90. b. reposition dislocations.—Additional skills the paramedic may utilize on patients who require an extensive evacuation time include: long-term hydration management, cleansing and care of wounds, removal of impaled objects, pain management, hypothermia management, and management of crush injuries and compartment syndromes.

Chapter 49: Hazardous Material Awareness and Operations

1. b. 473—Competencies for EMS Personnel Responding to Hazardous Materials Incidents—established two levels of EMS hazmat responders above the awareness level and was the first NFPA standard to specifically address EMS workers.

2. c. 704—The other choices relate to other NFPA standards.

3. b. First Responder operations—At this level, a trained person can also carry out basic decontamination procedures.

4. a. NFPA 472—Professional Competence of Responders to Hazardous Materials Incidents—this preceded and set the stage for the OSHA 1910.120 regulations.
5. b. five—First Responder awareness, First Responder operations, hazardous material technician, hazardous material specialist, and on-scene incident commander.
6. a. *North American Emergency Response Guidebook*—A well-known and used reference for identifying hazardous materials found in transport.
7. d. nonflammable.—Gases are classified as: poison A, flammable gas, nonflammable gas, and corrosive gas.
8. c. MSDS—material safety data sheets—a list of detailed information about a substance to be used when exposure occurs with that product. Employers are required to keep these on the work site.
9. d. adaptation.—The other choices are the three stages of the metabolism of a substance in the body.
10. a. Poison actions—The factors that affect poison actions are: dose, route of exposure, synergistic effects, and toxicity.
11. b. chemical—Training requirements are a significant factor that limits field decontamination.
12. a. two—Patient condition can limit the decontamination process. The more stable a patient is, the more thorough the decon that can be completed.
13. d. eight—Patient condition can limit the decontamination process. The more stable a patient is, the more thorough the decon that can be completed.
14. b. topical—Other common decon solutions are tincture of green soap, isopropyl alcohol, and vegetable oil.
15. d. milk—Milk may be used to transport a tooth that has been accidentally displaced.
16. d. reactivity.—The placards are colored and indicate specific hazards. Red = fire hazard; blue = health hazard; and yellow = reactivity hazard.
17. b. zones—These safety zones are designated as hot, warm, and cold.
18. d. Instruct the patient to remove contaminated shoes and clothing.—At this level of training, the paramedic can keep unnecessary people away from the hazard and provide first aid by having victims move into fresh air.
19. a. Dose response—Understanding this helps to determine the level of decontamination required.
20. d. critical patient condition.—The more stable a patient is, the more thorough the decon that can be completed.
21. d. threshold limit value-ceiling.—Exposure to higher concentrations must not occur.
22. c. Permissible exposure limit—The PEL is primarily intended as an exposure guide rather than as an absolute exposure limit.
23. b. access to MSDS.—Material safety data sheets are individual data sheets, rather than a manual or guidebook, used throughout the industry as a means of identifying chemicals.
24. d. Code of Federal Regulations (CFR)—EMS agencies must follow CFR 1910.1200 (the Right to Know Law) and CFR 1910.120 (Emergency Response to Hazardous Substance Releases).
25. d. Chemical Manufacturers Association—The telephone number is 1-800-424-9300.

Chapter 50: Crime Scene Awareness

1. c. Terrorism—Terrorism has become extremely heightened in recent years.
2. b. with information obtained from dispatch.—Attempt to use all available resources, such as law enforcement, prior to arrival at the scene, as well as on scene.
3. b. retreat right away.—When you are concerned for your safety, don't ever hesitate to run away.
4. c. Carbon monoxide poisoning—Poisoning from carbon monoxide can occur unknowingly and without violence.
5. d. Any of the above could cause the paramedic to be mistaken for law enforcement.—Avoid actions that make you look like a threat (law enforcement). This includes wearing a uniform similar to a police officer's.
6. c. out of sight of the scene.—Do not become an additional distraction for law enforcement.
7. a. Stand to the side of the door before ringing or knocking.—A simple form of concealment that could safe your life.
8. d. all the doors are locked.—Most vehicles have the self-locking feature which activates when the vehicle is put into gear.
9. a. exact location.—If you are struck by a vehicle, you may not be able to give the exact location.
10. b. driver would normally expect the police to approach on the driver's side.—Avoid actions that make you look like a threat (law enforcement).
11. c. have a portable radio in hand.—This way you can call for help. Many radios have an emergency button that can be activated with one finger.
12. b. it keeps them from looking like police officers.—Avoid actions that make you look like a threat (law enforcement). This includes wearing a uniform similar to a police officer's.

13. c. street gangs.—These are infamous gangs in cities and suburbs across the United States.

14. a. injuries from an explosion.—Meth labs contain highly flammable chemicals that can explode easily.

15. d. any of the above.—There are labs designed to do a variety of illegal drug processing.

16. c. booby traps to be set—The occupants of the labs are often armed and otherwise violent people.

17. c. potential for street violence.—Many of the gangs are heavily involved in drug trafficking and use underage children (minors) to conduct most of the violence.

18. c. colors—EMS providers must be careful to show respect to the colors or face deadly repercussions.

19. d. leave immediately and call law enforcement.—It is suggested that the incident command system be initiated and hazmat asked to respond, as well as the fire department.

20. b. the DEA—The local or state police may notify the Drug Enforcement Administration (DEA), which has responsibility for and expertise in this particular area.

21. c. economic—The other choices are not forms of domestic violence.

22. d. The patient has injuries that do not match her story.—Domestic violence occurs between people in a domestic relationship, such as spouses, boy- or girlfriends, or same sex relationships.

23. c. Protect the victim by getting between the victim and the abuser.—One of the most potentially dangerous situations to be in is the "middle" of a domestic disturbance. Always have a backup plan, radio in hand, and another unit at your side.

24. c. avoidance is always preferable to confrontation.—Be aware of the proper tactical response to avoid danger and know how to deal appropriately with danger in situations where it cannot be avoided.

25. b. make sure the EMD does not send any further EMS units directly into the scene.—Don't let your coworkers walk into a situation you are retreating from.

26. a. Concealment is positioning the paramedic or crew behind an object that hides them from the view of others.—Concealment offers no ballistic protection should the perpetrator begin firing a weapon at you.

27. d. Throw the equipment to slow or trip the aggressor.—Try to wedge the stretcher in the doorway to block the aggressor.

28. b. body armor does not offer protection against high-velocity rifle bullets.—It does not protect against thin or dual-edged weapons such as an ice pick either.

29. c. tactical EMS.—Tactical EMS is provided in a violent or tactically "hot" zone. This requires a working relationship with the law enforcement team, as well as special training.

30. a. CONTOMS—CONTOMS stands for Counter Narcotic and Terrorism Operational Medical Support program.

31. b. cutting along the seam of the clothing.—Protect the evidence by avoiding ripping or cutting through a knife or bullet hole.

32. a. a paper bag.—The moisture in plastic bags can break down the evidence. Better yet, have the law enforcement officer assist you so it is handled in the manner that she prefers.

33. d. cutting to avoid—The knot is evidence and must be preserved. Cut several inches above it.

34. c. destroying or "smudging" the perpetrator's prints.—Touch as little as possible.

35. c. keeping a safe stance with feet apart, ready to react.—This, together with keeping your hands out of the pockets and not hanging onto equipment, can help you to keep your balance and be ready to run.

Chapter 51: Basic Cardiac Life Support Resuscitation Issues

1. c. basic life support.—Together with advanced cardiac life support (ACLS), it is part of the emergency cardiac care provided to patients experiencing symptoms of a heart attack. BLS is used interchangeably with the old phrase basic cardiac life support (BCLS) when discussing cardiac care. BLS is often used to refer to the technique of cardiopulmonary resuscitation (CPR) when managing a cardiac arrest.

2. a. emphasizing that all rescuers should push hard and fast.—The better and faster the compressions, the more blood flow they will produce.

3. b. acute coronary syndrome.—An acute coronary syndrome (ACS) is a catch-all term devised to emphasize that many times it is impossible to tell the difference between unstable angina and infarction.

4. a. two—Studies have shown that the effectiveness of chest compressions deteriorate rapidly as the rescuer tires. The new recommendation is for the rescuers to switch, without interruption, every two minutes.

5. a. one second per breath.—When the adult patient has a pulse, but is not breathing, rescue breaths should be given over one second every five to six seconds.

6. a. 30:2 for all rescuers.—This change emphasizes the importance of maximizing chest compressions without interruptions for all rescuers.

7. c. based on scientific evidence.—This evidence was reviewed and scientific consensus obtained from the international resuscitation community.

8. b. IIa.—An example of a Class IIa treatment is that each rescue breath be given over one second.

9. c. IIb.—An example of a Class IIb treatment is for the healthcare provider to use the jaw-thrust without head extension in the patient with a suspected cervical spine injury.

10. d. Indeterminate.—Often these are ideas at a preliminary research stage, promising but in need of more research at a higher level. Thus, the AHA and resuscitation experts cannot make a recommendation for or against at this time.

11. a. all rescuers deliver one shock followed by immediate CPR for two minutes.—The new recommendation is for single shocks, followed by immediate CPR and rhythm checks assessed every two minutes.

12. b. IIb—EMS providers should be prepared to temporarily act as family advocates until additional help arrives for grief support (chaplain, family minister, or other family members) and management of the body (medical examiner, coroner, and police).

13. b. IIa—Another example of a Class IIa treatment is chest compressions delivered at a rate of 100 per minute.

14. c. every three to five seconds.—When the infant or child patient has a pulse, but is not breathing, rescue breaths should be given over one second every three to five seconds.

15. c. take less than ten seconds.—Interruptions in chest compression should occur as infrequently as possible and take no more than ten seconds.

16. d. allows the heart to fill with blood.—If the chest does not recoil, the heart will not receive adequate venous return and the subsequent compression will not produce adequate cardiac output.

17. a. it impedes blood return to the heart.—Overinflation of the lungs increases intrathoracic pressure, and this prevents adequate filling of the heart with blood.

18. b. DNAR order.—It is the responsibility of the healthcare provider to search for and honor a DNAR that is deemed valid.

19. c. consensus standards.—They are based on the ILCOR consensus and the science of resuscitation.

20. d. 360 J.—This is a change from the 2000 Guidelines. The recommended dose for initial and subsequent shocks using monophasic waveform is 360 J.

21. d. 360 J.—The recommended dose for initial and subsequent shocks using monophasic waveform is 360 J.

22. c. a low body temperature—In some instances hypothermia can mimic clinical death. The saying goes, "They are not dead until they are warm and dead."

23. b. two minutes of CPR—In the out-of-hospital setting, all rescuers should provide five cycles or approximately two minutes of CPR prior to using the AED.

24. b. defibrillation—Early defibrillation is the single acute intervention that really makes a difference in saving lives from sudden cardiac arrest.

25. d. one—Since 2003, the use of AEDs is recommended for children one year and older in sudden cardiac arrest.

26. c. removing barriers to implementing PAD—Limited funds are better spent on removing the barriers to training the lay public in CPR and public access defibrillation (PAD). Clearly, all the medications do not help save as many patients as getting the defibrillator operator there faster.

27. c. patients one year old to the onset of puberty.—The change applies to victims of cardiac arrest from about one year old to the onset of puberty or adolescence, as defined by the presence of secondary sex characteristics.

28. a. a child with previous ACS—The major exception to the phone-fast rule is those children under eight years old who are known to be at risk for ventricular fibrillation (VF) or ventricular tachycardia (VT), who have a history of cardiac dysrhythmias, or those with congenital heart disease who experience sudden witnessed collapse.

29. c. poisoning or drug overdose—These patients tend to be hypoxic and have the best chance of survival when CPR is provided in the first few minutes of sudden cardiac arrest.

30. d. supplemental oxygen is attached.—When the smallest tidal volumes are used, the chest should rise visibly and the oxygen saturation should be maintained at greater than 90%.

31. d. all of the above.—The technique of providing ventilations with a bag mask requires routine practice and is a fundamental skill that should be mastered by all healthcare providers.

32. b. about 18″ above the head of the patient—The ventilator should be positioned approximately 18″ above the head of the patient; hyperextend the airway and use the weight of the left arm, which is sealing the mask, to hold the airway in the hyperextended position. The other hand can be used to squeeze the bag against itself.

33. b. The jaw thrust can be used for one-rescuer bag mask technique on a trauma patient.—It is not possible to do a jaw thrust, jutting both sides of the jar anterior, with only one hand.

34. d. chest should rise visibly.—With supplemental oxygen attached to the bag mask, smaller tidal volumes

(400–600 ml) are acceptable. The rescuer should still be able to see the chest rise and maintain the patient's oxygen saturation at greater than 90%.

35. a. do mouth-to-nose breathing.—Close the mouth with one hand and provide ventilations through the nose.

36. a. two rescue breaths—After the two rescue breaths are given, the rescuer should immediately begin chest compressions in cycles of 30:2.

37. d. they were frequently wrong in their assessment—This step was taking too long to perform and was too often performed incorrectly. The goal now is to deliver chest compressions rapidly and without delays.

38. a. 150 J.—An initial dose of 150 J to 200 J is recommended when using a biphasic truncated exponential waveform, and 120 J for a rectilinear biphasic waveform.

39. b. reposition the neck and reattempt to ventilate.—Blind finger sweeps should not be used on any patient.

40. a. 2 J/kg.—Subsequent doses should be 4 J/kg.

41. b. chest compressions may be helpful.—Chest compressions generated at least as high or higher intrathoracic pressures than abdominal thrusts. Therefore, the chest compressions used in CPR are helpful in dislodging an FBAO in the unresponsive patient.

42. d. in the center of the chest between the nipples—This position has not changed in the new Guidelines.

43. c. 100—This rate has not changed in the new Guidelines.

44. b. 15:2.—For infants less than one year old, the compression to ventilation ratio is 5:1.

45. b. the heel of one or two hands to compress the lower half of the sternum.—The placement of the hand or hands should be at about the nipple line.

46. b. on adults and children.—The current recommendations are for abdominal thrusts on adults and children one year and older.

47. a. two-thumb-encircling-hands chest technique.—The Guidelines still recommends this as the primary method for compressions for the neonate.

48. c. compression-only CPR.—Compressions with or without ventilations are better than no compressions at all.

49. b. the LMA and Combitube® are better than bag mask.—Evidence shows that under certain clinical conditions, both the LMA and Combitube® are clinically equivalent to the ET tube.

50. d. the agency's Medical Director—Prior to making this decision, many factors must be considered by the Medical Director using the quality improvement process.

Chapter 52: Advanced Cardiac Life Support

1. b. evidence-based—The Guidelines were developed using an evidence-based rigorous review of the published scientific evidence and studies on resuscitation.

2. a. I—An example of a Class I treatment is giving aspirin to ACS patients.

3. c. Indeterminate—An example of a Class Indeterminate treatment is the use of AEDs in infants (below one year of age).

4. a. 1: six to eight—Once an advanced airway has been inserted, the rescuer delivers one ventilation every six to eight seconds, and the compressor continues without interruption.

5. a. bag mask—The bag mask provides effective ventilations when used by properly trained providers who practice the skill.

6. a. an IV or IO.—Medications administered through an IV or IO provide a more predictable delivery and pharmacologic effect.

7. c. resume CPR for five cycles, and then reanalyze the rhythm and check pulse.—Pulse and rhythm are not checked after the shock; rather, they are checked after five cycles of CPR, or about two minutes.

8. b. capnography—Capnography provides $EtCO_2$ readings in two forms; one is a number and the other is a wave form or graph.

9. d. This device requires extensive training to use.—This device is easy to use and does not require extensive training. The device is inserted blindly and does not require a mask seal to ventilate.

10. c. EMS dispatcher may instruct patients with symptoms of ACS to chew an aspirin.—The emergency medical dispatcher (EMD) may instruct the patient or caller to give the patient who is alert with symptoms of ACS an aspirin while awaiting the ambulance.

11. d. during CPR, as soon as possible after rhythm checks.—The emphasis is to minimize interruption of compressions. Therefore, medications should be administered during CPR, as soon as possible after rhythm checks.

12. b. Vasopressin—A single dose may be given to replace either the first or second dose of epinephrine in VF/pulseless VT, asystole, or PEA arrest.

13. d. all of the above.—There are possible benefits of induced hypothermia for twelve to twenty-four hours for patients who have an ROSC, but who remain comatose after a reversal of a cardiac arrest.

14. a. is very difficult to accurately dose to the patient's weight.—The use of high-dose epinephrine is not recommended (Class III) for all of the other reasons listed.

15. b. Amiodarone—Amiodarone is preferred (Class IIb), but lidocaine may be used when amiodarone is not available.

16. a. routine suctioning is no longer recommended.—The recommendation is to avoid routine suctioning of meconium staining.

17. c. the patient takes warfarin—Contraindications for fibrinolysis include: bleeding or clotting problems on blood thinners, pregnancy, history of serious systemic disease, recent surgery or trauma, and BP greater than 180 systolic or 110 diastolic.

18. a. diltiazem—Diltiazem, or Cardizem, is the first-line drug used to control the ventricular rate in atrial fibrillation and atrial flutter.

19. d. Magnesium sulfate—This drug is recommended for use in cardiac arrest when the rhythm is torsades de points or when you suspect the patient has hypomagnesemia.

20. c. Vasopressin—This drug may be used as an alternative vasopressor to epinephrine in adult cardiac arrest with shock-refractory VF. It may also be useful in cardiac arrest with asystole and PEA rhythms.

21. d. All of the actions listed above are appropriate and should be done.—If possible, one crew member or the EMS supervisor should talk with the family and explain what treatment is being provided, what the most likely outcome is, and answer questions, clarify information, and comfort the family.

22. b. the treatment is streamlined into one algorithm.—The goal was to simplify treatment for all providers, both in and out of the hospital setting.

23. a. acute coronary syndromes.—An acute coronary syndrome (ACS) is a catch-all term devised to emphasize that many times it is impossible to tell the difference between unstable angina and infarction.

24. c. primary angioplasty and intra-aortic balloon placement.—Patients with large anterior infarctions, systolic BP<100 mmHg, heart rates over 100, or rales greater than one-third of the lung fields should also be considered for transfer to these specialty facilities.

25. c. three hours of the onset of stroke symptoms.—These patients should be triaged with the same urgency as acute ST segment elevation MI (STEMI).

26. a. ventricular dysrhythmias.—Overdose of tricyclic antidepressants may also cause: tachycardia, bradycardia, impaired conduction, shock, and cardiac arrest.

27. a. systemic alkalosis.—The treatment of choice is the induction of a systemic alkalosis with a pH of 7.50 to 7.55.

28. a. ventricular dysrhythmias.—Cocaine has both alpha and beta stimulatory effects.

29. d. beta-blocking agents as a second-line therapy when the first-line treatment fails.—Beta-blockers are relatively contraindicated, and propranolol should definitely not be used for cocaine intoxication.

30. a. aspirin—All patients with signs and symptoms of ACS, including non-Q wave MI, should receive aspirin and beta-blockers in the absence of contraindications.

Appendix B:
Tips for Preparing for a
Practical Skills Examination

Paramedic courses are designed to cover specific objectives as outlined in the DOT National Standard Curriculum. The curriculum also suggests that EMS educators should take the option of enriching these courses with more material if they or their Medical Director choose. What prohibits many educators from enriching their courses is limited time and resources.

During a Paramedic course, many educators teach the core curriculum and provide enrichment material as time, resources, and experience permit. Near the end of a Paramedic course, it is typical for the educator to change his or her style of teaching and prep for the exam. That is to say, instructors will provide examples of the material to be tested on state and national exams, and give tips on how to take the written exams. He or she may hold one or more practice skills sessions and a mock practical exam to help the students prepare. Limited time and resources often do not allow for as much practice time for skills as some students would like. In preparing for the practical skills exam, I have included some tips to help you get ready.

If you haven't done so already, obtain a copy of the skills testing sheets to be used for *your* practical skills exam and carefully read the instructions well before the day of the practical skills exam. Note that each exam skills sheet has items that are identified as critical pass or fail items. These items are usually bolded for easy identification. These items include taking or verbalizing BSI or scene safety, as well as other critical tasks. National registry skills sheets will also list Critical Criteria at the bottom of each skills sheet. This is a list of items that were not performed and should have been. When an evaluator checks one of these items, the candidate will fail the station.

Often the course instructor will hand out a set of the skills testing sheets to be used for the state and/or registry exam during or near the end of the course, and you will be given an opportunity to practice the skills in lab using the testing sheets. I strongly recommend that you take every opportunity provided during the course to do this. In addition, find one or more students or experienced paramedics to practice skills with. While you demonstrate the skill, have another person use the testing sheet to evaluate your performance. Be tough on each other in a friendly way! Pay close attention to the critical failure items and then focus on obtaining every available point.

Prior to the day of the practical skills exam, make certain you are familiar with the location of the exam. Arrive fifteen minutes early on the day of the exam. Bring a copy of the skills sheets with you to review while you are waiting. On the testing day, be patient and prepare to be at the testing site for most of the day. As you already are aware, practical skills testing typically takes a lot of time. In addition to bringing the skills sheets to review, bring a book, a drink, lunch, and plenty of patience.

On the day of the practical exam, if you have the option of choosing the order of the testing stations, there are two theories I recommend. The first one is this: if you are a little nervous and you want to build your confidence, start with a short skill station like one of the EMT-B skills. This is a skill you have successfully completed in the past. From there, continue to build your confidence by selecting the stations that you feel you can complete without difficulty.

The second theory I recommend is selecting the most difficult stations and completing those first. For most people, the megacode and assessment stations seem the most difficult because they have the most steps and take the longest to complete. Once these stations are complete, you can breathe a little easier while completing the remaining stations.

If you do not have the option of choosing the order of skills to be tested, do not worry; at this point, you have prepared and are ready for each skills station. During the exam, the evaluators are instructed not to advise you if you have passed or failed a skills station until you have finished testing at all of the stations, so don't expect them to. If you fail a station early in the testing, you may become distracted and fail another.

Once in the station, you will be read a set of instructions and given the opportunity to ask questions for clarification and to check the equipment provided. I recommend that you do this, especially if you are the first candidate of the day coming into a station. The evaluator has been instructed to make sure that the equipment is functioning properly and that there are no distractions for the candidates. They are not there to trip you up, but occasionally a blood pressure cuff is broken and is not detected prior to starting the exam.

In the patient assessment station, I recommend that you ask if the injuries or significant signs that you are supposed to detect are going to be visible with moulage or by another method. This is a common area where problems can occur. Verbalize the steps and tasks you complete as if you are talking to a new partner. After a long day of testing, evaluators become fatigued just like you. If an evaluator happens to have his or her head turned while you are performing a critical step, he or she will hear you verbalizing it.

If you should have to repeat a station, know the retest policy and don't overreact. You have spent a lot of time training and should persevere rather than throwing in the towel over one bad day! Remember, we humans do make mistakes occasionally. The key is how you learn from your mistakes, correct them, and move forward.

Lastly, get some sleep before the examination. Try to get a good night's rest two nights before the exam, in addition to the night before. Many people are very nervous about test taking and do not sleep well the night before, no matter what. Getting good sleep two nights before does help.

Best of luck, and be prepared!

—Kirt and Bob

Appendix C:
Advanced Level Paramedic Exam Skill Sheets

National Registry of Emergency Medical Technicians
Advanced Level Practical Examination

BLEEDING CONTROL/SHOCK MANAGEMENT

Candidate: _____ Examiner: _____

Date: _____ Signature: _____

Time Start:_____	Possible Points	Points Awarded
Takes or verbalizes body substance isolation precautions	1	
Applies direct pressure to the wound	1	
Elevates the extremity	1	
NOTE: The examiner must now inform the candidate that the wound continues to bleed.		
Applies an additional dressing to the wound	1	
NOTE: The examiner must now inform the candidate that the wound still continues to bleed. The second dressing does not control the bleeding.		
Locates and applies pressure to appropriate arterial pressure point	1	
NOTE: The examiner must now inform the candidate that the bleeding is controlled.		
Bandages the wound	1	
NOTE: The examiner must now inform the candidate that the patient is exhibiting signs and symptoms of hypoperfusion.		
Properly positions the patient	1	
Administers high concentration oxygen	1	
Initiates steps to prevent heat loss from the patient	1	
Indicates the need for immediate transportation	1	

Time End: _____   **TOTAL**   10

CRITICAL CRITERIA

_____ Did not take or verbalize body substance isolation precautions
_____ Did not apply high concentration of oxygen
_____ Applied a tourniquet before attempting other methods of bleeding control
_____ Did not control hemorrhage in a timely manner
_____ Did not indicate the need for immediate transportation

You must factually document your rationale for checking any of the above critical items on the reverse side of this form.

National Registry of Emergency Medical Technicians
Advanced Level Practical Examination

DUAL LUMEN AIRWAY DEVICE (COMBITUBE® OR PTL®)

Candidate: _____ Examiner: _____

Date: _____ Signature: _____

NOTE: If candidate elects to initially ventilate with BVM attached to reservoir and oxygen, full credit must be awarded for steps denoted by "**" so long as first ventilation is delivered within 30 seconds.

	Possible Points	Points Awarded
Takes or verbalizes body substance isolation precautions	1	
Opens the airway manually	1	
Elevates tongue, inserts simple adjunct [oropharyngeal or nasopharyngeal airway]	1	
NOTE: Examiner now informs candidate no gag reflex is present and patient accepts adjunct		
**Ventilates patient immediately with bag mask device unattached to oxygen	1	
**Hyperventilates patient with room air	1	
NOTE: Examiner now informs candidate that ventilation is being performed without difficulty		
Attaches oxygen reservoir to bag mask device and connects to high flow oxygen regulator [12-15 L/minute]	1	
Ventilates patient at a rate of 10-20/minute with appropriate volumes	1	
NOTE: After 30 seconds, examiner auscultates and reports breath sounds are present and equal bilaterally and medical control has ordered insertion of a dual lumen airway. The examiner must now take over ventilation.		
Directs assistant to pre-oxygenate patient	1	
Checks/prepares airway device	1	
Lubricates distal tip of the device [may be verbalized]	1	
NOTE: Examiner to remove OPA and move out of the way when candidate is prepared to insert device		
Positions head properly	1	
Performs a tongue-jaw lift	1	

☐ USES COMBITUBE®	☐ USES PTL®		
Inserts device in mid-line and to depth so printed ring is at level of teeth	Inserts device in mid-line until bite block flange is at level of teeth	1	
Inflates pharyngeal cuff with proper volume and removes syringe	Secures strap	1	
Inflates distal cuff with proper volume and removes syringe	Blows into tube #1 to adequately inflate both cuffs	1	
Attaches/directs attachment of BVM to the first [esophageal placement] lumen and ventilates		1	
Confirms placement and ventilation through correct lumen by observing chest rise, auscultation over the epigastrium, and bilaterally over each lung		1	
NOTE: The examiner states, "You do not see rise and fall of the chest and you only hear sounds over the epigastrium."			
Attaches/directs attachment of BVM to the second [endotracheal placement] lumen and ventilates		1	
Confirms placement and ventilation through correct lumen by observing chest rise, auscultation over the epigastrium, and bilaterally over each lung		1	
NOTE: The examiner confirms adequate chest rise, absent sounds over the epigastrium, and equal bilateral breath sounds.			
Secures device or confirms that the device remains properly secured		1	
	TOTAL	20	

CRITICAL CRITERIA

_____ Failure to initiate ventilations within 30 seconds after taking body substance isolation precautions or interrupts ventilations for greater than 30 seconds at any time
_____ Failure to take or verbalize body substance isolation precautions
_____ Failure to voice and ultimately provide high oxygen concentrations [at least 85%]
_____ Failure to ventilate patient at a rate of at least 10/minute
_____ Failure to provide adequate volumes per breath [maximum 2 errors/minute permissible]
_____ Failure to pre-oxygenate patient prior to insertion of the dual lumen airway device
_____ Failure to insert the dual lumen airway device at a proper depth or at either proper place within 3 attempts
_____ Failure to inflate both cuffs properly
_____ **Combitube** - failure to remove the syringe immediately after inflation of each cuff
       PTL - failure to secure the strap prior to cuff inflation
_____ Failure to confirm that the proper lumen of the device is being ventilated by observing chest rise, auscultation over the epigastrium, and bilaterally over each lung
_____ Inserts any adjunct in a manner dangerous to patient

You must factually document your rationale for checking any of the above critical items on the reverse side of this form.

© 2000 National Registry of Emergency Medical Technicians, Inc., Columbus, OH
All materials subject to this copyright may be photocopied for the non-commercial purpose of educational or scientific advancement.

p304/8-003k

National Registry of Emergency Medical Technicians
Advanced Level Practical Examination

DYNAMIC CARDIOLOGY

Candidate: _____ Examiner: _____

Date: _____ Signature: _____

SET #_____

Level of Testing: □ NREMT-Intermediate/99 □ NREMT-Paramedic

Time Start:_____

	Possible Points	Points Awarded
Takes or verbalizes infection control precautions	1	
Checks level of responsiveness	1	
Checks ABCs	1	
Initiates CPR if appropriate [verbally]	1	
Attaches ECG monitor in a timely fashion or applies paddles for "Quick Look"	1	
Correctly interprets initial rhythm	1	
Appropriately manages initial rhythm	2	
Notes change in rhythm	1	
Checks patient condition to include pulse and, if appropriate, BP	1	
Correctly interprets second rhythm	1	
Appropriately manages second rhythm	2	
Notes change in rhythm	1	
Checks patient condition to include pulse and, if appropriate, BP	1	
Correctly interprets third rhythm	1	
Appropriately manages third rhythm	2	
Notes change in rhythm	1	
Checks patient condition to include pulse and, if appropriate, BP	1	
Correctly interprets fourth rhythm	1	
Appropriately manages fourth rhythm	2	
Orders high percentages of supplemental oxygen at proper times	1	

Time End: _____   **TOTAL** 24

CRITICAL CRITERIA

_____ Failure to deliver first shock in a timely manner due to operator delay in machine use or providing treatments other than CPR with simple adjuncts

_____ Failure to deliver second or third shocks without delay other than the time required to reassess rhythm and recharge paddles

_____ Failure to verify rhythm before delivering each shock

_____ Failure to ensure the safety of self and others [verbalizes "All clear" and observes]

_____ Inability to deliver DC shock [does not use machine properly]

_____ Failure to demonstrate acceptable shock sequence

_____ Failure to order initiation or resumption of CPR when appropriate

_____ Failure to order correct management of airway [ET when appropriate]

_____ Failure to order administration of appropriate oxygen at proper time

_____ Failure to diagnose or treat 2 or more rhythms correctly

_____ Orders administration of an inappropriate drug or lethal dosage

_____ Failure to correctly diagnose or adequately treat v-fib, v-tach, or asystole

You must factually document your rationale for checking any of the above critical items on the reverse side of this form.

p306/8-003k

INTRAVENOUS THERAPY

Candidate: _____ Examiner: _____

Date: _____ Signature: _____

Level of Testing: ❑ NREMT-Intermediate/85 ❑ NREMT-Intermediate/99 ❑ NREMT-Paramedic

Time Start: _____

	Possible Points	Points Awarded
Checks selected IV fluid for: -Proper fluid (1 point) -Clarity (1 point)	2	
Selects appropriate catheter	1	
Selects proper administration set	1	
Connects IV tubing to the IV bag	1	
Prepares administration set [fills drip chamber and flushes tubing]	1	
Cuts or tears tape [at any time before venipuncture]	1	
Takes/verbalizes body substance isolation precautions [prior to venipuncture]	1	
Applies tourniquet	1	
Palpates suitable vein	1	
Cleanses site appropriately	1	
Performs venipuncture -Inserts stylette (1 point) -Notes or verbalizes flashback (1 point) -Occludes vein proximal to catheter (1 point) -Removes stylette (1 point) -Connects IV tubing to catheter (1 point)	5	
Disposes/verbalizes disposal of needle in proper container	1	
Releases tourniquet	1	
Runs IV for a brief period to assure patent line	1	
Secures catheter [tapes securely or verbalizes]	1	
Adjusts flow rate as appropriate	1	

Time End: _____ **TOTAL** 21

CRITICAL CRITERIA
____ Failure to establish a patent and properly adjusted IV within 6 minute time limit
____ Failure to take or verbalize body substance isolation precautions prior to performing venipuncture
____ Contaminates equipment or site without appropriately correcting situation
____ Performs any improper technique resulting in the potential for uncontrolled hemorrhage, catheter shear, or air embolism
____ Failure to successfully establish IV within 3 attempts during 6 minute time limit
____ Failure to dispose/verbalize disposal of needle in proper container

NOTE: Check here (_____) if candidate did not establish a patent IV and do not evaluate IV Bolus Medications.

INTRAVENOUS BOLUS MEDICATIONS

Time Start: _____

Asks patient for known allergies	1	
Selects correct medication	1	
Assures correct concentration of drug	1	
Assembles prefilled syringe correctly and dispels air	1	
Continues body substance isolation precautions	1	
Cleanses injection site [Y-port or hub]	1	
Reaffirms medication	1	
Stops IV flow [pinches tubing or shuts off]	1	
Administers correct dose at proper push rate	1	
Disposes/verbalizes proper disposal of syringe and needle in proper container	1	
Flushes tubing [runs wide open for a brief period]	1	
Adjusts drip rate to TKO/KVO	1	
Verbalizes need to observe patient for desired effect/adverse side effects	1	

Time End: _____ **TOTAL** 13

CRITICAL CRITERIA
____ Failure to begin administration of medication within 3 minute time limit
____ Contaminates equipment or site without appropriately correcting situation
____ Failure to adequately dispel air resulting in potential for air embolism
____ Injects improper drug or dosage [wrong drug, incorrect amount, or pushes at inappropriate rate]
____ Failure to flush IV tubing after injecting medication
____ Recaps needle or failure to dispose/verbalize disposal of syringe and needle in proper container

You must factually document your rationale for checking any of the above critical items on the reverse side of this form.

p309/8-003k

National Registry of Emergency Medical Technicians
Advanced Level Practical Examination

PATIENT ASSESSMENT - MEDICAL

Candidate: _____ Examiner: _____

Date: _____ Signature: _____

Scenario:_____

Time Start: _____

	Possible Points	Points Awarded
Takes or verbalizes body substance isolation precautions	1	
SCENE SIZE-UP		
Determines the scene/situation is safe	1	
Determines the mechanism of injury/nature of illness	1	
Determines the number of patients	1	
Requests additional help if necessary	1	
Considers stabilization of spine	1	
INITIAL ASSESSMENT		
Verbalizes general impression of the patient	1	
Determines responsiveness/level of consciousness	1	
Determines chief complaint/apparent life-threats	1	

Assesses airway and breathing
    -Assessment (1 point)
    -Assures adequate ventilation (1 point)
    -Initiates appropriate oxygen therapy (1 point)
	3	

Assesses circulation
    -Assesses/controls major bleeding (1 point)   -Assesses skin [either skin color, temperature, or condition] (1 point)
    -Assesses pulse (1 point)
	3	

Identifies priority patients/makes transport decision	1	
FOCUSED HISTORY AND PHYSICAL EXAMINATION/RAPID ASSESSMENT		

History of present illness
    -Onset (1 point)   -Severity (1 point)
    -Provocation (1 point)   -Time (1 point)
    -Quality (1 point)   -Clarifying questions of associated signs and symptoms as related to OPQRST (2 points)
    -Radiation (1 point)
	8	

Past medical history
    -Allergies (1 point)   -Past pertinent history (1 point)   -Events leading to present illness (1 point)
    -Medications (1 point)   -Last oral intake (1 point)
	5	

Performs focused physical examination [assess affected body part/system or, if indicated, completes rapid assessment]
    -Cardiovascular   -Neurological   -Integumentary   -Reproductive
    -Pulmonary   -Musculoskeletal   -GI/GU   -Psychological/Social
	5	

Vital signs
    -Pulse (1 point)   -Respiratory rate and quality (1 point each)
    -Blood pressure (1 point)   -AVPU (1 point)
	5	

Diagnostics [must include application of ECG monitor for dyspnea and chest pain]	2	
States field impression of patient	1	
Verbalizes treatment plan for patient and calls for appropriate intervention(s)	1	
Transport decision reevaluated	1	
ON-GOING ASSESSMENT		
Repeats initial assessment	1	
Repeats vital signs	1	
Evaluates response to treatments	1	
Repeats focused assessment regarding patient complaint or injuries	1	

Time End: _____

CRITICAL CRITERIA   **TOTAL**   48

_____ Failure to initiate or call for transport of the patient within 15 minute time limit

_____ Failure to take or verbalize body substance isolation precautions

_____ Failure to determine scene safety before approaching patient

_____ Failure to voice and ultimately provide appropriate oxygen therapy

_____ Failure to assess/provide adequate ventilation

_____ Failure to find or appropriately manage problems associated with airway, breathing, hemorrhage or shock [hypoperfusion]

_____ Failure to differentiate patient's need for immediate transportation versus continued assessment and treatment at the scene

_____ Does other detailed or focused history or physical examination before assessing and treating threats to airway, breathing, and circulation

_____ Failure to determine the patient's primary problem

_____ Orders a dangerous or inappropriate intervention

_____ Failure to provide for spinal protection when indicated

You must factually document your rationale for checking any of the above critical items on the reverse side of this form.

PATIENT ASSESSMENT - TRAUMA

Candidate: _____ Examiner: _____

Date: _____ Signature: _____

Scenario # _____

Time Start: _____ NOTE: Areas denoted by "**" may be integrated within sequence of Initial Assessment	Possible Points	Points Awarded
Takes or verbalizes body substance isolation precautions	1	
SCENE SIZE-UP		
Determines the scene/situation is safe	1	
Determines the mechanism of injury/nature of illness	1	
Determines the number of patients	1	
Requests additional help if necessary	1	
Considers stabilization of spine	1	
INITIAL ASSESSMENT/RESUSCITATION		
Verbalizes general impression of the patient	1	
Determines responsiveness/level of consciousness	1	
Determines chief complaint/apparent life-threats	1	
Airway -Opens and assesses airway (1 point) -Inserts adjunct as indicated (1 point)	2	

Breathing
    -Assesses breathing (1 point)
    -Assures adequate ventilation (1 point)
    -Initiates appropriate oxygen therapy (1 point)
    -Manages any injury which may compromise breathing/ventilation (1 point)
	4	

Circulation
    -Checks pulse (1point)
    -Assesses skin [either skin color, temperature, or condition] (1 point)
    -Assesses for and controls major bleeding if present (1 point)
    -Initiates shock management (1 point)
	4	

Identifies priority patients/makes transport decision	1	
FOCUSED HISTORY AND PHYSICAL EXAMINATION/RAPID TRAUMA ASSESSMENT		
Selects appropriate assessment	1	
Obtains, or directs assistant to obtain, baseline vital signs	1	
Obtains SAMPLE history	1	
DETAILED PHYSICAL EXAMINATION		

Head
    -Inspects mouth**, nose**, and assesses facial area (1 point)
    -Inspects and palpates scalp and ears (1 point)
    -Assesses eyes for PERRL** (1 point)
	3	

Neck**
    -Checks position of trachea (1 point)
    -Checks jugular veins (1 point)
    -Palpates cervical spine (1 point)
	3	

Chest**
    -Inspects chest (1 point)
    -Palpates chest (1 point)
    -Auscultates chest (1 point)
	3	

Abdomen/pelvis**
    -Inspects and palpates abdomen (1 point)
    -Assesses pelvis (1 point)
    -Verbalizes assessment of genitalia/perineum as needed (1 point)
	3	

Lower extremities** -Inspects, palpates, and assesses motor, sensory, and distal circulatory functions (1 point/leg)	2	
Upper extremities -Inspects, palpates, and assesses motor, sensory, and distal circulatory functions (1 point/arm)	2	

Posterior thorax, lumbar, and buttocks**
    -Inspects and palpates posterior thorax (1 point)
    -Inspects and palpates lumbar and buttocks area (1 point)
	2	

Manages secondary injuries and wounds appropriately	1	
Performs ongoing assessment	1	

Time End: _____   **TOTAL**   43

CRITICAL CRITERIA
_____ Failure to initiate or call for transport of the patient within 10 minute time limit
_____ Failure to take or verbalize body substance isolation precautions
_____ Failure to determine scene safety
_____ Failure to assess for and provide spinal protection when indicated
_____ Failure to voice and ultimately provide high concentration of oxygen
_____ Failure to assess/provide adequate ventilation
_____ Failure to find or appropriately manage problems associated with airway, breathing, hemorrhage, or shock [hypoperfusion]
_____ Failure to differentiate patient's need for immediate transportation versus continued assessment/treatment at the scene
_____ Does other detailed/focused history or physical exam before assessing/treating threats to airway, breathing, and circulation
_____ Orders a dangerous or inappropriate intervention

You must factually document your rationale for checking any of the above critical items on the reverse side of this form.

National Registry of Emergency Medical Technicians
Advanced Level Practical Examination

PEDIATRIC INTRAOSSEOUS INFUSION

Candidate: _____ Examiner: _____

Date: _____ Signature: _____

Time Start:_____	Possible Points	Points Awarded
Checks selected IV fluid for: -Proper fluid (1 point) -Clarity (1 point)	2	
Selects appropriate equipment to include: -IO needle (1 point) -Syringe (1 point) -Saline (1 point) -Extension set (1 point)	4	
Selects proper administration set	1	
Connects administration set to bag	1	
Prepares administration set [fills drip chamber and flushes tubing]	1	
Prepares syringe and extension tubing	1	
Cuts or tears tape [at any time before IO puncture]	1	
Takes or verbalizes body substance isolation precautions [prior to IO puncture]	1	
Identifies proper anatomical site for IO puncture	1	
Cleanses site appropriately	1	
Performs IO puncture: -Stabilizes tibia (1 point) -Inserts needle at proper angle (1 point) -Advances needle with twisting motion until "pop" is felt (1 point) -Unscrews cap and removes stylette from needle (1 point)	4	
Disposes of needle in proper container	1	
Attaches syringe and extension set to IO needle and aspirates	1	
Slowly injects saline to assure proper placement of needle	1	
Connects administration set and adjusts flow rate as appropriate	1	
Secures needle with tape and supports with bulky dressing	1	

Time End: _____   **TOTAL**   23

CRITICAL CRITERIA
_____ Failure to establish a patent and properly adjusted IO line within the 6 minute time limit
_____ Failure to take or verbalize body substance isolation precautions prior to performing IO puncture
_____ Contaminates equipment or site without appropriately correcting situation
_____ Performs any improper technique resulting in the potential for air embolism
_____ Failure to assure correct needle placement before attaching administration set
_____ Failure to successfully establish IO infusion within 2 attempts during 6 minute time limit
_____ Performing IO puncture in an unacceptable manner [improper site, incorrect needle angle, etc.]
_____ Failure to dispose of needle in proper container
_____ Orders or performs any dangerous or potentially harmful procedure

You must factually document your rationale for checking any of the above critical items on the reverse side of this form.

p310/8-003k

PEDIATRIC (<2 yrs.) VENTILATORY MANAGEMENT

Candidate: _____ Examiner _____

Date: _____ Signature: _____

NOTE: If candidate elects to ventilate initially with BVM attached to reservoir and oxygen, full credit must be awarded for steps denoted by "**" so long as first ventilation is delivered within 30 seconds.

	Possible Points	Points Awarded
Takes or verbalizes body substance isolation precautions	1	
Opens the airway manually	1	
Elevates tongue, inserts simple adjunct [oropharyngeal or nasopharyngeal airway]	1	
NOTE: Examiner now informs candidate no gag reflex is present and patient accepts adjunct		
**Ventilates patient immediately with bag mask device unattached to oxygen	1	
**Hyperventilates patient with room air	1	
NOTE: Examiner now informs candidate that ventilation is being performed without difficulty and that pulse oximetry indicates the patient's blood oxygen saturation is 85%		
Attaches oxygen reservoir to bag mask device and connects to high flow oxygen regulator [12-15 L/minute]	1	
Ventilates patient at a rate of 20-30/minute and assures adequate chest expansion	1	
NOTE: After 30 seconds, examiner auscultates and reports breath sounds are present, equal bilaterally and medical direction has ordered intubation. The examiner must now take over ventilation.		
Directs assistant to pre-oxygenate patient	1	
Identifies/selects proper equipment for intubation	1	
Checks laryngoscope to assure operational with bulb tight	1	
NOTE: Examiner to remove OPA and move out of the way when candidate is prepared to intubate		
Places patient in neutral or sniffing position	1	
Inserts blade while displacing tongue	1	
Elevates mandible with laryngoscope	1	
Introduces ET tube and advances to proper depth	1	
Directs ventilation of patient	1	
Confirms proper placement by auscultation bilaterally over each lung and over epigastrium	1	
NOTE: Examiner to ask, "If you had proper placement, what should you expect to hear?"		
Secures ET tube [may be verbalized]	1	
TOTAL	**17**	

CRITICAL CRITERIA

_____ Failure to initiate ventilations within 30 seconds after applying gloves or interrupts ventilations for greater than 30 seconds at any time

_____ Failure to take or verbalize body substance isolation precautions

_____ Failure to pad under the torso to allow neutral head position or sniffing position

_____ Failure to voice and ultimately provide high oxygen concentrations [at least 85%]

_____ Failure to ventilate patient at a rate of at least 20/minute

_____ Failure to provide adequate volumes per breath [maximum 2 errors/minute permissible]

_____ Failure to pre-oxygenate patient prior to intubation

_____ Failure to successfully intubate within 3 attempts

_____ Uses gums as a fulcrum

_____ Failure to assure proper tube placement by auscultation bilaterally **and** over the epigastrium

_____ Inserts any adjunct in a manner dangerous to the patient

_____ Attempts to use any equipment not appropriate for the pediatric patient

You must factually document your rationale for checking any of the above critical items on the reverse side of this form.

p305/8-003k

National Registry of Emergency Medical Technicians
Advanced Level Practical Examination

SPINAL IMMOBILIZATION (SEATED PATIENT)

Candidate:_____Examiner:_____

Date: _____Signature:_____

Time Start: _____	Possible Points	Points Awarded
Takes or verbalizes body substance isolation precautions	1	
Directs assistant to place/maintain head in the neutral, in-line position	1	
Directs assistant to maintain manual immobilization of the head	1	
Reassesses motor, sensory, and circulatory function in each extremity	1	
Applies appropriately sized extrication collar	1	
Positions the immobilization device behind the patient	1	
Secures the device to the patient's torso	1	
Evaluates torso fixation and adjusts as necessary	1	
Evaluates and pads behind the patient's head as necessary	1	
Secures the patient's head to the device	1	
Verbalizes moving the patient to a long backboard	1	
Reassesses motor, sensory, and circulatory function in each extremity	1	

Time End: _____   **TOTAL**   12

CRITICAL CRITERIA

_____ Did not immediately direct or take manual immobilization of the head
_____ Did not properly apply appropriately sized cervical collar before ordering release of manual immobilization
_____ Released or ordered release of manual immobilization before it was maintained mechanically
_____ Manipulated or moved patient excessively causing potential spinal compromise
_____ Head immobilized to the device **before** device sufficiently secured to torso
_____ Device moves excessively up, down, left, or right on the patient's torso
_____ Head immobilization allows for excessive movement
_____ Torso fixation inhibits chest rise, resulting in respiratory compromise
_____ Upon completion of immobilization, head is not in a neutral, in-line position
_____ Did not reassess motor, sensory, and circulatory functions in each extremity after voicing immobilization to the long backboard

You must factually document your rationale for checking any of the above critical items on the reverse side of this form.

National Registry of Emergency Medical Technicians
Advanced Level Practical Examination

SPINAL IMMOBILIZATION (SUPINE PATIENT)

Candidate:_____Examiner:_____

Date: _____Signature:_____

Time Start: _____	Possible Points	Points Awarded
Takes or verbalizes body substance isolation precautions	1	
Directs assistant to place/maintain head in the neutral, in-line position	1	
Directs assistant to maintain manual immobilization of the head	1	
Reassesses motor, sensory, and circulatory function in each extremity	1	
Applies appropriately sized extrication collar	1	
Positions the immobilization device appropriately	1	
Directs movement of the patient onto the device without compromising the integrity of the spine	1	
Applies padding to voids between the torso and the device as necessary	1	
Immobilizes the patient's torso to the device	1	
Evaluates and pads behind the patient's head as necessary	1	
Immobilizes the patient's head to the device	1	
Secures the patient's legs to the device	1	
Secures the patient's arms to the device	1	
Reassesses motor, sensory, and circulatory function in each extremity	1	

Time End: _____　　　　　　　　　　　　　　　　TOTAL　　14

CRITICAL CRITERIA

_____ Did not immediately direct or take manual immobilization of the head
_____ Did not properly apply appropriately sized cervical collar before ordering release of manual immobilization
_____ Released or ordered release of manual immobilization before it was maintained mechanically
_____ Manipulated or moved patient excessively causing potential spinal compromise
_____ Head immobilized to the device **before** device sufficiently secured to torso
_____ Patient moves excessively up, down, left, or right on the device
_____ Head immobilization allows for excessive movement
_____ Upon completion of immobilization, head is not in a neutral, in-line position
_____ Did not reassess motor, sensory, and circulatory functions in each extremity after voicing immobilization to the device

You must factually document your rationale for checking any of the above critical items on the reverse side of this form.

National Registry of Emergency Medical Technicians
Advanced Level Practical Examination

STATIC CARDIOLOGY

Candidate: _____Examiner: _____

Date: _____Signature: _____

SET #_____

Level of Testing: ☐ NREMT-Intermediate/99   ☐ NREMT-Paramedic

Note: No points for treatment may be awarded if the diagnosis is incorrect.
Only document incorrect responses in spaces provided.

Time Start:_____

	Possible Points	Points Awarded
STRIP #1		
Diagnosis:	1	
Treatment:	2	
STRIP #2		
Diagnosis:	1	
Treatment:	2	
STRIP #3		
Diagnosis:	1	
Treatment:	2	
STRIP #4		
Diagnosis:	1	
Treatment:	2	
Time End: _____ TOTAL	12	

National Registry of Emergency Medical Technicians
Advanced Level Practical Examination

VENTILATORY MANAGEMENT - ADULT

Candidate:_____ Examiner:_____

Date: _____Signature: _____

NOTE: If candidate elects to ventilate initially with BVM attached to reservoir and oxygen, full credit must be awarded for steps denoted by "**" so long as first ventilation is delivered within 30 seconds.

	Possible Points	Points Awarded
Takes or verbalizes body substance isolation precautions	1	
Opens the airway manually	1	
Elevates tongue, inserts simple adjunct [oropharyngeal or nasopharyngeal airway]	1	
NOTE: Examiner now informs candidate no gag reflex is present and patient accepts adjunct		
**Ventilates patient immediately with bag mask device unattached to oxygen	1	
**Hyperventilates patient with room air	1	
NOTE: Examiner now informs candidate that ventilation is being performed without difficulty and that pulse oximetry indicates the patient's blood oxygen saturation is 85%		
Attaches oxygen reservoir to bag mask device and connects to high flow oxygen regulator [12-15 L/minute]	1	
Ventilates patient at a rate of 10-20/minute with appropriate volumes	1	
NOTE: After 30 seconds, examiner auscultates and reports breath sounds are present, equal bilaterally and medical direction has ordered intubation. The examiner must now take over ventilation.		
Directs assistant to pre-oxygenate patient	1	
Identifies/selects proper equipment for intubation	1	
Checks equipment for: -Cuff leaks (1 point) -Laryngoscope operational with bulb tight (1 point)	2	
NOTE: Examiner to remove OPA and move out of the way when candidate is prepared to intubate		
Positions head properly	1	
Inserts blade while displacing tongue	1	
Elevates mandible with laryngoscope	1	
Introduces ET tube and advances to proper depth	1	
Inflates cuff to proper pressure and disconnects syringe	1	
Directs ventilation of patient	1	
Confirms proper placement by auscultation bilaterally over each lung and over epigastrium	1	
NOTE: Examiner to ask, "If you had proper placement, what should you expect to hear?"		
Secures ET tube [may be verbalized]	1	
NOTE: Examiner now asks candidate, "Please demonstrate one additional method of verifying proper tube placement in this patient."		
Identifies/selects proper equipment	1	
Verbalizes findings and interpretations [compares indicator color to the colorimetric scale and states reading to examiner]	1	
NOTE: Examiner now states, "You see secretions in the tube and hear gurgling sounds with the patient's exhalation."		
Identifies/selects a flexible suction catheter	1	
Pre-oxygenates patient	1	
Marks maximum insertion length with thumb and forefinger	1	
Inserts catheter into the ET tube leaving catheter port open	1	
At proper insertion depth, covers catheter port and applies suction while withdrawing catheter	1	
Ventilates/directs ventilation of patient as catheter is flushed with sterile water	1	
TOTAL	**27**	

CRITICAL CRITERIA

_____ Failure to initiate ventilations within 30 seconds after applying gloves or interrupts ventilations for greater than 30 seconds at any time
_____ Failure to take or verbalize body substance isolation precautions
_____ Failure to voice and ultimately provide high oxygen concentrations [at least 85%]
_____ Failure to ventilate patient at a rate of at least 10/minute
_____ Failure to provide adequate volumes per breath [maximum 2 errors/minute permissible]
_____ Failure to pre-oxygenate patient prior to intubation and suctioning
_____ Failure to successfully intubate within 3 attempts
_____ Failure to disconnect syringe **immediately** after inflating cuff of ET tube
_____ Uses teeth as a fulcrum
_____ Failure to assure proper tube placement by auscultation bilaterally **and** over the epigastrium
_____ If used, stylette extends beyond end of ET tube
_____ Inserts any adjunct in a manner dangerous to the patient
_____ Suctions the patient for more than 15 seconds
_____ Does not suction the patient

You must factually document your rationale for checking any of the above critical items on the reverse side of this form.

p303/8-003k

Appendix D: Glossary

AAA (abdominal aortic aneurysm) Damage to the wall of the aorta, which causes a thinning of the wall and a large bubble that becomes a pulsatile mass in the patient's abdomen. If the AAA should leak or burst, it can be rapidly fatal.

abandonment Leaving a patient who requires medical care without turning him over to the proper medical care provider.

ABCD survey The survey that is taught in the ACLS course, which includes assessing and managing the airway, breathing, circulation, and defibrillation as needed.

abrasion Damage to the outermost layer of skin due to shearing forces.

abruption placenta The premature separation of the placenta.

absence seizure A type of seizure in which the patient stares off into space or seems to be daydreaming; common in children; once called petit mal.

accommodation The ability of the lenses of the eyes to adjust in order to focus on objects at different distances.

ACD-CPR Active compression-decompression CPR technique.

ACLS (advanced cardiac life support) Training required of medical professionals in the resuscitation of acute cardiac events and ECG dysrhythmias that may be life-threatening.

ACS See *acute coronary syndromes*.

acuity Clarity or sharpness of vision.

acute coronary syndrome (ACS) A broad category of cardiovascular disorders associated with coronary atherosclerosis that may develop a spectrum of clinical syndromes representing varying degrees of coronary artery occlusion. These syndromes include unstable angina, non-Q wave MI, Q wave MI, and sudden cardiac death.

acute life-threatening event (ALTE) An event that is a combination of apnea, choking, gagging, and change in skin color and muscle tone, and is not a sleep disorder.

acute mountain sickness See *AMS*.

acute myocardial infarction See *AMI*.

acute pulmonary edema (APE) A rapid onset of fluid in the alveoli and interstitial tissue of the lungs.

AD (affective disorders) Disorders that affect the patient's temperament.

adrenal gland disease A disease that affects the adrenal gland, such as Cushing's syndrome or adrenal insufficiency.

adrenal insufficiency The inadequate production of adrenal hormones (primarily cortisol and aldosterone).

advanced cardiac life support See *ACLS*.

advanced directive A document or order prepared at the request of the patient, an authorized family member or legal representative, or the physician to ensure that certain treatment choices are followed at a time when the patient is unable to speak for himself.

advanced life support See *ALS*.

adventitious Abnormal.

advocate Someone who looks out for the needs of others who are not in a position to look out for themselves for various reasons, such as ignorance, incapacity, underage, or misfortune; also, to look out for another.

AED (automated external defibrillator) A device designed to be applied by electrode pads to the chest of a pulseless patient, which will rapidly analyze if the ECG is a shockable rhythm and, if so, guide the user with voice prompts through clearing the patient and then administering a shock to the heart.

AEIOUTIPS The mnemonic used to remember the many possible reasons a person may experience an altered mental state: alcohol, epilepsy, infection, overdose, uremia, trauma, insulin, psychosis, stroke.

affect The emotional mindset prompting an expressed emotion or behavior.

agonal respirations Dying breaths; irregular and progressively slowing breaths.

air embolism A potentially life-threatening condition in which a bubble of air has collected in the patient's vessels. This can be caused by a SCUBA incident, a slashed neck vein, or accidental injection of air into a vein.

allergy A reaction from the body after an exposure to a foreign substance.

ALS (advanced life support) The care provided to patients with acute emergencies that involve invasive therapies such as medication administration and inserting an advanced airway device.

ALTE (acute life-threatening event) In the newly born, an event involving a combination of apnea, choking, gagging, and change in color and muscle tone, which is not a sleep disorder.

altered mental status (AMS) The mental status of a patient whose level of consciousness is anything other than alert (oriented to person, place, and day).

altitude illness Sickness brought on in high-altitudes where there is decreased atmospheric pressure. This condition is usually a result of flying in an unpressurized airplane or mountain climbing without first acclimatizing.

Alzheimer's disease A disorder that affects approximately four million Americans, involving cortical atrophy and a loss of neurons in the frontal and temporal lobes of the brain.

American Sign Language (ASL) A communication technique in which the hands and arms are used to sign words or phrases for individuals who are deaf or hard of hearing.

Americans with Disabilities Act (ADA) Federal legislation that regulates the rights of individuals with disabilities to ensure that these individuals have access to equipment and information that can improve their ability to function and interact.

AMI (acute myocardial infarction) The death of cardiac muscle tissue, usually due to a blockage of the blood flow through one of the coronary arteries.

amnesia Forgetting; usually the loss of short-term memory immediately after striking one's head.

amputation Complete loss of a limb or other body part.

AMS (acute mountain sickness) A combination of intracerebral edema and acute pulmonary edema, which is experienced by climbing very tall mountains without first acclimating.

anaphylaxis The most severe type of reaction to an allergen, involving cardiovascular collapse.

anemia of pregnancy An increase in the total blood volume that occurs during pregnancy without a proportionate increase in hemoglobin, creating a dilution effect.

angioedema Cutaneous swelling that most often affects the face, neck, head, and upper airways.

anisocoria Unequal pupils; normal in a small percentage of the population or may indicate a central nervous system disease.

antepartum factors Those medical history factors that may seriously affect pregnancy and labor. Some are controllable (e.g., drug use and smoking) while others are not (e.g., diabetes, placenta previa or abruptia).

anterior cord syndrome A partial transaction caused by bone fragments or pressure on spinal arteries. It involves loss of motor function and the sensation of pain, temperature, and heavy touch.

antibody A protein substance formed by the body in response to antigens that have entered the body.

antigen A foreign substance that, when introduced to the body, causes the production of antibodies.

antisocial behavior A period that some adolescents go through in which they have an identity crisis or act out against society and its rules. This typically peaks around the eighth or ninth grade.

aortic dissection A splitting of the wall of the aorta, usually due to systemic hypertension and a weakness in the wall.

This can lead to a tearing or leaking of the vessel, which can be rapidly life-threatening.

APCO Association of Public-Safety Communications Officials.

APE (acute pulmonary edema) Fluid that has rapidly gathered in the alveoli and interstitial tissue of the lungs from a backup of the blood in the left side of the heart. Primarily found in cardiac patients, but can also be found in patients with altitude sickness and narcotic overdose.

APGAR scoring system A well-accepted assessment scoring system for newborns that assigns a rating of 0, 1, or 2 to each of the following signs: color, pulse, reflex, muscle tone, and respirations. The APGAR score is measured at one minute and five minutes after birth.

aphasia A defect or loss of the ability to either say or comprehend words. The person may have difficulty reading, writing, speaking, or understanding the speech of others.

apical pulse The kick of the left ventricle, which can be felt at the point of maximal impulse on the lower left chest wall.

apnea A cessation of breathing.

apnea monitor A device that is designed to alert the family members or healthcare providers that a patient has stopped breathing. These devices are often used with premature infants and patients with sleep disorders.

apothecary system The system used prior to the metric system, involving units of measure such as minims, fluidrams, fluidounces, pints, and gallons.

arterial gas (air) embolism The most serious diving-related emergency, caused by failing to exhale on ascent with a resultant expansion of air in the lungs, causing alveoli to rupture and allow air to escape.

arterial tourniquet A band of cloth or bandage that is tied so tightly that it occludes the blood flow to an extremity. This is a form of bleeding control considered a last resort where the choice would be to potentially sacrifice the limb to save the life.

ascending nerve tracts Nerve tracts that carry impulses from body parts and sensory information to the brain.

ascites An abnormal accumulation of fluid in the peritoneal cavity.

aspirate To inhale vomitus, blood, or other secretions into the lungs.

assault and battery Striking out at someone or verbally accosting them with the intent to cause harm. In some states, these crimes are illegal against emergency service providers and carry higher penalties.

asthma A form of reversible obstructive lung disease; a multifactorial hypersensitivity reaction causing constriction of the bronchioles and difficulty breathing.

asystole The lack of a cardiac rhythm; cardiac standstill or flatline.

ataxia An abnormal gait that appears wobbly and unsteady, as when one is intoxicated or heavily medicated.

atelectasis Collapse of lung tissue.

atherosclerosis The plaque that forms on the inside of the arteries, also referred to as hardening of the arteries.

Cholesterol, fat, and other blood components build up in the walls of the arteries. As the condition progresses, the arteries to the heart may narrow, reducing the flow of oxygen-rich blood and nutrients to the heart.

atrial fibrillation An ECG dysrhythmia common in the elderly, which originates in the atria and is irregular; involving a fibrillating atria.

atrophy A decrease in cell size leading to a decrease in the size of the tissue and organ.

ATV (automatic transport ventilator) A positive pressure ventilation device that automatically cycles based on the setting of the volume and the rate per minute.

aura A sensation (e.g., color, lights) experienced just before a seizure.

auscultation To listen with a stethoscope, as in breath sounds, blood pressure, and heart sounds.

autoimmunity When a person's T cells or antibodies attack them, causing tissue damage or organ dysfunction.

automated external defibrillator See *AED*.

automatic transport ventilator See *ATV*.

automaticity The unique ability of the heart muscle tissue to generate impulses.

AVPU An abbreviation for the mini-neuro exam used by the EMS provider during the initial assessment of a patient: alert, verbally responsive, painful response, unresponsive.

avulsion Loose or torn tissue.

awareness-level training As specified in the OSHA regulation CFR 1910.120, the level of training for First Responders to hazardous materials incidents where the responders may come in contact with an incident but will be in the cold zone and have no responsibility for patient decontamination.

BAAM® (Beck Airway Airflow Monitor) A small device that fits onto the end of the tracheal tube and is designed to make a noise (like a kazoo) when the patient breathes or when the provider who is attempting to place a tracheal tube through the nasal route locates the glottic opening.

Babinski's reflex An abnormal response of dorsiflexion of the big toe and fanning of all the toes when the outer surface of the sole is firmly stroked from the heel to the toe; indicates a disturbance in the motor response in the central nervous system.

bag mask ventilation Formerly called the BVM, or bag-valve-mask, the Guidelines 2005 have standardized this terminology as the bag mask device or bag mask ventilation.

bag-valve-mask (BVM) See *bag mask ventilation*.

barrel chest The shape of the chest in a COPD patient who has chronically retained air in his lungs for an extended period of time.

baseline vital signs The first set of a patient's vital signs measured.

biological clock The term used to describe the time when a woman is approaching the end of her child-bearing years.

Biot's respirations An irregular but cyclic pattern of increased and decreased rate and depth of breathing, with periods of apnea.

black stool Dark, black, or tarry stool may indicate upper GI bleeding or the ingestion of iron or bismuth preparation, such as antacids.

blast injuries The injuries that occur as the result of an explosion, which are often compounded by occurring within a confined space, causing further injury from the pressure.

blood glucose A measurement of the sugar found in the patient's venous or capillary blood on a test strip or a glucometer.

blood pressure The pressure (systolic) within the arteries when the left ventricle pumps blood into the systemic system, and the pressure (diastolic) in the system during the relaxation of the left ventricle.

BLS (basic life support) 1. CPR; 2. The care provided by First Responders and EMT-Basics, which does not involve invasive interventions.

body language The expression of thoughts or emotions by means of posture or gestures.

body recovery A rescue effort in which it has been determined that the injuries to the patient are mortal wounds or the patient is obviously deceased. All safety must be taken, and this is not a rush that would ever put rescuers in jeopardy.

body surface area (BSA) The amount of skin surface on the body; used to measure the area burned on a person's body.

bone marrow The substance within the shaft of the long bones where red blood cells develop.

bones The strong, fibrous framework of the body. They protect vital organs and provide a structure for muscles to allow movement, as well as for red blood cells to develop.

bowel sounds The sounds of the bowel digesting food, which can be heard by listening with a stethoscope. This is rarely done in the out-of-hospital setting.

bradypnea Slow breathing.

brain abscess A serious condition that can develop within the brain, with signs and symptoms of fever, headache, and possibly sinusitis. The patient may also have a seizure, depending on the location where the abscess develops.

brain herniation A life-threatening injury to the brain, which causes a hematoma and swelling to push brain tissue through the tentorium.

brain stem Helps to connect the hemispheres of the brain. The parts of the brain stem include the midbrain, pons, and medulla oblongata.

Braxton Hicks contractions Irregular and inconsistent contractions; also called false labor.

breath sounds Upon auscultation with a stethoscope, the sound of the air flowing through the patient's lower airways. Depending on the specific location, the sounds can differ slightly.

bronchiolitis A viral infection of the bronchioles that causes swelling of the lower airways.

Brown-Sequard syndrome A syndrome caused by a penetrating injury that produces a partial transection of the spinal cord. It is referred to as a hemisection of the cord and involves only one side of the cord.

bruit A swishing turbulent sound heard over the arteries that indicates blockage of blood flow.

BS (blood sugar) A measurement of the sugar in the patient's bloodstream, as determined by a glucometer or chemical strip from a drop of blood.

BSI (body substance isolation) The level of precautions designed to protect the provider from body substances (e.g., blood, urine, vomit, saliva, etc.). This is used when the rescuer is not able to determine what a liquid substance might be, to which he could potentially be exposed.

CAD (computer-aided dispatch) system A dispatch system where the computer has digitalized locations in the response area and is able to make recommendations to the dispatcher based on available units and their specific locations.

CAD Coronary artery disease.

cancer Includes a large number of malignant neoplasms. The prognosis depends on the extent of its spread when found, metastases, and the effectiveness of treatment.

capillary refill time The amount of time it takes for the capillaries in the fingertips to fill with blood after being temporarily squeezed. Normal capillary refill time is less than two seconds.

capnography A measurement of the level of carbon dioxide exhaled by the patient.

capnometer A device that has a digital readout of end-tidal carbon dioxide.

cardiac enzyme testing When cardiac muscle dies, enzymes are released in the blood stream. The measurement of CK-MB (creatine kinase; M, muscle; B, brain) over a twelve- to twenty-four-hour period.

cardiac muscle The heart is a muscle that has the unique ability to generate and conduct electrical impulses.

cardiac tamponade An accumulation of fluids or a loss of blood into the pericardial sac.

cardiac valves The valves between the chambers, and at the entry and exit of the heart. Designed to prevent backflow of blood into the chamber or vessel from which it came.

cardiogenic shock Hypotension due to a massive ACS or the cumulative effect of multiple MIs, leaving a critical mass of ineffective pumping muscle.

cardiomegaly An increase in heart size, for any number of reasons.

cardiomyopathies Incurable diseases of the heart that ultimately lead to congestive heart failure, ACS, or death.

cardiopulmonary resuscitation (CPR) The technique of providing a combination of high-quality chest compressions and artificial ventilations on a pulseless patient.

carotid artery disease (CAD) Deterioration in the carotid artery as a result of blockage or breakdown in the vessel that can result in inadequate blood flow and blood supply to the organs of the body.

carpopedal spasms Spasmodic contractions of the hands, wrists, feet, and ankles associated with alkalosis and hypocapnia.

cartilaginous joints Joints in which there is cartilage connecting the bones.

catacholamines Various substances that function as hormone or neurotransmitters, or both (e.g., epinephrine or norepinephrine).

CE (continuing education) Updates, reviews, and new training on relevant topics for the healthcare provider. Some providers renew their licenses or certifications based on a specific number of CE hours and topics.

cellular adaption When cells are exposed to adverse conditions, they go through a process of adaption. In some situations, they change permanently; in others, they change their structure and function only temporarily.

cellular environment The distribution of cells throughout the body; the change in cell distribution with aging and disease.

cellular immunity Also known as cell-mediated immunity, the portion of our immune system that primarily involves cells.

cellular injury May result from various causes, such as hypoxia (the most common cause), chemical injury, infectious injury, immunological injury, and inflammatory injury.

central cord syndrome Partial transaction usually occurs with a hyperextension of the cervical region. The patient may have weakness or paresthesia in the upper extremities but normal strength in the lower extremities.

central nervous system (CNS) The brain and spinal cord.

cerebellum The portion of the brain responsible for balance, coordination, and equilibrium.

cerebrospinal fluid (CSF) A clear body fluid, manufactured in the ventricles of the brain, that bathes the brain and spinal cord.

cerebrovascular accident (CVA) A stroke in which there is an interruption of blood flow to an area of the brain, caused by an embolus, hemorrhage, or thrombus.

cerebrum The portion of the brain responsible for thought and higher cognition.

CHD (coronary heart disease) The development of atherosclerosis in the coronary arteries.

chemical injury Chemicals injure and ultimately destroy cells. Chemical carcinogens, cancer-causing agents, can be found everywhere in our environment.

chemical restraint The use of a sedative medication to calm a violent patient.

chemoreceptors Receptors found in the aortic arch and carotid sinus, which analyze the chemistry of the blood and report the findings to the brain.

CHEMTREC A resource that emergency responders to a chemical spill can call for consultation and advice. This hotline, which is open 24 hours a day, 365 days a year, was developed by chemical manufacturers.

Cheyne-Stokes respirations A rhythmic pattern of gradually increased and decreased rates and depths of breathing, with periods of apnea.

CHF (congestive heart failure) Heart failure in which the heart is unable to maintain an adequate flow of blood through the body. Excess fluid collects in the dependent parts of the body, such as the ankles or sacral area, if the patient is bedridden.

chief complaint (CC) The reason EMS was called; best told in the patient's own words.

cholesterol An odorless, white, waxy, powdery substance, needed by the body in small quantities; found in foods.

cholinergic receptor Activated by the involvement of the neurotransmitter acetycholine.

chronic bronchitis An inflammation of the bronchial tubes causing a productive cough that lasts at least three months and reoccurs for two or more years.

chronic obstructive pulmonary disease (COPD) A form of obstructive lung disease (e.g., emphysema, chronic bronchitis, asbestosis, or black lung) that is progressive and irreversible.

Cincinnati Prehospital Stroke Scale A prehospital stroke assessment tool.

circadian rhythms Regular changes in mental and physical characteristics that occur in the course of a day (*circadian* is Latin for "around the day").

CISM (critical incident stress management) A technique for defusing and debriefing stress in emergency responders as a result of major incidents such as the death of a coworker, pediatric catastrophies, or MCIs.

clarification A communication technique in which the EMS provider asks the patient for more information to determine whether his interpretation is accurate.

clean accident An incident that involves an explosion or spill, which does not involve hidden hazards (such as radioactive particles) that could easily spread to those exposed.

cleft lip A birth defect; a cosmetic problem that appears as a separation in the lip.

cleft palate A birth defect; a split in the palate that creates an opening between the mouth and the nose. The opening may be unilateral, complete, or incomplete.

closed fracture A broken bone that has not, as yet, punctured the skin.

closed question A type of question that requires only a "yes" or "no" response or a one- or two-word response; also known as a direct question.

clotbusters Drugs designed to rapidly thin the blood; typically called fibrinolytics or thrombolytics.

CNS (central nervous system) The brain and spinal cord.

CO (cardial output) The stroke volume times the heart rate.

Combitube® A dual-lumen airway that is considered one of the few acceptable advanced airway devices used by out-of-hospital personnel.

communication process The process by which a sender encodes a message to be decoded by an intended receiver, who in turn provides feedback.

compartment syndrome The edema and ischemia caused to the soft tissue by pressure or heavy weight on top of it. The tissue pressure rises above the capillary hydrostatic pressure, resulting in ischemia to the muscle.

compensated shock The early phase of the shock syndrome, in which the patient is able to sustain her systolic BP and adequately perfuse the brain.

comprehensive examination and health assessment An examination of the body as a whole.

compression-ventilation (CV) ratio The number of chest compressions administered to the patient during CPR compared to the number of rescue breaths. For adult, children, and infants, during single-rescuer CPR, this ratio is 30:2.

concealment Positioning oneself behind an object that hides one from the view of others. This offers no ballistic protection.

concussion An injury that shakes up the brain but usually does not involve long-term injury to the brain itself.

conductivity The ability of tissues, such as heart muscle tissue, to allow electrical current to flow through.

confidentiality Keeping the private information that was shared with you about a patient private.

confined-space rescue Access and removal of a patient from a space that is often a low-oxygen environment. A confined space is not designed for people to be in it, and the rescue requires specialty equipment and training.

congenital bleb A birth defect causing a weak spot on the surface of the lung that can burst, causing a pneumothorax.

congenital heart defects Problems with the heart that a patient is born with (e.g., valves not operating properly, holes in the wall of the chambers).

conjugate gaze The normal position of the eyes.

connective tissue Stellate or spindle-shaped cells with interlacing processes that support and bind together other tissues of the body.

consensual light reflex Constriction of both pupils when a light is shone into one eye; a normal response.

consent Permission from an adult to treat a patient.

contained incident A hazmat or MCI that is an isolated area, where all the patients are in one place and not spread out. An example would be an incident on a ferry boat, where all the patients are currently on the boat.

contamination That which is soiled, stained, or containing a potentially hazardous material that could be a danger to the patient and others.

CONTOMS program Counter Narcotic and Terrorism Operational Medical Support program.

contra coup An injury to the brain that develops on the opposite side of the point of impact.

contusion A closed, soft-tissue injury in which cells are damaged and blood vessels are torn.

converge To move closer together; normal movement of the eyes as an object comes closer to the face.

COPD (chronic obstructive pulmonary disease) A lung disease, such as emphysema, chronic bronchitis, asbestosis, or black lung, which involves progressive deteriorating of the lung tissue.

coronary heart disease (CHD) Caused by the narrowing of coronary arteries. In time, the inadequate supply of oxygen-rich blood and nutrients damages the heart muscle and can lead to chest pain and heart attack, and possible death.

coup An injury to the brain that develops directly beneath the point of impact.

coup-contra coup A type of head injury that results when the head is struck on one side, and the force of the impact causes injury to the side that was struck as well as to the opposite side.

cover To hide behind something that conceals a person as well as provides protection from bullets (e.g., a brick wall as opposed to a curtain).

CPR (cardiopulmonary resuscitation) The technique of providing a combination of high-quality chest compressions and artificial ventilations on a pulseless patient.

CQI (continuous quality improvement) A process designed to review and attempt to improve the work or product provided to your customers.

crackles A sound similar to that made by the crumpling up of a candy wrapper, usually heard on expiration; also called rales.

cranial nerves The twelve pairs of nerves that come directly out of the brain, which innervate mostly the head, face, and shoulders, and control sensory and motor functions.

crepitation The sound or sensation of broken bone ends grating on each other.

Cricoid pressure See *Sellick maneuver.*

crisis An internal experience that can create reactions such as severe anxiety, panic, paranoia, or some other brief psychotic event.

croup A viral respiratory infection often caused by other types of infection, such as an ear infection, that results in swelling of the vocal cords, trachea, and upper airway tissues and, thereby, a partial obstruction of the airway.

crushing injury A closed, soft-tissue injury resulting in organ rupture and severe fractures from a crushing force.

CSF (cerebrospinal fluid) Fluid manufactured in the brain's ventricles that circulates around the outer coverings of the brain and spinal cord.

Cullen's sign Ecchymosis in the periumbilical region (around the belly button), indicating internal bleeding.

CUPS A system used in EMS to prioritize patients by severity of presenting problem: critical, unstable, potentially unstable, and stable.

Cushing's triad Three assessment findings that, when displayed together, indicate increasing intracranial pressure (ICP): rising blood pressure, decreasing pulse rate, and changes in the respiratory pattern.

Cystitis An inflammation of the urinary bladder.

DAI (diffuse axonal injury) The effect of acceleration or deceleration on the brain. Often a mild or classic concussion, though it can be moderate or severe.

DAN® The Diver's Alert Network; a resource for injured divers and those who provide emergency care for them.

DCAP-BTLS A mnemonic for assessment points in the examination of soft tissue: deformities, contusions, abrasions, penetrations or punctures, burns, tenderness, lacerations, and swelling.

DCI (decompression illness) A sickness occurring during or after ascent, secondary to a rapid release of nitrogen bubbles. Also called the bends.

DDC (defensive driving course) A course for the general driving public designed to help improve their awareness of how crashes occur, and how to prevent them from occurring.

DEA (Drug Enforcement Agency) Part of the Homeland Security Agency; responsible for enforcing the drug laws.

decerebrate A form of neurological posturing characterized by the patient's stiffly extending both the arms and legs and retracting the head.

decode To interpret a message.

decompensated shock The late phase of shock, when the body is no longer able to maintain the systolic blood pressure and adequately perfuse the brain.

decon To remove a hazardous material from a patient who has been exposed by washing and rinsing him with the appropriate agent in the warm zone of a hazmat.

decorticate A form of neurological posturing characterized by the patient's flexing the upper extremities to the torso, or core of the body, while extending the lower extremities.

degenerative disc disease A common disk problem in patients over fifty years of age. It is a narrowing of the disk that results in variable segments of instability.

degloving Type of open, soft-tissue injury in which the epidermis is removed.

delegation of authority The granting of medical privileges by a physician, either online (direct) or off-line (indirect), to an EMS provider to perform skills or procedures within the EMS provider's scope of practice.

delusion A false personal belief or idea that is portrayed as true.

demand valve A ventilator with a valve that opens to allow self-administered oxygen when the patient creates a negative pressure against the valve or "demands" oxygen by inhaling through the mask. This device is not used for resuscitation of a nonbreathing patient unless it has a positive pressure feature with a triggering device for the healthcare provider to use to ventilate the patient.

dementia A condition of decaying mentality that is characterized by marked decline from the individual's former intellectual level and often by emotional apathy.

depression 1. A depression downward and inward; 2. a psychiatric disorder marked by sadness, inactivity, and difficulty with thinking and concentration.

dermatomes The areas on the surface of the body that are innervated by afferent fibers from one spinal root.

descending nerve tracts The tracts that carry motor impulses from the brain to the body. There are three groups: the corticospinal, reticulospinal, and rubrospinal tracts.

detailed physical examination (DPE) A component of the patient assessment, to be conducted on trauma patients who have significant MOI; this should be done only while en route to the hospital.

developmentally disabled Term used to describe an individual with impaired or insufficient development of the brain, resulting in an inability to learn at the usual rate.

diabetic ketoacidosis (DKA) During hypoglycemia, the inability of patients with diabetes to metabolize fat.

diagnosis The identification of a specific disease or condition; usually made after the medical team has evaluated the entire situation; the determination, by a physician, of the medical problem that a patient is experiencing.

dialysis A general term for a method, involving a semipermeable membrane, used to separate smaller particles from larger ones in a liquid mixture.

diarrhea Abnormally frequent intestinal evacuations with liquid stool.

diastolic The residual blood pressure in the arterial system as the left ventricle relaxes.

diffuse axonal injury (DAI) Injury to brain tissues that results from rapid acceleration or deceleration on the brain.

diffusion The process where particles of liquids, gases, or solids intermingle as a result of their spontaneous movement caused by thermal agitation; in dissolved substances, the movement from regions of higher to lower concentrations.

digital intubation A blind form of intubation that involves using the fingers.

diplopia Double vision.

dirty accident An incident involving a bomb or chemical spillage that is laced with radioactive particles that are extremely hazardous.

disentanglement To carefully remove the parts of a vehicle that a patient is wrapped around or pinned underneath in order to release the patient.

disinfection To free from infection and destroy harmful microorganisms.

dislocation Displacement of one or more of the bones at a joint.

distress Pain or suffering affecting the body.

diverge To move apart; normal movement of the eyes as they focus on a distant object.

diving emergencies Any one of a number of injuries or illnesses that can occur during underwater diving (e.g., the bends, nitrogen narcosis, overpressurization injuries).

dizziness The sensation of unsteadiness and the sensation of movement within the head.

DKA See *diabetic ketoacidosis*.

DNAR (do not attempt resuscitation) order An order in a patient's chart that was prepared after consultation with the patient or her legal proxy and physician, based on the wishes of the patient that a resuscitation not be attempted should she go into cardiac arrest.

DNR (do not resuscitate) order The current terminology is DNAR.

domestic violence Violence that occurs, either physical, sexual, or emotional, within an adult partner relationship.

doppler ultrasound A device used for physical examination that monitors the Doppler effect. The Doppler effect is a change in frequency during which waves (sound or light) from a given source reach an observer, while the source and the observer are in rapid motion with respect to each other, so that the frequency increases or decreases according to the speed at which the distance is decreasing or increasing.

DOT-KKK-1822 The Federal Ambulance Specifications.

Down syndrome Moderate to severe mental retardation caused by trisomy of the human chromosome 21, in which a person often has slanting eyes, a broad, short skull, and broad hands with short fingers.

DPE (detailed physical examination) The head-to-toe examination that is done on the trauma patient with significant MOI en route to the hospital.

DPL (diagnostic peritoneal lavage) A procedure that is done on patients with abdominal trauma and suspected internal organ injury to see if there is bleeding into the abdomen.

drowning To suffocate in water or some other liquid.

due regard A legal term found in most state's motor vehicle laws describing the level of responsibility of an operator of an emergency vehicle (i.e., with *due regard* for the safety of all other motorists).

duty to act A legal term that describes the level of responsibility of an EMT or paramedic when on duty and receiving a call.

dysarthria An abnormal articulation of speech due to disturbances in muscle control.

dysphagia Difficulty swallowing.

dysphasia Abnormal speech due to lack of coordination and failure to arrange words in the proper order.

dysphonia Discomfort when speaking due to laryngeal disease.

dysplasia Abnormal growth or development of cells.

dyspnea Difficulty breathing.

dysrhythmias An irregular electrocardiogram.

dysuria Difficulty urinating.

eclampsia An attack of convulsions due to toxcemia of pregnancy.

ECF (extracellular fluid) The fluid outside the cells.

ECG (electrocardiogram) The tracing made by an electrocardiograph of the electrical potential occurring within the heart.

edema An abnormal collection of serous fluid in a connective or serous tissue.

EGTA (esophageal-gastric tube airway) An advanced airway device that is a Class III device and may be harmful to use in the field.

Einthoven's triangle Dr. William Einthoven, the inventor of the ECG machine, described the placement of the first three standardized leads (lead I, II, and III) as a triangle over the body and around the heart.

electro-mechanical disassociation (EMD) A lack of an association between the electrical activity and the mechanical activity of the heart, resulting in a cardiac standstill or lack of perfusion. The terminology was changed to pulseless electrical activity, or PEA.

emancipated minor A child under the age of eighteen who has legally declared himself free of his parents. In most states, this also includes a pregnant female or one who is the mother of a child.

EMD Emergency medical dispatcher.

emergency doctrine The type of consent given for emergency intervention for a patient who is physically or mentally unable to provide expressed consent; also called implied consent. This type of consent remains in effect for as long as the patient requires lifesaving treatments.

Emergency Medical Services Systems Act The law enacted by each state to allow for a designated lead agency (e.g., health, emergency management, DOT, etc.) to supervise and coordinate the development of the EMS system.

emotional disorder Also called a "mental disorder," any disturbance of emotional balance manifested by maladaptive behavior and impaired functioning (e.g., depression).

empathy A sensitivity to and an understanding of another person's feelings.

emphysema A chronic lung disease that results from a destruction of the walls of the alveoli.

EMS-C (Emergency Medical Services for Children) Act Passed in 1983, this act (PL-98-555) was designed to improve the care of children.

EMS Command The overall leader of the EMS response at the scene of an MCI.

EMT-Basic One of the four national levels of EMS provider (FR, EMT-B, EMT-I, EMT-P) that has training curriculum developed by the U.S. Department of Transportation. The EMT-Basic is the program designed as the minimum training level required to work or volunteer on an ambulance; skills involved in the training revolve around that role.

encode To determine what terms to use to convey a message.

endocrinology The study of the endocrine glands.

endometriosis The presence and growth of functioning endometrial tissue in places other than the uterus, which often results in severe pain and infertility.

Endotrol® tube A specialized endotracheal tube that has a small ring with a connection to the tip of the tube. This is particularly helpful, when doing a blind nasal intubation, in directing the tip of the tube into the glottic opening.

end-tidal carbon dioxide (EtCO₂) The concentration of carbon dioxide (CO_2) in the exhaled gas at the end of the exhalation.

enhanced 911 A system of alerting emergency services by the public in communities where the 911 uniform access number is in place. In the enhanced version, the software places the caller's location (based on the phone he or she is calling from) on the dispatcher's CRT screen.

enteral drug administration Administering medicine that is swallowed and then passes through the stomach and intestines.

environmental emergencies A group of illnesses that relate to extreme conditions of the weather or activities that occur outdoors (e.g., drowning, submersion, heat-related illness, hypothermia and frostbite, diving accidents, etc.).

EOA (esophageal obturator airway) A Class III airway device that may be considered harmful to use in the field.

epidemiology A study of the causes and trends of injury or illness and disease.

epidural hematoma An injury to the brain that involves an arterial tear resulting in increased intracranial pressure.

epiglottitis A rare, life-threatening infection causing severe inflammation and swelling of the epiglottis.

epilepsy A disease that involves convulsions that can be controlled by taking anticonvulsants.

Epi-pen® Designed for patients who are highly allergic, the pen is a self-injector of epinephrine for anaphylaxis.

epistaxis A nose bleed.

error of commission or omission Negligent acts, for which a provider could be sued, that involve going beyond the scope of practice (commission) and not providing treatment at the level of the standard of care by eliminating vital steps (omission).

escharotomy A surgical incision into necrotic tissue of a burn to expand the tissue and decrease ischemia from a circumferential burn.

esophageal intubation detector (EDD) device An airway tool with either a bulb syringe or a rigid syringe that is used to determine whether an endotracheal tube is in the trachea or esophagus.

esophageal tracheal combitube (ETC; see Combitube®) The esophageal-tracheal combitube is referred to as the Combitube® throughout the Guidelines 2005 publication.

ethics The study of hard decisions that are not defined by laws but are considered the right thing to do, involving values and morals.

etiology The cause of a disease or condition.

ET tube A clear plastic tube that is designed to be passed through the vocal cords and glottic opening to assist with ventilations directly into the patient's lungs.

eupnea Normal breathing.

eustress The normal stress of life that is necessary to function.

EVOC (emergency vehicle operator course) A training program that involves both a didactic and lab (hands-on) component, developed by the U.S. DOT and designed to improve the driving skills of the operator of an emergency vehicle. There are three versions of the course, each focused on a specific audience and type of vehicle (e.g., police, firefighters, EMS workers).

exacerbation An increase in the seriousness of a disease or disorder.

extracorporal CPR The technique of cardiac compressions that are employed when a patient arrests during open chest surgery.

extraocular muscles (EOMs) Muscles that produce movement of the eyes.

extravasate Escape of fluid, such as blood from a vessel into the surrounding tissues.

extubation The removal of a tube, such as the ET tube, from the trachea or when incorrectly inserted from the esophagus.

facilitation The method in which EMS providers speak and use posture and actions to encourage the patient to say more.

false imprisonment To take someone someplace and keep him or her there against his or her will, without consent (e.g., kidnapping).

FAS (fetal alcohol syndrome) A group of birth defects, including mental retardation, deficient growth, and defects of the skull, face, and brain, that tends to occur in the infants of women who consume a large amount of alcohol during pregnancy.

FAST Abbreviation used in stroke assessment to remind the provider of facial droop, abnormal speech, smile, and time, which are components of the Cincinnati Prehospital Stroke Scale.

fat One of the essential nutrients that supplies calories to the body. Fat provides nine calories per gram, more than twice the number provided by carbohydrates or protein. Small amounts of fat are necessary for normal body function.

FCC (Federal Communications Commission) The federal agency responsible for allocating and supervising the radio airwaves and frequencies.

febrile seizures The convulsions in an infant, which are a result of the rapid rise in temperature from a fever.

feedback A receiver's response to a message.

festination An abnormal gait that appears uneven and hurried, as seen in Parkinson's patients.

fetal alcohol syndrome See *FAS*.

fetal distress A fetus may be stressed while in the uterus due to a number of reasons (e.g., post-term gestation over forty-two weeks, maternal supine hypotensive syndrome, eclampsia, umbilical cord obstruction or prolapse, placental insufficiency, hypoxia, drug effects, or bacterial sepsis).

fetal heart rate (FHR) The heart rate of a fetus.

fetal heart tones (FHTs) The heartbeats of a fetus.

fibrinolysis The body's natural and normal way of preventing excess blood clot formation.

fibrous joints Joints that are connected by fibrous tissue, such as the immovable sutures that are located in the skull.

Fick principle Oxygen transport principle that states that adequate cellular perfusion requires four components to be present and working: an adequate oxygen supply, oxygen exchange in the lungs, the circulation of oxygen to the cells, and an adequate number of red blood cells.

field impression A working diagnosis to determine the cause of a patient's condition.

"fight or flight" response The hormonal response to stress that can affect the EMS provider's decision-making ability both positively and negatively.

first-party caller An emergency call to the EMS dispatcher or 911 operator that comes directly from the patient.

First Responder awareness level Level at which an EMS provider is trained to recognize a hazardous materials incident, back off, and call for help.

First Responder operations level Level at which an EMS provider is trained to perform risk assessment, to select and don appropriate personal protective equipment, and to contain the scene and carry out basic decontamination procedures.

flail segment A section of the rib cage that has two or more ribs broken in two or more places, creating a paradoxical movement of the broken section as the patient breathes; also called a flail chest.

flow-restricted, oxygen-powered ventilation device (FROPVD) Used for mechanical positive pressure ventilation of a patient in the out-of-hospital setting. The Guidelines 2005 refer to these devices as manually triggered, oxygen-powered, flow-limiting resuscitators.

FLSA (Fair Labor Standards Act) The FLSA is the federal law that regulates minimum wages and overtime in the workplace.

flu Influenza, or the flu, is a specific type of viral infection that may affect both the upper (e.g., dry, hacking cough with diffuse muscle aches) and lower respiratory tracts (e.g., pneumonia).

fluid wave test A special procedure that is performed on the abdomen to test for ascites.

focal head injury Injury to the brain tissues resulting in lesions.

focused history and physical examination (FH&PE) A component of patient assessment that varies depending on whether the patient has a medical or trauma complaint. If trauma, the MOI is determined, vital signs are taken, and a history of presenting illness is determined on the basis of OPQRST.

FOIA (Freedom of Information Act) A law that allows the general public to obtain copies of government documents.

food poisoning Gastroenteritis or a more severe infection caused by pathogens in spoiled or improperly prepared food.

foreign body airway obstruction (FBAO) The blockage of the upper airways due to the inhalation of objects such as a large bolus of meat, a coin, or a balloon. These are classified as mild or severe.

fractures Broken bones.

frontal lobotomy A surgical procedure designed to disconnect the frontal cerebral lobe, which houses inhibition and extreme emotional reactions, from the rest of the brain. This is a last resort in the psychiatric patient prone to fits of anger.

FROPVD See *flow-restricted, oxygen-powered ventilation device.*

frostbite A local cold injury ranging from superficial to partial thickness to full thickness. At risk are the very old and very young, as well as those who are outdoors in very cold and windy temperatures with hands or face exposed.

fundus The top of the uterus.

gallstones Also referred to as cholelithiasis, these are caused by the precipitation of substances contained in bile such as cholesterol and bilirubin.

GAS (general adaptation syndrome) GAS is a long-term physiological response pattern to adaption. The response is mediated by cortisol release from the adrenal cortex.

gastric distention The bloating of the stomach with air and food, which leaves the patient prone to regurgitation.

gastric ulcers Ulcerations of the stomach caused by the bacterium *Helicobacter pylori* (*H. pylori*).

gastroenteritis A general term that includes many types of infections and irritations of the digestive tract.

gastroenterology The study of the digestive system and its workings.

GCS (Glasgow Coma Scale) A numerical score to quantify the severity of an altered mental status resulting from head injury, utilizing the sum of the following three variables: best eye opening response (4 to 1), best verbal response (5 to 1), and best motor response (6 to 1). Scores can range from 3 to 15.

general impression The EMS provider's first impression of the patient to determine the priority of care, taking into consideration the environment and the patient's chief complaint.

generalized seizure A type of seizure that involves the entire brain and is classified as complete motor seizure, absence seizure, or atonic seizure; once called grand mal.

geriatrics The study of the elderly.

gerontology The study of the problems of all aspects of aging.

GI bleed Hemorrhaging from an ulceration of the stomach or other GI tract structures.

glaucoma A disease in which elevated pressure in the eye, due to an obstruction of the outflow of aqueous humor, damages the optic nerve and causes visual defects.

Global Med-Net A medical information service with a toll-free phone number EMS providers can call to obtain a patient's complete medical profile using the patient's member identification number.

glucose meter A hand-held glucose meter, which is a relatively accurate method to determine the range of a person's glucose.

golden hour The optimum limit of one hour between time of injury and surgery at the hospital.

Good Samaritan law A state law designed to provide legal protection and limited immunity from civil suits for individuals who stop at the scene of an accident to render first aid.

governmental immunity A specific state law designed to provide legal protection and limited immunity for local government employees.

gravida The total number of pregnancies a woman has had.

gray matter The gray fibers of the CNS including the cerebral cortex, basal ganglia, and parts of the brain and spinal cord.

Grey-Turner's sign Ecchymosis in the flanks and periumbilical areas that is a late sign of internal bleeding.

grieving A process in response to the death or dying of a loved one, which includes the stages of shock, denial, anger, bargaining, depression, and acceptance.

grunting A sound that results from breathing out against a partially obstructed epiglottis.

guarding A particular position of comfort to protect a body part from pain.

Guidelines 2005 The American Heart Association's latest issue of the resuscitation and emergency cardiovascular care treatments, which are based upon the latest science as well as the consensus of the International Liaison Committee on Resuscitation (ILCOR) councils.

gynecology The study of problems associated with the female reproductive system and its structures.

HACE (high-altitude cerebral edema) Swelling of the brain caused by failing to properly acclimate to high altitudes.

HAPE (high-altitude pulmonary edema) Swelling and fluid collected in the lungs caused by failing to properly acclimate to high altitudes.

hazardous material (hazmat) Any substance that can cause injury or death to an individual who has been exposed to the substance.

HDL cholesterol High-density lipoprotein, which helps carry the "bad cholesterol" away from the walls of the arteries and returns it to the bloodstream, thus preventing buildup of cholesterol in the artery walls.

headache Pain in the head that may be caused by one of a number of conditions such as: cerebral aneurysm, glaucoma, meningitis, migraine, stress, subarachnoid, temporal arteritis, temporomandibular joint syndrome, trauma, and trigeminal neuralgia.

healthcare power of attorney A durable power of attorney or healthcare proxy allows a person to designate an agent to act in cases where the person is unable to make decisions for him- or herself.

healthcare professional (HCP) One who confirms to the standards of a healthcare profession to provide quality patient care.

healthcare proxy The person who has the legal authority to make medical decisions for a patient should he or she become incapacitated.

heart sounds The sounds of the valves closing, heard through a stethoscope, during the pumping phases of the heart.

heat illness Medical condition sustained from exposure to extremely hot weather conditions or environmental conditions, such as heat exhaustion or heat stroke.

HEENT An acronym for head, eyes, ears, nose, and throat.

HELP position The heat-escape lessening position, which involves floating with the head out of the water and the body in a fetal tuck.

hematocrit The number of red blood cells (RBCs) in the peripheral blood.

hematology The study of the blood and its medical conditions.

hematoma A collection of blood beneath the skin.

hematopoietic system The system that produces blood cells.

hemoglobin and hematocrit (H&H) Hemoglobin is the part of the red blood cell that contains iron and carries oxygen to the lungs and tissues. Hematocrit is the percentage of the whole volume of blood contributed by cells.

hemophilia Hereditary deficiency of clotting factors IVVV (hemophilia A) or IX (hemophilia B).

hemoptysis Coughing up blood from the respiratory tract.

hemothorax Blood in the chest cavity.

hepatitis An inflammation of the liver causing an acute or chronic potentially life-threatening condition.

hepatojugular reflux Observing the jugular veins while simultaneously performing a deep palpation on the upper-right quadrant of the abdomen for thirty to sixty seconds.

herniated intervertebral disk Damage to the disk that can allow leakage of the fluid in the disk. This is a very painful injury or condition that can easily be aggravated by simply bending the wrong way.

HHNC (hyperosmolar hyperglycemia nonketotic coma) Results from a relative insulin deficiency that leads to marked hyperglycemia and the absence of ketones and acidosis.

high-frequency chest compressions An experimental type of CPR involving over 120 chest compressions per minute.

history of the present illness (HPI) Specific patient information about the current illness or condition.

HIV (human immunodeficiency virus) The virus that has been found to be the cause of acquired immunodeficiency syndrome (AIDS).

homeostasis The effort and mechanisms of the body to keep its environment "normal."

hospice The psychological, physical, spiritual, and pain management support for a terminally ill patient and his or her family.

HPV Human papillomavirus.

HTN Hypertension.

humane restraints Wide leather or cloth restraints that are used to tie a patient in the supine or seated position onto a stretcher. It is not appropriate to use handcuffs to restrain a patient with a medical or psychiatric problem, as they can cause injury to the patient.

humoral immunity Also known as antibody-mediated immunity, primarily involves antibodies that are produced by a specialized WBC, the B lymphocyte.

Huntington's disease A rare hereditary disorder involving chronic progressive chorea, psychological changes, and dementia.

hypercapnia An abnormally high concentration of carbon dioxide in the blood.

hypercarbia Carbon dioxide retention.

hydrocephalus An increase in the amount of CSF due to either a blockage or decreased reabsorption.

hydrophobia Another name for rabies, a viral infection of the central nervous system.

hyperbaric chamber therapy A chamber used to treat conditions brought on by SCUBA accidents and carbon monoxide poisoning. Under pressure, it is possible to help the oxygen attach to the hemoglobin receptor sites on the red blood cells.

hyperglycemia An elevated blood sugar level often found in diabetics or patients who have problems with their pancreas or insulin production.

hypernatremia A high sodium level.

hyperplasia An increase in the number of cells due to hormonal stimulation. The excess growth often causes tumors that may be malignant or benign.

hypersensitivity Any bodily response to any substance to which a patient is abnormally sensitive.

hypertensive emergency A life-threatening, sudden, and severe increase in BP that can lead to serious, irreversible end-organ damage within hours if left untreated.

hypertrophy An increase in the size of the cell leading to an increase in tissue and organ size.

hyperventilation A respiratory rate greater than that required for normal body function.

hyphema Bleeding into the anterior chamber of the eye.

hypocapnia An abnormally low concentration of carbon dioxide in the blood.

hypoglycemia A low blood sugar level, often found in patients with a history of diabetes after a period of exercising or not eating.

hyponatremia A low sodium level.

hypothermia A generalized low body temperature and the associated condition it causes.

hypothyroidism Also called myxedema, a clinical syndrome due to a deficiency of thyroid hormone.

hypoventilation Irregular and shallow breathing.

hypovolemic shock Poor peripheral perfusion due to a loss of blood volume.

hypoxemia A lack of oxygen in the blood (e.g., carbon monoxide taking up all the oxygen receptor sites on the hemoglobin).

hypoxia Inadequate oxygenation of the blood cells.

IAC-CPR Interposed abdominal compressions CPR technique.

iatrogenic disorder A medical condition that is caused by the care provided by a healthcare provider.

IBS (irritable bowel syndrome) A condition characterized by recurrent abdominal pain, usually crampy in nature, and diarrhea, often alternating with periods of constipation.

ICF (intracellular fluid) The fluid within the cells. Water moves between the ICF and the extracellular fluid by osmosis.

ICS (incident command system) See *IMS*.

ictal phase The period during a seizure attack.

ILCOR (International Liaison Committee on Resuscitation) The group of resuscitation councils and experts who develop the Consensus on Science, on which the American Heart Association's Guidelines are based.

illusions Misperceptions of actual existing stimuli by any sense.

immune system The body's complex system that acts to fight off foreign substances and disease-causing agents.

immunizations Injections of medications designed to prevent infectious diseases (e.g., tetanus, diphtheria, hepatitis B).

immunologic injury When cellular membranes are injured by direct contact with the cellular and chemical components of the immune or inflammatory process, such as phagocytes, histamine, antibodies, and lymphokines.

impaled object An object that has pierced and become fixed in the skin and tissues.

IMS (incident management system) The system used to coordinate the efforts at a disaster or major incident. It involves command and the four key functional areas of finance, logistics, operations, and planning, as well as a module design for escalation and de-escalation as the incident warrants. Previously called incident command system, or ICS.

incident command system (ICS) See *IMS*.

incident report The appropriate documentation, aside from the PCR, that EMS agencies prepare in unusual instances or for reportable cases (e.g., infectious disease exposure, work injury or fatality, multiple casualty incident).

incision A clean break in the skin, usually made by a knife.

index of suspicion Injury patterns associated with specific mechanisms of injury from which the EMS provider can anticipate the potential for shock or other problems.

infants According to the American Heart Association, a child is considered an infant from the release of the initial hospitalization to one year of age.

infectious and communicable diseases Conditions that can be transmitted from person to person. A communicable disease can be transmitted directly or indirectly from one person to another. An infectious disease is an illness caused by an invasion of the body by an organism such as a virus, bacteria, or fungus.

inflammatory injury Inflammation is a protective response that can occur without bacterial invasion. This occurs when cellular membranes are injured by direct contact with the cellular and chemical components of the inflammatory process.

initial assessment (IA) The second component of patient assessment; an orderly and sequential examination with correction of life-threats and determination of the patient's priority.

injury Blunt or penetrating trauma that has damaged a body part.

inspection The first step in the examination of a patient, which involves looking at the body part and comparing it to the other side (e.g., right leg to left leg).

interstitial fluid The fluid that is found between the cells of the body.

intracranial hemorrhage Bleeding into the head, usually developing a collection of blood that is named in relation to the meninges (e.g., subdural, epidural).

involuntary commitment Each state law may differ on this, but a patient can be committed to a mental health facility for an evaluation, against his or her will, on the order of a county mental health physician.

IPPB (intermittent positive-pressure breathing) Indicated when a conscious or unconscious adult patient needs a high volume of high-concentration oxygen. It is not indicated with noncompliant patients who are breathing but fight the device.

IQ (intelligence quotient) One of the standardized tests commonly used to identify mental retardation. When the IQ exam is administered, a tested IQ of seventy is considered the upper line for those needing special care and training.

irreversible shock The phase of shock when the patient has attempted to compensate but his mechanisms have been overwhelmed, and the damage occurring at the cellular level is irreversible.

ischemia Tissue that is starved of oxygen but the damage is not yet permanent.

isoimmunity Formation of antibodies or T cells directed against antigens on another person's cells.

isotonic fluid volume The fluid in the extracellular compartment that can shift into the cells or vascular space. An isotonic fluid excess represents an increase in both sodium and water in the ECF compartment. This is commonly caused by kidney, heart, or liver failure.

ITD (impedance threshold device) A valve that is designed to improve coronary perfusion and is easily employed during CPR.

jaundice Caused by an excess of bilirubin, this is a yellowish pigment to the skin. This condition is common with liver disease and in premature infants during their initial hospitalization.

JVD (jugular vein distention) The external, noninvasive measurement of CVP. With the patient placed in the semi-Fowler's position, distension indicates increased CVP.

KE (kinetic energy) Energy that is absorbed by the body in a car crash or a penetrating or blunt injury. It is calculated by multiplying half the mass by the velocity squared.

Kehr's sign Abdominal pain that radiates to the left shoulder, which may be an indication of intraperitoneal bleeding.

keloid scar formation The excessive accumulation of scar tissue that extends beyond the original wound border is called a keloid scar.

kinesthetic Refers to the sense of body position.

Kussmaul's respirations Air hunger.

labor The pain and contractions of the uterus while the cervix dilates to allow expulsion of the fetus. It is divided into three stages.

laceration A break in the skin; can be deep or superficial and usually has uneven edges.

lactose intolerance A very common GI abnormality affecting almost half the world's population. Patients get bloating, pain, and diarrhea, sometimes violent, within minutes to hours after eating the sugar lactose that is found in milk and cheese.

laryngeal spasm A closure of the vocal cords and surrounding muscles. It may be caused by the trauma of an overly aggressive intubation attempt.

laryngectomy A surgical removal of the larynx, often due to cancer of the throat.

latex A natural sap from the rubber tree used to make natural rubber products.

LDB-CPR CPR compressions that employ a load-distributing band or vest CPR device.

LDL cholesterol The "bad cholesterol" or low-density lipoprotein that carries the largest amount of cholesterol in the blood and is responsible for depositing cholesterol in the artery walls. An elevated LDL cholesterol level is associated with risk of heart disease.

LeFort classifications Named after French surgeon Leon LeFort, a classification of facial fractures.

leukocytes Includes the two white blood cell types: granulocytes and monocytes.

leukotriene blockers Produced during asthma attacks, these are the anti-inflammatory drugs that either block the leukotriene receptor or the substance that synthesizes leukotrienes.

Levine's sign Presentation of a sick-looking patient who places a clenched fist over the sternum to describe chest pain.

libel An act in which a person's character or reputation is injured by the false or malicious written words of another person.

life expectancy The amount of time remaining before a person is expected to die.

life span The total duration of one's life from birth to death.

lightning injuries An electrical burn injury from a strike, or from being very close to a strike, of a lightning bolt.

limbic system Located in the diencephalon, the limbic system is comprised of several brain structures that are involved with emotions.

lipids Fatty substances that are present in blood and body tissues and include cholesterol and triglycerides.

lipoproteins Protein-coated packages that carry fat and cholesterol through the body. Lipoproteins are classified by their density.

living will An advanced directive that states the type of life-saving medical treatment a patient wants or does not want to be employed in case of terminal illness.

LMA (laryngeal mask airway) An advanced airway device that is used on unconscious or non-breathing patients to improve ventilation. Its use is recommended for patients with an empty stomach, as aspiration is a concern if the patient regurgitates.

loaded bumper A shock-absorbing bumper on a motor vehicle that has been compressed and can release suddenly without warning.

LOC (level of consciousness) The patient's mental status, usually described using the acronym AVPU.

Los Angeles Prehospital Stroke Screen (LAPSS) An out-of-hospital ministroke assessment tool.

Lyme disease An infection that is transmitted by ticks. Flu-like symptoms and muscle joint aches follow, with or without a rash. The infection can lead to AMS, paralysis, paresthesia, stiff neck, sensitivity to light, dysrhythmias, and chest pain.

LZ (landing zone) The location where a helicopter can safely land. It needs to be flat, wide, or obstruction free, and approximately $100' \times 100'$.

malpractice Dereliction of professional duty.

manic-depressive disorder A major mental disorder characterized by fits of mania and periods of depression.

manual spinal motion restriction (MSMR) Instead of using the terminology "spinal immobilization," this phrase is now used in the Guidelines 2005, as it is more accurate.

Marfan's syndrome Inherited disease of the connective tissue characterized by elongated long bones and ocular and circulatory defects.

MAST/PASG Military antishock trousers/pneumatic antishock garment.

McBurney's point A landmark on the abdomen associated with the late pain of appendicitis; an imaginary triangle on the anterior lower right quadrant, from the navel out to the right superior iliac spine.

MCI (multiple casualty incident) An incident involving many patients.

MD (muscular dystrophy) Any of a group of hereditary diseases characterized by progressive muscular wasting.

mechanical piston device A device used for CPR, such as the life vest or the Thumper®.

meconium The greenish, tar-like substance that an infant may be covered with at birth. It is thought to be the result of fetal distress.

medical command At a major incident, the leader of the EMS personnel who should be working with the incident commander in the command post.

medical direction Either online or off-line input or physician direction of EMS providers in their care of patients.

MedicAlert® Foundation An organization that maintains a twenty-four-hour emergency response center with a toll-free phone number that EMS providers can call to obtain information on patients who wear medical identification necklaces or bracelets with an identifiable symbol.

medical monitoring At a hazmat incident or fire rehab sector, the monitoring of the firefighter's vital signs or the hazmat team prior to suiting up and after removing the suits. This is conducted in the cold zone.

Medical Practice Act The state law that specifies exactly what a healthcare provider is allowed to do in his or her work environment.

melena Blood in stool.

meninges The three layers that cover the brain and spinal cord.

meningitis An inflammation of the meninges that can be caused by a bacteria or virus. Bacterial meningitis is highly communicable and may be fatal if not aggressively treated in the hospital setting.

menopause The period of natural cessation of menstruation occurring between the ages of forty-five and fifty.

menstrual cycle The entire cycle of physiological changes from the beginning of one cycle to the beginning of the next.

mental retardation Sub-average intellectual ability that is equal to or below an IQ of seventy and is present from birth.

mental status (MS) Determination of whether a patient is alert and oriented.

message The points being conveyed by a sender to a receiver.

metabolic acidosis A shift in the body's pH caused by the metabolic processes, producing a pH under 7.35.

metabolic alkalosis A shift in the body's pH caused by the metabolic processes, producing a pH over 7.45.

metaplasia The transformation of one tissue into another (e.g., cartilage into bone); the abnormal replacement of cells by another type of cell.

MI (myocardial infarction) A heart attack where cardiac cells are deprived of oxygen for a long enough time that they begin to die.

middle meningeal artery The artery in the temporal skull that is usually the cause of an epidural hematoma, due to a blow to the temporal skull.

minimum data set The data elements defined by the federal government to be placed on all standardized prehospital care reports in the United States.

minute volume The amount of gas inspired in a minute.

mitral valve prolapse Also referred to as a floppy mitral valve, which has been associated with Marfan's syndrome, osteogenesis imperfecta, and other connective tissue disorders.

mittelschmerz Abdominal pain in the middle of the menstrual period usually associated with ovulation.

MODS (multiple organ dysfunction syndrome) This is a new diagnosis (since 1975) that involves the progressive failure of two or more organ systems after severe illness or injury.

MOI (mechanism of injury) The forces that caused an injury, which can be predictive of the extent of the injury patterns (e.g., type of collision, speed and type of penetrating projectile, distance of fall).

monocyte A large leukocyte with finely granulated chromatin dispersed throughout the nucleus.

monounsaturated fat Slightly unsaturated fat that is found in greatest amounts in foods from plants, including olive and canola oil. When substituted for saturated fat, monounsaturated fat helps to reduce blood cholesterol.

morbidity The extent of injury in groups of patients caused by trauma or medical conditions.

Morgan lenses® A special contact lens that is designed to allow flushing of the eye that has been exposed to chemicals or a burn injury.

mortality The death rate of patients caused by injuries or medical conditions.

MS (mental status) The state of a patient's level of consciousness as described using AVPU.

MS (multiple sclerosis) A demyelenating disease marked by patches of hardened tissue in the brain or spinal cord. It is associated with paralysis and muscular jerking or tremors.

MS-ABC The plan for the initial assessment of a patient involving an assessment of the mental status, airway, breathing, and circulation.

multiparous Term used to describe a woman who has given birth.

musculoskeletal trauma An injury to the bones or muscles such as a sprain, strain, dislocation, or a fracture.

myelin A soft, white, fatty sheath around the protoplasmic core of the mylenated nerve.

myxedema Severe hypothyroidism characterized by a firm, inelastic edema, dry skin and hair, and loss of mental and physical vigor.

NAERG (North American Emergency Response Guidebook) The book that should be carried in every emergency vehicle to identify the most commonly found hazardous materials in transport on the highways.

NALS (neonatal advanced life support) A training program focused on the initial hospitalization of an infant.

narrow complex SVT A category of rapid ECG rhythms presumably originating from the atria.

nasal cannula A basic oxygen-administration device used on patients who will not tolerate a mask or who require only small percentages of oxygen.

nasal flaring Widening of the nostrils during breathing.

nasal pharyngeal airway (NPA) A basic airway adjunct designed to be lubricated with a water-soluble gel and then inserted into the nares.

nasotracheal intubation An advanced procedure that involves a blind insertion of a tube down the nares, listening for air movement, while attempting to insert the distal end into the glottic opening.

nature of the illness (NOI) The condition or chief complaint of the patient.

nausea The sensation that a patient describes of feeling like he or she could vomit.

near drowning A patient who was submersed under water for a long enough period of time to need emergency medical care and possibly rescue breathing or CPR.

needle cricothyrotomy The last-resort technique in a patient with a complete airway obstruction or in whom tracheal intubation is otherwise impossible.

needle stick injuries A potentially serious exposure if the needle or sharps has been contaminated with a patient's blood. Work practices should be engineered to minimize these injuries by placing the sharps immediately into a container as part of the procedure.

neglect A form of abuse where necessary care is not provided.

negligence Providing care improperly or eliminating essential steps. To prove negligence, the plaintiff must show that the provider had a duty to act, breached his or her duty, an injury occurred, and the breach of duty caused the injury.

neonatal sepsis Severe, overwhelming infection in a neonate (birth to one month).

neoplasm A new growth of tissue serving no physiological function.

neurogenic shock A form of shock, often called fainting or syncope, due to disorders of the nervous system with an absence of sympathetic response. Three assessment findings that, when displayed together, indicate neurogenic shock are decreasing blood pressure, decreasing pulse rate, and decreasing respiratory rate.

neurological posturing Positioning of the patient as a reflex in response to pain. Examples include decorticate and decerebrate posturing, or the fetal position.

neurology The study of the nervous system and its components and function in sickness and health.

neurons The basic unit of the nervous system.

NHTSA (National Highway Traffic Safety Administration) A division of the U.S. Department of Transportation where the EMS initiatives are coordinated at the federal level.

nitrogen narcosis (rapture of the deep) A state of euphoria or exhilaration occurring when nitrogen enters the blood stream at approximately seven times the atmospheric pressure during a diving incident.

non-rebreather mask A basic oxygen-therapy appliance used by all levels of out-of-hospital and in-hospital providers to administer high concentrations of oxygen to the breathing patient.

North American Emergency Response Guidebook (NAERG) A book that provides responders instructions and information on how to handle the first thirty minutes of a hazmat spill.

nosocomial disorder A medical condition that originates in the hospital setting.

NPA (nasal pharyngeal airway) A basic airway adjunct designed to be lubricated with a water soluble gel and then inserted into the nares.

NPO (nothing by mouth) A hospital order for patients who are going to surgery or have a medical condition that does not allow them to take in any food or drink.

NREMT (National Registry of EMTs) The organization that provides a standardized examination and practical skills examination for the First Responders, EMT-Basics, EMT-Intermediates, and Paramedics of many states.

NSTEMI An acute myocardial infarction that does not show ST-segment elevation on the ECG.

nulliparous Term used to describe a woman who has never given birth.

nutrition The act or process of being nourished with food and drink required to survive.

nystagmus A fine motor twitching of the eyeball, normal during extreme lateral gaze but not in any other position.

obesity A condition characterized by excessive body fat.

objective information Data representing the clinical signs that can be observed and measured by the examiner, such as the pulse, respiratory rate, and blood pressure.

obstetrics The branch of medical science that deals with birth, pregnancy, and its complications.

obstructive airway disease A medical condition that causes constriction, spasms, or thick secretions and inflammation of the airways.

occlusive dressing A covering to apply to a puncture wound that will not allow air to pass through the hole. Many services use Vaseline gauze for this purpose.

ongoing assessment (OA) The assessment of the patient that is normally conducted en route to the hospital involving serial vital signs, reassessment, and checking on interventions.

OPA (oropharyngeal airway) A basic airway adjunct used on patients with no gag reflex to help keep the tongue away from the back of the throat.

opacification The forming of cataract cloudiness, impairing vision.

open-ended question A type of question that requires a narrative form of response.

open fracture A break in a bone that has punctured the skin with the bone ends.

open pneumothorax Air in the chest due to a penetrating wound, allowing air to enter the chest cavity.

OPQRRST An elaboration of the chief complaint, including: onset; provocation; quality; region, radiation, relief, recurrence; severity; time.

ophthalmoscope A tool used by healthcare personnel to perform a detailed examination of the eye.

organ donors Patients who have agreed to donate their organs should they die in a fatal accident or from a fatal medical condition, so others may benefit from them.

orthopnea The abnormal condition in which a patient must sit or stand to breathe comfortably.

orthostatic changes An increase in heart rate and a decrease in blood pressure when a patient rises from a supine or sitting position.

orthostatic hypotension A drop in the patient's blood pressure when he or she stands up; usually due to internal bleeding.

OSHA (Occupational Safety and Health Administration) A program of the U.S. Department of Labor that is designed to protect the employee from the employer and assure that the workplace is a safe environment.

osmosis Movement of a solvent across a semipermeable membrane into a solution of higher-solute concentration to equalize the concentrations of solute on the two sides of the membrane.

osteoporosis A condition, primarily affecting older women, that causes decreased bone mass and density, resulting in bones that break more easily.

otorrhea A discharge from the ear.

otoscope A tool used by health personnel to perform a detailed examination of the ear.

out-of-hospital care This term has replaced prehospital care in the Guidelines 2005. This seems to be the direction of most of the national organizations in respect to care provided outside of the hospital.

overdose An excessive and dangerous, potentially lethal, dose of a drug.

oxyhemoglobin saturation curve A sigmoid-shaped curve that represents the percentage saturation of hemoglobin by oxygen on the vertical axis and the partial pressure of oxygen (PO_2) in arterial blood on the horizontal axis.

pacemaker An implanted device that is designed to provide an electrical impulse to pace the heart when the normal conduction cells are not functioning properly.

pacemaker cells The cells in the heart that generate the electrical impulses. Typically assembled in nodes (e.g., SA node, AV node).

palliative care Treatment that reduces the violence of a disease without actually curing the disease.

PAR (primary area of responsibility) The territory in which a roving ambulance is assigned to stay within when not assigned to an actual call.

paradoxical motion Seen when a free-floating section of the rib cage moves in the opposite direction of the rest of the rib cage during respirations.

paralytic ileus A twisted and paralyzed bowel.

paraplegia The inability to move the legs after an injury or illness involving the spine.

parenteral drug administration The introduction of a medication to the body outside of the GI tract (e.g., IV medications).

parity The total number of births a woman has had.

Parkinson's disease A chronic, progressive nervous disease involving tremors and muscular weakness.

paroxysmal nocturnal dyspnea (PND) A form of transient pulmonary edema that wakes the patient during the night with severe shortness of breath; associated with heart failure.

partial seizure A type of seizure that occurs only in a particular area of the brain, so the patient remains conscious and the effects are apparent only in a specific area of the body.

pathogenesis The origination or development of a disease.

pathologic fracture A break in a bone weakened by disease.

pathology The study of disease and its effect on the anatomy and physiology of the organism.

pathophysiology The study of the irregular or abnormal functioning of the body or its organ systems.

patient advocacy A key part of the EMS provider's role in lobbying for the most appropriate care for his or her patient in a busy healthcare facility.

patient assessment The methodical process by which a patient's condition is evaluated.

PCC (poison control center) A resource of information on poisons and their management.

PCI Percutaneous coronary intervention, such as coronary catheterization for the diagnosis and management of ACS.

PE (pulmonary edema) The collection of fluid in the lungs usually due to heart failure or pump failure, although it is occasionally found in narcotic overdoses and high-altitude sickness.

PEA (pulseless electrical activity) An ECG found on a patient in cardiac arrest that shows some electrical activity but not enough to cause sufficient pumping to move the blood. Previously called electromechanical dissociation, or EMD.

peak flow A measurement of how rapidly a patient can exhale.

pediatrics The study of the care of healthy and sick children.

penetration A break in the skin due to an object's being forced into and tearing the skin and internal organs.

pepper spray Used by the police as an irritant to the eyes to disperse a potentially violent crowd without doing any long-term, serious medical damage to the victims.

percussion A step in the examination of the patient that involves tapping the body to listen for dull or hollow sounds.

perfusion Blood flow to the tissues of the body.

peritonitis Inflammation of the peritoneum.

PERRLA An acronym for documenting normal findings related to the eyes: pupils equally round, reactive to light and accommodation.

personal protective equipment (PPE) Items that can be worn to protect the EMS provider from harm from bodily fluids or hazardous substances, such as disposable gloves, eye shields or goggles, masks, and gowns.

pertinent negatives Symptoms the patient does not have that may be relevant to the case (e.g., a patient struck his head but did not lose consciousness).

PFDs (personal flotation devices) A life preserver that should be worn whenever rescue personnel are near or around water.

pH The scale of a chemical's acidity or alkalinity (acid or base), where the body's normal pH is defined as between 7.35 and 7.45.

pharmacodynamics The division of pharmacology dealing with reactions between drugs and organisms.

pharmacokinetics The study of bodily absorption, distribution, metabolism, and excretion of drugs.

pharmacology The study of drugs, their functions, and their medical applications to treatment.

phlebitis The inflammation of a vein.

phobia An exaggerated and often incapacitating fear.

PID (pelvic inflammatory disease) An infectious disease in the female reproductive and surrounding organs that can lead to complications including sepsis and infertility.

piloerection A reflexive response to cold; also known as goose pimples.

placenta previa Abnormal attachment of the placenta near the opening of the birth canal, which can cause the placenta to precede the delivery of the infant.

plague An acute febrile, infectious, and highly fatal disease caused by a gram positive bacteria.

plantar reflex A reflex that is assessed on both conscious and unconscious patients with suspected spinal cord injury. With the end of a capped pen, a light stroke is drawn up the lateral side of the sole of the foot and across the ball of the foot, like an upside-down letter J. The normal response is plantar flexion of the toes and foot.

plasma A combination of 91% water and 9% proteins found in the blood.

platinum ten minutes The optimum limit of ten minutes at the scene with a critical trauma patient; used in both Montana's and New York State's Critical Trauma Care courses.

platelets Particles in the blood responsible for forming the initial blood clot.

pleural friction rub A grating sound in the chest caused by inflamed pleural surfaces.

pleurisy Inflammation of the lining of the lungs.

pleuritic pain Pain caused by any condition that causes inflammation in the lung or heart that extends to the pleural surfaces of the lung.

PMH (past medical history) Relevant recent surgeries, illnesses, trauma, periods of immobilization or hospitalizations, changes in mental status or physical ability, and changes in medication or daily routine/activity.

PMS (premenstrual syndrome) Varying symptoms manifested by some women prior to menstruation that may include emotional instability, irritability, insomnia, fatigue, anxiety, or depression. Previously referred to as premenstrual tension syndrome, this is now called premenstrual dysphoric disorder.

PMS (pulses, motor function, and sensory function) When evaluating the distal circulation and nervous system function, especially before and after applying a splint, the PMS should be evaluated.

PND (paroxysmal nocturnal dyspnea) The shortness of breath that occurs during the night, often waking the patient up.

pneumonia An inflammation of the lungs commonly caused by bacteria, a virus, or other pathogens.

pneumothorax A collection of air or gas in the pleural space of the chest, causing one or both lungs to collapse.

PNS (peripheral nervous system) The twelve pairs of cranial nerves and thirty-one pairs of peripheral nerves existing between each vertebrae of the spinal column.

point of maximal impulse (PMI) The point on the chest where the impulse of the left ventricle is felt most strongly.

poisoning Connotes exposure to a substance that is generally only harmful and has no usual beneficial effects.

polypharmacy (polymedication) The administering or taking of many medications concurrently, often for the same condition.

polyunsaturated fat Highly unsaturated fat that is found in food products derived from plants, including sunflower, corn, and soybean oils. Like monounsaturated fat, this is a healthier alternative to saturated fat.

positive findings Information obtained in the focused history and physical examination that is clearly relevant to the chief complaint.

post-ictal The third phase of a seizure, during which the patient is extremely exhausted and confused while slowly regaining consciousness.

preeclampsia A disorder of the last trimester marked by edema, hypertension, and proteinuria. Formerly called toxicemia of pregnancy.

preexcitation syndrome See *WPW (Wolf-Parkingson-White) syndrome*.

prehospital care The term "out-of-hospital setting" has replaced "prehospital care."

prehospital care report (PCR) A report that should be completed on every call; an accurate and thorough documentation of the assessment findings and field management of the patient.

pre-ictal phase The period before a seizure attack.

prejudice Preconceived notions, judging patients by stereotypes, and intolerance to cultural diversity.

preload The degree of stretch in a cardiac contraction.

premature infant An infant born prior to full term (i.e., before thirty-six weeks).

presbycusis Normal hearing loss that occurs with aging.

Pressure dressing A sterile gauze applied to a soft-tissue injury designed to provide continuous bleeding control to assist in the clot formation.

preterm labor True labor that occurs before thirty-eight weeks' gestation.

Prinzmetal's angina An atypical form of angina caused by the vasospasm of otherwise normal coronary arteries.

profession A "calling" requiring specialized and specific academic preparation.

prognosis Prediction of the outcome of the problem.

pronator drift A test used to assess focal weakness. The patient is asked to extend both arms out in front of him, with palms up, while both eyes are closed. If one arm "drifts" lower or the palm turns down, this is considered a deficit.

proprioception The perceptions concerning movements and position of the body.

protected airway Rather than saying "secure the airway" or "protect the airway," the phrase "insert or pass an advanced airway" is used, since terminology like "secure" or "protect" may give a false sense of security to the provider.

protective custody When police take someone into custody for the purpose of protecting that person from him- or herself, or others, or to have the person evaluated.

protocol The treatment guidelines that are agreed upon for a typical patient presentation. These are a form of indirect or off-line medical control.

PSVT See *reentry SVT.*

psychosis A serious mental disorder characterized by a loss of contact with reality.

PTACD-CPR CPR employing a device to provide phased thoracic-abdominal compression-decompression.

PTL (pharyngotracheal lumen airway) A dual lumen airway that is blindly inserted into the patient when other forms of advanced airways are not available. These are no longer commonly used by out-of-hospital providers.

pulmonary circulation The circuit of blood flow between the heart and the lungs.

pulmonary contusion A common serious injury from blunt thoracic trauma.

pulmonary edema The filling of the lungs with fluid in the interstitial space, the alveoli, or both.

pulmonary embolism (PE) A serious condition caused by a foreign body (e.g., a clot) that lodges in the pulmonary capillary bed.

pulse deficit A result of the irregular filling of the ventricles; present when there is a slower distal pulse compared to the core pulse (apical).

pulse oximetry A technique used to measure the percentage of hemoglobin saturated with oxygen.

pulseless ventricular tachycardia (VT) An ECG generating in the ventricles, which is generally over 180 beats per minute and is not able to produce effective cardiac pumping. It is considered a shockable rhythm.

pulsus differens A condition in which the pulses on either side of the body are unequal.

pulsus paradoxus (also called **paradoxical pulse**) A pulse that diminishes during the inspiration phase of breathing.

puncture A break in the skin as a result of an object's being forced into the skin.

pursed-lip breathing Exhaling past partially closed lips to build up air pressure in the lungs.

quadriplegia The inability of a patient to move his or her four extremities due to an injury or medical condition affecting the cervical spine.

quality assurance (QA) A program that looks closely at the medical care given to assure that the highest quality is provided and to make improvements to the care on an ongoing basis.

quality improvement (QI) A program that looks closely at the medical care provided in order to strive to improve the quality of care so excellence can be achieved on a regular basis.

rabies (also see **hydrophobia**) A viral infection transmitted through saliva of an infected animal. It is fatal in humans if not aggressively treated.

radiating pain Pain or discomfort that spreads from the source to another area (e.g., ischemic chest pain radiating down the left arm).

radiation exposure Injuries and medical ailments caused by excessive exposure to ionizing radiation. The extent of the injury is a function of the duration of exposure and the types of particles to which a person is exposed (e.g., alpha, beta, or gamma).

rales See *crackles.*

range of motion (ROM) The area and span of motion of the joints.

rapid extrication The procedure for removing a patient found in the seated position from a vehicle using only a long backboard, a rigid cervical collar, and three to four trained EMS providers. This is only done if the patient is unstable, as in all other cases the vest-type device (i.e., KED) should be utilized.

rapid physical examination (RPE) A systematic, quick examination of the major body sections (head, neck, chest, abdomen, pelvis, back, buttocks, and extremities) for injuries, conducted on the medical patient who is not responsive (e.g., hypoglycemia, hypothermia, or post-ictal state).

rapid takedown technique The procedure for carefully moving a patient who has a suspected spine injury from the standing position to the supine position on a long backboard. This procedure requires a rigid cervical collar, a long backboard, and three trained EMS providers.

rapid trauma assessment (RTE) A quick head-to-toe assessment conducted on a trauma patient with significant mechanism of injury involving the major body sections (head, neck, chest, abdomen, pelvis, back, buttocks, and extremities).

rapid trauma examination (RTE) A systematic, quick examination of the major body sections (head, neck, chest, abdomen, pelvis, back, buttocks, and extremities) for injuries.

rapture of the deep See *nitrogen narcosis.*

reciprocity The ability of one's certification or license to be utilized between one state and another. This is a function of the use of a standardized training curriculum (e.g., DOT) and the specific rules of each state.

reentry SVT Previously called PSVT, a tachycardic rhythm caused by a reentry circuit originating from above the ventricles, as depicted on the ECG.

referred pain Pain that originates in one area of the body that is also sensed in another area.

reflection A communication technique in which the EMS provider repeats the patient's words to encourage further discussion.

reflex arc An involuntary or immediate response to a stimulus.

refractory period Not responding or yielding to treatment.

regurgitation Backward flow, as in the return of stomach contents into the esophagus.

respiration The chemical and physical processes in which an organism acquires oxygen and eliminates carbon dioxide.

respiratory acidosis A condition in which the body's pH falls below 3.35, primarily as a result of not breathing enough.

respiratory alkalosis A condition in which the body's pH rises above 3.45, primarily from breathing too much.

respiratory distress The sensation of dyspnea or the signs of difficulty breathing (e.g., tripod position, intercostal separations, grunting, cyanosis, etc.).

restraints Supplies or devices used to tie a patient for the purpose of protecting the patient or others from violence. When dealing with injured or medical patients, humane restraints (e.g., wide bands of cloth, sheets, leather restraints) are used instead of handcuffs.

retraction A pulling in of skin in the suprasternal, subclavicular, and intercostal areas during inhalation.

revised trauma score (RTS) A numerical grading system used for triage and to predict patient outcomes, developed by Howard Champion, MD; see also trauma score.

Reye's syndrome An acute, frequently fatal childhood syndrome marked by encephalopathy, hepatitis, and fatty accumulations in the viscera; thought to be caused by excess administration of salicylates to children.

Rh A factor in the blood, derived from the rhesus monkey, that is inherited.

rhabdomyolysis An acute, potentially fatal disorder involving disintegration of skeletal muscles and urine excretion of the muscle pigment myoglobin.

rheumatic heart disease A manifestation of rheumatic fever consisting of inflammatory changes and damaged heart valves.

rhonchi Rattling noises in the upper airways caused by mucus or other secretions; singular rhoncus.

right-sided heart failure A potential backup of fluid into the systemic system that is also referred to as cor pulmonale.

RMA (refusal of medical assistance) The term used when a patient does not want to give consent to a specific treatment (e.g., an IV or cervical collar) or transport to a hospital.

rotavirus A virus that causes acute gastroenteritis in children.

RSI (rapid sequence induction) The use of medications to paralyze and cause amnesia when it is medically necessary to rapidly intubate a patient.

rubberneckers Individuals who pose a traffic hazard when passing the scene of an accident so they can get a look at the damage and rescue taking place.

rule out Process by which a diagnosis is made in the cardiac care unit in order to determine a definitive diagnosis.

S1 A normal heart sound; the first sound heard, which is produced by the atrioventricular valves.

S2 A normal heart sound; the second sound heard, which is produced by the semilunar valves.

safety A key concern at any EMS or rescue operation to assure that procedures are done in the least potentially harmful manner possible. Some agencies appoint a safety officer at major incidents.

SAMPLE history An acronym for the information needed to assess and manage an incident or complaint: signs and symptoms, allergies, medications, pertinent past medical history, last oral intake, events leading up to this incident.

saturated fat Usually solid at room temperature. This is commonly found in animal products, such as meat, poultry, egg yolks, and dairy products. It is also found in a few vegetable products, such as coconuts and cocoa. Saturated fat raises blood cholesterol more than anything else in the diet.

scalp The skin and hair on the outside of the cranium; provides a protective layer against minor blunt trauma to the head.

scaphoid abdomen A sinking, or concave, shape to the abdomen.

scene choreography An important element of the management of the healthcare providers who are administering care to a patient.

scene size-up The first component of patient assessment, which involves determining whether the location, or environment, is safe for the responders and the patient.

SCI (spinal cord injury) A laceration, bruise, cut, or compression injury to the spinal cord that can have devastating implications for the patient.

SCIWORA (spinal cord injury without radiographic abnormalities) A potential problem in children, where the vertebrae can slip out of place and then return on their own to the appropriate positioning, leaving a damaged or severed cord behind.

scope of practice As usually defined in state laws, the extent to which healthcare providers can practice within their specific state.

SCUBA (self-contained underwater breathing apparatus) The tank and regulator that allows an underwater diver to breathe for extended periods of time without returning to the surface.

second-party caller A call for emergency services made by the bystander or family member and not the patient.

seizure An attack or sudden onset of disease. A convulsion or epileptic attack classified into different types (e.g., absence, clonic, focal motor, generalized tonic-clonic, or partial focal seizure).

Sellick's maneuver See *cricoid pressure*.

semantics The study of the meanings in language.

serial vital signs All measurements after, or comparisons against, the baseline measurements.

sexual abuse Abuse of a sexual nature.

shaken baby syndrome Bleeding into the skull of an infant from damage to the bridging veins on the outside of the brain, due to picking up the child and shaking him or her continuously.

sharp A device, such as a needle, that could puncture the skin and may transmit pathogens.

shipping papers The documentation of potentially hazardous materials on a ship, train, truck, or plane.

shock 1. The body's response to low perfusion states, which involves an initial compensation phase followed by decompensation, and then an irreversible or terminal phase, if not properly managed early on; 2. an electrical injury; 3. treatment of a "shockable" ECG in a pulseless patient.

SIDS (sudden infant death syndrome) The sudden death of an otherwise healthy infant.

sign A finding that can be measured accurately by hand or with a measuring device such as a blood pressure cuff.

silent myocardial infarction (MI) An ACS with atypical signs and symptoms; common among elderly and diabetic patients.

simple pneumothorax An injury or medical condition that causes air to enter the chest cavity. The simple pneumothorax is a respiratory problem; because it does not continue to suck air into the chest, it does not proceed to move the mediastinum or turn into a tension pneumothorax.

sinus arrhythmia A cardiac rhythm, typical in children and healthy adults, characterized by a regular rate that increases and decreases rhythmically with breathing.

skeletal muscle The voluntary (striated) muscle that moves the long bones.

skin CTC (color, temperature, and condition) Assessment that the EMS provider can do to determine circulatory status.

skin lesions Breaks or injuries to the skin, such as papule, scale, crust, patch, plaque, wheal, cyst, bulla, pustule, fissure, ulcer, vesicle, and macule.

skin turgor An indication of the patient's state of hydration.

skull The outer cover of bone that encases the brain; consisting of the bones of the face and the cranium.

skull fracture Isolated linear, nondepressed fractures with an intact scalp that are common and do not require treatment. However, life-threatening intracranial hemorrhage may result if the fracture causes disruption of the middle meningeal artery or a major dural sinus.

small-volume nebulizer Another form of administering oxygen combined with medicine (e.g., Albuterol).

smooth muscle Found in the lower airways, vessels and intestines can relax or contract to alter the inner lumen of the vessels.

sniffing position A position of the head and neck used to help visualize the vocal cord during intubation.

soft spots The fontanelles are the membrane-covered spaces between the incomplete ossified cranial bones of an infant.

soft tissue trauma Injuries to the skin, which are open or closed.

somatic pain Pain caused by irritation of pain fibers in the parietal peritoneum; tends to be localized to the area of pathology.

SOPs (standard operating procedures) The policy that an agency uses to define the steps they would like personnel to take when confronted with a particular situation or operating a specific device (e.g., SOP on wearing seat belts).

span of control In the incident command system, it is recognized that emergency managers can effectively lead and communicate with approximately five to seven people each. Keeping this in mind, the Incident Commander at a school bus rollover should not attempt to talk to all fifty emergency personnel at the scene; rather, he or she should communicate with the staging officer, the triage officer, the transport officer, the treatment officer, and the other service leaders (police and FD) at the command post.

spastic hemiparesis An abnormal gait with unilateral weakness and foot dragging.

spina bifida A birth defect where the infant is born with exposed spinal structures.

spinal immobilization See *manual spinal motion restriction*.

sprain An injury to the ligaments around a joint; marked by pain, swelling, and the dislocation of the skin over the joint.

staging Effectively parking resources (e.g., emergency vehicles) within a few minutes of the incident rather than cluttering up the actual incident site. This way, they can be moved in as they are needed, and traffic flow may be maintained.

START An acronym for simple triage and rapid treatment; a system used to triage patients in a multiple-casualty incident.

status asthmaticus A severe, prolonged asthma attack that does not respond to standard medications.

status epilepticus Two or more seizures occurring without full recovery of consciousness between attacks, or continuous seizure activity for ten minutes or more.

STDs (sexually transmitted diseases) Common examples include AIDS, bacterial vaginosis, chancroid, clamydial infections, cytomegalovirus infections, genital herpes, genital warts, gonorrhea, granuloma inguinale, hepatitis, leukemia, lymphoma, mylopathy, lymphogranuloma venereun, molluscum contagiosum, pubic lice, scabies, syphilis, trichomoniasis, and vaginal yeast infections.

STEMI An acute myocardial infarction that show ST-segment elevation on the ECG.

steppage An abnormal gait in which the person appears to be walking up steps when on an even surface.

sterilization To disinfect equipment in a manner that kills all germs.

stethoscope A device that is used to listen to the patient's heart or lung sounds.

stings Punctures made by an insect.

Stokes-Adams syndrome Syncope or convulsions caused by complete heart block and a pulse rate of forty or less.

stress A factor that induces bodily or mental tension.

striae Atrophic lines or streaks from a rapid or prolonged stretching of the skin.

stridor A high-pitched sound associated with upper airway obstruction.

stroke The result of any process that causes disruption of blood flow to a particular part of the brain.

stroke volume The normal amount of blood ejected from the left ventricle with each contraction of the heart (approximately 70 cc in the adult).

subcutaneous emphysema Air bubbles under the skin resulting from a pneumothorax; sometimes exhibits as crackling like Rice Krispies® or the sensation of plastic packing bubbles.

subdural hematoma An injury to the brain resulting in bleeding from the rupture of bridging vessels between the cortex and dura mater.

subjective information Data obtained from the patient and commonly referred to as the symptoms; this cannot be measured by the EMS provider.

subluxation Partial dislocation of a joint that usually has a great amount of damage and instability.

substance abuse Abuse of drugs, including alcohol and tobacco.

substance dependence A psychological craving for, or a psychological reliance on, a chemical agent resulting from abuse or addiction.

suctioning The use of an aspirator or suction device to remove fluid or small solid particles from a patient's airway.

suicide An attempt to take one's life.

supine hypotension A drop in blood pressure that occurs during the third trimester of pregnancy, when the mother is supine, because the weight of the fetus lies on the inferior vena cava.

supplemental See *supplementary*.

supplementary Increasing the percentage of inspired oxygen. The previous term used was "supplemental," though the correct term, "supplementary," is now used throughout the Guidelines 2005.

sympathy An expression of sorrow for another's loss, grief, or misfortune; implies having feelings and emotions similar to or shared with another person.

symphysis pubis The area of the anterior pelvis where the two pubic bones grow together.

symptom A subjective finding that the patient tells the EMS provider.

symptomatic bradycardia A heart rate below sixty in an adult patient, in which the patient has an altered mental status, difficulty breathing, hypotension, or chest pain. This may include an AV block on the ECG.

syncope Fainting.

synovial joints A joint filled with fluid that lubricates the articulated surfaces.

system status management A method of deploying ambulances that involves assigning them to very specific locations and reassigning their locations as the call volume changes throughout the day.

systolic The peak blood pressure in the arterial system as the left ventricle contracts.

tachypnea rapid, shallow breathing.

tactile fremitus A vibration of the chest wall during breathing that can be felt by the examiner, often associated with inflammation, infection, or congestion.

tactile intubation Involves placing the first two digits into the mouth to push the tongue down.

TB (tuberculosis) An infection of the lungs that presents as a severe cough, a hemoptysis, chest pain, fever and night sweats, chills, weakness, loss of appetite, and weight loss.

tear gas The chemical used by police to gain control of an angry crowd. Causes a burning sensation that usually lasts for about an hour.

technical terminology Language or professional jargon that has meaning only for the medical community or professional group.

temperature The measurement of the degree of hot or cold in the body. The core temperature is the most accurate, and is approximately 98.6° F.

tension pneumothorax A life-threatening condition resulting from air or gas trapped in the pleural space of the chest and causing collapse of one or both lungs, movement of the mediastinum, and a dramatic decrease in cardiac output.

tenting Characteristic of skin that has poor turgor or a connective tissue disease; the skin remains in a tent position when pinched and does not return to normal.

terminal illness Usually means that the patient has a condition that, regardless of any currently available treatment, will result in her death in the next six to twelve months.

testicular torsion Occurs when a testicle twists on its pedicle, leading to acute ischemia.

tetanus A ubiquitous bacteria that pops up in many places at the same time and is potentially fatal. Prophylaxis is recommended every ten years.

thalidomide A sedative that was banned in the 1960s because it caused severe birth defects.

thermal regulation The process by which the body controls its heat loss and gain.

third collision When the internal organs strike against the inside of the body in a motor vehicle crash.

thoracic trauma Injury, either blunt or penetrating, that occurs to the chest cavity or chest wall.

thyroid disease Entropy and the over- or underproduction of hormones produced by the thyroid gland can lead to hypothyroidism, hyperthyroidism, a goiter, or thyroid cancer.

thyrotoxicosis A general term for the overactivity of the thyroid gland, or hyperthyroidism.

TIA (transient ischemic attack) A ministroke; a temporary occlusion of an artery to the brain caused by a blood clot.

tiered response A response to an EMS incident that involves multiple units of different training levels arriving at different times.

tilt test A test used to assess heart rate and blood pressure for orthostatic changes when a patient rises up from a lying position.

toddler A child between the ages of two and four years.

tolerance The capacity to assimilate a drug continuously in large doses.

tonicity 1. The normal condition of tension during the slight continuous contraction of skeletal muscles; 2. the effective osmotic pressure.

tonsils A small mass of lymphoid tissue, especially the palatine tonsil.

total cholesterol The total of the HDL cholesterol, LDL cholesterol, and VLDL cholesterol.

toxicology The study of the harmful effects of chemicals on the body.

transfer of command The passing of the command function to a more superior or experienced leader in such a way as to minimize the interruption in the flow of the incident; occurs at a major incident, where the incident command system has been implemented.

transient ischemic attack (TIA) A temporary interruption of blood flow to an area of the brain; may be a precursor to a major cerebrovascular accident.

trauma center A hospital that has the capability of caring for the acutely injured patient.

trauma registry A computer database with relevant data elements for research on the trauma care provided by regional trauma centers.

trauma score An assessment tool that assigns a numerical value to represent the extent of injury on the basis of respiratory rate and chest expansion, capillary refill, and blood pressure ranges; also known as the revised trauma score.

traumatic asphyxia Sudden compression to the chest that causes the blood to rush backward into the systemic circulation. These patients often appear blue above the chest.

traumatic brain injury (TBI) A blunt or penetrating injury to the brain.

Trendelenberg position The shock position where the patient is lying down with his legs raised approximately eighteen inches above the rest of the body.

trending Changes over time observed by the comparison of multiple sets of vital signs and/or assessments to establish a diagnostic picture of the patient's status.

triage A French word that means "to sort."

triglycerides Fat-like substances that are carried through the bloodstream to the tissues. Much of the body's fat is stored in the form of triglycerides for later use as energy.

trimester One of the three-month segments of pregnancy.

tripod position A sitting position often assumed by patients who are having difficulty breathing; leaning forward, with elbows outward and hands on knees.

trismus Difficulty in opening the mouth due to tonic spasm of the muscles of mastication.

true labor Persistent, regular contractions.

turnout gear Protective personal gear used for fire rescue (e.g., boots, pants, helmet, coat, gloves).

tunnel vision The making of judgments or determinations on the basis of history and past experiences with an individual or an event.

tympany A drum-like sound.

unified command The command of a major incident that involves the police, fire, and EMS leadership working together to resolve the situation.

universal precautions Taking the appropriate precautions as a standard procedure when handling all patients, in order to protect the rescuer from body substances.

unsaturated fat Usually liquid at refrigerator temperature. This is primarily found in vegetable products and includes either monounsaturated or polyunsaturated fats.

up triaging A concept used in medicine that means that if a patient's presenting problem could be either more or less serious, the patient should be managed as having the more serious of the two possibilities until the patient's condition has been absolutely determined.

URI Upper respiratory infection.

urology The study of the urinary system and excretion of fluids from the body.

urticaria The hives that develop as a sign of a severe allergic reaction.

U.S. Pharmacopoeia The book that lists all official drug names.

UTI Urinary tract infection.

VADs Vascular access devices.

ventilation The physiological process where air in the lungs is exchanged with atmospheric air.

vertigo A vestibular disorder that includes motion sickness, in which the patient expressed a false sensation of motion.

Vial of Life® A rolled piece of paper with pertinent medical information about the patient that is kept in a plastic tube similar to a prescription drug container. Patients are often told to keep this in their refrigerator for ease of EMS providers locating them.

virulence How strong a virus is; the degree of disease-producing capability of a microorganism.

visceral pain Pain caused by the stretching of nerve fibers surrounding either solid or hollow organs in the abdomen; this type of pain is often poorly localized and diffuse.

vital signs Pulse, blood pressure, and respirations, often considered the starting point for assessment and a gauge of a person's health status.

VLDL cholesterol Very-low-density lipoprotein that carries cholesterol and triglycerides for later use as energy.

vomiting The active process of expelling the contents of the stomach.

Waddell's triad An injury pattern seen in children that involves the legs, chest, and head.

wheezing A continuous whistling sound caused by narrowing of the lower airways, usually heard at the end of exhalation.

withdrawal 1. The act of removing or discontinuing; 2. a pathologic detachment or retreat from emotional involvement with people or the environment.

WPW (Wolf-Parkinson-White) syndrome Congenital heart condition with an anomalous AV excitation that is marked by irregular heartbeat and distorted patterns of ECG (e.g., shortened P-R and prolonged QRS). Also called preexcitation syndrome.

THOMSON DELMAR LEARNING END USER LICENSE AGREEMENT

IMPORTANT-READ CAREFULLY: This End User License Agreement ("Agreement") sets forth the conditions by which Delmar Learning, a division of Thomson Learning Inc. ("Thomson") will make electronic access to the Thomson Delmar Learning-owned licensed content and associated media, software, documentation, printed materials and electronic documentation contained in this package and/or made available to you via this product (the "Licensed Content"), available to you (the "End User"). BY CLICKING THE "I ACCEPT" BUTTON AND/OR OPENING THIS PACKAGE, YOU ACKNOWLEDGE THAT YOU HAVE READ ALL OF THE TERMS AND CONDITIONS, AND THAT YOU AGREE TO BE BOUND BY ITS TERMS CONDITIONS AND ALL APPLICABLE LAWS AND REGULATIONS GOVERNING THE USE OF THE LICENSED CONTENT.

1.0 SCOPE OF LICENSE

1.1 <u>Licensed Content</u>. The Licensed Content may contain portions of modifiable content ("Modifiable Content") and content which may not be modified or otherwise altered by the End User ("Non-Modifiable Content"). For purposes of this Agreement, Modifiable Content and Non-Modifiable Content may be collectively referred to herein as the "Licensed Content." All Licensed Content shall be considered Non-Modifiable Content, unless such Licensed Content is presented to the End User in a modifiable format and it is clearly indicated that modification of the Licensed Content is permitted.

1.2 Subject to the End User's compliance with the terms and conditions of this Agreement, Thomson Delmar Learning hereby grants the End User, a nontransferable, non-exclusive, limited right to access and view a single copy of the Licensed Content on a single personal computer system for noncommercial, internal, personal use only. The End User shall not (i) reproduce, copy, modify (except in the case of Modifiable Content), distribute, display, transfer, sublicense, prepare derivative work(s) based on, sell, exchange, barter or transfer, rent, lease, loan, resell, or in any other manner exploit the Licensed Content; (ii) remove, obscure or alter any notice of Thomson Delmar Learning's intellectual property rights present on or in the License Content, including, but not limited to, copyright, trademark and/or patent notices; or (iii) disassemble, decompile, translate, reverse engineer or otherwise reduce the Licensed Content.

2.0 TERMINATION

2.1 Thomson Delmar Learning may at any time (without prejudice to its other rights or remedies) immediately terminate this Agreement and/or suspend access to some or all of the Licensed Content, in the event that the End User does not comply with any of the terms and conditions of this Agreement. In the event of such termination by Thomson Delmar Learning, the End User shall immediately return any and all copies of the Licensed Content to Thomson Delmar Learning.

3.0 PROPRIETARY RIGHTS

3.1 The End User acknowledges that Thomson Delmar Learning owns all right, title and interest, including, but not limited to all copyright rights therein, in and to the Licensed Content, and that the End User shall not take any action inconsistent with such ownership. The Licensed Content is protected by U.S., Canadian and other applicable copyright laws and by international treaties, including the Berne Convention and the Universal Copyright Convention. Nothing contained in this Agreement shall be construed as granting the End User any ownership rights in or to the Licensed Content.

3.2 Thomson Delmar Learning reserves the right at any time to withdraw from the Licensed Content any item or part of an item for which it no longer retains the right to publish, or which it has reasonable grounds to believe infringes copyright or is defamatory, unlawful or otherwise objectionable.

4.0 PROTECTION AND SECURITY

4.1 The End User shall use its best efforts and take all reasonable steps to safeguard its copy of the Licensed Content to ensure that no unauthorized reproduction, publication, disclosure, modification or distribution of the Licensed Content, in whole or in part, is made. To the extent that the End User becomes aware of any such unauthorized use of the Licensed Content, the End User shall immediately notify Delmar Learning. Notification of such violations may be made by sending an Email to delmarhelp@thomson.com.

5.0 MISUSE OF THE LICENSED PRODUCT

5.1 In the event that the End User uses the Licensed Content in violation of this Agreement, Thomson Delmar Learning shall have the option of electing liquidated damages, which shall include all profits generated by the End User's use of the Licensed Content plus interest computed at the maximum rate permitted by law and all legal fees and other expenses incurred by Thomson Delmar Learning in enforcing its rights, plus penalties.

6.0 FEDERAL GOVERNMENT CLIENTS

6.1 Except as expressly authorized by Delmar Learning, Federal Government clients obtain only the rights specified in this Agreement and no other rights. The Government acknowledges that (i) all software and related documentation incorporated in the Licensed Content is existing commercial computer software within the meaning of FAR 27.405(b)(2); and (2) all other data delivered in whatever form, is limited rights data within the meaning of FAR 27.401. The restrictions in this section are acceptable as consistent with the Government's need for software and other data under this Agreement.

7.0 DISCLAIMER OF WARRANTIES AND LIABILITIES

7.1 Although Thomson Delmar Learning believes the Licensed Content to be reliable, Thomson Delmar Learning does not guarantee or warrant (i) any information or materials contained in or produced by the Licensed Content, (ii) the accuracy, completeness or reliability of the Licensed Content, or (iii) that the Licensed Content is free from errors or other material defects. THE LICENSED PRODUCT IS PROVIDED "AS IS," WITHOUT ANY WARRANTY OF ANY KIND AND THOMSON DELMAR LEARNING DISCLAIMS ANY AND ALL WARRANTIES, EXPRESSED OR IMPLIED, INCLUDING, WITHOUT LIMITATION, WARRANTIES OF MERCHANTABILITY OR FITNESS OR A PARTICULAR PURPOSE. IN NO EVENT SHALL THOMSON DELMAR LEARNING BE LIABLE FOR: INDIRECT, SPECIAL, PUNITIVE OR CONSEQUENTIAL DAMAGES INCLUDING FOR LOST PROFITS, LOST DATA, OR OTHERWISE. IN NO EVENT SHALL DELMAR LEARNING'S AGGREGATE LIABILITY HEREUNDER, WHETHER ARISING IN CONTRACT, TORT, STRICT LIABILITY OR OTHERWISE, EXCEED THE AMOUNT OF FEES PAID BY THE END USER HEREUNDER FOR THE LICENSE OF THE LICENSED CONTENT.

8.0 GENERAL

8.1 <u>Entire Agreement</u>. This Agreement shall constitute the entire Agreement between the Parties and supercedes all prior Agreements and understandings oral or written relating to the subject matter hereof.

8.2 <u>Enhancements/Modifications of Licensed Content</u>. From time to time, and in Delmar Learning's sole discretion, Thomson Thomson Delmar Learning may advise the End User of updates, upgrades, enhancements and/or improvements to the Licensed Content, and may permit the End User to access and use, subject to the terms and conditions of this Agreement, such modifications, upon payment of prices as may be established by Delmar Learning.

8.3 <u>No Export</u>. The End User shall use the Licensed Content solely in the United States and shall not transfer or export, directly or indirectly, the Licensed Content outside the United States.

8.4 <u>Severability</u>. If any provision of this Agreement is invalid, illegal, or unenforceable under any applicable statute or rule of law, the provision shall be deemed omitted to the extent that it is invalid, illegal, or unenforceable. In such a case, the remainder of the Agreement shall be construed in a manner as to give greatest effect to the original intention of the parties hereto.

8.5 <u>Waiver</u>. The waiver of any right or failure of either party to exercise in any respect any right provided in this Agreement in any instance shall not be deemed to be a waiver of such right in the future or a waiver of any other right under this Agreement.

8.6 <u>Choice of Law/Venue</u>. This Agreement shall be interpreted, construed, and governed by and in accordance with the laws of the State of New York, applicable to contracts executed and to be wholly preformed therein, without regard to its principles governing conflicts of law. Each party agrees that any proceeding arising out of or relating to this Agreement or the breach or threatened breach of this Agreement may be commenced and prosecuted in a court in the State and County of New York. Each party consents and submits to the non-exclusive personal jurisdiction of any court in the State and County of New York in respect of any such proceeding.

8.7 <u>Acknowledgment</u>. By opening this package and/or by accessing the Licensed Content on this Website, THE END USER ACKNOWLEDGES THAT IT HAS READ THIS AGREEMENT, UNDERSTANDS IT, AND AGREES TO BE BOUND BY ITS TERMS AND CONDITIONS. IF YOU DO NOT ACCEPT THESE TERMS AND CONDITIONS, YOU MUST NOT ACCESS THE LICENSED CONTENT AND RETURN THE LICENSED PRODUCT TO THOMSON DELMAR LEARNING (WITHIN 30 CALENDAR DAYS OF THE END USER'S PURCHASE) WITH PROOF OF PAYMENT ACCEPTABLE TO DELMAR LEARNING, FOR A CREDIT OR A REFUND. Should the End User have any questions/comments regarding this Agreement, please contact Thomson Delmar Learning at delmarhelp@thomson.com.